BRUKNER&KHAN'S

# CLINICAL SPORTS MEDICINE

6TH EDITION

## FOUNDATIONS OF CLINICAL PRACTICE

# BRUKNER & KHAN'S
# CLINICAL SPORTS MEDICINE
## 6TH EDITION

## FOUNDATIONS OF CLINICAL PRACTICE

Peter Brukner
Clare Ardern
Roald Bahr
Paul Blazey
Ben Clarsen
Kay Crossley
Bruce Forster
Mark Hutchinson
Anne Lasinsky
Karim Khan

This sixth edition published 2025
First published 1993; Second edition 2001; Revised second edition 2002; Third edition 2006; Revised third edition 2009; Fourth edition 2012; Fifth edition 2017

Text © 2025 McGraw-Hill Education (Australia) Pty Ltd
Additional owners of copyright are acknowledged in on-page credits.

A catalogue record for this book is available from the National Library of Australia

Authors: Brukner, Peter; Khan, Karim
Title: Brukner & Khan's clinical sports medicine: foundations of clinical practice
Edition: 6th edition
ISBN: 9781761000010
MHID 1761000012

Published in Australia by
**McGraw-Hill Education (Australia) Pty Ltd**
Publisher: Rochelle Deighton
Copyeditor: Caroline Hunter
Proofreader: Sue Jamieson
Permissions manager: Rachel Norton
Cover designer: Simon Rattray, Squirt Creative
Cover image: © 2012, Darren J Wilkinson (darrenjw.github.io)
Internal designer: Simon Rattray, Squirt Creative
Typeset by Straive
Printed by MARKONO PRINT MEDIA PTE LTD

# Brief contents

## PART A  The sport and exercise clinician

1   The patient                                    2
2   Providing quality clinical care                8
3   Clinical reasoning                            16
4   Shared decision making                        24

5   The multidisciplinary team approach           32
6   Working with sporting teams                   42
7   Career development                            54

## PART B  Clinical sciences

8   Acute injuries                                68
9   Overuse injuries                              90
10  How does pain work? Using contemporary
    neuroscience to understand pain,
    performance and recovery                     126
11  Managing pain                                138
12  Introduction to clinical biomechanics        164

13  Biomechanical aspects of injury in
    nine specific sports                         178
14  Training principles, programming
    and prescription                            216
15  Load management                             228
16  Recovery                                    240

## PART C  The clinical approach

17  Preventing injury                            256
18  Periodic health assessment of athletes       278
19  Diagnosis: history and physical examination  292
20  Diagnosis: imaging                           306
21  Diagnosis: phases of clinical assessment     318
22  Red flags                                    328

23  Using PROMs in clinical practice             342
24  Treatment of sports injuries                 356
25  Athlete education                            402
26  Surgery in sports and exercise medicine      418
27  Principles of sports injury rehabilitation   438
28  Return to sport                              450

# Contents

Preface     x
About the authors     xii
Editors     xiv
Contributors     xv

Reviewers and illustrator     xix
Acknowledgments     xx
Special features     xxi

## PART A   The sport and exercise clinician

### 1   The patient     2

Context: patients' voices     3
Becoming a patient     3
What we hope for in the clinical encounter     4
The clinical encounter as a relationship     5
We're all in this together     5

### 2   Providing quality clinical care     8

Putting the patient first and establishing boundaries     9
Practising people skills     9
Getting governance right     10
Medical equipment and ergonomics     12
Maintaining skills     12
Being civil     12
Embracing human factors in sports and exercise medicine     13

### 3   Clinical reasoning     16

What is evidence-based practice?     17
What information do you prioritise for clinical decisions?     19
Can research help answer your clinical question?     19
Can you trust the results of research you are reading?     20
How do you know whether the athlete has improved?     20
Do the results apply to the person in front of you?     21
Bringing it together: shared decision making     21

### 4   Shared decision making     24

What is shared decision making?     25
The three-talk model of shared decision making     25

Key principles for making shared decisions     26
Shared decision making in practice     27

### 5   The multidisciplinary team approach     32

Introduction: why sports and exercise medicine?     33
Athlete, coach and clinician: the tripartite nucleus     33
High-performing clinical teams     34
Injury and illness management and athlete performance: a delicate balancing act     36
Top teamwork tips from the frontline     38
"Love thy sport" (and physical activity!)     38

### 6   Working with sporting teams     42

The role of the sport and exercise clinician in a team setting     43
Pre-season     45
In-season     48
Travel     49
Off-season     52

### 7   Career development     54

The clinician's journey     56
The heart of clinical practice: the office consult     56
Goal setting and time management     57
Building referrals: relationship marketing     58
Other skills that make you a better clinician     58
Take control of your career     59
Choose an empowered workplace     61
Common concerns     63

## PART B  Clinical sciences

**8  Acute injuries**  68

Mechanisms of acute injury  69
Pathophysiology and initial management  70
Bone  71
Joint  73
Hyaline cartilage  74
Fibrocartilage  75
Ligament  77
Muscle  77
Tendon  86
Fascia  87
Bursa  87
Nerve  87
Fat pad  88
Skin  88

**9  Overuse injuries**  90

Have we made progress with the challenges
of overuse injuries?  91
Bone stress injuries: nomenclature and
pathophysiology  91
Bone stress injuries: management principles  102
Other overuse conditions of bone  108
Articular cartilage  109
Joint  109
Ligament  109
Muscle  109
Tendon  110
Tendon management principles  116
Other tendon pathologies  120
Bursa  122
Nerve  122
Skin  122
But it's not that simple  124

**10  How does pain work? Using
contemporary neuroscience to
understand pain, performance and
recovery**  126

What is pain?  127
What is nociception?  127

The "fit for purpose/play/performance" model  131
Always a nano step ahead: our internal models,
predictions and corrections  132
The brain is different in those with persistent pain  135
Treating someone in pain: a complex system
requires a comprehensive approach  136

**11  Managing pain**  138

The pain spectrum  139
Contextualising pain for the individual  140
Neuropathic pain or neuropathic
"contribution" to pain?  146
Somatic and radicular referred pain  146
Rethinking models of care: biomedical versus
biopsychosocial  147
Managing acute and subacute pain  150
Managing persistent pain  152
Other treatment tools  158
Bringing it all together  161

**12  Introduction to clinical biomechanics**  164

Key concepts in biomechanics  165
Measurement of muscle performance  170
Tissue-specific tolerance to loads  171
Tissue homeostasis and mechanotherapy  172
How do we obtain biomechanical data?  175

**13  Biomechanical aspects of injury
in nine specific sports**  178

Baseball  179
Climbing  186
Cricket (fast bowling)  188
Cycling  192
Golf  196
Rowing  199
Swimming  204
Tennis  208
Volleyball  211
Running shoes  213

# Contents

## 14 Training principles, programming and prescription 216

Principles of training 217
Conditioning training 218
Endurance training 218
Speed training 219
Agility training 220
Resistance training 220
Flexibility training 225
Putting it all together: designing the training program 227

## 15 Load management 228

Collecting training load data 229
Analysing training load data 233

Decision making with training load data 234
Why load management remains more art than science 235

## 16 Recovery 240

Cooling 241
Heating 241
Contrast therapy 243
Hydrostatic pressure 243
Compression 243
Nutrition 244
Mental recovery 248
Sleep 250
Practical strategies: putting it all together 252
Conclusion 254

## PART C The clinical approach

## 17 Preventing injury 256

What has sport learned from injury-prevention science? 257
Reducing injury risk in your team 259
Sport policy and rules 266
Personal protective equipment 268
Embedding injury prevention in coach-led programs 272
The role of playing surfaces in injury prevention 276
Stretching 276

## 18 Periodic health assessment of athletes 278

Why perform the health assessment? 279
Who to assess 286
When to perform a PHA 287
What to include in the template 287
Other things to consider 288

## 19 Diagnosis: history and physical examination 292

Diagnosis isn't limited just to tissue diagnosis 293
Keys to accurate diagnosis 293
History 294

Physical examination 297
Differential diagnoses 304

## 20 Diagnosis: imaging 306

Five imaging habits of top clinicians 307
Conventional radiography 310
Magnetic resonance imaging 310
Ultrasound 314
Computed tomography 315
Radionuclide bone scanning 316
Artificial intelligence (AI) in imaging 316

## 21 Diagnosis: phases of clinical assessment 318

Clinical assessment 319
Phase 1: gathering clinical data 319
Phase 2: making the diagnosis and sharing the prognosis 319
Phase 3: choosing the treatment plan 324

## 22 Red flags 328

What is a red flag? 329
Three tips to spot red flags 330
Conditions that often come with red flags 330

## 23 Using PROMs in clinical practice    342

What are PROMs?    343
Using PROMs to benefit the injured athlete    344
Choosing which PROM to use    344
Interpreting the PROM score    349
Examples of commonly used PROMs    351
Clinical case    352

## 24 Treatment of sports injuries    356

Overview of Chapters 24–28    357
Acute injury management    358
Therapeutic exercise    362
Manual treatments    368
Taping    376
Bracing    378
Electrophysical agents    380
Dry needling and acupuncture    383
Therapeutic medication    386
Nutraceuticals and nutrition    394
Autologous blood, blood products and cell therapy    396
And finally …    398

## 25 Athlete education    402

Why educate the athlete?    403
Theories, models and frameworks relevant
to athlete education    404
Common topics covered in education programs    408
Preparing successful education sessions
for athletes    411
Using external learning resources: choose wisely    414
Evaluating the success of your education    416
When your education program isn't working    417

## 26 Surgery in sports and exercise medicine    418

Identifying surgical candidates    419
A surgical approach to two current controversies    421
Communication for better surgical outcomes    424
Common surgeries in sports and exercise medicine    425
Post-surgical complications    433
Return-to-sport decisions post-surgery    433

## 27 Principles of sports injury rehabilitation    438

General principles    440
Understanding the patient: build a working
alliance    440
Goal setting and targeted interventions    441
Phases of rehabilitation    443
Knowing when to progress the exercises    446
When rehabilitation does not go according
to plan    447

## 28 Return to sport    450

The return-to-sport continuum    451
Progressing from out (injured) to outstanding
(performance)    451
Testing the athlete's readiness to return    452
Gathering and synthesising information to
support shared return-to-sport decisions    452
What to work on today to avoid poor
return-to-sport outcomes tomorrow    459
Data science supporting high-quality
return-to-sport decisions    460

*Index*    462

# Preface

Every page of *Clinical Sports* Medicine has a purpose and this preface introduces you to three new characters in the *Clinical Sports Medicine* story. In 1993, *Clinical Sports Medicine* was one book—one character. Sport has changed dramatically in the past 30 years—and the new three-book format of the 6th edition parallels how our profession has adapted—and now provides much to benefit the health of our communities.

The goal of *Clinical Sports Medicine* is to provide value for (a) students learning our craft, (b) those who manage injuries and (c) those who address the medical issues related to sport and health. Three audiences—three books of manageable size at a reasonable price. *Clinical Sports Medicine* is meant to be used—let's name that price is important for access.

- Book 1, *Clinical Sports Medicine: Foundations of Clinical Practice:* If you are beginning your career in sports and exercise medicine and rehabilitation, you need a foundational comprehensive text that introduces you to the principles of our field and spells out things that experienced clinicians know. Making the implicit explicit. Book 1 will help you get through your exams and get your licence so you can deliver athlete care. More details below.
- Book 2, *Clinical Sports Medicine: Managing Injuries:* If you have a clinical licence and want to know what those with many years of experience might be thinking about the patient in front of you, Book 2 is for you. By moving the foundational concepts into their own book (Book 1), we can pack more expert tips into Book 2. The book begins with emergency management and then guides your management of patients who present with conditions from head to toe. Yes—via shoulder, knee, ankle—of course! The go-to manual for the practising clinician. Practical, illustrated, multimedia. More than 100 authors have been pouring their expertise into this. This book will be available in 2025.
- Book 3, *Clinical Sports Medicine: The Medicine of Exercise:* Sports and exercise medicine is much more than managing injuries alone. Active people complain of breathlessness, dizziness, bloody urine—a gamut of symptoms that don't arise from the musculoskeletal system. Internal medicine, health promotion, public health related to physical activity and sport . . . generally not well covered in traditional medical texts. This body of work is captured in Book 3, scheduled to be published in 2026.

In sum, across the three books, you'll benefit from more than 300 experts sharing their wisdom. But just engage with the material you need—in one or more of the three books.

Now let's dive into the details of Book 1—which we affectionately call "Foundations". Sticking with the rule of threes (!)—this first book has three key parts!

## Part A: The sport and exercise clinician

"Part A: The sport and exercise clinician" has seven very practical chapters, four of which are completely new. We open with patient voices (Chapter 1), we discuss the elements of quality care (Chapter 2) and clinical reasoning (Chapter 3), and we introduce shared decision making to our field (Chapter 4). We are delighted with how the chapters on *working as* a (multidisciplinary) team and *working with* a team (Chapters 5 and 6) came together. And working on those reminded us that it's essential to think about career development from day one—hence we include the experiences of one of the great mentors, Mike Kenihan (Chapter 7). What does it take to get that job you really want?

## Part B: Clinical sciences

"Part B: Clinical sciences" provides the knowledge base that underpins our clinical work. What are the common pathologies in acute (Chapter 8) and overuse (Chapter 9) injuries? Two chapters (Chapters 10 and 11) explain pain science—a field with remarkable advances in recent years. Two chapters provide the foundation for biomechanics—the clinically relevant terms and principles (Chapter 12) and then wisdom from the great clinicians in nine specific sports (Chapter 13). This is an example of where you will benefit from 20–30 years of the authors' clinical experience at the highest levels by reading, reviewing the images and, where appropriate, following the QR codes to additional content.

Part B closes out with chapters on training and recovery: the definitions and core concepts in the applied setting (Chapter 14), an all-new chapter on training load management (Chapter 15) and the latest on the ever-changing science of recovery (Chapter 16). How much is too much? Mid-career and older clinicians all wish they'd had the benefit of these experts—their advice beautifully illustrated and in one place—when they were at your stage!

## Part C: The clinical approach

"Part C: The clinical approach" guides you in the clinic. As a learner with supervision, or as a junior clinician, this part is your handbook for three key "how-to" elements of practice that you must master before prescribing treatment. First, how to prevent injuries and how to do a health assessment (Chapters 17 and 18). Second, how to listen, how to examine, how to interpret imaging and how to spot red flags (Chapters 19–22). Third, one of our favourite new chapters (Chapter 23) guides you as to why and how to use patient-reported outcome measures in the clinical setting. The images of the clinician's thought bubbles, the case studies and the specific tools mean you can turn one night's reading into your next day's clinical practice.

The last five chapters in the print version focus on the athlete's journey after diagnosis. This is what you have been preparing for: learning the rationale for various treatments (Chapter 24), educating the athlete—definitely an important part of treatment (Chapter 25)—and the principles of surgery in the context of sport (Chapter 26). We have revisited principles of skilful rehabilitation (Chapter 27) and are delighted that Dr Clare Ardern agreed to helm a new chapter—return-to-sport participation and performance (Chapter 28). In that way, we close the circle that began with the athlete and their clinical presentation.

We are quietly confident that you will find yourself spending a lot of time with *Foundations of Clinical Practice*. Like athletes confident in their training, our confidence stems from the quality of the 88 stars who joined us to create this book. It was a privilege to work with them.

We wish you every success in your training with this first book of the 6th edition, *Foundations of Clinical Practice*.

Peter Brukner
Karim Khan
August 2024

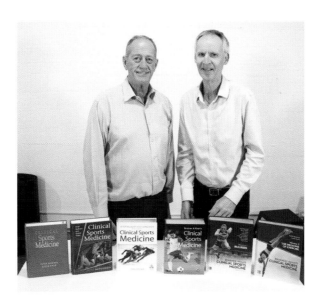

# About the authors

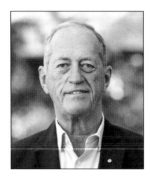

## Peter Brukner

OAM, MBBS, DSc (honoris causa), DRCOG, FACSEP, FASMF, FACSM, FFSEM (Ireland, Hon), FFSEM (UK, Hon)

### Sport and exercise physician

Professor of Sports Medicine, La Trobe Sports and Exercise Medicine Research Centre, La Trobe University, Melbourne, Australia

Founding Partner, Olympic Park Sports Medicine Centre, Melbourne, Australia

Founding Partner, Imaging @ Olympic Park, Melbourne, Australia

Head, Sports Medicine and Sports Science, Liverpool Football Club, UK, 2010–2012

Editor, *Sport Health,* 1990–1995

Associate Editor, *British Journal of Sports Medicine,* 2010 – present

Founder and Chair, SugarByHalf, 2016 – present

Founder and Chair, Defeat Diabetes, 2021 – present

### Team physician

Australian Cricket Team, 2012–2017, World Cup 2015

Socceroos, 2007–2010, Asian Cup Finals 2007, World Cup Finals 2010

Australian Olympic team, Atlanta 1996, Sydney 2000

Australian Commonwealth Games team, Edinburgh 1986, Kuala Lumpur 1998

Australian team, World Student Games, Edmonton 1983, Kobe 1985, Zagreb 1987

Australian Athletics team 1990–2000, World Championships Tokyo 1991, Gothenburg 1995, Seville 1999

Australian team, World Cup Athletics, Havana 1992

Australian Men's Hockey team, 1994–1995

Australian team, World Swimming Championships, Madrid 1986

Melbourne Football Club (AFL), 1987–1990, 2020–2021

Collingwood Football Club (AFL), 1996

University Blues Football Club, 1972 – present

### Books

*Food for Sport,* 1987

*Stress Fractures,* 1999

*Drugs in Sport—What the GP Needs to Know,* 1996, 2000

*The Encyclopedia of Exercise, Sport and Health,* 2004

*Essential Sports Medicine,* 2005

*Clinical Sports Anatomy,* 2010

*A Fat Lot of Good,* 2019

*The Diabetes Plan,* 2023

### Selected awards

Medal of the Order of Australia, 2006

Inaugural Honour Award, Australian College of Sports Physicians, 1996

Citation Award, American College of Sports Medicine, 2000

Honorary Fellowship, Faculty of Sport and Exercise Medicine (UK), 2010

Honorary Fellowship, Faculty of Sports and Exercise Medicine (Ireland), 2012

Life Membership, Melbourne University Football Cub, 1979

Life Membership, Athletics Australia, 2023

Honorary Doctorate, DSc (honoris causa), La Trobe University, 2022

State Government of Victoria Outstanding Contribution to Sport in Victoria Award, 2023

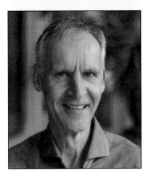

# Karim Khan

AO, MD, PhD, MBA, FACSEP, FSMA, FCAHS, DipSportMed (CASEM), FACSM, FFSEM (Ireland, Hon), FFSEM (UK, Hon)

## Sport and exercise physician

Professor, University of British Columbia (Department of Family Practice and School of Kinesiology), Vancouver, Canada

Scientific Director, Canadian Institutes of Health Research (CIHR), Institute of Musculoskeletal Health and Arthritis (IMHA), Ottawa, Canada

Adjunct Professor, School of Allied Health, College of Science Health and Engineering, La Trobe University, Melbourne, Australia

Visiting Professor, School of Human Movement Studies, The University of Queensland, Brisbane, Australia

Exercise is Medicine Committee, American College of Sports Medicine, 2009–2011

Director of Research and Education, Aspetar Orthopaedic and Sports Medicine Hospital, Qatar, 2013–2015

Sports Medicine Advisory Board to the International Olympic Committee, 2015–2020

Scientific Committee Member, IOC World Conference on Prevention of Injury and Illness in Sport, 2012–2024

Academic Advisory Board: IOC Diplomas in Sports Medicine and Sports Physical Therapies

## Team physician

Olympic Games Sydney 2000, Basketball Competition Venue

Australian Women's Basketball (The Opals) 1991–1996

The Australian Ballet Company, 1991–1996

The Australian Ballet School, 1991–1996

Australian team, World Student Games, 1993

Australian team, Junior World Cup Hockey, 1993

## Editor-in-chief

*British Journal of Sports Medicine,* 2008–2020

*BMJ Open Sport and Exercise Medicine,* 2015–2019

*Sport Health,* 1995–1997

## Books (co-author)

*The Encyclopedia of Exercise, Sport and Health,* 2004

*Physical Activity and Bone Health,* 2001

## Board member

Governance Council, *Canadian Medical Association Journal (CMAJ)* 2024–

## Selected awards

Officer of the Order of Australia, 2019

Honorary Doctorate, LLB (honoris causa), University of Edinburgh, 2019

Honorary Doctorate, PhD (honoris causa), Norwegian School of Sports Sciences, 2018

Honorary Fellowship, Faculty of Sport and Exercise Medicine (UK), 2014

Honorary Fellowship, Faculty of Sports and Exercise Medicine (Ireland), 2011

Sports Medicine Australia Fellows' Citation for Service, 2005

Prime Minister's Medal for Service to Australian Sport, 2000

# Editors

**Clare L Ardern** BPhysio (Hons), PhD

Assistant Professor, Department of Physical Therapy, Faculty of Medicine, The University of British Columbia, Vancouver, Canada; Editor-in-Chief, *Journal of Orthopaedic & Sports Physical Therapy;* Editor-in-Chief, *JOSPT Open*

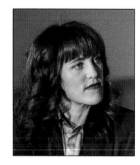

**Roald Bahr** MD, PhD

Professor and Chair, Oslo Sports Trauma Research Center, Department of Sports Medicine, Norwegian School of Sport Science; Chief Medical Officer, Olympiatoppen and Norwegian Olympic Training Center; Director, Aspetar Injury and Illness Prevention Program, Aspetar Orthopaedic and Sports Medicine Hospital, Doha, Qatar

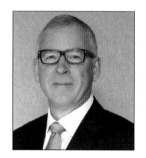

**Paul Blazey** PT, MSc, PGCE

Research Manager, Faculty of Medicine, University of British Columbia, Vancouver, Canada; Physiotherapist, Restore Physiotherapy, Vancouver, Canada; Editor, *Journal of Orthopaedic & Sports Physical Therapy*

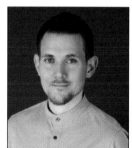

**Ben Clarsen** PT, MSc, PhD

Medical Researcher, Fédération Internationale de Football Association; Associate Professor, Oslo Sports Trauma Research Center, Norwegian School of Sport Sciences; Specialist Sports Physiotherapist, Norwegian Olympic Training Centre (Olympiatoppen), 2011–2019

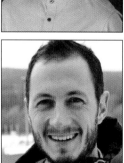

**Kay Crossley** AM, BAppSci, PhD

Professor and Director, La Trobe Sport and Exercise Medicine Research Centre, School of Allied Health, Human Services and Sport, La Trobe University, Melbourne, Australia; Australian Olympic Team Physiotherapist, Sydney 2000

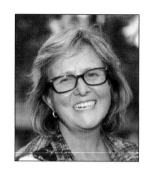

**Bruce B Forster** MSc, MD, FRCPC, FCAR, FFRRCSI (Hon)

Professor, Department of Radiology, University of British Columbia, Vancouver, Canada; Member, IOC Medical and Scientific Games Group

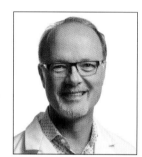

**Mark R Hutchinson** MD, FACSM, FAANA, FAAOS

Distinguished Professor of Orthopaedic Surgery and Sports Medicine, Head Team Physician and Division Chief of Sports Medicine, University of Illinois at Chicago, Chicago, USA

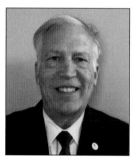

**Anne Lasinsky** BSc (ATC), MA, MSc, PhD

Senior researcher, School of Kinesiology, University of British Columbia, Vancouver, Canada. Senior educational editor—*Clinical Sports Medicine.*

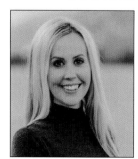

# Contributors

**Elanna K Arhos** PT, DPT, PhD

Postdoctoral Scholar, School of Health and Rehabilitation Sciences, The Ohio State University, Columbus, USA

**Ummukulthoum Bakare** PT, BSc, MSc, PhD

Member, Medical and Scientific Commission, Nigeria Olympic Committee, Nigeria

**Joletta Belton** MSc

Fraser, USA

**James Broatch** PhD, ESSAM AES ASpS1

Senior Research Fellow, Institute for Health and Sport, Victoria University, Melbourne, Australia

**Garrett Bullock** PT, DPT, DPhil

Assistant Professor, Department of Orthopaedic Surgery, Wake Forest University School of Medicine, USA

**Darren Burgess** BSpSci (Hons), PhD

General Manager High Performance – Adelaide Crows FC, Adelaide, Australia

**Graeme L Close** BSc (Hons), PhD, SENr, FBASES, FECSS

Professor of Human Physiology, Liverpool John Moores University, Liverpool, UK

**Natalie J Collins** BPhty (Hons), M Sports Physio, PhD

Associate Professor in Physiotherapy, School of Health and Rehabilitation Sciences, The University of Queensland, Brisbane, Australia

**Chad Cook** PT, PhD, FAPTA

Professor and Director of Clinical Research Facilitation, Department of Orthopaedics, Department of Population Health Sciences, Duke Clinical Research Institute, Duke University, Durham, USA

**Sean Cumming** PhD

Professor of Paediatric Exercise Science, University of Bath, UK

**Torstein Dalen-Lorentsen** MSc, PhD

Research Manager, Department of Health Research, SINTEF Digital, Oslo; Researcher, Oslo Sports Trauma Research Center, Department of Sports Medicine, Norwegian School of Sports Sciences, Oslo, Norway

**Faraz Damji** BKin, MSc, MD

Family Medicine Resident Physician, Department of Family & Community Medicine, Temerty Faculty of Medicine, University of Toronto, Toronto, Canada

**Stefano Della Villa** MD

President, Isokinetic Medical Group, Italy and UK

**Robert-Jan de Vos** MD, PhD

Sports Medicine Physician and Associate Professor, Department of Orthopedics and Sports Medicine, Erasmus MC University Medical Center, Rotterdam, The Netherlands

**H Paul Dijkstra** MBChB, BSc (Hons), MPhil, FFSEM, DPhil

Specialist Sport and Exercise Medicine Physician; Director of Medical Education at Aspetar Orthopaedic and Sports Medicine Hospital, Doha, Qatar; Nuffield Department of Orthopaedics, Rheumatology and Musculoskeletal Sciences, University of Oxford, Oxford, UK

**Matthew Driller** SpExSci (Hons), PhD, ASpSc2

Associate Professor, School of Allied Health, Human Services and Sport, La Trobe University, Melbourne, Australia

**FC du Toit** BA (Hons), MSc, PhD

Lecturer, Senior Biokineticist and Practice Manager, Sport, Exercise Medicine and Lifestyle Institute and Division of Biokinetics and Sports Science, Department of Physiology, Faculty of Health Sciences, University of Pretoria, South Africa

**Carolyn A Emery** PT, PhD

Canada Research Chair (Tier 1); Professor and Chair, Sport Injury Prevention Research Centre, Faculty of Kinesiology and Cumming School of Medicine, University of Calgary, Calgary, Canada

**Sharron Flahive** MBChB, Dip Sp Med, FACSEP

Sport and Exercise Physician; Chief Medical Officer, NRL; Team Doctor, Sydney Swans AFL, Australia

**Dale Forsdyke** BA (Hons), MSc, PGCE, PhD, MSST, SFHEA

Senior Lecturer and Programme Lead, School of Science, Technology and Health, York St John University, York, UK

**Kal Fried** MBBS, FACSEP

Sports & Exercise Physician, Chief Medical Advisor, Pain Revolution Local Pain Educator Program, Melbourne, Australia

**Daniel J Friedman** MBBS (Hons)

Sport and Exercise Medicine Registrar (ACSEP), Australian Institute of Sport, Canberra, Australia

**Cas Fuchs** PhD

Postdoctoral Researcher and Lecturer, Department of Human Biology, Maastricht University Medical Centre+, Maastricht, The Netherlands

**Phil Glasgow** PhD, MTh, MRes, BSc (Hons), FFSEM (Hon)

Head of Performance Support, Irish Rugby Football Union, Dublin, Ireland

**Adam Gledhill** PhD, FHEA, FBASES

Course Director, Sport, Exercise and Health Sciences, Carnegie School of Sport, Leeds Beckett University, Leeds, UK

**Anthony Goff** BSc, MSc, PhD

Assistant Professor, Singapore Institute of Technology, Health and Social Sciences, Singapore

**Robert Granter** BSocSci, AdDipRemMass (Myotherapy)

Myotherapist, Head of Soft Tissue Therapy Services Australian Olympic Team, 1996 and 2000; Head of Massage Therapy Services, Melbourne 2006 Commonwealth Games

**Steffan Griffin** MBChB, BSc (Hons), DipMSKMed, MFSEM, PGCert (MSK US)

Moray House School of Education and Sport, University of Edinburgh, UK

**Shona Halson** BAppSci (Hons), PhD

Professor and Deputy Director, SPRINT Research Centre, School of Behavioural and Health Sciences, Australian Catholic University, Australia

**Jonathan Hanson** FFSEM, FRCEM, FFSEM (I)

Consultant Physician in Sport and Exercise Medicine, NHS Fife, Scotland; Team Doctor, Scotland Rugby (Men)

**Kimberly G Harmon** MD

Professor, Departments of Family Medicine and Orthopaedics and Sports Medicine; Head Football Physician, University of Washington, USA

**Roger Hawkes** MB ChB, Dip Sports Med, FFSEM (UK)

Founder Member of the DP World, Golf Science and Health Committee, Virginia Water, UK

**Lina Holm Ingelsrud** MSc, PhD

Physiotherapist; Senior Researcher, Clinical Orthopaedic Research Hvidovre, Department of Orthopaedic Surgery, Copenhagen University Hospital, Hvidovre, Denmark

**Sabeena Jalal** MBBS, MScPH, SM, PhD

Senior Researcher, University of British Columbia, Vancouver, Canada

**Steven Kamper** BSc (Hons), BAppSc, PhD

Professor of Allied Health, University of Sydney and Nepean Blue Mountains Local Health District, Australia

**Emma Kavanagh** BSc, MSc, PhD, FBASES, CSci, HCPC Registered Sport and Exercise Psychologist

Associate Professor in Sport Psychology and Safe Sport, Bournemouth University, Bournemouth, UK

**Michael Kenihan** Dip Tech Phys, MAPA, FASMF, FFIMS

Director, Magellan Stem Cells; Director and GM of Melbourne Stem Cell Centre Research; Director of MK Healthcare Business Consulting, Australia

**Paul Kirwan** BSc Physio (Hons), MSc, PhD, MISCP

Assistant Professor, Discipline of Physiotherapy, School of Medicine, Trinity College Dublin, Ireland; Clinical Specialist Physiotherapist, Connolly Hospital, Dublin, Ireland

**Ash Kolstad** MSc

PhD Candidate, Sport Injury Prevention Research Centre, Faculty of Kinesiology, University of Calgary, Calgary, Canada

**Vasileios Korakakis** BPhysio, PhD, OMPT

Research Associate, Department of Health Sciences, School of Life Sciences and Health Sciences, PhD in Physiotherapy Program, University of Nicosia, Cyprus

**Alex Kountouris** BAppSci (Physio), PostGradDip Sports Physio, PhD

Sports Science and Sports Medicine Manager, Cricket Australia

**Jeremy Lewis** PhD, FCSP

Consultant Physiotherapist, Therapy Department, Central London Community Healthcare National

Health Service Trust, Finchley Memorial Hospital, London, UK; Professor of Musculoskeletal Research, School of Health Sciences, University of Nottingham, Nottingham, UK; Professor of Physiotherapy, School of Life and Health Sciences, University of Nicosia, Cyprus

**Behnam Liaghat** PT, PhD, RISPT

Assistant Professor, Department of Sports Science and Clinical Biomechanics, University of Southern Denmark, Odense, Denmark

**Christoph Lutter** MD, PhD, MSc, MHBA

Professor for Sports Orthopaedics, University Medical Center Rostock, Rostock, Germany

**Kerry MacDonald** PhD, ChPC

High Performance Manager, Volleyball Canada

**Erin M Macri** MPT, PhD

Senior Researcher, Department of Orthopaedics and Sports Medicine, Erasmus MC University Medical Center Rotterdam, Rotterdam, The Netherlands

**Håvard Moksnes** PhD

Sports Physiotherapist, The Norwegian FA Sports Medicine Clinic (Idrettens Helsesenter), The Norwegian Olympic Training Center and Oslo Sports Trauma Research Center, Oslo, Norway

**G Lorimer Moseley** AO, DSc, PhD, FAAHMS, FACP

Bradley Distinguished Professor of Clinical Neurosciences & Foundation Chair in Physiotherapy, University of South Australia, Adelaide, Australia

**Margo Mountjoy** MD, PhD, CCFP (SEM), FCFP, FACSM, FCAHS, Dip Sport Med

Clinical Professor, Department of Family Medicine (Sport & Exercise Medicine), McMaster University, Hamilton, Canada; IOC Medical & Scientific Commission Games Group, ASOIF (Association of Summer Olympic International Federations) Medical & Scientific Consultative Group Chair

**Andrew Murray** MRCGP, FRCP(G), PhD, FFSEM

Chief Medical and Scientific Officer, European Tour Group/DP World Tour Golf, Virginia Water, UK

**Dustin Nabhan** PhD, DC, FACSM

Consultant, Tucson, USA

**James O'Donovan** MB BCh, BaO, MICGP, FFSEM (Ire), MSc (SEM) DipSportMed (CASEM)

Sports and Exercise Medicine Consultant; Sport Ireland Institute, National Sports Campus, Dublin,

Ireland; Assistant Professor Sports & Exercise Medicine, Dublin City University, Ireland; Chief Medical Officer, Team Ireland Olympic Team

**Kieran O'Sullivan** Postgrad Dip Teaching and Learning, B Physio, M Manip Ther, PhD, FISCP

Professor, School of Allied Health, University of Limerick, Ireland

**Brooke Patterson** BPhysio (Hons), PhD

Research Fellow, La Trobe University Sport and Exercise Medicine Research Centre, La Trobe University, Melbourne, Australia

**Babette Pluim** MD, PhD, MPH, FFSEM (UK), FFSEM (Ire)

Extraordinary Professor, Section Sports Medicine, Faculty of Health Sciences, University of Pretoria, Pretoria, South Africa; Chief Medical Officer, Royal Netherlands Lawn Tennis Association (KNLTB), Amstelveen, The Netherlands

**Emily Powell** MBBS, iBSc (Hons)

Anaesthetics Department, Chelsea and Westminster Hospital NHS Foundation Trust, UK

**Dawn Richards** BSc (Hons), PhD

Founder, Five02Labs Inc., Toronto, Canada

**Suzanna Russell** BExSS (Hons), PhD, ESSA ASpS

Postdoctoral Research Fellow, Sports Performance, Recovery, Injury and New Technologies Research Centre, Faculty of Health Sciences, Australian Catholic University, Australia

**Annina Schmid** PhD, MManipTher, MMACP, MCSP

Professor of Pain Neurosciences, Nuffield Department of Clinical Neurosciences, University of Oxford, UK

**Volker Schöffl** MD, PhD, MHBA

Department of Orthopedic and Trauma Surgery, Sportsmedicine, Klinikum Bamberg, Bamberg, Germany

**Isla Shill** MSc

PhD Candidate, Sport Injury Prevention Research Centre, Faculty of Kinesiology, University of Calgary, Calgary, Canada

**Kevin Sims** Dip Phyty, M Phyty St, PhD, FACP

National Physiotherapy Manager, Tennis Australia

**Christopher Skazalski** PT, DPT, ATC, PhD

Researcher/Consultant, Skazalski Sports Medicine and Performance, Michigan, USA

**Alicia Tang** B Physio, PG Dip Sports Physio, MSc

APA Sports Physiotherapist; Head of Academy Medicine, Derby County Football Club, UK

**Stephen Targett** MB ChB, FACSEP

Sport and Exercise Medicine Physician, Aspetar Hospital, Doha, Qatar; Assistant Professor of Clinical Medicine Weill Cornell Medical School, Qatar

**Athol Thomson** BAppSci (Podiatry), BBiomedSci, PhD

Adjunct Associate Professor, Discipline of Podiatry, School of Allied Health, Human Services and Sport, La Trobe University, Australia

**Jane S Thornton** MD, PhD, CCFP (SEM), Dip Sport Med (IOC), Dip Sport Med (CASEM), OLY

Medical Director, International Olympic Committee; Associate Professor and Canada Research Chair in Injury Prevention and Physical Activity for Health, Western University, London, Canada

**Elsbeth van Dorssen** MD

Sports Medicine Physician, UMC Utrecht and Sportgeneeskunde Rotterdam, Utrecht University, Utrecht and Rotterdam, The Netherlands

**Nicol van Dyk** BSc (Phys), MSc, PhD, MICSP

Assistant Professor (Ad Astra Fellow), School of Public Health, Physiotherapy and Sport Science, University College Dublin, Dublin, Ireland

**Dina (Christa) Janse van Rensburg** MBChB, MSC, MMed, DMed (PhD), FACSM

Professor and Head of Department, Sports and Exercise Medicine, Section Sports Medicine, Faculty of Health Sciences, University of Pretoria, Pretoria; Specialist Rheumatologist, Eugene Marais Hospital, Pretoria, South Africa; Chair, Medical Advisory Panel, World Netball

**Stuart Warden** BPhysio (Hons), PhD, FACSM

Professor and Associate Dean for Research, School of Health and Rehabilitation Sciences, Indiana University, Indianapolis, USA

**Liam West** BSc (Hons), MBBCh, MSc, FACSEP

Sport and Exercise Medicine Physician; Head Doctor and Head of Health, Hawthorn Football Club, Melbourne, Australia

**Stephen West** BSc, PhD

Lecturer in Injury Prevention, Department for Health, University of Bath, Bath, UK

**Chris Whatman** PT, PhD

Associate Professor, School of Sport and Recreation, Auckland University of Technology, Auckland, New Zealand

**Rich Willy** PT, PhD

Associate Professor, School of Physical Therapy and Rehabilitation Sciences, University of Montana, Missoula, USA

**Fiona Wilson** BSc, MSc, PhD, MA, FTCD, MISCP

Professor and Chartered Physiotherapist, Discipline of Physiotherapy, School of Medicine, Trinity College Dublin, University of Dublin, Ireland

**Mara Yamauchi** BA, MSc

Former elite athlete, coach, UK

**Kate Yung** BSc Physio (Hons), MSc Sports Med & Health Sci, PhD

Director, Medical and Performance Innovations, Kitchee Sports Club, Hong Kong SAR; Lecturer, Department of Orthopaedics and Traumatology, Faculty of Medicine, The Chinese University of Hong Kong, Hong Kong SAR, China

## Reviewers

**Indiana Cooper** MD

Team Doctor, Richmond Football Club (VFL), Melbourne, Australia

**Craig Engstrom** BHMS (Ed) (Hons), MSc, PhD

Program Convener, Master of Sports Medicine, School of Human Movement and Nutrition Sciences, Faculty of Health and Behavioural Sciences, University of Queensland, Australia

**Daniel J Friedman** MBBS (Hons)

Sport and Exercise Medicine Registrar (ACSEP), Australian Institute of Sport, Canberra, Australia

**Benedict Tan** MBBS, MSpMed, DFD, FAMS, FACSM, DUniv

Head, SingHealth Duke-NUS Sport & Exercise Medicine Centre, Singapore

## Medical illustrator

**Vicky Earle** BSc, MEdTech, AFC

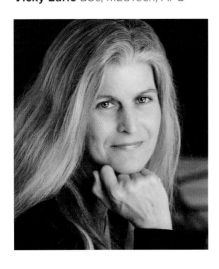

Vicky, an international award-winning medical illustrator, has worked with renowned authorities around the globe. She has created thousands of illustrations for medical and scientific textbooks and journals, as well as artwork for legal litigation, videos, animations and websites. She has co-created many of the most-recognisable images in key sports and exercise medicine publications. Vicky's keen interest in *Clinical Sports Medicine* stems not only from a great appreciation of the human body and its capabilities, but also from years of race experience as a championship rower, a world-class paddler and a rock climbing enthusiast. She knows first-hand the many injuries that accompany these activities.

# Acknowledgments

"It takes a village ..." is often used because many worthwhile projects do. More recently, you may have come across the African proverb: "If you want to go fast, go alone—if you want to go far, go together." Importantly, the concept of going far together is very familiar to those in our community—not only for those in team sports but of course also for individual athletes who rely on a team to help them get far.

We use this page to thank those who have taken *Clinical Sports Medicine* reasonably far to date. Far in age (32+ years), far in reach (all continents other than Antarctica), far in copies in the hands of clinicians, far via the Access Physical Therapy platform, far via social media shares and the www. ClinicalSportsMedicine.com website. Most of all, we hope far in quality—a trusted source of clinical advice anchored, wherever possible, in evidence— that clinicians and patients can use to make shared decisions.

We thank our eight colleagues and friends—Clare Ardern, Roald Bahr, Paul Blazey, Ben Clarsen, Kay Crossley, Bruce Forster, Mark Hutchinson and Anne Lasinsky—who have helped co-create this book. Their long-standing support and wisdom have been invaluable. Vicky Earle, the internationally renowned medical illustrator, extends her unique contribution that first poured into *Clinical Sports Medicine* 25 years ago and keeps making the book more and more useful. Specific thanks for *Clinical Sports Medicine: Foundations of Clinical Practice* go to the 88 chapter co-authors listed, with their affiliations, on pages xix–xxiii.

A book of this size, full of information as it is, is a complex task and we are grateful to our reviewers— Indiana Cooper, Craig Engstrom, Daniel Friedman and Benedict Tan—who have undertaken this thankless task with dedication and expertise. We have been fortunate to have benefitted from Amelia Choy as the art and permissions manager as well as project coordinator. Alisa Ribeiro provided design advice and created visual assets. Maya Lima was the lead reference researcher along with Adrianne Chow and Nejat Hassen.

The University of British Columbia (Department of Family Practice—Faculty of Medicine; Faculty of Education—School of Kinesiology) provided essential support (KK), as did La Trobe University's Sport and Exercise Medicine Research Centre (LASEM).

We thank Rochelle Deighton from McGraw Hill for her patience and understanding, and Caroline Hunter for her astute copy editing, eye for design and project management. This has made *Foundations* much, much better for the reader.

# Special features

*Clinical Sports Medicine* is designed as a manual to help you solve clinical problems. Here's a list of features that help you get quick answers. Four are completely new to this edition; six others are features you told us you loved.

## Chapter outline

What's a chapter about? The chapter outline lists the major headings within the book. This allows you to quickly find the information that you need.

### CHAPTER OUTLINE

Putting the patient first and establishing boundaries
Practising people skills
Getting governance right
Medical equipment and ergonomics
Maintaining skills
Being civil
Embracing human factors in sports and exercise medicine

## Learning objectives

Learning objectives provide a snapshot of what you will learn in the chapter.

### LEARNING OBJECTIVES

By the end of this chapter you should be able to:
- discuss the basic principles that facilitate quality clinical care
- explain how systems and processes can facilitate high-quality clinical care
- take action to facilitate a work environment conducive to safe and effective clinical care
- recognise human factors and how to incorporate them into good clinical care.

## Key points

The key points close off the chapter. Together with the learning objectives, they form the two ends of the bridge of new knowledge, and are another quick way to review (or preview!) a chapter.

### KEY POINTS

- Always put the patient first, even if that means protecting them from themselves.
- Athletes and clinicians spend much time together. This creates familiarity, which can be an advantage, but also requires you to develop formal boundaries to stop this strength becoming a pitfall.
- Developing people skills is an investment in providing better clinical care and delivering better patient care.
- The nature of high-performance sport entails the pursuit of marginal gains, which can involve expensive, novel or experimental interventions. Prioritise patient care and good governance.

## QR codes

With hours of additional trusted content, QR codes provide quick links to valuable and vetted resources. These resources elaborate on the content within the book in your learning.

 JOSPT

# Figures

With 383 expertly crafted figures, many by international award-winning medical illustrator Vicky Earle, this book includes illustrated concepts, photographs of assessment techniques, and algorithms that explain clinical phenomena (such as injury occurrence).

## Practice pearls

Practice pearls reflect expert clinicians' experience and provide advice key tips

> **PRACTICE PEARL**
>
> "One of the essential qualities of the clinician is interest in humanity, for the secret of the care of the patient is in caring for the patient." (Francis Peabody)

## Feature boxes

Feature boxes are included to highlight and address advanced clinical issues and areas of debate.

## Tables

Tables allow you to access clinically relevant information at a glance.

TABLE 22.1 Examples of conditions that can mimic one other

| "Obvious" (but incorrect) diagnosis | Alternative (correct) diagnosis, based on red flags |
|---|---|
| Migraine headache | Upper cervical facet joint hypomobility/cervicogenic headache |
| Rotator cuff tendinopathy | Glenohumeral joint instability (in a younger athlete) Acromioclavicular joint osteoarthritis (in an older athlete) |
| Tennis elbow | Cervical disc abnormality |
| Wrist "tendinitis" | Cervical abnormality |
| Hip osteoarthritis | Upper lumbar spine disc degeneration |
| Persistent hamstring strain | Abnormal neuromechanical dynamics |
| Patellofemoral pain/knee osteoarthritis | Referred pain from hip |
| Bucket handle tear of the meniscus | Referred pain from a ruptured L4–5 disc |
| Patellar dislocation | Anterior cruciate ligament rupture |
| Osgood-Schlatter lesion | Osteoid osteoma tibial tuberosity |
| "Shin splints" (periostitis, tendinopathy) | Chronic compartment syndrome or stress fracture |
| Achilles tendinopathy | Posterior impingement Retrocalcaneal bursitis |
| Plantar fasciitis | Medial plantar nerve entrapment |
| Morton's neuroma | Referred pain from an L5–S1 disc prolapse |
| Shoulder pain | Scapular pain caused by rib dysfunction or referred pain from the cervical spine |
| Compartment syndrome | Popliteal artery entrapment syndrome |
| Persistent lateral midfoot pain following sprain | Cuboid subluxation |

## References

A comprehensive list of carefully chosen references for each chapter can be found here: www.mhprofessional.com/CSM6e.

## www.clinicalsportsmedicine.com

Please visit the authors' website for more on clinical sports medicine. We aim to make this a community hub—a place for two-way interaction.

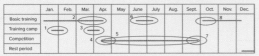

**BOX 17.2** An example risk profile for a college basketball team

Risk profiling (Fig. 17.6) works best when the clinical team truly engages with coaches and players. Including them allows you to draw on their past experiences with the team; this is especially important if there are no injury surveillance data available from the past. Coaches and players are key for interventions—implementing preventive measures.

**Risks 1–8**

1. Change in time zone, off-court training surface, climate and altitude during training camp in Colorado. Emphasis on defensive stance training and quick lateral movements could lead to several groin injuries. Players should not increase the amount or intensity of training too much.
2. Transition to greater amount of on-court training and intensity, combined with several practice games. Floor surface quite hard. Risk of lower limb injuries such as Achilles tendinopathy, medial tibial stress syndrome.
3. New training camp before beginning the competitive season; practice games on unusually slippery courts.

Training and practice matches are intense as players try to avoid being cut from the squad.
4. Beginning of the competitive season. A higher tempo and packed competitive schedule to which the player is unaccustomed. Risk of gradual-onset injury (e.g. patellar tendinopathy, tibial stress fracture) compounded by heavy academic periods (e.g. exams) leads to additional fatigue.
5. High risk of acute injuries during the competitive season, and a tough competition schedule at full intensity.
6. Interposed period of hard basic training with strength exercises to which the player is not accustomed and plyometric training increases risk of tendinopathy and muscle strain.
7. The end of the competitive season. Worn out and tired players? This is an important time to aggressively treat low-level "grumbling" injuries. Waiting for the injury to heal with rest alone is not recommended.
8. Transition to basic training period with running on trails.

|  | Jan. | Feb. | Mar. | Apr. | May | June | July | Aug. | Sept. | Oct. | Nov. | Dec. |
|---|---|---|---|---|---|---|---|---|---|---|---|---|
| Basic training | | 2 | | | 6 | | | | | | 8 | |
| Training camp | 1 | | 3 | | | | | | | | | |
| Competition | | | | 4 | 5 | | | | 7 | | | |
| Rest period | | | | | | | | | | | | |

**Figure 17.6** One way of depicting the elements of training (rows) and the rhythm of the season (months/columns). The circles represent the injury risks outlined in this box.

Scan here to access additional resources for this topic and more provided by the authors

# The sport and exercise clinician

# CHAPTER 1

# The patient

by **DAWN RICHARDS** and **JOLETTA BELTON** (patient authors)

*Work with us, rather than on us. The first step is building a relationship.*

DAWN RICHARDS AND JOLETTA BELTON

## CHAPTER OUTLINE

Context: patients' voices
Becoming a patient
What we hope for in the clinical encounter
The clinical encounter as a relationship
We're all in this together

## LEARNING OBJECTIVES

By the end of this chapter you should be able to:

- identify ways that you can improve the patient experience in healthcare
- recognise areas that patients can find frustrating
- reframe common clinical questions to avoid placing blame or judgment on the patient
- outline strategies to better incorporate the patient voice/perspective into clinical research and practice.

## Introduction to the chapter authors, Dawn Richards and Joletta Belton, by Peter Brukner and Karim Khan

The first edition of *Clinical Sports Medicine* (1993) began by explaining what our profession did and why it was needed. In Chapter 1, a figure depicted the athlete (patient) at the centre of a team of clinicians who provided clinical care. But that athlete didn't have a voice in our first edition, or in the second, third, fourth or fifth editions.

We have always had the athlete at the core of our work—our raison d'être—but we didn't spell that out in a chapter. We (along with all the book chapter authors) are delighted that Dr Dawn Richards and Joletta Belton agreed to open this sixth edition with the patient's perspective. And patient voices are prominent in many chapters in this book (and in *Clinical Sports Medicine 6e: Managing Injuries*).

As we turn this chapter over to Dawn and Joletta (Fig. 1.1), please note that for this chapter "we" means patients. Other chapters of this book are written by clinicians and scientists—in those chapters, "we" refers to clinicians and scientists.

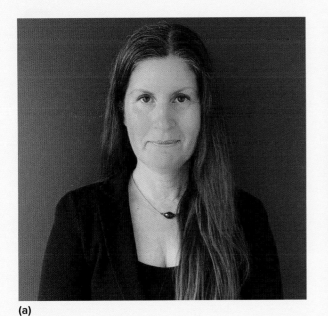
(a)

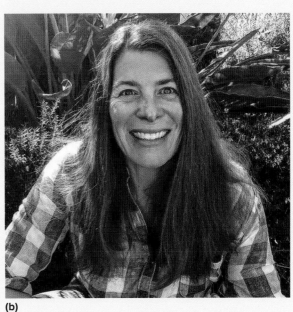
(b)

**Figure 1.1** Providing the patient perspective. Chapter authors (a) Dr Dawn Richards and (b) Joletta Belton.

## CONTEXT: PATIENTS' VOICES

We are writing this from our perspective as people—people who lead fulfilling lives, who have careers, families, friends and more, even though we may live with pain or a chronic disease.[1,2] People who sometimes find themselves as patients. And we recognise that the healthcare professionals who work with us are also people—people who may one day find themselves as patients.[3,4] We hope to emphasise our shared humanity in this chapter.

This chapter is not about blame or shame, or taking things personally. It is about learning how you (the clinician) can provide excellent care to anyone who is a patient. The same kind of care you would probably appreciate when you are a patient one day too. Or when you have a loved one who is a patient, and you are advocating for them or helping them to navigate through what may be a difficult and distressing time. This chapter aims to help you to learn from our patient experiences. And our experiences are just that, ours alone. Yet these experiences may also reflect the experiences of millions of people throughout the world, perhaps even yours.

## BECOMING A PATIENT

Imagine that you are a lifelong athlete, whether you are competitive or not. You have always been active. You lift weights, run, play sports. Your idea of a holiday is to go on an adventure where you can hike, climb, swim, surf, snowboard, ski or otherwise play outside. Or imagine that you work in a physically active profession. You are always on the move and don't feel like yourself if you're not doing something.

And then, suddenly, musculoskeletal pain, injury or disease stops you in your tracks. You can no longer do the things you love to do or need to do. The things that make you feel like you. And because you can no longer do the things that make you feel like yourself, you are no longer yourself.

You're probably not too worried at first. You expect to recover in due course, why wouldn't you? But things don't go as you expected. The pain, injury or illness lingers, and you don't know why. It becomes a bit more worrisome, and you have questions: How long will this last? Will it get better, or will it get even worse? What does it mean, not just in terms of a diagnosis—what does it mean for my future? For me? What will change if this doesn't get better?

It is understandably distressing to have your life altered by pain or illness. Especially when things don't make sense, when the path forward is unclear, and you don't have answers to all of your questions. So, reasonably, you continue to seek care, to seek answers, to seek a way forward. It is common to consult many different health professionals when pain or illness lingers. Imagine you are about to see the next clinician along your healthcare journey. What do you hope for in the clinical encounter? What do you want from the health professional in that encounter?

## WHAT WE HOPE FOR IN THE CLINICAL ENCOUNTER

What type of healthcare do patients want? What do all of us want for our loved ones? What do all of us want for our fellow beings?

There are a few things we think are fairly universal, things we've learned from our own experiences as active people who became patients because of musculoskeletal pain, injury or conditions:

- Set the stage with a calm, welcoming, non-judgmental environment. It might sound hokey, but it's not. It can make or break the relationship.
- Listen. Full stop. Listen to us when we are seeking your care. Invite us to tell our story and listen intently, without judgment.[5] The "without judgment" part is important. Be neutral. Let us share our experiences as we see and understand them. Help us to tell you our story, not the story you expect or want to hear. It may not be a story you can relate to or easily make sense of, and that's ok.
- Listen to understand, not to respond. Take it all in. So often we are rushed to get to the "important stuff",

which means that what is actually important to us is never shared.
- Allow time and space for silence. Sometimes we need a pause to find the words to express our experiences without feeling rushed.
- Be curious. Show us that you're interested in our story, in us as people, not just as a puzzle to be solved or a problem to be fixed.
- Ask relevant questions to gain context. Follow up with questions related to or relevant to our story. Not only does this show you're listening, you're curious and that you care, it will also help you to figure out what's going on.

> **PRACTICE PEARL**
>
> Validate our experiences, feelings and knowledge.[6] Acknowledge our challenges and distress. Of course we feel and think this way! You don't have to agree with or completely understand us to validate us.

- Recognise that we are experts of our own bodies and context: our environment, our culture, our goals, our values, our lives.
- Learn from us, just as we will learn from you. Understand that it's ok to say things like "I don't know", "I'll find you the answer" and "We'll work together to find the solution". Admitting you don't know and that we will find the answers together can help establish trust and show us that we've found a partner in our care who isn't afraid to be honest with us and work alongside us.
- Create a shared understanding of our experiences or diagnosis with us, rather than delivering a diagnosis to us. Invite us to combine our knowledge and expertise with yours to come up with explanations that make sense to us and for us and are about us and our unique lives and contexts. Ensure that we understand what you are saying and that you understand what we are saying.
- Work with us to develop a treatment plan that is acceptable, realistic and appropriate, and is aligned with our goals, values, culture and life. This plan may not be what you would do, and that's ok. These decisions need to be made for and with us, because it is our lives and health we are talking about here. Being a "patient" is just a slice of our identities. Most of our life is lived outside the clinic where we are not patients, we are just people, trying to get by like everybody else.[7] We have a lot going on that makes us fully rounded individuals beyond this part of us. We have to consider this as we make our own decisions about our care.

**A**

• Don't fret that this will take too much time. Some of us are long-winded, but most of us are not and are able to share our stories and what most concerns us in just a few minutes. With relevant follow-up questions you may actually be able to make a more accurate diagnosis more quickly, saving time in the long run.

That is our ideal clinical scenario, for us and for you. We hope that this is the type of encounter you have if ever you, or one of your loved ones, becomes a patient. We hope that you can be that clinician for your patients, too.

In Box 1.1, Dr Ben Darlow, a physiotherapist and Associate Professor at the University of Otago in Wellington, New Zealand, shares his thoughts on his approach to working with patients.

---

**BOX 1.1** Lessons I've learned from patients: Ben Darlow

"Conducting qualitative research gave me the opportunity to explore and consider patient stories without having to reach conclusions or find solutions. This experience influenced my clinical practice more than anything else.

I learned that allowing patients to present their story in their way helps me to hear what is most important. I learned to listen with curiosity, focusing on the story not my interpretation. I learned to value patients as experts in their field.

Sharing who I am (outside of my clinical role) and learning who the person is (outside of their patient role) allows us to develop our relationship as people, as well as partners with complementary expertise and shared goals. Exploring how the person makes sense of their condition and their experience helps me to ensure that my contribution is sensible."

REPRODUCED WITH PERMISSION FROM DR BEN DARLOW

---

## THE CLINICAL ENCOUNTER AS A RELATIONSHIP

Our ideal scenario doesn't always happen, for a variety of reasons. We have both seen a great many clinicians who we know cared about us as they cared for us, yet there was still something missing from the encounter. We have felt blamed and shamed for not getting better when we *should* have, and we know clinicians who have also felt ashamed or blamed when their patients didn't get better, too. It is understandable that patients want what ails them to be fixed, and understandable that clinicians want to fix people.

Patients and clinicians can have very similar feelings when working together. We may be frustrated in the clinical relationship when we are not responding to treatment the way we think we should. We can be frustrated with each other in terms of communication, not having enough time, not having a clear diagnosis or prognosis, not being aligned in the treatment plan or when facing other barriers to what we think of as "good care".

To alleviate this frustration, perhaps it would help to view our work together as a relationship. A relationship where we both play an important part, without "sides", and where we can both have emotions—similar or different. In this patient–clinician relationship, it is important that we speak a shared language, which we can only do when we come to together.

Miscommunication is very common, especially when musculoskeletal symptoms have lasted longer than expected.[8-10] Some commonly used, well-meaning phrases and questions from clinicians can take on a different meaning altogether for a distressed patient. Table 1.1 shares some of these phrases, and how they may be heard in ways you don't intend. We've also shared some possible ways you might reframe these behaviours and phrases. We are not clinicians, so these suggestions come from our experience as patients and what would have helped us better understand the clinicians' message.

## WE'RE ALL IN THIS TOGETHER

The thing we hope for most from this chapter is a sense that there is no "us versus you". We're all just humans trying to figure out this musculoskeletal health stuff. We all want answers that make sense to us. We all want to be able to act on what we learn. We all want what's best for ourselves, within our own particular contexts, whether we are patients or clinicians, or both.

To get to a relational frame within the clinical encounter, clinicians need to consider the lived expertise of patients. There is a lot you can learn from people who live with musculoskeletal pain or conditions. Not just hearing and learning from patient stories in the clinical encounter, which is incredibly important, but outside of the encounter as well. As Ben Darlow shared in Box 1.1, reading qualitative research was one way he learned more about patients' experiences. Another way is to work directly with patient and public partners in your own research,[11] in guideline development, clinical program development or when you are discovering the best ways to implement research into practice. There is a growing body of such work from which you can also learn.[12]

**TABLE 1.1    Common things clinicians do or say and what patients hear or feel**

| When clinicians do or say ... | Patients hear or feel ... | Suggestions for clinicians |
|---|---|---|
| Clinicians interrupt the patient's story to get to the "important stuff" | *The things that are important to me don't matter.* | Don't interrupt. Listen with curiosity and follow up with relevant questions once we've finished talking or made a particular point. If we've said something that doesn't make sense to you, ask us to clarify. Simply asking "Can you tell me more about that" may be very helpful and it shows us you're listening. |
| "What is your pain on a scale of 0–10?" | *A scale of 0–10? Does that mean at this moment? This morning? At its worst? At its best? Typically? On average over the last week?* | "Let's talk about the pain you are feeling. Can you tell me in your own words about your pain? What is most concerning to you about it? Are there times of day when it is worse? Better?" |
| "Good news, we didn't find anything wrong!" | *"Your experience isn't real, it's all in your head, you're making this up, you're exaggerating, it's not as bad as you're making it out to be."* | "These tests didn't show us anything, so a lot of scary things have been ruled out, which is good news. Your pain and symptoms are very real, but these tests cannot help us to work out what to do, so we will have to do some things differently to sort out what's going on and figure this out together. Are you ok with that?" |
| "How is the [hip/knee/shoulder, etc.] today?" | *The only thing that matters is the body part that is symptomatic (which reinforces that all that matters is the tissues).* | "How are you doing today—and how have things gone since we last met? Are you able to do what you'd like to? What have you been prevented from doing that you'd like to do?" |
| "Do you understand? Do you have any questions?" | *I feel like this is a quiz or I'm at school. Do they think I'm not smart enough to get what they're saying?* | "What questions do you have? What questions did you have after your last appointment or that have come up since?" |
| "Did you do your exercises?" | *Judgment. Even if I did my exercises! "What possible excuse do you have for not doing your exercises? Why aren't you better if you did them?"* | "Did you get a chance to try any of the things we suggested at your last appointment? Did they change how you feel at all? What questions do you have? What can I help you with—whether it's with the exercises we've talked about, or other things?" |
| "Pain is in the brain [or pain is psychological, or psychosocial]" | *"It's all in your head, you're making this up, you're exaggerating."* | "Pain can be really tough. It's often influenced by a whole range of interacting things that are unique to you. By working together, we can work out what's important for your pain and how we can change these." |
| "Your goal for the next visit is ..." | *My goals don't matter in any clear way, what matters most is what the clinician says.* | "What are your priorities between now and your next visit? What do you want to be able to do? What can you do to work towards this? What can I do to help? We will align your rehabilitation goals with what matters most to you." |
| "Recovery will take 6–8 weeks." | *"You'll be back to who you were before 6–8 weeks."* | "Recovery is individual. It might take [xyz] or it might take [abc] ... I'm committed to helping you get back to doing what is important to you in the time it takes you." |

The overarching theme is collaboration and relationship-building between clinicians and patients, inside and outside of the treatment environment. The more we work together to find the best ways forward, the better the outcomes will be for patients and clinicians alike.

We are grateful for the opportunity to share our experiences and insights in this chapter. We hope you feel validated by seeing all the good things you already do in the clinical encounter, and that you can take away something new to bring to your work as well.

## KEY POINTS

- Clinicians can create a better patient experience by demonstrating good listening skills, being curious about their patients, and acknowledging there are many things that they don't know.

- Patients are experts on themselves. Clinicians should bring together the patient's knowledge and expertise with their own clinical knowledge and expertise to co-create the treatment plan. (See also Chapters 3 and 4.)

- Miscommunication is a common source of frustration in the clinical encounter. Clear communication is critical to good clinical care.

- The patient and clinician share the goal of improving the patient's health. The patient–clinician relationship should be viewed as cooperative, not adversarial.

- By reframing common clinical questions to avoid blaming or presumptive language, the patient experience (and therefore, clinical care) may be improved.

- Clinician-researchers should incorporate the patient experience/voice into research, guideline/program development and knowledge translation efforts.

## REFERENCES

References for this chapter can be found at www.mhprofessional.com/CSM6e

## ADDITIONAL CONTENT

 Scan here to access additional resources for this topic and more provided by the authors

## CHAPTER 2

# Providing quality clinical care

with **STEFFAN GRIFFIN, JONATHAN HANSON, EMILY POWELL** and **SHARRON FLAHIVE**

*Time, sympathy and understanding must be lavishly dispensed, but the reward is to be found in that personal bond which forms the greatest satisfaction of the practice of medicine.*

DR FRANCIS PEABODY (1881–1927)

## CHAPTER OUTLINE

Putting the patient first and establishing boundaries

Practising people skills

Getting governance right

Medical equipment and ergonomics

Maintaining skills

Being civil

Embracing human factors in sports and exercise medicine

## LEARNING OBJECTIVES

By the end of this chapter you should be able to:

- discuss the basic principles that facilitate quality clinical care
- explain how systems and processes can facilitate high-quality clinical care
- take action to facilitate a work environment conducive to safe and effective clinical care
- recognise human factors and how to incorporate them into good clinical care.

A

You are probably reading this book to learn how to assess, diagnose and manage patients with a wide range of medical or musculoskeletal pathologies. In so doing you should feel armed with the theory to better manage patients with tendinopathies or traumatic injuries. However, patients don't exist as a theoretical construct. You might be caring for a patient as part of a wider network of professionals, and there are many factors beyond your immediate clinical knowledge that can have a substantial effect on a patient's health and outcomes.

In this chapter we introduce you to factors relevant to all healthcare settings and professionals—tips that will affect the quality of care you provide to your patients (Fig. 2.1). From ergonomics to communication, we hope that you will be able to apply what you learn here to your own professional setting. We believe that these factors are crucial for the health and wellbeing of those who trust you with their medical care.

## PUTTING THE PATIENT FIRST AND ESTABLISHING BOUNDARIES

A pillar of medicine is the notion of "primum non nocere": first, do no harm. In sports and performance settings, where clinicians are likely to be around their patients more often, familiarity can breed informality. While informality can be good for building trust, enabling patients to feel more comfortable disclosing pertinent information relating to their health, it can also place clinicians in a conflicting position.

It is naturally more difficult to rule an athlete out of a competition or match when you know the impact of participating on their finances, reputation and legacy, regardless of the clinical justification. Recognising this, clinicians and departments should make a concerted effort to establish clinical and ethical boundaries with their athletes, by explicitly making these known and/or through a consistent set of behaviours.

These boundaries might extend to procedural or medical principles around pre-match analgesia or communication of an athlete's medical status to external stakeholders (agents, coaches, press, etc.). They should be concrete and at the forefront of the clinician's mind. Although professional athletes may have better access to medical services than the general public, they too deserve to be treated in a safe clinical environment reinforced by the principles, concepts and systems designed to keep all patients safe and at minimal risk of harm, regardless of their occupation.

## PRACTISING PEOPLE SKILLS

The clinician–patient relationship can impact patient outcomes and is known to greatly influence patient satisfaction with their care. Communication and empathy

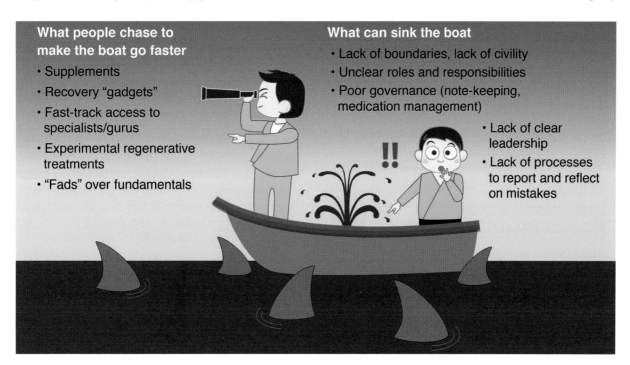

**Figure 2.1** There are many factors that some clinicians may consider contribute to quality health care. We recommend being explicit about the ones you feel are most important and monitoring your performance on those. Beware of behaviours that can sink the boat.
ARTWORK BY VICKY EARLE. PHOTO CONTRIBUTOR: ISTOCK/AOMVECTOR

**TABLE 2.1**   Examples of people skills that we suggest are essential skills—they can be developed

| People skills | How you can practise them well |
|---|---|
| Create a positive first impression | • Be punctual<br>• Have the patient's background information to hand (where possible)<br>• Make eye contact and give them your full attention, with no distractions |
| Communicate well | • Be a better listener than a talker<br>• Ask open questions<br>• Use language appropriate for the patient<br>• Don't interrupt! On average, research indicates that patients have just 11 seconds to explain their concerns before the clinician interrupts them<br>• Give them a chance to open up:<br>  • "Is there anything else you'd like to tell me?"<br>  • "Have I addressed the things you wanted to get out of the appointment today?" |
| Display empathy | • Get to know how this issue impacts their life, hobbies and mental wellbeing |
| Show humility | • Don't act as if you are the smartest person in the room; have the self-awareness to admit you don't know something, would like to check or get someone else's perspective |
| Share decision making (see Chapter 4) | • Involve the patient in their plan and give them ownership of it<br>• Give them the chance to repeat the plan back to you to ensure understanding, and the opportunity to ask questions |
| Work with other members of the multidisciplinary team (see also Chapter 5) | • Interdisciplinary care is vital: encourage broad involvement in the management plan<br>• Outline who else you would like to involve in their care, and why<br>• Invite them to bring others into the consultation, or the opportunity to provide their input |

are essential clinical attributes that contribute to the patient feeling respected, safe and listened to. Agreeableness is a personality trait that modestly reduces the risk of a doctor being sued.

As sport and exercise clinicians, we come across fewer life-and-death situations than colleagues in emergency or intensive care departments, but that doesn't mean the patients we see are any less scared or vulnerable. When sport, exercise or physical activity is the key that holds their life together—what pays their bills or is their lifeline in terms of social support—being faced with a spell of inactivity can be incredibly frightening.

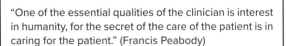

**PRACTICE PEARL**

"One of the essential qualities of the clinician is interest in humanity, for the secret of the care of the patient is in caring for the patient." (Francis Peabody)

Treat the people skills that you need to build a rapport with patients as "essential" skills. Invest in upskilling in these domains and take pride in performing them to a high standard. Given that these skills are sometimes overlooked and underappreciated, Table 2.1 outlines some people skills that you can practise.

## GETTING GOVERNANCE RIGHT

In elite sport, athletes, coaches and the wider performance team often chase the "marginal gains" to get ahead of the competition. As a clinician in this high-performance environment, there is pressure to facilitate the team's performance goal. There is absolutely nothing wrong with this—many clinicians have played an integral (and often invisible) role to support successful teams and individuals.

While you should be alert to "things that make the boat go faster", there are ethical boundaries and too many clinicians have overstepped these and become embroiled in controversy and criticism (see Chapter 30). Striving for the marginal gains to help make the boat go faster should not come at the expense of core medical practice and governance principles. Neglecting them can sink the boat (Fig. 2.1).

Although you may find yourself in settings where clinical governance hasn't been considered, or where appropriate note-keeping and governance systems are not in place, this is not an excuse to adopt sloppy practices. You should see yourself as a leader in implementing this into your working environment, not with a view or pretence that this will help make the boat go faster, but to minimise the risk of the boat sinking due to medical or governance issues. Communicating this to those with a performance

**TABLE 2.2**  Governance principles in sports and exercise medicine

| Governance principles | Practical examples |
| --- | --- |
| Recording work clearly, accurately and legibly | Putting in place a secure, encrypted system to keep medical notes |
| Contributing to and complying with systems to protect patients | Conducting, sharing and acting on risk assessments for various training and competition venues; putting in safeguarding protocols and policies |
| Responding to risks to safety | Creating a culture of reporting near-misses/critical incidents, with clear outcomes and action points |
| Teaching, training, supporting and assessing | Leading intra- and interdepartmental teaching and research, and leading or organising pitchside simulation practices |
| Having clear roles and responsibilities | Ensuring who is responsible and accountable for each area of governance and practice is clear and visible |

Source: General Medical Council. Good medical practice, 2023 [Available from: https://www.gmc-uk.org/ethical-guidance/ethical-guidance-for-doctors/good-medical-practice]

lens can often be a challenge, but by providing examples of the consequences of poor governance and how they can negatively impact whole organisations and shadow various achievements, they can often be convinced.

Table 2.2 outlines some governance principles to consider when working in sport, with examples of ideas and initiatives that feed into each principle.[1]

Unlike in hospitals or some clinic settings, within the sports setting clinical teams are often small and lack administrators to ensure equipment and medications are available, in date and functional. Therefore, the responsibility to check that equipment is appropriate and functioning and medications align with relevant standards set by governing/regulatory bodies falls on busy clinicians.

Measures such as logging a timetable of regular checks are valuable to ensure that items are functional when needed. Items such as medications may only need to be checked once or twice a season, but others such as defibrillators may need to be checked more frequently, such as at every home fixture as part of a specific matchday checklist.

## Safe prescribing and dispensing

Modern pharmaceuticals management requires a system to ensure that prescribing and dispensing are legal and safe. Many sports teams and events do not have a full-time on-site doctor and remote prescribing may take place via a therapist in some countries. The therapist may not be trained in safe legal dispensing to minimise errors relevant to the intended preparation, the suitability of the preparation (e.g. checking for allergies) and dosing schedules. When the prescriber is not present, they should provide the dispenser with written guidance to minimise the risk of overprescribing or inadvertently doping (a version of which can also be provided to the athlete to ensure clarity).

Clinical leaders should outline a pharmaceuticals management policy as a reference standard, with clear roles assigned to relevant team members. The policy should cover:

- prescribing practice in detail including record-keeping responsibilities, preferred dispensers, storage of medications, disposal of expired medications, methods of assessment for common situations (e.g. acute contusions, viral upper respiratory tract infections)
- evidence-based pain management (e.g. Oxford analgesia table)
- policies on drug use in certain pathologies
- methods of communication between prescriber and dispenser
- that safe dispensing means giving the patient only labelled packaged medication with written dosing instructions.

## Incident reporting, reflection and learning

Any human system will suffer from errors occasionally. By reporting such incidents via a robust process, they will be less likely to recur. Incidents must be taken seriously and reporting is encouraged when they are processed in a non-judgmental way and seen as an opportunity for further learning and training. Significant events thought to be more serious (e.g. a near-miss) or where actual patient harm occurs should follow a formal process with deeper analysis known as a significant event analysis.

Debriefs of a specific incident can be "hot" or "cold", and both should be undertaken following significant events:

- Hot debriefs are usually an opportunity to create a shared mental model of what happened for all concerned and to make any immediate essential changes as a result. Follow the STOP mnemonic:

  **S**ummarise what happened
  **T**hings that went well
  **O**pportunities to improve
  **P**oints to action

- A cold debrief may be done a few days later, when everyone involved can go through the events in detail and ask questions.
- Teams should also consider facilitating an independent review by external practitioners from the same or different sports to help provide a different lens for reflection.

## MEDICAL EQUIPMENT AND ERGONOMICS

Ergonomics is the science of how a person interacts with their environment. Many sports teams work in a mobile fashion, so equipment is often stored and transported from venue to venue. Sports teams spend 90% of their working week in training and 10% in competition. During that 90% you may be the only first responder, unlike on matchdays when paramedics and specialist doctors may be present.

Most clinicians do not have a background in dealing with emergencies or the critically injured, although sports pre-hospital immediate care courses are now available worldwide. Clinicians are often called upon to respond to a situation in a time-critical manner, be it a minor illness or injury at a key moment relative to performance, or a seriously unwell or injured athlete. This is a stressful time that may saturate your cognitive capacity and move your thought processes from a state of "flow" to "frazzle" or even "freeze".[2]

Several measures can reduce the stress of this situation:

- Organise equipment so that you do not lose time searching through pockets or containers to find something. There are medical bags available (Fig. 2.2)

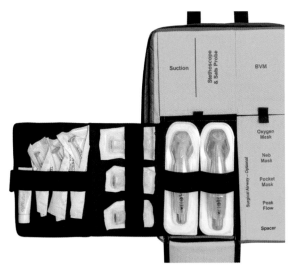

**Figure 2.2** An example of a standardised ergonomic emergency bag
PROMOTE MEDICAL (HTTP://PROMOTEMEDICAL.COM)

that lay out equipment in a visible and logical fashion. Alternatively, you can include a laminated photo guide within the equipment bags to show where various pieces of kit are stored.
- To ensure that equipment is present and functional, seal bags once equipment has been checked and provide a way to rapidly open them (e.g. cable-tied zips and tuff-cut scissors attached to the bag). Also include a clear visible label of when the bag was last checked and when it is next due for checking.

## MAINTAINING SKILLS

Up to 90% of new skills may be lost after just one year if those skills aren't regularly reinforced. For medical practitioners, avoiding the degradation of infrequently used skills is thus a significant challenge. As with equipment checks, having a formal logged commitment to regular simulated practice of on-field situations improves the automaticity of those skills and ensures everyone's shared understanding.

This could apply to regular on-field situations such as assessment and strapping of joints, so that the quality and speed of practice remains high irrespective of which practitioner is involved. It also applies to emergency situations such as cardiac arrest or spinal extrication where regular practice is an opportunity not only to review the usability of equipment but also to think about leadership skills under pressure.

## BEING CIVIL

Excellent outcomes rely on effective teamwork. Research across healthcare settings has shown that when staff perceive themselves to be in a good team, it leads to a range of beneficial outcomes, including:

- reduced hospital standardised mortality rates
- fewer patient complaints
- improved staff satisfaction and performance.[3]

Civility between team members creates a sense of psychological safety and is a key ingredient of great teams. Incivility includes rude or unsociable speech or behaviour, as interpreted by the recipient.

High performance will always require individuals and teams to challenge themselves and each other. Organisations should take steps to ensure the psychological safety to facilitate this in a civil fashion.

Having an environment where everyone feels they can voice their opinion, challenge others and contribute can make a significant difference to overall performance, as well as job satisfaction.

Incivility within teams has been shown to reduce team functioning, clinical decision making and patient outcomes,

A

with patients potentially being less likely to ask for help or to report a symptom.

One randomised controlled trial compared the outcomes of resuscitation scenarios in teams with perceived rudeness and those without. When rudeness was present, there was an increase in diagnostic and procedural errors and the researchers were able to attribute more than 50% of these errors to rudeness.[4]

Considering the impact of incivility is the first step. The next steps are recognising it, acknowledging it and taking steps to address it. Whether that is within the clinical team, within the department or within the wider organisation, be brave to call it out and address it, for the good of patients as well as those around you.

## EMBRACING HUMAN FACTORS IN SPORTS AND EXERCISE MEDICINE

The concept of human (or non-technical) factors is a key part of modern healthcare systems and patient safety,

coming to medicine from industries such as aviation. Human factors include the effects of communication, teamwork, equipment, workspace and culture on people's behaviour and abilities.[5]

As the sports and exercise medicine environment is very different from hospital or clinic services, it is important that these factors are considered in the design of our systems. Some factors have already been outlined in the chapter (leadership, teamwork and communication). Here we discuss several sport-specific factors that you might find useful.

### Emergency action plan

All events and teams should have a documented, reviewed and easily accessible emergency action plan detailing key processes, roles and responsibilities and equipment in the event of an emergency (Fig. 2.3). This should be sent to all relevant medical personnel ahead of events, including the medics of any visiting teams or organisations.

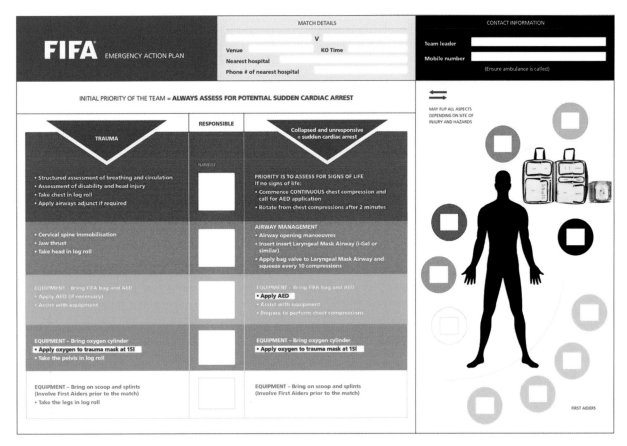

**Figure 2.3** FIFA poster for emergency action planning: the name of the person responsible should be entered into the coloured space
Source: Reproduced with permission from Federation Internationale de Football Association (FIFA).

## Advanced medical information

As athletes and teams compete at multiple venues, it is important to have for each venue a readily accessible database of advanced medical information with key contacts and services such as hospitals. For sports involving home and away teams, making the provision of this database the responsibility of the home team is easier for everyone.

## Pre-event "safety huddle"

A "flash team" is a team of individuals without previous connections who are put together to work on a problem or an event (e.g. a medical team at a sports event). Having a pre-event meeting or "safety huddle" can reduce any challenges that arise from unfamiliarity by making introductions, clarifying skill mixes and roles and responsibilities, explaining protocols, and agreeing modes of communication (e.g. hand signals).

## Positioning and skill mix relevant to the team

The optimal place to position yourself during a competition or event will depend on the sport. Some sports allow access only by invitation (e.g. soccer or martial arts), some allow free access (e.g. rugby union) and in others, due to the nature of the event, clinicians are often remote from the participants (e.g. road running). Having a mixed skill base across the pitchside responders is often valuable (e.g. one physio, one doctor) and will enable rapid accurate assessment and intervention for most problems, as well as allowing each rescuer to focus on a single task—assessing or communicating, rather than both.

## Radio skills

Performance teams may use radios for logistical, operational and tactical reasons. However, unless the whole team has an established radio etiquette and understands how to use the system, messaging can get lost, with people talking over each other or using drawn-out language to make their point. This also increases the chances that messages will not be interpreted correctly.

The military and organisations such as Mountain Rescue use several systems to ensure that messages are clear and concise and to minimise radio traffic. Examples include "PRESS, PAUSE, SPEAK" to ensure that the radio is activated after pressing the button, and three-point messaging using concise language.

For sport, this could translate to NAME, BODY PART, FITNESS TO CONTINUE, with some teams employing a traffic light system of red (immediate removal), amber (continue to observe) and green (no concerns). Certain words can be double-emphasised to ensure clarity—for example, "Green, green", or in Formula 1 "Box, box" is used when the engineer wants the driver to perform a pitstop.

## Available video technology

Real-time rewindable video technology is increasingly evident in our work. While this is an extremely valuable tool to review events, robust systems are needed to reduce the risks of error. For example, a reviewer may feel rushed and not review all angles, or a non-trained observer may inadvertently comment if the environment is not private. Breaking incidents down into immediate, early and late behaviours and using a checklist to ensure that the reviewer comments on each area may minimise absent or random comments.

## Drill practice

Drill practice of specific skills on-field will improve the quality of assessment and intervention by standardisation and creating a shared model of situations and actions. Practising skills such as spinal board extrication or advocating behaviours such as the second rescuer preparing the tape rolls or holding scissors ready to cut in direct anticipation of what the first rescuer needs will improve the speed and quality of the intervention.

## Maintaining cognitive breadth and situational awareness

It is possible that despite an injury to a player or athlete, the competition will continue and it is important that you are aware of surrounding events and do not become too focused on the incident in front of you. If everyone "honeypots" to the incident, other players may be at risk while play continues elsewhere. If you focus too heavily on worrying about the injured player, you may lose focus on other areas, such as remembering how many replacements you have, which may be important for future on-field medical decision making.

## KEY POINTS

- Always put the patient first, even if that means protecting them from themselves.
- Athletes and clinicians spend much time together. This creates familiarity, which can be an advantage, but also requires you to develop formal boundaries to stop this strength becoming a pitfall.
- Developing people skills is an investment in providing better clinical care and delivering better patient care.
- The nature of high-performance sport entails the pursuit of marginal gains, which can involve expensive, novel or experimental interventions. Prioritise patient care and good governance.

- Be proactive in putting systems in place that will protect both you and your patients. One particular area of focus is the management of medications, particularly when the prescriber and dispenser are remote from each other.
- Documentation and record keeping are critical. This applies to adverse incidents, the maintenance and upkeep of equipment and supplies, and the rehearsal of infrequently performed skills and procedures.
- Consider the role of human factors in your working environment and what steps you can take to address them.

## REFERENCES

References for this chapter can be found at www.mhprofessional.com/CSM6e

## ADDITIONAL CONTENT

Scan here to access additional resources for this topic and more provided by the authors

# CHAPTER 3

# Clinical reasoning

with **CLARE ARDERN** and **STEVE KAMPER**

*Effective clinical reasoning requires the integration of science and humanity, evidence and empathy, logic and intuition.*

DR PETER L. TANGUAY

## CHAPTER OUTLINE

What is evidence-based practice?
What information do you prioritise for clinical decisions?
Can research help answer your clinical question?
Can you trust the results of research you are reading?
How do you know whether the athlete has improved?
Do the results apply to the person in front of you?
Bringing it together: shared decision making

## LEARNING OBJECTIVES

By the end of this chapter you should be able to:

- discuss the evolution of healthcare in terms of evidence-based practice and shared decision making
- weigh the relative contributions of clinical information, research and a patient's values and preferences in a clinical scenario
- explain the elements of scientific research that you should consider when deciding how to apply it in practice
- recognise bias in clinical research and list strategies that could be used to mitigate that risk
- identify ways that you can stay up to date with current scientific research.

Most clinicians work within an evidence-based practice paradigm.[1] Sometimes called evidence-based medicine, evidence-based practice is the dominant model in healthcare teaching and practice. We prefer the term *evidence-based practice* as we include all professions that contribute to supporting athletes to stay healthy and perform at their best.

## WHAT IS EVIDENCE-BASED PRACTICE?

Professor David Sackett is credited with defining a widely accepted model of evidence-based practice (Fig. 3.1).[2] Evidence-based practice is a framework for considering information from various sources (the patient's values and preferences, research, and clinical practice) when making clinical decisions. This model has been criticised as being a slave of research but this misrepresents the model: evidence-based practice does not mean doing something because "that's what the research said".[3]

If you embrace evidence-based practice you decide how much weight to assign to each of the elements of research, clinical practice and patient values and preferences and how to synthesise them. Rarely will the three information sources contribute equally to a decision. Instead, the clinician works with the athlete to gather and consider the evidence, and make an informed decision about what to do next. How much weight you place on information from each source will depend on how trustworthy the evidence is (see Box 3.1 for two cases that illustrate how the weighting changes between different clinical settings).

Evidence-based practice aims to prioritise trustworthy information. Clinicians need reliable and efficient ways to find and critique evidence before deciding what

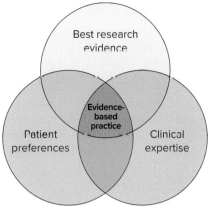

**Figure 3.1** The three elements of David Sackett's model of evidence-based practice[2]

information to incorporate into clinical decisions. Knowing how to appraise research will help you decide which of the millions of new research articles published each year are worth spending time on.[4]

In this chapter, we describe five broad concepts to help you understand and use research evidence. The chapter draws on the Evidence in Practice series in the *Journal of Orthopaedic and Sports Physical Therapy.* We encourage you to read the series for broader and more in-depth coverage of the topics we cover here, and more.

Evidence in Practice series

---

**BOX 3.1** How to apply the principles of evidence-based practice to real-life clinical decisions

### Clinical case 1: Knee arthroscopy for managing osteoarthritis

Sonya is an active, middle-aged accountant who asks for your help to manage her right knee pain (Fig. 3.2).

She has stopped her regular CrossFit and running activities (approximately 20 km per week) due to knee pain, and the pain is now limiting how far she can walk.

Sonya hands you some radiographs that her general practitioner ordered, and you observe the cardinal signs of substantial joint space narrowing in the medial tibiofemoral compartment plus osteophytes, which characterise radiographic osteoarthritis. Sonya asks whether she should have a knee arthroscopy to manage her knee pain.

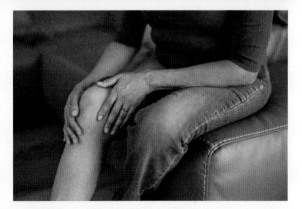

**Figure 3.2** Sonya is an accountant with right knee pain
ISTOCK/AZMANJAKA

*continues*

### What is your answer?

You have read the 2017 BMJ Rapid Recommendation summarising the evidence for knee arthroscopy to treat knee pain in adults.[5] There is strong evidence that knee arthroscopy delivers no additional benefit for pain and function at long-term follow-up, and non-surgical treatment is the recommended approach.[5] The consistent, trustworthy research evidence should factor heavily in your evidence-based practice approach (Fig. 3.3).

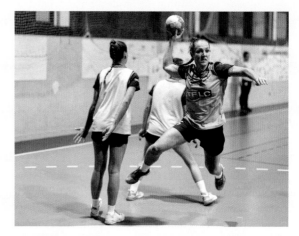

**Figure 3.4** Kianna is a school-girl handball player with shoulder pain
ISTOCK/ANCHLY

### What is your answer?

While there is debate about the content of an exercise program (few trials with limited certainty evidence), the GRASP trial[6] found similar outcomes for pain and function whether the program was delivered as a home-based exercise therapy program or in the clinic. Your clinical judgment and Kianna's preferences should factor heavily in your evidence-based approach (Fig. 3.5).

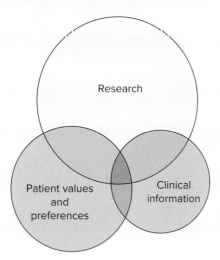

**Figure 3.3** The size of each circle reflects the relative weight that each evidence source contributes to the clinical decision. The strong and trustworthy (i.e. low risk of bias) evidence, represented by the largest circle for research, carries most weight when making the clinical decision in this osteoarthritis case.

### Clinical case 2: Supervised versus home exercises for shoulder pain

Kianna plays handball for her school team, area age-group representative team and the senior women's team at her club, where you are also the team physiotherapist (Fig. 3.4). After one mid-season training session, Kianna comes to you for help to manage chronic pain in her right (throwing) shoulder. You work with Kianna to design a rehabilitation program based on progressive loading. Kianna has limited time outside of her academic and sport commitments and asks whether she could do her exercise program at home rather than coming to the physiotherapy clinic 4 days per week.

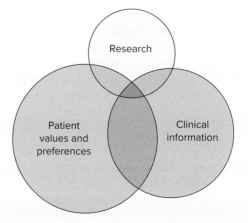

**Figure 3.5** In contrast to the osteoarthritis case, where you had the benefit of strong research evidence, in this case your clinical judgment and the patient's values and preferences carry most weight in the clinical decision. The absence of research evidence provides limited population-level guidance on which specific exercise program to prescribe.

## WHAT INFORMATION DO YOU PRIORITISE FOR CLINICAL DECISIONS?

Clinical practice demands that clinicians consider, appraise and prioritise information from different sources and then synthesise that information as they discuss the management plan with the athlete. Information sources may include:

- foundational knowledge of anatomy and human systems
- previous experience with similar patients
- conversations with colleagues
- professional and social media
- formal and informal training
- professional development
- practice audits
- published research.

It is the clinician's task to decide how to prioritise (and effectively weigh up) this information, especially when information is conflicting. A barrier to effective clinical practice is bias. A *bias* is a particular tendency or inclination, especially one that prevents unprejudiced consideration of a question.[7] The implication of relying on biased information—whether the information itself is biased or the reader's interpretation of it—is that clinical decisions might be made on the basis of false information. Bluntly, a diagnosis may be mistaken or missed, incorrect advice about prognosis provided or an ineffective treatment delivered.

With respect to research, bias means that the sample estimate differs systematically from the population parameter. In plain language, this means that results reported in a study are wrong; estimates, associations and effects are overestimated.[8]

### PRACTICE PEARL

Prioritise information that is at the lowest possible risk of bias. This requires you to assess the bias in all the sources of information that you are considering.

## CAN RESEARCH HELP ANSWER YOUR CLINICAL QUESTION?

A research question is the foundation of any study. A research question needs to be clear, specific and answerable if it is to support a trustworthy and useful study.[9] The same features are necessary to ensure that you can interpret the findings and decide whether to apply them to your practice.

A clear question is one that a reader can understand and describe simply in their own words to a colleague. Without this level of clarity, the reader cannot judge whether the methods are appropriate or correctly interpret the results.

The study methods flow from the question. Recruiting the research participants, choosing how and when to measure outcomes (including which tools to use), and how to analyse the results map directly to the research question. The research question must be specific and well-defined. If the question is too broad or ambiguous, the reader cannot determine whether the recruitment, data collection and analysis methods are appropriate.

Research questions in the sports medicine field fall into one of three categories—questions that are best answered by (1) a description, (2) a prediction (equation) or (3) a decision as to whether a factor may be the cause of a phenomenon (see examples in Table 3.1).[10]

With these three categories front of mind, it will be easier to understand a study, appraise its quality and interpret the results. Different participant inclusion, recruitment, data collection, analysis and interpretation methods apply to the different categories of question. Questions about cause and effect are the most difficult for researchers to answer well and questions about describing are the simplest.

### Describing

Descriptive questions aim to paint a picture of the landscape regarding an aspect of health. Common examples of descriptive questions include those regarding prevalence, incidence, case mix, patterns of health services, patient views or experiences, clinical or natural courses of health conditions, diagnostic test accuracy and costs of illness.

**TABLE 3.1**    Research questions in the sports medicine field fall into one of three categories

| Category | Example |
| --- | --- |
| 1. Studies that describe clinical populations and phenomena | A study of the knee health of former athletes (football players, Olympians, recreational players) |
| 2. Studies that predict an outcome based on past data | A study that uses clinical test results to predict the likelihood of a new ankle injury after returning to sport |
| 3. Studies that address whether factor A is a cause of phenomenon B | A 3-arm randomised trial of surgery, rehabilitation and placebo treatment of a condition (shoulder, knee, ankle condition) |

Studies that address descriptive questions may be qualitative or quantitative, and cross-sectional or longitudinal.

## Predicting

Predictive questions aim to tell the reader something about what will happen in the future given some information available at present. These studies develop and test prediction models or assess the predictive capacity of individual risk or prognostic factors. The studies require longitudinal data (i.e. taking repeated measures over a period of time).

## Estimating

Causal questions are usually one of two types: estimating the causal effect of one treatment versus another; or estimating the causal impact of a particular clinical or demographic factor on an outcome. Studies addressing causal questions need to be longitudinal. Sports medicine and sports science researchers may make mistakes in the methods and language they use, especially when attempting to answer predictive or causal questions.[11]

> ### PRACTICE PEARL
>
> A clear, specific, answerable and relevant question is fundamental to research. If you cannot clearly describe the research question in your own words, there is no point in reading the article. Different research methods apply to descriptive, predictive and causal questions; a reader should be able to categorise the question.

## CAN YOU TRUST THE RESULTS OF RESEARCH YOU ARE READING?

Research involves a process of specifying a question, gathering data, analysing the data and applying the analysis results to answer the question. The numerous tools and features that researchers use during the process comprise the research methods.

How a study is designed and what happens during the study (research methods) help to ensure that information is as unbiased as possible. The better a study is designed to reduce bias, the higher quality the study will be.

Different types of research questions are at risk from different types of bias. How bias is assessed depends on the type of study. A study that estimates the effectiveness of treatment A compared with treatment B (causal question) is at risk of confounding bias,[12] whereas a study that assesses the clinical course of people with a health condition (descriptive question) or a study testing whether a clinical feature predicts outcome (predictive question) is not at risk

of confounding bias. Randomisation, which is a technique to reduce the risk of confounding bias, is a key indicator of quality for the first study but not relevant to the other two.[13]

There are tools to assess the risk of bias associated with studies of different types. These tools are usually a checklist that identifies which of the different design features a study includes.[14] Examples include the PEDro scale[15] and Cochrane risk of bias tool[16] for treatment effectiveness studies; QUIPS[17] for prognostic studies; and QUADAS[18] for diagnostic test accuracy studies.

By understanding the types of bias relevant to a particular study question, the reader can identify the design features that are important, the tools to assess risk of bias and study quality offer a short cut to help.

>
>
> ### PRACTICE PEARL
>
> The methodological features of clinical research studies are designed to reduce the risk of bias. To effectively appraise research, you need to know what common types of bias are relevant to a particular study and what research methods help mitigate the risk of this bias.

## HOW DO YOU KNOW WHETHER THE ATHLETE HAS IMPROVED?

A question can only be answered to the extent that the relevant outcomes can be accurately measured. Regarding measuring outcomes, the "construct" is *what is being measured* and the "measure" (or tool or instrument) is *what is being used* to quantify the construct.[19] For example, a study focused on the outcome of health-related quality of life (construct) may use the SF-36 (measure) to measure quality of life.

Readers often assume that objective measures are superior to subjective measures. This assumption does not hold because:

- many constructs themselves are subjective (e.g. pain, quality of life) and can only be measured using a questionnaire or similar self-report tool
- objective measures are not always more reliable and valid than subjective measures.

## Reliability

*Reliability* is the degree to which a measure is free from random error. A reliable measure would give the same score if it was applied twice with the same person (in the absence of change in the construct). This would be the case regardless of whether it was scored by the participant themselves or applied by one or several researchers. If an outcome is measured with an unreliable measure, it is not possible to know whether any change in score was due to clinical improvement or to error.

## Validity

*Validity* is the degree to which the score on a measure reflects the construct it is supposed to quantify. Validity is difficult to assess for many of the constructs relevant to sports medicine, particularly patient-reported outcomes that are the focus of clinical research and practice. Selecting reliable and valid outcome measures is a key component of high-quality research, and researchers should justify their choice with reference to evidence supporting their chosen measures.[20]

### PRACTICE PEARL

Place more trust in studies that provide evidence to support the reliability and validity of the outcome measures.

## DO THE RESULTS APPLY TO THE PERSON IN FRONT OF YOU?

The study population includes all people who meet the inclusion criteria for the study. The study sample is the people selected from the population who participate in the study. After a study has been completed, the value of the findings extends only as far as they can be applied to everyone in the study population. The degree to which the results from a study sample can be applied to the study population is known as generalisability.[21] You need to decide how well the findings in a study apply to your patient.

A key factor in determining whether the results from research apply (generalise) to the person in front of you is the "representativeness" of the sample. A representative sample is the same as the study population in terms of the proportions of all the important characteristics. For example, the proportion of younger and older people is similar, the mean severity of symptoms is similar, and the

distribution of socioeconomic disadvantage is similar. Perfect representativeness is practically impossible, so generalisability is best thought of as a continuum: study findings are *more* or *less generalisable,* rather than generalisable or not.

Study features that help determine generalisability:

- how the researchers identified and enrolled participants into the study (e.g. through GP clinics, posters in a hospital, social media)
- inclusion and exclusion criteria
- baseline demographic and clinical characteristics, usually presented in Table 1 of the published paper.

These features can be compared with your own patient to help judge generalisability. Box 3.2 has suggestions to help you keep up to date with research evidence.

### PRACTICE PEARL

To assess how study findings apply to your patient, look at the study recruitment methods, inclusion and exclusion criteria, and participant characteristics.

## BRINGING IT TOGETHER: SHARED DECISION MAKING

Healthcare practice is slowly transitioning from a paternalistic way of delivering care (doing *to* the patient) to a shared decision-making model (doing *with* the patient). Health systems, clinical professions and individual clinicians are at different points along this transition.

Understanding how to appraise and communicate the findings of research to patients offers an opportunity for you to bring credible and relevant information to a clinical encounter. Open and transparent conversations about your own biases, and guard rails that research puts in place to try to overcome bias, build trust in healthcare. Clear communication about the findings of research studies, along with honest appraisal of limitations and issues of generalisability, can underpin a shared approach to management decisions.

## BOX 3.2 Timesavers for staying up to date with research evidence

- *Read clinical practice guidelines developed by trusted professional organisations.* High-quality practice guidelines summarise the evidence related to a specific clinical area or question. Look for (1) a detailed search, (2) a clear system for synthesising the evidence and making a recommendation about what to do in practice (e.g. GRADE[22]), (3) patients and clinicians from several professions involved in the guideline panel and (4) any funding and potential conflicts of interest declared and managed to avoid bias.
- *Learn more about reading and understanding research:* see, for example, the Evidence in Practice series from JOSPT.[23]

JOSPT Evidence in Practice series

- *Consult the Physiotherapy Evidence Database (PEDro)* for summaries of treatment effectiveness studies and evidence-based practice tools.

PEDro

- *Use the PubMed Clinical Queries algorithm* to organise the results of PubMed searches.

PubMed Clinical Queries algorithm

- *Search for trustworthy evidence using the Translating Research Into Practice (TRiP) database.*

TRiP database

- *Sign up for email alerts from academic journals* to receive an alert when new research is published.
- *Listen to podcasts:* leading journals like BJSM and JOSPT (Fig. 3.6) have well-established and popular podcasts. Apply the same criteria to find trustworthy information disseminated in audio format as you would when reading research.
- *Start a discussion group (sometimes called a "journal club") with colleagues.*

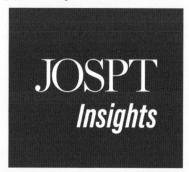

REPRODUCED WITH PERMISSION FROM THE JOURNAL OF ORTHOPAEDIC & SPORTS PHYSICAL THERAPY

JOSPT

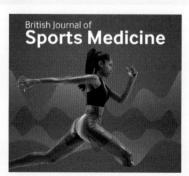

BJSM

**Figure 3.6** Free podcasts with more than 700 episodes of largely clinical content generally based on sound clinical reasoning

## KEY POINTS

- Evidence-based practice does not mean that you indiscriminately base your practice on research evidence. Instead, it involves a careful balance of research evidence, clinical information and a patient's values and preferences.

- Applying evidence in clinical practice can be guided by several questions that you should ask yourself when determining the value of a given research study. These questions assess the risk of bias, try to identify the research question being asked and attempt to determine the trustworthiness, validity, reliability and generalisability of the results.

- If authors of a research paper have been unable to give you a clear idea of the research question, we suggest there is no point in you trying to interpret the results.

- The ease with which a research study can address a question relates to the category of research question being asked: descriptive, predictive or establishing cause and effect (in order of ascending difficulty). There are certain risks of bias associated with each category.

- Historically, objective measures of patient improvement have been seen as superior to subjective measures. However, subjective measures are not necessarily less reliable or valid. Each tool should be assessed individually.

- The shared decision-making model requires you to communicate clearly the strengths and limits of available evidence.

- There are helpful tools to assist you in identifying risk of bias in research and strategies to help you stay up to date with clinical research.

## REFERENCES

References for this chapter can be found at www.mhprofessional.com/CSM6e

## ADDITIONAL CONTENT

 Scan here to access additional resources for this topic and more provided by the authors

## CHAPTER 4

# Shared decision making

**with SABEENA JALAL and CLARE ARDERN**

*They (the clinicians) didn't bring an ego at all to the table. They were really helpful in giving me all the information I needed to make an informed decision. They truly wanted the best for me, and I get the same feeling from all the physios. It makes a big difference when they know what your goals are and they remember what you're trying to do ... your timeline. I have that extra layer of confidence in them.*

CANADIAN FREESTYLE SKIER COURTNEY HOFFOS SPEAKING ABOUT HER CLINICIANS AS SHE PREPARED FOR HER ACL RECONSTRUCTION. INTERVIEW WITH ATHLETE BRIAN WALLACK IN 2023.

## CHAPTER OUTLINE

What is shared decision making?
The three-talk model of shared decision making
Key principles for making shared decisions
Shared decision making in practice

## LEARNING OBJECTIVES

By the end of this chapter you should be able to:

- outline the goals of shared decision making in the sports and exercise setting
- describe factors to consider and incorporate when implementing shared decision making
- use the three-talk model as a guide to practising shared decision making
- reflect on your own approach to shared decision making with athletes
- prioritise treatment options based on their risks and benefits.

## WHAT IS SHARED DECISION MAKING?

In the process of shared decision making, clinicians, athletes and appropriate others collaborate to make a health related decision.[1-4]

- As a *process,* shared decision making provides a scaffold for the athlete's values, preferences and circumstances to be given primacy when discussing options, benefits and risks.[5-7]
- As a *mindset,* shared decision making is a standard of excellence in clinical practice; it ensures that the clinician's focus centres on the athlete with the aim of supporting the athlete to authentically engage in their healthcare decisions.[8-11]

In fully embracing a shared decision-making mindset, clinicians, athletes and coaches foster an athlete-centred and evidence-based approach.[1,12,13] Some members of the clinical community might assert that sports practitioners have yet to fully, or formally, embrace shared decision making in their practice.[7] The nature of the clinician's work—with its emphasis on return to sport—requires clinicians to share opinions with the athlete and for the athlete to engage with those opinions.[1,4,13-15] For shared decision making to work well in practice, members of the shared decision-making team need to trust each other, share accurate information and communicate in a transparent and timely way.[1,9]

In this chapter, we outline Dr Glyn Elwyn's foundations of shared decision making[16-19] as a framework to guide how you practise effective shared decision making. We consider possible roadblocks and share ways that experienced clinicians have overcome barriers. Let's dive in and see how this chapter influences the way you think about shared decision making in your practice.

## THE THREE-TALK MODEL OF SHARED DECISION MAKING

Shared decision making transforms healthcare interactions by engaging clinicians and patients in collaborating to make a decision. This approach prioritises the patient's values and preferences, marking a shift away from clinician-dominated decisions to a balanced partnership. In shared decision making, the clinician and athlete consider the athlete's values and preferences alongside the best available research and clinical practice to guide their decisions.[3-5]

Elwyn's three-talk model of shared decision making (Figure 4.1) has been developed, studied and refined to improve healthcare decisions in general practice.[2,12,16-23] Elwyn's work in patient-centred care and shared decision making spans decades and the three-talk model is a culmination of research and clinical experience. The model

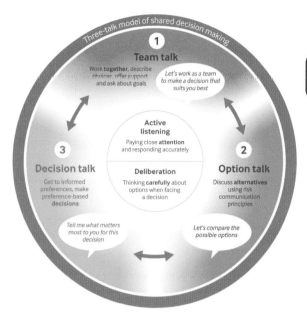

**Figure 4.1** The three-talk model of shared decision making
Source: Elwyn G, Durand MA, Song J, et al. A three-talk model for shared decision making: multistage consultation process. *BMJ* 2017;359.

depicts an iterative process for making decisions and has been adapted and applied in almost every medical specialty.

The three "talks" represent how clinicians can work with athletes to reach a healthcare decision:

- In *team (partner) talk,* the clinician works to establish a partnership with the athlete—inviting them to participate in making decisions, and emphasising that their values and preferences are important.[2] Partner talk lays the groundwork for trust, transparent communication and respect.
- In *option talk,* the clinician presents detailed information about all reasonable options, including the risks and benefits.[2] The information is tailored to the athlete's specific health complaint and context. Option talk supports the athlete to consider options in their specific context.
- In *decision talk,* the athlete and clinician consider the options together, taking into account the athlete's preferences.[2] They work towards the athlete making an informed choice and reaching a decision that best aligns with their goals and lifestyle, with the clinician providing support and guidance throughout the process.

### Pulse check: where are you at in your shared decision-making practice?

Consider how a shared decision-making mindset figures in your current practice. Use the matrix in Table 4.1 to self-diagnose your shared decision-making practice and consider ways to integrate the shared decision-making process and mindset into your clinical practice.

TABLE 4.1    Self-diagnose your shared decision-making practice

| | Experienced proponent | On-board and keen to learn more to improve practice | Need a nudge to get going |
|---|---|---|---|
| **Process** | • You collaborate with all members of the multidisciplinary team (including the athlete, other clinicians and coaches) to support the athlete to make an informed decision.<br>• You focus on building trust and sharing information.<br>• You are a clear and open communicator, and have a strong understanding of the latest evidence for managing the common complaints you encounter.<br>• You use regular check-ins as a strategy to monitor athletes' progress and address queries and concerns as they arise. | • You try to work with members of the multidisciplinary team where you can.<br>• As your practice is developing, you are getting better at knowing the reasonable options to share in the option talk.<br>• You are starting to try different ways of communicating with athletes and coaches to understand their values and preferences.<br>• You have started to implement strategies to check in with athletes and are working on making the check-ins more regular. | • You make unilateral decisions on the athlete's behalf.<br>• Making a decision as fast as possible is your number 1 priority.<br>• You often make decisions without seeking or considering input from others.<br>• You rely on the athlete coming to you to raise issues or concerns. |
| **Mindset** | • You do not take the decision an athlete makes personally. You see the decision as reflecting what's best for the athlete, rather than your ability as a clinician. | • You sometimes find it hard not to share with athletes what you would do if you were in their shoes.<br>• You are working on supporting athletes to consider their options and make a decision instead of telling them what to do. | • You know what is best for the athlete. You expect the athlete to take your advice whenever you offer it, and see the decision as a reflection of your worth and ability as a clinician. |

## KEY PRINCIPLES FOR MAKING SHARED DECISIONS

When supporting athletes to make decisions about their health, there are at least three core principles to keep in mind:

1. *Allocate sufficient time to consider information and make decisions.* Rushing is the enemy of effective shared decision making. You need to make time for meetings to discuss options, review best practice evidence and consult with colleagues, coaches and others to seek additional information and/or guidance. Take time to ensure that decisions are well-considered. Jumping to a quick decision may overlook crucial details and athlete perspectives. Thoughtful, informed discussions that respect the complexities of each individual case are vital.

2. *Know what the reasonable options are, and their key details.* If you are uncertain, let the athlete know that you need some time to find out. Ensure that everyone contributing to the shared decision-making team is fully informed of the options, including the potential risks and benefits associated with each. Understanding all the options facilitates a balanced discussion and helps the athlete to weigh the options against their values, preferences and goals.

3. *Support the athlete to make the best decision for them.* Build an environment where athletes feel psychologically safe to make decisions that align with their best interests. Provide enough support, information and time for the athlete to reach the decision they feel comfortable with and that reflects their values, preferences and goals.

> **PRACTICE PEARL**
>
> Shared decision making is all about supporting the athlete to make an informed decision, rather than you (the clinician) making a decision on the athlete's behalf.

## Snakes and ladders in shared decision making

Shared decision making is focused on delivering care that has the athlete at its centre. Athlete-centred care respects the athlete's agency and capacity to collaborate with clinicians, while making their own decisions about their health care. Figure 4.2 illustrates some key ingredients for shared decision making to work well (the ladders) and some potential barriers that can throw you and the athlete off course (the snakes).

A

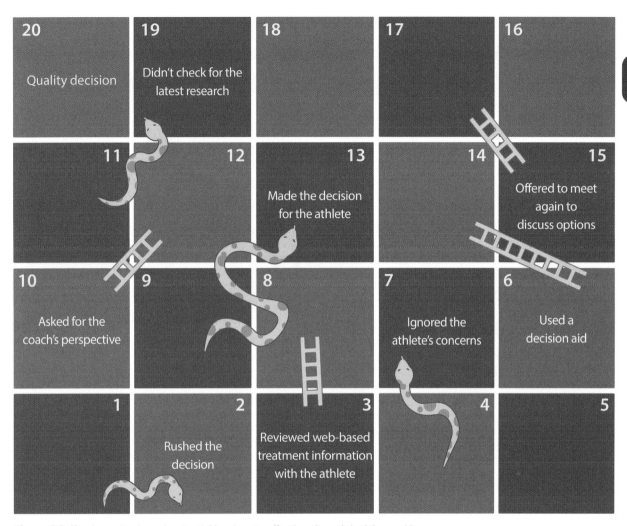

**Figure 4.2** Key ingredients and potential barriers to effective shared decision making

> **PRACTICE PEARL**
>
> Practising efficient and effective shared decision making relies on frequent and clear communication.

## SHARED DECISION MAKING IN PRACTICE

Shared decision making brings benefits for athletes and clinicians—it helps deliver high-value care[24, 25] by supporting strong relationships. Athletes may feel more satisfied with the outcome when they are involved in the decisions about treatment plans.[26, 27] A shared decision-making approach helps athletes stay informed about their health and recovery, and facilitates communication from clinicians to athletes and coaches.[1, 14, 15, 28]

If you are new to the practice and mindset of shared decision making, it is easy to feel overwhelmed by how to implement it. The shared decision-making approach is complex, yet it does not have to be complicated. To help illustrate the principles of shared decision making in practice, the two clinical scenarios in Boxes 4.1 and 4.2 outline how experienced clinicians can support an athlete to make an informed decision.

In each scenario, you will see how the decision-making team can differ, depending on the athlete's specific needs and circumstances. The roles of each team member will change and adapt according to the specific context. Shared decision making is flexible and responds to the needs of each athlete.

## BOX 4.1 Clinical scenario: supporting a youth athlete and his parents to make an informed decision about hip surgery

### Context for shared decision making

Ali is a sports-mad 15-year-old who enjoys playing Xbox when he is not training with his soccer academy or playing for his school team. He has been with the academy since the age of 8. He lives with his parents, who are considering whether Ali should move to living full-time on the academy campus to give him the best environment to progress to professional soccer.

When you meet Ali, he has been experiencing increasing right-sided groin pain (in the anterior hip region) over the previous 12 months. Initially he felt the pain after training and matches, and it settled within 24 hours. In the last 6 months, the pain has been lasting longer, and Ali feels the pain during training and matches. The pain has restricted his training, especially his running load. Ali also reports feeling a sharp pain when he takes corner kicks or makes crosses from his typical playing position on the right wing. Ali's typical training load is 7 training sessions per week plus matches.

### Gathering information

You perform a clinical assessment and find:

- negative flexion abduction external rotation (FABER) test
- positive flexion adduction internal rotation (FADIR) test
- negative Thomas test
- positive adductor squeeze test with hips in 45° flexion and in neutral (long lever)
- reduced hip flexion, adduction and internal rotation range of motion
- reduced hip abductor and adductor muscle strength.

Based on Ali's history and the clinical assessment findings, you consider 5 differential diagnoses: (1) femoroacetabular impingement syndrome with primary cam morphology, (2) slipped capital femoral epiphysis, (3) adductor tendinopathy, (4) acetabular labrum tear and (5) stress fracture to the neck of the femur.

You liaise with the academy physician to obtain hip radiographs and magnetic resonance imaging (MRI). For the radiographs, AP pelvis and Dunn 45° views are taken of both hips to assess the alpha angle and rule out slipped capital femoral epiphysis. For the MRI, the radiologist performs standard soft-tissue sequences to assess for intra-articular pathology (including labral tear) and stress fracture, and to visualise the soft tissues surrounding the hip.

When you review the radiographs, you note a "bump" on Ali's right hip, characteristic of primary cam morphology. You note the same morphology on his left hip. The radiologist reports the right alpha angle as 57° and the left alpha angle as 60°. There is no sign of slipped capital femoral epiphysis, and nothing additional to note on the MRI.

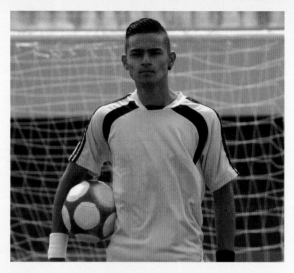

**Figure 4.3** Ali is a junior soccer player with hip pain
ISTOCK/HAMMARBY STUDIOS

### Shared decision making

You diagnose femoroacetabular impingement syndrome with primary cam morphology. You arrange to meet with Ali and his parents to explain the diagnosis and start planning what to do next (partner talk), discuss the reasonable treatment options (option talk) and make a decision about how to manage Ali's short-term hip health (decision talk).

#### Partner talk

During your first meeting (partner talk 1), Ali's parents share their concerns about what the imaging findings might mean for his long-term hip health (both hips have primary cam morphology). They also want him to have the best chances of a successful professional soccer career. All Ali wants to do is to play without pain. At a training session later in the week (partner talk 2), Ali shares with you how worried he feels about letting his parents down if he can't play enough soccer to progress his career.

Here, the focus is on how you implement shared decision making to support Ali and his parents to make a decision about the best way to manage Ali's hip pain. It is common (and appropriate) to schedule follow-up meetings as part of a shared decision-making approach to discuss new issues and make additional decisions as needed (e.g. managing Ali's long-term hip health).

#### Option talk

To manage Ali's main complaint of hip pain, you discuss the options: active rehabilitation alone[29,30] and hip arthroscopy plus active rehabilitation. Hip arthroscopy is an invasive treatment that carries small risks of infection

A

and complications with anaesthesia. Best practice rehabilitation advocates for a minimum 6 months of active (i.e. progressive exercise-based) treatment. Ali might need hip arthroscopy later if his hip pain does not improve with active rehabilitation, and there is no guarantee that hip arthroscopy will resolve his pain. There is uncertainty in the research about which treatment approach produces superior results. The most recent analysis suggests similar results for pain relief and physical function; return to sport outcomes are also similar.

### Decision talk

Ali muses that if he tries active rehabilitation first, and if he needs surgery later, his body and mind will be in as good condition as possible to recover from hip arthroscopy and he will know what he is facing for post-operative rehabilitation. Ali's parents are hesitant for their son to have invasive treatment given his young age and that there is a viable alternative in active rehabilitation. Ali gives his assent, and his parents give their consent, to begin active rehabilitation.

---

**BOX 4.2**   Clinical scenario: deciding how to manage acute patellar tendinopathy on the eve of a major tournament

In this scenario, the athlete, team physician (you) and physiotherapist work together to decide how best to manage patellar tendinopathy in the high-pressure and time-limited context of a major tournament.

### Context for shared decision making

Lia is the starting point guard for her country's national basketball team. The Olympic Games competition starts in 5 days. The team will play games every 2 days, with a recovery day in between, and they are expected to challenge for a medal.

Lia has been managing her patellar tendinopathy flare-ups over the past 6 years, sometimes by reducing her training load and match minutes, and has never missed a game at a major tournament because of tendinopathy.

Lia seeks your help after an acute flare-up of her anterior knee pain when landing from a rebounding duel with other players during training. She felt a sudden sharp pain when she landed and stopped training to get immediate treatment. You are the team physician and Lia and the team physiotherapist ask for your input. Lia's typical training load is 6 days per week, including 3 days of on-court training (basketball drills), 2 days of strength and conditioning, and 1 day of active recovery (light jogging, stretching).

### Gathering information

You and the team physiotherapist perform a clinical assessment and find:

- mild tenderness at the lower pole of the patella
- positive jump test (evaluating patellar tendon loading), with pain on landing
- positive single-leg decline squat test, with pain at 30° of knee flexion
- Victorian Institute of Sport Assessment-Patella (VISA-P) score of 47 out of 100 (indicates moderate impairment).

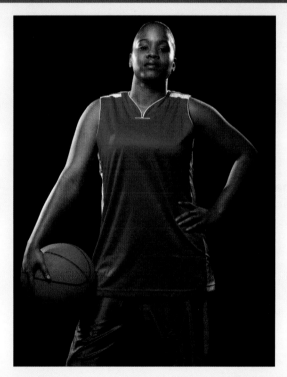

**Figure 4.4**   Lia is a starting player for her country's national basketball team. She had a flare-up of patellar tendinopathy 5 days before the Olympic Games
ISTOCK/NICKP37

Based on Lia's history of patellar tendinopathy and the clinical assessment findings, you consider 4 differential diagnoses: (1) patellar tendinopathy, (2) meniscus tear, (3) patellofemoral pain syndrome and (4) patellar subluxation.

*continues*

In the Olympic Games village, you request plain radiographs, ultrasound and MRI. The radiographs show calcific deposits along the patellar tendon. On the ultrasound, there is thickening of the patellar tendon with a 9 mm × 4 mm hypoechoic region in the sagittal plane. On the MRI, you observe an abnormally thickened patellar tendon. There is increased signal intensity on T1 and T2 sequences consistent with patellar tendinopathy.

### Shared decision making

You diagnose patellar tendinopathy. You arrange to meet with Lia and the team physiotherapist to start planning what to do next (partner talk), discuss the available treatment options (option talk) and make a decision about how to manage Lia's tendinopathy for the duration of the tournament (decision talk).

You all agree that managing load is core to your approach (partner talk). Because the tournament starts in 5 days and the competition schedule is so compressed, there is no time to implement an effective resistance training program (option talk 1). Lia and the team physiotherapist have worked together to tailor Lia's training load with her past tendinopathy flare-ups and feel confident they can do the same this time. They involve the coaching and performance staff to plan Lia's training and match minutes throughout the tournament (decision talk 1).

To manage Lia's main complaint—her knee pain—you discuss 2 options (option talk 2): oral non-steroidal anti-inflammatory drugs (NSAIDs) and local corticosteroid injection. Lia has not felt much benefit from NSAIDs with her previous flare-ups. There is a small risk of gastrointestinal and cardiovascular system side effects when taking NSAIDS. You consider the corticosteroid injection a better option for short-term pain relief, especially given the timeframe you are all working in. There is research evidence supporting the short-term effects of corticosteroid injection for reducing tendon pain.[31] You aim to ensure that Lia understands the absolute risk of tendon rupture after corticosteroid injection is low, yet tendon rupture is a potential harm of the injection.[31] You carefully explain the risks so Lia can make an informed decision.[32]

Lia considers the benefits and risks and indicates that she understands the risk of tendon rupture. You answer her follow-up question about whether the risk of rupture increases if she has more than one corticosteroid injection. You advise against repeated injections. Lia is determined to compete in the Olympics and thinks a corticosteroid injection today plus the load management plan throughout the tournament is the best way for her to reach her performance goal (decision talk 2).

## The complex elements of effective shared decision making in practice

Effective shared decision making requires you to:

- *Acknowledge the athlete's preferences.* Understand each athlete's preferences, values, goals and risk tolerances—listen to the athlete.
- *Navigate perspectives from different contributors.* Shared decision-making teams may include athletes, clinicians, coaches, nutritionists, psychologists, family and team management. Ensuring that their diverse perspectives and interests are heard and respected requires active listening skills and time.
- *Integrate information from different sources.* Data to inform shared decision making might come from medical records, imaging, clinical tests, patient-reported outcome measures, performance data and research. Knowing who to turn to for help in interpreting and applying these data helps you to support the athlete to make an informed decision.

- *Overcome barriers to clear and effective communication.* Understanding the athlete's knowledge of their health, performance and recovery helps you to meet the athlete at their level.
- *Address ethical and legal considerations.* Seeking consent and assent and maintaining confidentiality are foundation skills of clinical practice.
- *Keep up to date with the latest research evidence.* Trustworthy clinical guidelines, consensus statements and systematic reviews can help you keep on top of new research. (See Chapter 3 for more ideas on ways to keep your knowledge up to date.)
- *Consider psychological factors.* Assess the mental impact of injuries and decision making on the athlete.
- *Use technology to your advantage.* Smartphone apps can deliver exercise programs and measure performance. Digital capture and storage of athlete data facilitates efficient analysis.

**A**

## KEY POINTS

- The practice of shared decision making is a standard of excellence in clinical practice that prioritises the athlete's goals, respects their preferences and values, and incorporates their input in constructing a treatment plan.

- Practising shared decision making involves communicating and incorporating the best available clinical evidence throughout the decision-making process.

- The three-talk model is a helpful framework for structuring discussions during shared decision making.

- You should reflect on the extent to which you are currently adopting the values and practices of shared decision making in your clinical work.

- Shared decision making requires an investment of time. Rushing through clinical interactions is the enemy of quality shared decision making.

- There are instances in which you may need more time to explore the benefits, risks, effectiveness and contraindications for a treatment option. Communicate that need transparently.

- Athletes need to feel safe and respected to fully engage in the shared decision-making process. Building this trust and respect is an important precursor to practising shared decision making.

- Factors that can derail quality shared decision-making practice include lack of time, trust, respect or knowledge of treatment options. Overloading an athlete with information and pre-existing paternalistic team structures are other roadblocks.

## REFERENCES

References for this chapter can be found at www.mhprofessional.com/CSM6e

## ADDITIONAL CONTENT

Scan here to access additional resources for this topic and more provided by the authors

## CHAPTER 5

# The multidisciplinary team approach

with **PAUL DIJKSTRA, UMMUKULTHOUM BAKARE, STEFANO DELLA VILLA** and **MARA YAMAUCHI**

*You can have the nine greatest individual ball players in the world, but if they don't play together the club won't be worth a dime.*

BABE RUTH (1895–1948)

## CHAPTER OUTLINE

Introduction: why sports and exercise medicine?

Athlete, coach and clinician: the tripartite nucleus

High-performing clinical teams

Injury and illness management and athlete performance: a delicate balancing act

Top teamwork tips from the frontline

"Love thy sport" (and physical activity!)

## LEARNING OBJECTIVES

By the end of this chapter you should be able to:

- describe the key characteristics of a high-performing sports and exercise medicine team
- develop an athlete health and performance care plan based on the integrated performance health and coaching model
- describe the benefits and challenges of clinical (athlete health) case management.

# INTRODUCTION: WHY SPORTS AND EXERCISE MEDICINE?

Sports and exercise medicine is now an established core medical specialty in many countries, including Australia, South Africa and the UK.[1] In North America, sports medicine is a 1-year Accreditation Council for Graduate Medical Education (ACGME) subspecialty (as Sports Medicine or Orthopaedic Sports Medicine Fellowships) following core medical specialty training in one of five disciplines: family medicine,[2] physical medicine and rehabilitation, emergency medicine, paediatrics and orthopaedic surgery. A few years ago, some of us developed a syllabus for the sports and exercise medicine medical specialty.[3,4] Although not formal specialty training programs, several sporting organisations, including the IOC[5] and FIFA,[6] deliver online or hybrid courses in sports medicine and related disciplines.

Whether practising as a core medical specialist, as a sports medicine subspecialty or as one of many clinicians in the sports medicine ecosystem, your work could include a variety of tasks and responsibilities,[7-13] including:

- injury and illness prevention
- injury diagnosis, treatment and rehabilitation
- management of medical problems
- performance enhancement through training
- nutrition and psychology
- exercise prescription in health and in chronic disease states
- exercise prescription in special subpopulations
- medical care of sporting teams and events
- medical care in situations of altered physiology, such as at altitude, in environmental extremes or at depth
- dealing with ethical issues, such as the problem of drug abuse in sport
- administrative tasks related to WADA anti-doping code compliance
- research and injury/illness surveillance.

Sports and exercise medicine has been defined as the scope of (medical) practice that focuses on:

1. prevention, diagnosis, treatment and rehabilitation of injuries that occur during physical activity
2. prevention, diagnosis and management of medical conditions that occur during or after physical activity
3. promotion and implementation of regular physical activity in the prevention, treatment and rehabilitation of chronic diseases of lifestyle.[14]

Because of the ever-growing breadth of content and skill, sports and exercise medicine is usually practised by a multidisciplinary team of clinicians with specialised knowledge and skills. They provide optimal care for the athlete and improve each other's knowledge and skills. The sporting adage that a "champion team" would always beat a "team of champions" applies to sports and exercise medicine too. This team approach can be implemented in a multidisciplinary sports and exercise medicine clinic or by individual clinicians of different disciplines collaborating by cross-referral.

However, the real-world application of this multiskilled team approach poses significant challenges, including leadership and communication. A symphony orchestra cannot play well without a conductor. Similarly, high-performance teamwork pivots on skilful and eloquent clinical case management (athlete health case management).

The "conductor" of the orchestra should ideally be a specialist sport and exercise physician, focusing on—and taking the responsibility for—athlete wellbeing in the context of performance. We elaborate on this key principle later in this chapter.

We explore the following important elements of teamwork that will set you up for success:

1. athlete, coach and clinician—the tripartite nucleus of any sports and exercise medicine team
2. high-performing sports and exercise medicine teams
3. injury/illness management and athlete performance—a delicate balancing act
4. top tips from experienced clinicians on the frontline
5. love thy sport (and physical activity).

## ATHLETE, COACH AND CLINICIAN: THE TRIPARTITE NUCLEUS

The athlete, coach and clinician form the tripartite nucleus that makes or breaks any sports and exercise medicine team (Fig. 5.1). Clinicians must earn the athlete and coach's trust. Mutual trust and confidence underpin any shared decision-making journey when navigating athlete health challenges—especially when the rubber hits the road (or track!) in a major event like the Olympics.[15] Let's briefly explore the gold-standard tripartite nucleus:

- Athletes feel empowered to contribute to informed preference decisions about their readiness to perform (train or compete). The athlete's contribution is subjective, asking the question: "What is best for me now and for the rest of my athletics career?" Shared decision-making decisions—sometimes very complicated—are therefore influenced by the athlete's personal circumstances (e.g. the type of injury and level of competition) and experience, their view on risk-taking, and other contextual factors (e.g. sponsorship deals, media/family pressure).

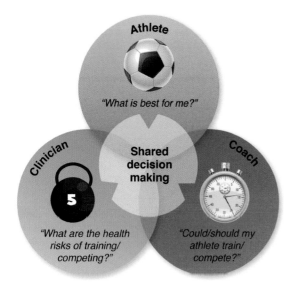

**Figure 5.1** The tripartite—athlete, coach and clinician—shared decision-making nucleus of every sports and exercise medicine team. This requires shared responsibilities. Different factors (athlete health status, participation risk, level of competition, other decision modifiers) influence the size of the contributing circles to the process. The position of the shared decision-making circle would therefore differ for a concussed athlete with "no capacity" to take part in the shared decision-making process: the decision would be firmly within the clinician circle. When athlete and coach travel alone to training camps or competitions, the clinician's role is different (or even absent, though not ideal).
Source: Adapted from Dijkstra HP, Pollock N, Chakraverty R, et al. Return to play in elite sport: a shared decision-making process. *Br J Sports Med* 2016;51:419–20. © 2016 BMJ Publishing Group Ltd & British Association of Sport and Exercise Medicine. All rights reserved.

- As the coach is directly responsible for the athlete's training and performance, they bring context to the table: "Could/should my athlete train or compete?" It is therefore important to involve the coach in clinical shared decision making. The coach holds the key for athlete compliance and adherence. They often supervise treatment or exercise rehabilitation programs and are seen as authority figures. Furthermore, discussion with the coach might spotlight a possible technique- or training-related cause for an injury. Unfortunately, some coaches distrust clinicians, particularly when they feel the clinician inhibits rather than supports their work or tells them what to do. They sometimes perceive clinicians as too risk-averse; however, it is essential for coaches to understand that clinicians are also aiming to maximise performance while balancing that with protecting athlete health. Professional athletes' agents could also be confidentially involved in discussions, especially when major injuries occur.

- The clinician (usually a sport and exercise physician or a physiotherapist, depending on the context) evaluates the athlete's health status and provides objective advice on management options and the possible clinical outcomes of training or competing. Their contribution is objective: they base their decision on the clinical situation, the best (scientific) evidence and their professional experience—often supported by a team of professionals working with the athlete.

In sum, it is crucial that athletes, coaches and clinicians understand the health *and* performance environment. They should develop transferable knowledge and skills (e.g. in communication and leadership) to complement optimal share decision making in challenging situations (see also Chapter 4).

## HIGH-PERFORMING CLINICAL TEAMS

High-performing clinical teams trust one another, embrace conflict, commit to a common goal, accept accountability and focus on results.[16] However, what a high-performing team looks like also depends on context. Clubs and sporting bodies increasingly employ specialist sport and exercise physicians.

Their primary role, with other team members, is the comprehensive health management of athletes to facilitate optimal performance.[17] This includes the diagnosis and treatment of injuries and illnesses associated with exercise to ultimately facilitate and improve performance.

In other contexts, the clinical team may consist of a family physician/general practitioner or a physiotherapist/physical therapist alone. In a populous city, or in the polyclinic of a major sporting event like the Olympics serving thousands of athletes, the team may consist of several clinicians and sports scientists working together. They might include:

- specialist sport and exercise physician
- family physician/general practitioner
- physiotherapist/physical therapist
- soft-tissue therapist
- exercise specialist for exercise prescription
- other medical specialists with an interest in sports and exercise medicine (orthopaedic surgeon, rheumatologist, radiologist, cardiologist)
- podiatrist
- dietitian/nutritionist
- psychologist
- sports trainer/athletic trainer
- other clinicians such as osteopaths, chiropractors, exercise physiologists, biomechanists, occupational therapists, nurses, orthotists, optometrists, dentists
- coach
- fitness adviser.

Irrespective of the context, the athlete and their wellbeing should always be central. And, as described above, the coach often plays a pivotal role.

## Roles, responsibilities and communication

There are, of course, distinct differences in roles and responsibilities when clinicians are employed by sporting organisations or clubs (as opposed to providing care as a "one-off expert opinion" for a specific athlete's injury or illness). Loyalty to club or athlete tug-of-war is real for many clinicians, and an ethical dilemma for some. Equally, medical teams contracted by the local organising committees of sporting events have very specific roles and skills depending on the size of the event.

> **PRACTICE PEARL**
>
> The clinician's first responsibility is *always* the health and wellbeing of their patient.[18]

Team multiskilling (where a diverse group of clinicians each has skills in a particular area) is important but may pose challenges like role or responsibility creep among team members. This can be either a real or perceived overlap of roles and responsibilities; for example, coaches acting as "soft-tissue therapists" for their athletes. The key is always effective teamwork with clear roles and responsibilities, ethical practice guidelines, leadership and communication. Individual multiskilling may be of use when a clinician is geographically isolated or is travelling alone with a team, but telemedicine (or TeleSEM[19]) is changing this perceived isolation.

Here is an example of high-performance teamwork. When an athlete presents with a lower limb overuse injury, the specialist sport and exercise physician (or other physician) usually has diagnostic responsibility. Other team members such as the sport-specific therapist, podiatrist or biomechanist might have a better knowledge of clinical biomechanical assessment, the functional relationship between abnormal biomechanics and the development of the injury, and how to correct any biomechanical causal factor. However, it is essential in this context that all clinicians are able to perform a clinical assessment and have a basic understanding of lower limb anatomy, injury pathogenesis and biomechanics.

Similarly, for an athlete who complains of excessive fatigue and underperformance, the sports dietitian is best able to assess the athlete's nutritional status and unravel possible nutritional factors that could play a role

in their symptoms. However, other team members should also appreciate the role of nutrition in fatigue or delayed recovery, and briefly assess the athlete's nutritional status.

## The sports and exercise medicine model

Like other healthcare fields, sports and exercise medicine is increasingly focused on individualised health care (note the difference between "healthcare" and "health care") and clinical case management. In the traditional sports medicine model, the doctor was seen as the primary contact practitioner, with subsequent referral to other medical and paramedical practitioners. This has now changed: the athlete's primary contact could be, for example, a physiotherapist, coach, sport and exercise physician or soft-tissue therapist.

All members of the team understand their own strengths and limitations, and embrace and amplify other team members' strengths when making treatment plans. Although this improved sports and exercise medicine model recognises the multidisciplinary nature of the athlete's "primary contact", it may still reinforce a reductionist approach to health care. Clinicians may operate in their own specialist silos and their actions, although well-intended, may be fractured: fractured because they don't communicate well, because they don't integrate holistic athlete healthcare, and because the spotlight is not on athlete wellbeing and performance.

The athlete and coach are often ill-equipped to integrate the different contributions in this setting of increasing complexity and multi-specialists. They need to rely on an expert case manager with sport-specific understanding (in bigger teams the specialist sport and exercise physician) to provide "health leadership".

The clinical case manager fosters interprofessional collaboration. Interprofessional collaboration in healthcare is "an active and ongoing partnership between professionals from diverse backgrounds with distinctive professional cultures and possibly representing different organizations or sectors working together in providing services for the benefit of healthcare users".[20] The case manager bridges gaps in athlete health care, negotiates overlaps in the roles and tasks of the sports and exercise medicine team, and creates open environments for honest and constructive communication. They skilfully integrate the contributions of all key players in the so-called integrated performance health management and coaching model (Fig. 5.2).[21]

This model pivots on skilful interprofessional collaboration underpinned by athlete health case management—when an athlete is healthy as well as when they are injured or ill. The focus is to integrate health

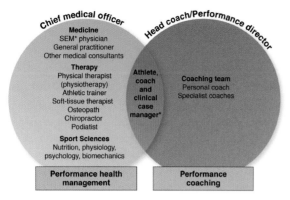

*Personal sport and exercise physician or chief medical officer case-managing athlete health

**Figure 5.2** The integrated performance health management and coaching model

Source: Adapted from Dijkstra HP, Pollock N, Chakraverty R, et al. Managing the health of the elite athlete: a new integrated performance health management and coaching model. *Br J Sports Med.* 2014;48:523–31. © 2014 BMJ Publishing Group Ltd & British Association of Sport and Exercise Medicine. All rights reserved.

management and coaching to improve performance while protecting the athlete's health. One accountable clinical case manager is *the* key. In what follows, we explore some of the affordances and challenges of athlete health case management.

## Affordances and challenges of athlete health case management

As mentioned earlier, the sports and exercise medicine orchestra will play out of tune without a conductor. So a skilful athlete health case manager–ideally a sport and exercise physician–is worth their weight in gold! Here's why.

First, specialist sport and exercise physicians invest years (often more than 12 years) in formal training programs. Second, as clinical case managers they usually know the athlete, coach and sporting context really well. They know what it takes to perform at a high level under pressure. Third, unlike one-off external clinicians, clinical case managers embrace the burden of ongoing responsibility for optimal athlete health management–when things go well, and as part of the powerful athlete, coach, clinician trio in the trenches of high-level performance. It is important to emphasise that responsibility for athlete health case management is far more than case-managing, say, a hamstring injury. An effective sport and exercise physician takes all aspects of optimal athlete health into account.

However, clinical case management has its challenges:

- Too many cooks in the kitchen: athletes and coaches–more so at the elite level–often shop around for health care when they suffer from significant illness or injury.

This can lead to several clinicians (who don't talk to each other or who give mixed messages) "managing" the injury or illness. This is disastrous.

- No cook in the kitchen (or worse, a "guru" cook working far away): this happens when the athlete and coach "cook" without attending to injury warning signs. They work in isolation, only to jump on a plane to a world "guru" when their kitchen is on fire … This happens more at the elite level but the message is important for every athlete in competitive sport: don't eat from a kitchen with no cook.

- A cook with limited knowledge and skills: clinical case managers should have the medical and sport-specific knowledge and skills to manage (and prevent) injury *and* illness.

The key message to athletes and coaches is that, for success, they should invest in *one* clinical case manager who they trust–preferably a sport and exercise physician with the knowledge, skills and sport-specific experience to manage and prevent athlete injury and illness. A clinical case manager is vital to protect the athlete's health–including their emotional health.

## INJURY AND ILLNESS MANAGEMENT AND ATHLETE PERFORMANCE: A DELICATE BALANCING ACT

The secret of success in sports and exercise medicine is to take a holistic view of the patient and their condition. The narrow view may provide short-term symptom relief but will ultimately lead to failure. For example, a narrow view would be a slapdash rest-until-pain-free approach to a runner who presents with shin pain and is diagnosed with a tibial stress fracture. Although it is likely that in the short term the athlete will improve and return to activity, there is a high likelihood of recurrence of the problem on resumption of activity.

The clinician should always ask "Why has this injury/illness occurred?" The cause may be obvious (e.g. a sudden doubling of training load) or subtle and, in many cases, multifactorial.

The greatest challenge of sports and exercise medicine is to identify and correct possible injury/illness causal factors. The runner with a tibial stress fracture may have abnormal biomechanics, inappropriate footwear, a change in their training surface or a change in the quantity or quality of training. In sports and exercise medicine, there are two main challenges: diagnosis and treatment. In our profession, we must aim to diagnose both the problem and the cause. Treatment then needs to focus on both these areas.

## Diagnosis

Every attempt should be made to diagnose the precise anatomical, pathological and functional cause of the presenting problem. Knowledge of anatomy (especially surface anatomy) and an understanding of the pathological and functional processes likely to occur in athletes can facilitate a more precise diagnosis. Thus, instead of using a purely descriptive term such as "shin splints", you should attempt to diagnose the underlying cause—bone stress injury/stress fracture, chronic compartment syndrome or medial tibial stress syndrome (periostitis)—and use the specific term. An accurate diagnosis guides more precise treatment.

Some clinical situations do not allow a precise anatomical and pathological diagnosis. For example, for most athletes with low back pain, it is clinically impossible to differentiate between potential sites of pathology. If red flags (see Chapter 22) signalling a more sinister diagnosis are absent, it is necessary to establish a functional diagnosis, monitor symptoms and signs through careful clinical assessment and reassessment, and correct any contributing factors present (e.g. hypomobility) using appropriate treatment techniques.

Diagnosis of the presenting problem should be followed by identifying a possible causal factor. American orthopaedic surgeon Ben Kibler coined the term "victim" for the presenting problem and "culprit" for the causal factor.[22] To identify causal factors often requires a good understanding of biomechanics, technique, training, nutrition and psychology. Just as there may be more than one pathological process contributing to the patient's symptoms, a combination of causal factors might contribute to the problem.

As with any branch of medicine, diagnosis depends on careful clinical assessment, which consists of a history, physical examination and special investigations. The most important of these is undoubtedly the history but, unfortunately, this is often neglected.

---

**PRACTICE PEARL**

"Listen: the patient is telling you the diagnosis." (William Osler, 1849–1919)

---

Once a thorough history has been taken, an examination can be performed. It is essential to develop systematic examination routines for each joint or region and to include an assessment of any potential causal factor. The *British Journal of Sports Medicine* has excellent (and free!) clinical examination videos.[23]

BJSM knee examination video

**A**

Special investigations should be evidence-based and regarded as an adjunct to, rather than a substitute for, thorough history and examination.[24] The investigation should be appropriate to the athlete's problem, cost-effective and aimed at providing additional information. Special investigations should be performed only if they will affect the diagnosis and/or treatment.

## Treatment

Apart from being evidence-based, treatment has at least three other components: discussion ("deliberation" is an effective term used in the literature[25]) of the proposed treatment plan with the athlete, coach and key role players (in the context of immediate and future performance goals); treatment of the presenting injury/illness; and treatment aimed at the causal factors. Generally, no single form of treatment can "cure" the majority of sports and exercise medicine problems. A combination of forms—usually with clinician-led incremental exercise rehabilitation as the foundation—will likely give the best results.

Therefore, it is important for you to be aware of the evidence base for a variety of treatments and to appreciate when their use may be indicated. It is also important to develop as many treatment skills as possible or, alternatively, to ensure access to others with particular skills. It is essential to regularly evaluate the effectiveness of treatment. If a particular treatment does not seem to work, it is important to reconsider the diagnosis. If the diagnosis appears to be correct, other treatment options should be considered.

## Meeting the individual athlete's needs

Every patient is a unique individual with very specific needs. Without an understanding of this, it is not possible to manage athlete health appropriately. One size does not fit all, even though there is a guidance framework. The patient may be: (1) an Olympic athlete whose selection depends on peak performance at their forthcoming trials; (2) a business executive who jogs to cope with the stresses of everyday life; or (3) a tennis player whose weekly club game is as important to them as a Wimbledon final is to a professional. Alternatively, they may be someone for whom sport is not at all important but whose low back pain causes discomfort at work.

Treatment should also be cost-effective. Does the athlete merely require a diagnosis and reassurance that they have no major injury? Or do they require twice-daily treatment sessions to prepare for an important game? Treatment depends on the patient's context, not purely on the diagnosis.

## TOP TEAMWORK TIPS FROM THE FRONTLINE

In Box 5.1, four experienced clinicians share their top tips for high-performance sports and exercise medicine teamwork. These are summarised in Table 5.1.

In keeping with this book's emphasis on the patient/athlete (see Chapter 1), the final word goes to Dame Kelly Holmes, double Olympic gold medallist. We quote from a 2015 interview in the *Aspetar Sports Medicine Journal:*[26]

"The most important thing is communication. If an athlete is very successful, all of those people [physiotherapist, doctor, physiologist, coach etc.] have had a part to play in it, but they have to be able to communicate well to achieve that. When I was a younger athlete I had scenarios where the coach would set the training, while the physio advised different training to treat an injury and the nutritionist would come in and say they weren't considering my diet properly. If the team doesn't communicate, it can cause friction and at the end of the day the athlete just wants to run fast and stay fit. I learned over time that my whole team needed to know each other and speak to each other to become an integrated team. A mature athlete who is at an Olympic standard has dedicated their life to the sport and they are relying on their team to help them achieve their goals."

For effective high-performance teamwork (an "integrated team"), communication is key!

Effective teamwork can make a significant difference to the health and wellbeing of athletes and the broader community. Applying and adapting these excellent tips will help you to provide better clinical care and to excel as a high-performing team member.

## "LOVE THY SPORT" (AND PHYSICAL ACTIVITY!)

Finally, to be a successful sport and exercise clinician it is essential that you are an advocate for physical activity too. As a clinician who understands sport you have at least two advantages:

- by appreciating the physical demands and technical aspects of a particular sport, you will understand the possible causal factors of injury and can better contribute to sport-specific exercise rehabilitation and prevention programs
- athletes and coaches will have more confidence in you.

The best way to understand a sport (and its demands) is to attend training sessions and competitions, and ideally to participate! The advice from the experts is to not only be available when injuries occur, but also to embrace the sport and its culture. Confucius and Mark Twain are both attributed as saying: "Choose a job you love, and you will never have to work a day in your life." We're not sure if they were referring to sports and exercise medicine though.

---

**BOX 5.1**　Top teamwork tips from clinicians who've walked the walk

### Professor Christa Janse van Rensburg

Professor Christa Janse van Rensburg is a South-African sport and exercise physician and current chair of the World Netball Medical Advisory Panel. She has travelled with many teams across the globe: "Don't try anything new during travel", she emphasises, and "always have a Plan B, and C, and so on …"

When travelling, Professor Janse van Rensburg is prepared to assist in any challenge, not only medically related, and always plans carefully before leaving the country. This may include "travel and medical insurance for athletes and support staff, knowledge of required vaccinations, and medicine to treat support staff, not just athletes".

### Dr Andrea Mosler

Dr Andrea Mosler is an Australian specialist sports physiotherapist. She has travelled extensively with teams, including as team physiotherapist for the 2000, 2004 and 2008 Olympic Games:

"The most successful sports and exercise medicine teams work together with athletes and their coaches to facilitate optimal sporting performance.

… they work collaboratively, respecting each member as an expert within their field, and an integral part of the performance team. The team shares the vision of performance success, balanced with a culture of care, integrity and fairness. Effective delivery of performance team support requires understanding and meeting of the athlete/coach needs, and those of the other team members, and the high-performance environment in which they all operate."

## Dr Celeste Geertsema

Dr Celeste Geertsema is a New Zealand trained sport and exercise physician. Dr Geertsema was team physician for the New Zealand national men's football team for 7 years and the first female team physician at a FIFA World Cup when she accompanied the team to the 2010 FIFA World Cup in South Africa:

"Remember to stay within your professional boundaries. It is important to become an equal part of the team and share in some light-hearted banter and jokes, but never lose sight of the fact that you are not one of the players, or one of the coaching staff. Your job is to provide professional medical care to all members of the team. This requires you to keep your professional distance and allow players to trust you as an independent member of the group. This is even more important if you are a female doctor of a male team, or the other way around."

Dr Geertsema stresses the importance of documenting every medical encounter—even a quick corridor conversation: "If it isn't documented, it never happened—at least from a medico-legal point of view." She has three more tips:

1. Develop a modular system of bags, which each have a purpose on their own, but together make up your entire medical kit: "Ensure you are able to carry all your own gear—and label them very clearly, so that they are easy to find on a luggage carousel. My bags consist of essentials kit (always on me, the size of a small handbag), field of play bag (with AED in it, the size of a medium backpack), sideline/changing room bag (with diagnostics, suturing etc., the size of a small sports bag) and hotel bag (the "pharmacy", the size of a carry-on trolley bag). Mine are all black bags, but next time I will buy them in bright red!"
2. When travelling a lot with your team, build a professional network of colleagues you trust in the places where you travel: "These colleagues can be invaluable if you need medical assistance with your team in another city and especially in another country"
3. Enjoy your job: "Remember to pause every now and then and reflect on how much you are enjoying this job, how fortunate you are and what it means to you. And when you don't enjoy such a moment any longer, it is time to let someone else have this opportunity ..."

## Dr Ummukulthoum Bakare

Dr Ummukulthoum Bakare is a sports physiotherapist from Nigeria with more than two decades' experience on the African continent:

"In low-resource settings and developing countries, sport and exercise clinicians face unique challenges when providing care to athletes and individuals involved in physical activity. In these contexts, teamwork is crucial to ensure that patients receive the best possible care despite limited resources. Often, you have to 'wear many hats' to support athletes and their supporting cast."

Dr Bakare emphasises four key teamwork tips from the frontline for those in charge of providing athlete care in such settings:

1. *Foster collaboration*—work together to maximise the impact of limited human resources: "Foster a culture of collaboration among all members of the healthcare team, including physicians, physiotherapists, nurses, first aiders as well as volunteers who are keen to support operations."
2. *Provide training and education, including continuing professional development*—provide ongoing training and education to team members and volunteers, focusing on the specific needs and challenges of the local population and sports culture: "The high cost of attending international conferences or workshops or accessing leading journals is a real barrier for practising clinicians. Some organisations like Isokinetic Medical Group have made it possible for those from low- and middle-income countries to attend conferences at significantly reduced costs. Other ways to build capacity include virtual workshops and webinars as well as following sports and exercise medicine content on social media that share information."
3. *Engender cultural sensitivity*—understand local customs and beliefs: "Cultural sensitivity can help you to build trust and improve patient compliance with treatment plans."
4. *Build value-alliances with coaches*—"Coaches are often on the defensive when it comes to discussing player health and availability. There is a delicate balance between protecting a player's long-term health and short-term availability to train or compete. As sport and exercise clinicians we need to think carefully about our messages to coaches; emphasise that we are invariably on the same team!"

**TABLE 5.1**   Top tips on high-performance sports and exercise medicine teamwork

| Tip | Context |
| --- | --- |
| Foster a culture of intra-team collaboration | Foster a culture of collaboration among all members of the healthcare team, including physicians, physiotherapists, nurses, first aiders and volunteers who are keen to support operations. Many settings have limited (human resources) options for diversity in sports and exercise medicine teams. Therefore, we should work together to maximise the impact of available resources. |
| Delegate tasks | Identify the strengths and expertise of each team member and delegate tasks accordingly. For example, nurses and physiotherapists can handle routine assessments and follow-up care, while physicians focus on more complex cases. |
| Communicate clearly | Establish clear communication channels within the team and ensure that everyone understands their role and responsibilities. Encourage open and honest communication to address challenges and share knowledge. |
| Stay on top of your game through training and continuing education | Provide ongoing training and education for team members and volunteers focusing on the specific needs and challenges of the local population and sports culture (e.g. workshops on injury prevention, health promotion, basic first aid and rehabilitation techniques). Continuing professional development—to stay on top of the latest information and best practices—could be challenging. Cost is a burden—it is expensive to attend international conferences or workshops or to access peer-reviewed journals. Find ways to mitigate this (e.g. opportunities to attend conferences at significantly reduced costs for students or clinicians from low-resourced countries; free education materials such as *Aspetar Sports Medicine Journal*; and online education including workshops and webinars).<br><br>*Aspetar Sports Medicine Journal* |
| Optimise your resources | Learn to make the most of limited resources by improvising and adapting equipment and treatment protocols, and sharing innovative solutions within the team to optimise resource use. |
| Engage with the local community | Engage with the local community to raise awareness about sports and exercise medicine and the importance of injury prevention. Encourage community involvement in sports events and health-promotion initiatives. |
| Prepare for emergencies | Develop clear protocols for handling sports-related emergencies, including on-field injuries. Regularly practise these protocols where feasible as a team to ensure a coordinated response in high-pressure situations. Know your environment: for example, where the nearest local hospital is, what services they provide and how to contact them. |
| Keep detailed records | Maintain accurate and organised patient records, even when struggling with limited resources. Electronic health records or simple paper-based systems can help track patient progress and improve continuity of care. |
| Continuously assess and adapt | Regularly assess the effectiveness of your team's interventions and adjust your approach based on the latest evidence, patient outcomes and feedback from others. Be willing to adapt to changing circumstances and needs. |
| Advocate and raise funds | Advocate for increased sports and exercise medicine resources and funding with government entities at all levels. Collaborate with local organisations and government bodies to secure support for sports medicine programs. |
| Collaborate with other individuals and teams | Establish connections with other healthcare providers and sports medicine experts nationally, regionally and globally. Sharing experiences and knowledge with colleagues from different regions can lead to valuable insights and solutions. Engage and mentor students to provide them with support and stimulate their interest in being part of the sports and exercise medicine ecosystem when they graduate. |

**A**

## KEY POINTS

- The formalised practice of sports and exercise medicine is relatively new. In its short history, there has already been an evolution of the clinicians practising in this specialty and how they manage care for athletes and physically active individuals.

- With the expanding number of care providers who may interact with an athlete, it is important to clearly define roles and responsibilities within the team and maintain clear communication about the athlete's care.

- The process of decision making in sports and exercise medicine is often shared among three core members: the athlete, their coach and the clinician. In certain contexts, other individuals (e.g. the athlete's agent) may be involved.

- The clinical case manager plays a pivotal role in coordinating care across team members while prioritising the athlete's health and performance.

- The sport and exercise clinician should focus on diagnosing the problem and the cause of the problem. Treatment and prevention of re-injury depend on a firm grasp of both.

- Having a personal interest in and passion for sport and physical activity is an asset for the sport and exercise clinician.

## REFERENCES

References for this chapter can be found at www.mhprofessional.com/CSM6e

## ADDITIONAL CONTENT

Scan here to access additional resources for this topic and more provided by the authors

CHAPTER 6

# Working with sporting teams

with LIAM WEST, KIMBERLY HARMON and ALICIA TANG

*Patients don't care how much you know until they know you care.*

## CHAPTER OUTLINE

The role of the sport and exercise clinician in a team setting
Pre-season
In-season
Travel
Off-season

## LEARNING OBJECTIVES

By the end of this chapter you should be able to:

- develop a clinical practice that prioritises athlete care and respects your professional boundaries
- implement a set of pre-season actions that prepare you and athlete for the competitive season
- construct a series of travel-related policies and procedures for athletes
- prepare an end-of-season plan to finalise athlete treatment plans and prepare for the next season.

A

Working with athletes, in both individual and team settings at any level of competition, can be extremely rewarding yet challenging (Fig. 6.1). Your role may allow you to travel both nationally and internationally, have a pitchside seat to witness sporting history and remunerate you at the same time! Working as part of a sports medicine multidisciplinary team will help you to learn new skills and techniques that can be adapted for other clinical roles. You will work outside of a typical clinic or office setting and develop lifelong friendships with like-minded colleagues.

Regular attendance at training sessions and competitions gives you a relatively unique opportunity to observe mechanisms of injury and monitor progress during rehabilitation. It enables you to develop an in-depth understanding of the biomechanical, physical and psychological demands of a particular sport. Above all else, it can be a fun experience contributing towards individual and team athletic achievements!

Working within a team environment poses challenges that are not usually experienced in a clinic setting. Clinicians are often expected to be on call for medical and injury advice every hour of every day. Travelling with a team may require the clinician to: fulfil a variety of unfamiliar roles, as not all team members will be able to travel; work long hours; cancel clinic/office sessions at minimal notice; and spend time away from their family/loved ones. These unsociable hours are not exclusive to travel—often training sessions and competitions are scheduled in the evenings or on weekends.

Working in the spotlight can be stressful and working with high-profile athletes can increase medico-legal risk. Job insecurity is prominent in team environments. Clinicians may lose their job not because of clinical competency, but due to coach preference or a new external team sponsorship with fixed medical arrangements. Unfortunately, these challenges are not always reflected in the remuneration offered for such roles.

## THE ROLE OF THE SPORT AND EXERCISE CLINICIAN IN A TEAM SETTING

As discussed in Chapter 5, a wide range of responsibilities are bestowed upon you as a clinician working in a sports team. You may be required to demonstrate clinical leadership and subsequently act as an active team player, recognising you are a small cog in a very large wheel that often values athletes and coaches as the key people.[1]

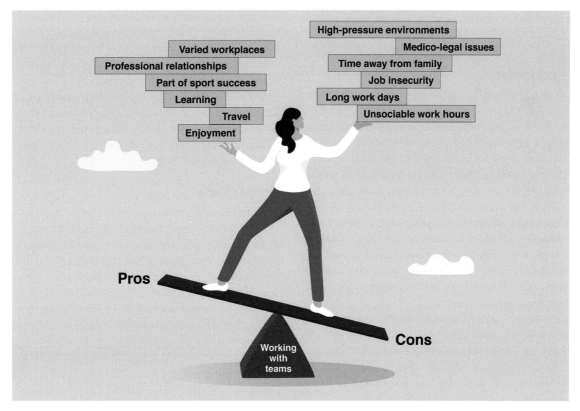

**Figure 6.1** Balancing the pros and cons of working in sport can be both challenging and rewarding
ADAPTED FROM ISTOCK/NUTHAWUT SOMSUK

You will interact with athletes multiple times over any given week and get to know them and their families on a more personal level than occurs within a typical patient–clinician relationship. As highlighted in Chapter 2, this can lead to a blurring of boundaries with athletes and you must actively be aware of this so that you can establish boundaries. When required, you need to be able to remove the emotion from difficult medical and performance decisions to ensure that you best serve your athletes. You are there to do your job: be friendly, but not their friend. This is a difficult balancing act.

Athletes need to know that you care before they care how much you know. Show an understanding of the pressures they are under and acknowledge the goals they want to achieve within their sport. This is also true of your interaction with coaches. To be an effective team clinician, you need to earn respect and trust to implement your medical decisions.

A key element of this is effective and timely communication of medical decisions. Having situational awareness is important in sport.[2] Behind every injury or illness, no matter how big or small, is an athlete under stress, with emotions and aspirations at risk. Avoid being so fixated on an injury that you forget there is an athlete attached to it. A balance must be made between educating athletes on their injuries and making them question the physical resilience of their body as it is the main tool of their trade. Chapter 11 can help you here.

## Core principles

Several core principles underpin quality sports medicine care (see also Chapter 2). The athlete's right to privacy and confidentiality should be strictly adhered to. All healthcare interactions, even corridor conversations (which should be avoided where possible), should be documented in a secure password-encrypted electronic medical record. Being able to access this record remotely is useful when travelling with a team. Ideally the electronic medical record should separate confidential medical and mental health notes, accessible only to nominated staff, from non-confidential musculoskeletal notes. If this is not possible, two systems should be used.

You should keep up to date with the relevant evidence base and attend regular continuing professional development to help achieve this.

There is emerging evidence of the potential for interpersonal violence that can occur in sporting environments. Ensure that you are competent to safeguard those under your care and are upskilled to recognise suspicious behaviour (in person and also online). Practising in a culturally safe and inclusive manner is important.

Sport and exercise clinicians often have responsibilities that go above just caring for athletes. You may need to communicate decisions directly to coaches or the team media department, have an in-depth knowledge of anti-doping processes so that you can attend drug testing to provide support to athletes while monitoring the integrity of the process, attend board meetings or sit on risk and medical integrity committees acting as a health and wellbeing advocate. To be a highly effective team clinician you need to develop a diverse set of skills.

## It's not about you

You may find yourself being televised or photographed providing medical care, or you may be asked to provide commentary for different news media. It is important to remember that this exposure is not about you—it is about the athletes.

In most instances it is advisable to remain in the background, unless you are specifically asked by the communications and media manager to comment on an injury, in which case you should stick to the facts, respect confidentiality and ask to access the transcript prior to publication. "No comment" is an acceptable answer!

Remember you are there to work, not to be a fan. Your role is often to protect the athlete from themselves and their coach (or agent) while prioritising their psychological and physical health, and simultaneously optimising their performance. Focus on what is best for the athlete, considering their preferences and risk tolerance, rather than on what is best for team success.

Do not accept a contract with a "win bonus"—your focus should be on providing holistic care rather than aggressive risk-taking to enhance player availability. It is better to risk losing your job doing the right thing, than to lose your professional licence doing the wrong thing.

## Social media

Social media is an increasingly valuable education tool. It can direct followers to tools and resources, as well as help build your professional profile and increase referrals.

However, social media has the potential to blur the professional patient–clinician boundary—avoid becoming "friends" with or "following" your athletes online. Before posting, or indeed socialising in person, ask yourself, "Would I interact with this patient from my clinic/hospital?"

---

**PRACTICE PEARL**

Do not interact with any content your athletes/patients produce (i.e. replying to, reposting or liking posts).

---

Consider having separate social media accounts for your work and personal content. Ensure that your accounts are set to the maximal privacy settings and remember that anything you post online could be used by your current employer or in a future job application or interview process—avoid posting controversial or negative comments about other athletes, coaches or teams! You are a medical professional and should act accordingly.

## Mentor

Put no speed limit on the rate you can improve as a clinician within team sports. Actively reflect on your own experiences so that learning lessons do not pass you by. To help accelerate your development, you should also learn from the experiences of your colleagues.

A mentor is a fantastic benefit for all clinicians, especially for those starting their careers. Create a peer review group where you can regularly discuss difficult and challenging cases/scenarios. Chapter 7 details career development.

## Self-care

Working in a sporting environment naturally means that you will be surrounded by people exercising—while this can be inspiring, it can also be challenging if you don't find time to perform regular physical activity yourself. Team clinicians often work under pressure, outside of normal office hours, and their decisions may be discussed by media outlets and on social media, causing further stress. Aim to develop a work-life balance; for example, by prioritising your own and family time, taking holidays when your schedule allows (with appropriate medical cover for your athletes so that you can properly relax) or putting your phone on "do not disturb" during dinner. Consider having your own GP and checking in with them periodically to discuss your physical and mental health.

The more you get involved in sports and exercise medicine, the more opportunities will present themselves to you. Before committing ask yourself, "Is this a 'need to do' for my career or is it a 'nice to do' that I sadly don't have time to commit to?" If you take on an opportunity, be prepared to leave one of your current commitments to maintain your work-life balance.

## PRE-SEASON

During the pre-season period, aim to accomplish various tasks to set up for a safe and successful campaign ahead.

## Medical equipment

Medical equipment such as defibrillator pads/batteries, needles and medications often has an expiry date and needs to be replaced. All medications should be stored safely at the appropriate temperature in a locked cabinet in the treatment room. You need to be aware of, and adhere to, any regulations associated with storing, dispensing or travelling with medications, including acquiring import/export licences if required by the destination authorities.

> **PRACTICE PEARL**
>
> It is useful to add a warning sticker to any medications that may breach the WADA code if used in excess (e.g. salbutamol) or without a therapeutic use exemption (e.g. prednisolone).

Dispose of expired medications and blood-stained equipment appropriately. Check equipment such as defibrillators, oxygen cylinders, spinal boards, cervical collars, ultrasound or shockwave machines to ensure that it is functioning properly.

The treatment room needs to be fit for purpose. If performing injections, optimising sterility, safe disposal of sharps and an ability to wash your hands are a minimum requirement. The room must provide space for confidential consultations; if this is not possible, an alternative room should be identified. It is often useful to have a skeleton or relevant anatomical model to help explain injuries and their biomechanics to athletes, although these can be found on the internet.

Every sport has different requirements given the inherent risk of acute versus overuse injuries, lacerations or concussions—the medical equipment will need to reflect this. Table 6.1 contains a comprehensive list of equipment that could be used across a season, including where there is no immediate access to more sophisticated facilities—you can use this to help plan for your individual requirements. Ensure that the contents of your medical bag are clearly labelled and ideally arranged in an ABC (Airway, Breathing, Circulation) manner, so that other staff can be easily directed to obtain equipment in an emergency.

## Medical team

A wide variety of disciplines make up the medical team and the pre-season period is the perfect time to develop professional relationships with any new members. Ensure that all members are given appropriate team apparel to feel included—this is often forgotten!

It is important to develop clearly defined roles and duties within the medical team and to establish boundaries of care. Should the team doctor be treating an athlete's children?

**TABLE 6.1**   An extensive list of things to consider including in your medical bag (will vary by the sporting context)

**Diagnostic instruments**
- Oral/rectal thermometer
- Stethoscope
- Blood pressure cuff
- Ophthalmoscope
- Otoscope (auroscope) and earpieces
- Pencil torch
- Tongue depressors
- Pulse oximeter
- Blood glucose monitor
- SCAT6 paperwork (up to date)
- Tendon hammer
- Portable ultrasonography device
- Snellen eye chart and Ishihara plates

**Medications**
- Oral analgesics (e.g. paracetamol [acetaminophen], aspirin, codeine, tramadol)
- Intravenous analgesics (ketorolac, morphine, tramadol)
- Adrenaline (epinephrine) for anaphylaxis (and hydrocortisone)
- NSAIDs (non-steroidal anti-inflammatory drugs)
- Antibiotics (e.g. amoxicillin clavulanate, erythromycin, flucloxacillin, doxycycline, metronidazole)
- Antacid tablets
- Anti-nausea tablets (e.g. prochlorperazine [oral/IM], metoclopramide)
- Antidiarrhoeal agent (e.g. loperamide)
- Faecal softeners
- Antihistamines
- Bronchodilators (e.g. salbutamol inhaler, beclomethasone inhaler)
- 50% glucose solution
- Sedatives and hypnotics
- Throat lozenges
- Cough mixture
- Creams/ointments: antifungal, antibiotic, corticosteroid, anti-inflammatory
- Tetanus toxoid
- GTN (glyceryl trinitrate)
- Corticosteroid injections (e.g. Cortisone/Kenacort)
- Tranexamic acid

**Sutures/dressings**
- Needle holders
- Forceps
- Scissors: nail clippers, small sharp scissors and tape scissors
- Syringes (various sizes)
- Needles (various sizes)
- Sutures: various sizes, absorbable and non-absorbable
- Suture cutters
- Scalpels
- Local anaesthetics: lignocaine (lidocaine) with and without adrenaline (epinephrine)
- Steri-strips (various sizes)
- Alcohol swabs
- Gauze swabs
- Dressing packs
- Antiseptic solution
- Tincture of benzoin
- Dressing pads (various sizes)
- Low adherent dressing (Jelonet)
- Band-aid plastic strips
- Crepe bandages
- Tube gauze (Tubigrip)
- Sterile gloves, goggles and mask

**Resuscitation/emergency equipment**
- Defibrillator (see also Chapter 48)
- Resuscitation medications (e.g. adrenaline [epinephrine], amiodarone)
- Oropharyngeal and nasopharyngeal airways (various sizes)
- i-gel®
- Bag valve mask (BVM)
- Oxygen with suitable masks
- Emergency cricothyroid set
- Portable suction device
- Cannulation equipment
- IV sodium chloride
- IV giving set
- Rectal diazepam (for seizures)
- EpiPen
- Vacuum split/stretcher

**Blood management**
- Gauze swabs
- Klatostat for lacerations
- Klatostat strings and Rapid Rhino for epistaxis
- Blood tape (Coban)
- Co-phenylamine/tranexamic acid nasal spray
- Betadine spray
- Vaseline

**Equipment**
- Bolt cutters/screwdriver
- Air/box splints
- Triangular bandages (sling)
- Cotton-tipped applicators
- Rigid sports tape (various sizes)
- Elastic adhesive tape (various sizes)
- Compression bandages (various sizes)
- Adhesive foam pad
- SAM splint
- Blister pads
- Coolant spray
- Deep-heat muscle warming spray
- Finger splints
- Adjustable cervical collar (soft and hard)
- Spinal board with straps
- Eye kit: irrigation solution, fluorescein, eye patches, local anaesthetic/dilating eye drops, contact lens container
- Sunscreen
- Bonjela
- Massage oil/heat rubs
- Electrotherapy (e.g. TENS, portable laser)
- Portable examination table
- Alarm clock
- Plaster of Paris/thermoplastic casting equipment
- Portable slit lamp
- Bluetooth ECG/EKG device

**Other**
- Pen and paper
- Urine reagent strips and urine sample pots
- Safety pins
- Tampons and other period products
- Condoms
- Face masks, including N95s
- Sharps container
- Acupuncture needles
- Foam rollers and rehabilitation equipment
- Spare shoelaces
- Spare mouth guard
- Flexible orthoses
- Batteries
- Safety razor
- Plastic bags and clingfilm for ice
- Heel raises
- List of banned substances
- Transformer and dual voltage connector (if appropriate)
- Glucose sweets (for hypoglycaemia)
- Alcohol hand gel

Should the physiotherapist be managing the head coach's back pain? Should the dietitian be providing nutritional strategies to the operations manager who is trying to lose weight? Care within the sporting environment should be limited to the athletes; all other individuals should be managed externally.

All medical team members must ensure that their medical indemnity and working with children or vulnerable people certificates are up to date and cover the full scope of their practice, including if interstate or overseas travel is planned for the season. The medical team should be up to date with an official sports trauma course, and regularly practise trauma scenarios (log roll, spinal board, CPR etc.) throughout the season to maintain these skills.

While all staff play a role in protecting athletes' mental health, it is advisable to create a "wellbeing" team, consisting at a minimum of the doctor and psychologist, to formally manage difficult situations regarding confidential information. Mental health first aid courses are a valuable addition for those medical staff without formal training in the area.

## Health screening

The clinical team should identify what comprehensive physical screening data will be collected in the pre-season to use for comparison during future rehabilitation and to help address issues identified from the previous season. Minimum health screening standards set by the sporting body must be adhered to, but you may look to be more comprehensive in your approach, including external specialist input to cover areas such as cardiac (ECG $\pm$ echocardiogram), lab work (blood tests), dental, dermatology, optometry, sleep, disordered eating, relative energy deficiency, sexual health, concussion baseline testing, neuropsychology and mental health screening.

Whatever you choose to screen, you need to have the budget to offer it to all athletes and to have expedited pathways for abnormal findings (e.g. hypertrophic cardiomyopathy— sports cardiologist and psychologist in case of sport exclusion).[3] Also check with each athlete that nothing has changed in the off-season, such as new medications, allergies, family medical history or musculoskeletal injuries you may not be aware of.

## Relationships

As a sport and exercise clinician, you should build trust and rapport at various levels within your sporting environment to maximise outcomes for your athletes—getting to know coaches and other key personnel on at least a professional level will help later in the season when you need to make difficult decisions, such as ruling out a star athlete with a

concussion in a crucial match. Investing in developing the cohesion and trust of the healthcare team will help down the track so that robust discussions can be held in a safe, innovative and non-judgmental space to improve athlete care.

It is also important to develop relationships with external medical specialists to whom you can refer athletes, or with whom you can discuss cases urgently—this includes medical imaging and reports: 1–2 days is a long time in sport and any delay in optimal treatment may lead to matches/ competitions missed. You should also get to know your athletes and allow them to get to know you and realise that you care for them as people, not just athletes.

## Communication

Clear, open and effective communication is crucial. Communication protocols should be developed in the pre-season to ensure that the relevant information gets to the right people, including both full- and part-time staff. Remember to engage the end users of your communications, such as coaches or fitness staff, to ensure that your information meets their needs. You need to be aware of cybersecurity if using email or apps such as WhatsApp, and consider whether it is appropriate to message adolescent athletes without including their parents or to use your personal mobile number for such communications.

## Education

Health education for athletes is usually mandated, and sometimes provided, by the relevant sporting body. In addition to such sessions, consider talking to your athletes as a group and on an individual basis about your medical policies and protocols, as well as issues such as concussion, illicit substances and alcohol, anti-doping, supplements (especially changes in the WADA code) and mental health. It can be advantageous to include coaches and other club personnel in these sessions. Education should also be provided opportunistically: managing injuries and illnesses provides a space to educate athletes, coaches and other support personnel.

## Continuing professional development

The medical and performance team should plan continuing professional development for the upcoming season via journal clubs, conferences or engaging external specialists. If you travel with a team, this can be a good time to meet with a specialist at your destination for this development. Also consider conducting research during the season, potentially linked with a local university or other academic institution. If you are new to the sport, look to educate yourself on its required biomechanics, physiology and rules.

## Policies and protocols

Developing and reviewing policies and protocols that involve the medical team are crucial aspects of the pre-season. Ensure that you have an appropriate electronic medical record system to document all medical care involving athletes. The system should be password protected, ideally accessible online to allow use when travelling and have stratified access so that confidential notes can be created. Your phone and laptop should also be password protected to increase security.

You should have an emergency action plan for your training facility and any competition venues—template examples can be found online.[4] Illness and infection control policies should detail how athletes report issues to medical staff, when they should stay at home (i.e. gastroenteritis), vaccinations required (influenza, hepatitis B etc.) and how the training facility will be cleaned to reduce the transmission of infection.

You should also have a medication and supplement policy that informs athletes of the risks of ingesting prohibited substances, the need to follow WADA guidance and how to manage drugs with a risk of addiction (i.e. sleeping tablets or strong painkillers). Global Drug Reference Online[5] is an international database that athletes can use to ensure a medication is safe for use within their sport.

Global Drug Reference Online

Protocols should be developed for how athletes are expected to initially manage injuries such as significant muscle contusions and the club's individual alcohol policy for those rehabilitating an injury, for example. These protocols should detail that athletes are not to enter pools, saunas or spas with open wounds and should report these to medical staff for appropriate management.

If your athletes compete in environmental extremes, policies should be developed on how to prepare for air pollution (consider air quality apps), altitude (consider training camps) or temperature (consider heat or cold acclimation).

## IN-SEASON

### Scheduling/planning

Elite sport has numerous competing time pressures, and daily scheduling can be a fine balance trying not to overload athletes and staff, with burnout when travelling a particular

risk. A daily process to assess injuries, discuss wellbeing data and meet with coaching staff will prevent unnecessary stress and miscommunication. It is also important to have protocols on how to communicate match availability, including what details are released to the media.

Having strong relationships with your multidisciplinary team will ensure that you can raise any medically related concerns and have difficult conversations when you feel schedules may compromise health and wellbeing. Unlike private practice or one-to-one rehabilitation, prioritising medical input becomes a joint decision with the multidisciplinary team and must be justified in comparison to other needs, meetings, commercial/media commitments, and so on.

Combatting your own fatigue during a long season is important to ensure that you can complete your role to the best of your ability. Clinicians are at risk of burnout as athlete rest periods are not your downtime—you are still required to be available for assessments and treatments. Ensure you make time for paperwork and schedule time off. Resources we often share with athletes, such as the HeadSpace meditation app, can be equally as valuable for staff.

If you are away from your regular facilities, the logistics of accessing them can affect the schedule and tough decisions may need to be made for the overall benefit of the athlete; for example, travelling an hour on a bus to access a pool for recovery may negate the benefits. When faced with difficult decisions about recovery, Chapter 16 will help prioritise the best decision.

### Treatment room

While in the treatment room, the athlete's wellbeing is your primary concern, irrespective of pressures such as team expectations, program timings or coaching demands. Be aware of sensitivities if the room is in view of the manager's office, as athletes may be worried that "being in the treatment room" could affect their selection. Ensure that the room has adequate privacy (both visual and auditory) and can be locked to help facilitate private examinations or discussions.

Have clear standards for behaviour, such as no phones, and be mindful of the room not becoming a storage facility that impacts your ability to assess or treat unhindered.

### Equipment and consumables

If appropriate to your role, match day radios need to be charged before a competition and checked for regional operation. To avoid confusion, ensure good earpieces that ideally "unlock" (so that you don't hear incidental conversations), check that staff understand radio etiquette and that specific use in your emergency action plan is understood. It is also important to consider whether radios should only be allowed for permitted users and to check their operation from pitch to the changing room—especially when a mobile phone is not an optional backup due to restricted use for safeguarding, gambling or match fixing control.

Consider separating and labelling equipment that you will take to the pitch from equipment that will stay in the treatment room. Ensure your pitchside bag is not left in direct sunlight or rain, which may damage its contents.

## Other important considerations

Religious and cultural beliefs may influence medical practices or treatments and should be considered in an environment of cultural safety. Cultural or wellbeing officers can be a great source of advice above and beyond discussing with the athlete or staff member how to best support them. Examples include observing periods of fasting and using an appropriate chaperone when removing religious garments or examining intimate areas.

Deciding when to keep an athlete on the field and when to definitively treat an injury can be difficult—especially with additional factors such as athletes at the end of their career, loan players or upcoming transfer windows. This creates a grey zone and in this setting of uncertainty leaning on the multidisciplinary team for shared decision making regarding return-to-sport decisions is best practice. Where there is disagreement between the athlete and multidisciplinary team, or members of the team, the medico-legal responsibility lies with the sport and exercise physician to make a decision in the best interests of the athlete.

## TRAVEL

Travel adds to the challenges of caring for athletes as the usual medical support structure is temporarily unavailable and the level of medical support services at the destination may vary substantially. To become self-sufficient, create a detailed plan before travelling. You may find it useful to split preparation into before travel, during travel, arrival and journey home.

## Before travel

### Travel destination

You need to know the climate, altitude, level of pollution, water supply, security, recent health epidemics and natural disasters at the destination.[6-8] This includes any medication import restrictions and consideration of language barriers, especially in a medical emergency. Players carrying their own medications should be advised of travel and local requirements (e.g. a medical letter to take needles on a plane). Having a good understanding of local culture and expectations can help avoid any issues with local authorities—such as athletes being aware of how much skin they expose, especially when not in official training gear. Having an interpreter on hand is advantageous, especially should an emergency occur.

### Accommodation

Encourage athletes to take home comforts to minimise home sickness, as well as their own pillows or a preferred mattress topper to improve sleep. (Further sleep hygiene information can be found in Chapter 16.) In a hot climate, having air conditioning may be advantageous for comfort, but it can delay heat acclimatisation and cause respiratory issues if used excessively as it can dry out the upper respiratory tract mucosa. Particularly tall athletes will require extra-long beds. In-room safes are useful for important personal or valuable items. If financially viable, athletes should have separate rooms to reduce the spread of illness and promote better sleep.

### Treatment room

Try to have a dedicated treatment room within the hotel to allow for privacy and confidentiality, especially from public guests and media. Be aware that ballrooms or meeting rooms may not have toilets, sinks or suitable doors/curtains or may be situated a long distance from bedrooms. If equipment is stored a significant distance from bedrooms, you may need to take emergency equipment to your room overnight to minimise time lost in an emergency.

If budget allows, a spare room on the same floor as team bedrooms can be used for storage and as an emergency isolation room if athletes are sharing rooms. Enquire about any major events at the hotel during your stay and request rooms away from these areas to minimise noise disturbance and to plan for situations of busy elevators/hotel reception that can impact transit times.

If you will need to set up your treatment space within the athlete's changing room, develop a protocol whereby players only undress and shower once staff have been given time to examine any injuries post competition and then leave the changing room—this is especially important when working with athletes of the opposite sex.

### Vaccinations

Specific vaccinations or malaria prophylaxis may be needed before embarking on travel to certain destinations. Liaise with your local travel clinic to help plan these requirements.

### Equipment and travel logistics

Deliveries can be delayed and products may not be available, especially when travelling abroad, so planning is key. Detailed lists save time when shipping items or if import documents must contain itemised information. Equally, duplicating equipment can save on costs as items can be sent ahead via cheaper transportation.

Consider the size of items/medical bags to ensure that they fit in the aeroplane hold, can be lifted safely and repeatedly by staff and offer flexibility (e.g. battery-operated recovery pumps allow use on buses and aeroplanes). Checking pre-clearance for certain items in the hold (e.g. oxygen) and pre-screening items at check-in will save valuable time. Clearly label all items and bags. Insurance for expensive items should cover transit too in case of damage during on-/offloading in vans or buses.

When moving large amounts of equipment, it is important to have foldable trolleys or wheeled cases to make it easier for all involved. If you are planning to source medications, consumables or equipment locally on arrival, ensure that equivalents are available (e.g. some countries may not stock portable oxygen tanks for pitch use, sunscreen may not be the same UVA/UVB standards or certain sanitary items may not be sold). The preference is to take all potentially required medications given the anti-doping risk of purchasing medications overseas. Electrical equipment will need extension cords and travel adapters and to be checked to ensure that it can be used with the voltage at the destination.

Timings for arrival of any equipment not travelling with you must be factored in if you are expecting to be able to immediately assess or treat athletes on arrival and if any branding needs to be removed due to restrictions at competition venues. With reliance on an internet connection for communication apps, EMR systems and concussion assessment apps, a strong wi-fi signal is key; portable hotspot devices can reduce costs and prevent any connectivity concerns. This is extremely important if you need to access medical information urgently. In some cases, a folder of printed key medical information stored securely may be the best option.

Charging stations for laptops/iPads, a kettle, rolls of garbage bags, whiteboard markers and whiteboard sheets, hot-water bottles and blankets are just a few important items for the treatment room that often aren't available in hotels or at stadiums.

---

> **PRACTICE PEARL**
>
> Speaking to clinicians who have travelled to the same venue previously is invaluable when packing.

---

It is important to note that medications may have different compositions in other countries. There are formulas that can assist in estimating the pharmacological needs for a trip,[9] and it is important that all medications are accompanied by a prescription or doctor's letter, as well as being kept in the original container. Any bags of medications should go through customs with the medical team rather than being carried by other staff. If medications are in freight or with kit staff on alternative transport you should have a clear "controlled drugs" process, logbook and security tagging.[10]

### Reconnaissance

The local destination hotel/medical services should be researched and ideally visited in advance during team reconnaissance to decide whether medical facilities are equivalent, kitchens are clean and to make a local connection who speaks your language. This also includes checking the training and match venues to ensure that evacuation locations/equipment are available and pre-scouting the toilet/treatment room/shower setup in changing rooms to help manage expectations of cleanliness, establish ease of use or consider additional privacy with screens or curtains. Understanding the rules for using facilities, such as pools that require swimming caps or gyms that require individual towels, means you can purchase these items in advance and brief players and staff.

### Emergency action plans

The emergency action plan created for your home training facility may not be suitable when travelling. It may need to be translated into the destination language (in case you need to give it to local medical staff), involve local medical care or follow a specific competition action plan. If an athlete needs to be extricated to a local healthcare setting, try to ensure that your equipment (i.e. spinal collar or SAM splint) doesn't go with them so that you don't need to replace it while away. Decide in advance who will go to the hospital with the athlete and how to arrange prepayment for care, if needed.

### Medical travel assessments

Contact all team members, including coaches and officials, to establish any past or present injuries and illnesses. Coaches and officials with chronic medical conditions such as coronary artery disease should be reminded to bring their own medications. If there is no doctor in the travelling party, it is wise to develop safe practices around medication dispensing for athletes by officials or non-medical healthcare professionals. For example, while athletes can carry regular over-the-counter medications, prescribed medications should be taken in sufficient quantities to last the entirety of travel and it is advantageous to arrange access to a "home-based" doctor for telehealth consults.

Injuries and illnesses, including dental care, should ideally be treated prior to departure. Ensure that your employer has appropriate travel insurance and repatriation for all athletes and staff. Additional screening may be warranted to help identify those who require extra wellbeing support, especially young athletes unaccustomed to travel or individuals with mental health diagnoses or disordered eating. Screening should also identify individuals with allergies to medications/foods/animals and those with food intolerances/restrictions, so that appropriate measures can be taken before departure.

### Nutrition

It is challenging for athletes to maintain good dietary habits when travelling and they should be counselled on wise food choices before they travel.[11] At large competitions, athletes often eat in village communal restaurants where buffet-style dining may lead to overeating or risk illness.

In addition to food intake, adequate hydration is important, especially when travelling to warm climates. Traveller's diarrhoea is very common,[12] and while the infection is usually self-limiting, team physicians should institute oral fluid replacement as the mainstay of treatment, in addition to isolation. To minimise the risk of traveller's diarrhoea, athletes should only eat food that has been cooked, and should avoid raw shellfish, salads, unpasteurised milk products and unpeeled fruit. In countries where water quality is poor, they should also consider drinking and brushing their teeth with bottled water.

### Jet lag

Jet lag can detrimentally affect performance for athletes and staff alike. Before travel, exposure to sunlight can be planned to maximise phase shifting towards the destination time zone. Some athletes may benefit from using melatonin (or prescribed hypnotics) to promote sleep or caffeine to induce daytime alertness. See Chapter 16 for sleep monitoring systems and further information.

### Insurance and indemnity

Your policies must cover you to practise at the destination. If any minors are in attendance, it is important that they travel with the appropriate guardian consent to treat them, as well as their guardian's contact information.[13]

### SAMPLE forms

It is useful to create a history and treatment sheet for each athlete prior to travel, in case they need to be transferred to hospital during the trip. The sheet can be pre-filled with details such as past medical history, regular medications, allergies, personal details and next of kin.

The SAMPLE format is useful for this: Signs and symptoms, Allergies, regular Medications, Past medical history, Last meal/drink and Events (including examination and treatment/intervention).

### Injury prevention

While expectations and processes are often clear at home, when travelling it is important to ensure that the team still conduct proper warm-ups, stretching/yoga and strength maintenance, receive regular soft-tissue therapy and use recovery strategies (Chapter 16), adapting as required to the facilities, fewer staff or minimal equipment. Athletes should be reminded to try to replicate their daily recovery practices as on tour they may be faced with a significant increase in options, which can be overwhelming.

## During travel

Create a medical travel bag that contains medications to deal with travel sickness, sickness bags, basic blood management items (nosebleeds etc.), facemasks and simple analgesic medications. Your controlled drugs policy may require you to carry this with you rather than in the hold. Consider having an emergency grab-bag in your carry-on luggage with the equipment needed to conduct vitals examinations during travel (i.e. stethoscope, pulse oximeter, manual sphygmomanometer, thermometer, otoscope, Bluetooth 6-lead ECG/EKG). Only carry items you are comfortable using.

Athletes and officials can become sick during travel so having masks, personal protective equipment and alcohol hand gel may help contain infection outbreaks. In addition, consider managing seating plans on buses/planes so that the entire team will not be affected by one infectious individual.

It may be useful to provide athletes with a simple travel pack that contains some basics: paracetamol, lip salve, ear plugs, eye mask, saline nasal spray, ice bag etc. Defibrillators should always be carried by the medical team and if players are split across two modes of transport, the process for locating medical staff/emergency equipment discussed. Ensure that athletes have sufficient water and food for the duration of their trip, especially if they are to compete soon after reaching their destination—simply ensuring the bus always has a supply of water bottles is an easy win.

If travelling long distances via road or aeroplane, using thromboembolism-deterrent (TED) stockings, electronic calf stimulators, battery-operated recovery pumps/ice therapy, earplugs, eye masks, facemasks and air humidifiers can help athletes to sleep in comfort and reduce the risk of venous thrombosis. Consideration should be given to stops to stretch or break up a trip overnight might be more beneficial than long transits. If no toilets are available during transport factor in time for toilet stops and consider hand sanitisation on buses/trains if they are not equipped with a private food preparation/kitchen area and sink.

## Arrival

A treatment room should be established soon after arrival or if kit/early setup staff are travelling ahead give clear instructions and diagrams for what you want where. Having spare towels/pillows from the hotel available in advance can be invaluable, especially if you need to start treating immediately to attempt to balance recovery against sleep schedules the day before competition.

The room can be at risk of becoming a "social hub" so it is important to consider confidentiality and set up a private space just as you would at your club/clinic. Plan the best route for any equipment that needs to be taken in/out daily to buses and lean on your multidisciplinary team or hotel staff to support this. Hotel management may agree to you using "staff only areas" to help aid quicker movement of gear and unnecessary walking.

Ensure that athletes know the room numbers of the medical staff in case of emergencies and that the treatment room is locked when not in use or is monitored accordingly, especially if it contains medications. It is important that the team manager knows how to contact medical staff if the room is unattended. It is also helpful to obtain an athlete room list from the team manager.

Ensuring that players know where to access ice/clean drinking water and ideally having it available in the treatment room, along with a method to transport it to player rooms, can help athletes to be self-sufficient and save you time logistically, especially for ice baths. Pre-ordering this with the hotel will prevent you running out, especially if you are sharing the hotel with other teams.

---

### PRACTICE PEARL

Treatment hours should be specified using an appointment sheet or online booking system so that you have adequate time for meals, administration tasks and wellbeing (i.e. to exercise). This must be strictly enforced as athletes tend to extend these hours.

---

A repeat or advanced visit to the training and competition venues means that one final safety check can be done for cleanliness, availability of emergency equipment and treatment tables and access such as the pitchside emergency room being unlocked or sharps bins available.

A pitch check should be conducted just as it would be when you are at your home venue, and especially if it is accessible to the public, to ensure safety such as sprinkler heads covered and no signs of glass. If there are multiple venues, the advantage of bringing your own treatment table must be weighed against the inconvenience of transporting it everywhere; borrowing one locally may be a solution.

## Journey home

Preparing for the return journey is important as some injuries or illnesses incurred while away may need specialist arrangements for travel or referral for follow-up.[14] Thought must be given to the thromboembolic risk of various injuries, such as fractures, and whether anticoagulation should be used prior to return travel. Once back at the home destination, medical staff should have a debriefing session to review any issues during the trip and enable changes to be implemented for future medical care.[15]

## OFF-SEASON

### Exit screening

At the end of the season, many teams or leagues recommend or require an exit screening or physical. Understanding the purpose of the examination is the first step to performing it properly. Is it to document ongoing injuries for future teams in case of a trade or change of team? Is it to establish injuries that your organisation will remain responsible for and need to manage in the off-season? Is it to recommend treatment or rehabilitation strategies for the off-season?

You should also communicate clearly to athletes where your duty of care lies. In professional leagues your duty of care may be to the team or league, especially for exit screenings.

You need to plan how and when these screenings will be conducted. Will they be done the day after the season ends? Players may wish to leave for another location as soon as a season is over, and this timing may be unpredictable (e.g. after a loss in an end-of-season tournament or championship play), so you will need to plan for any contingencies. Is there a standard form or method for the screenings? Depending on the size of your team and the timeframe allowed to complete the screenings, you may need to arrange for additional help.

### Trades

You need to know what information you are required to provide to other teams that your athletes may be going to. Likewise, you should develop a proforma to help gather information and clinical examination requirements for potential trades for your club.

**A**

Use established and approved channels of communication. Over the years you will get to know medical staff on other teams but despite this familiarity you should ensure that you gain athlete consent before sharing any confidential medical information.

### Other considerations

Have a system in place that can expedite any surgeries or consultations that were intentionally postponed until the off-season. Expedient scheduling of surgeries provides athletes more time to recover before the next season.

Establish procedures for athletes to contact you during the off-season. Will you see them at the club or in a clinic?

How will these visits be paid for? If you are working with a national/international team whose athletes will be going to a home club, establish channels of communication with medical staff to discuss injuries, illnesses and ongoing rehabilitation needs. Make sure you have appropriate documentation that can be provided to home clubs via established approved methods.

If you will be away from the club for a period, this may be a good time to dispose of expired medications or supplies and order for the next season. And finally, the end of the season is a great opportunity for you to take a holiday, rest, recharge and thank your family/loved ones for their support over the season before you get ready to do it all again.

## KEY POINTS

- Establishing a good relationship with your athletes is important, but this must remain within professional boundaries.

- Navigating social media is an important skill to develop. Be cautious about interacting with athletes on social media and consider maintaining separate professional and personal accounts.

- The pre-season period is a good time to check equipment, orient new staff, screen athletes and review emergency procedures.

- Among other in-season tasks, preparing for travel is critically important.

- Travel requires extensive planning, athlete education, emergency preparedness and coordination with numerous parties and venues.

- At the end of the season, you should coordinate the exit screening of athletes, schedule off-season procedures and prioritise your own time off before the next season.

## REFERENCES

References for this chapter can be found at www.mhprofessional.com/CSM6e

## ADDITIONAL CONTENT

 Scan here to access additional resources for this topic and more provided by the authors

## CHAPTER 7

# Career development

with **MICHAEL KENIHAN**

*It is the greatest of all mistakes to do nothing because you can only do little.*

(SYDNEY SMITH, *ELEMENTARY SKETCHES OF MORAL PHILOSOPHY,* 1849, "LECTURE XIX: ON THE CONDUCT OF THE UNDERSTANDING, PART II")

## CHAPTER OUTLINE

The clinician's journey
The heart of clinical practice: the office consult
Goal setting and time management
Building referrals: relationship marketing
Other skills that make you a better clinician
Take control of your career
Choose an empowered workplace
Common concerns

## LEARNING OBJECTIVES

By the end of this chapter you should be able to:
- provide an athlete or patient with a high-quality consultation
- identify skills you can develop to progress your career
- discuss the importance of good listening skills in the clinical workplace
- outline a career development plan
- create habits to remain up to date with emerging science
- recognise the characteristics of an empowering workplace.

## Introduction to Mike Kenihan by Peter Brukner and Karim Khan

This chapter is written for everyone who is considering a career in one of the many health professions that involve sport, exercise or physical activity. We are biased, of course, but contend that working to promote physical activity and to help people obtain the benefits of exercise is one of the most rewarding careers one can undertake.

This chapter outlines a trajectory—a journey—to achieve the career you choose, irrespective of which health discipline you are currently training in. You'll see we use the word "clinician" in an inclusive way in this chapter, as we do throughout this book. Do you love sport, exercise or physical activity? Do you love health? If you answered "yes" to any part of these questions, this chapter is for you.

We invited Mike Kenihan (Fig. 7.1) to helm the chapter because of his diverse and extensive experience in mentoring so many people who have achieved great heights in our field. He has been an elite athlete, an expert physiotherapist, a multidisciplinary clinic owner, a partner in an integrated health delivery company and a personal coach. He has held major leadership roles in national and international sports medicine organisations. He contributes to his community and is a committed partner and parent. In short, he has a lot to offer and we are grateful that he has summarised the key elements of his 2024 book, *The Health Practitioner's Journey,* here.[1]

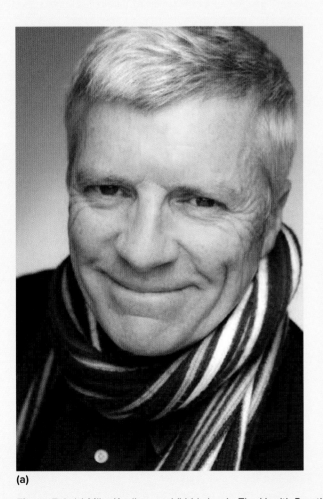

(a)

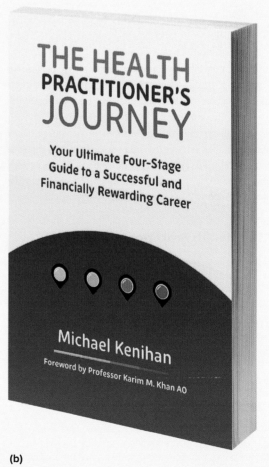

(b)

**Figure 7.1** (a) Mike Kenihan and (b) his book, *The Health Practitioner's Journey*

## THE CLINICIAN'S JOURNEY

My career was primarily as a sports physiotherapist in the days before postgraduate sports medicine courses were available. Back then, a clinician could work with elite sporting teams without any additional qualifications and the roles were very part-time. Of course, the workload in elite sport has grown exponentially. Both extra study and time are needed to be devoted to a career that includes roles with professionals and other teams.

In this chapter, I share the necessary elements to develop your career. The attributes presented apply whether you are a sport and exercise physician, sports physiotherapist, podiatrist, massage therapist, strength and conditioning coach or another clinician in sport.

There is a pathway for your career, and it will require you to explore, learn, watch and listen. Expert clinicians:

- read widely
- listen intently
- think deeply
- speak lightly.

The time it takes you to achieve your goals may be shorter or longer than you envisage. Some clinicians pause their careers to be more clinic-based or to explore an academic interest without team attachment. As you grow in your career you will be "harvesting knowledge" in your journey that should enable you to grow and seek new opportunities.

I have developed a model that outlines the journey of a clinician in practice (Fig. 7.2). The model is based on my experience and not everyone will follow this journey in a linear fashion. The four stages build on each other and you harvest knowledge while on that journey.

To become an excellent clinician, it's critical that you invest in your clinical skills. To achieve this, you need to be able to understand, develop and apply sound clinical reasoning and problem solving, learn solid manual tests and techniques, seek out the right training processes that suit you, and develop your learning and experience.

Successful sport and exercise clinicians have high-level time management and planning skills, including being able to set realistic goals. They are very good communicators and demonstrate excellent communication skills—verbal, non-verbal and written. All of these attributes contribute to a fulfilling career path.

The path is a challenge and a very personal one and you will need to be proactive. The pathway will not always be linear, and you should be open to take opportunities that arise, often unexpectedly, to progress your career.

## THE HEART OF CLINICAL PRACTICE: THE OFFICE CONSULT

In my book, *The Heath Practitioner's Journey,* I recommend an eight-step approach to the office consultation. This sounds more complex than how you were taught to approach the consult, but after using the approach for even a few days you will find it very natural. This approach will make your patients realise that you care greatly about them. The steps are outlined in Table 7.1.

Once you have completed the consultation, made the observations from your examination, reasoned solutions and shown the benefit of your treatment interventions, you will have demonstrated value to the athlete.

### Advice

What you say to an athlete is immensely powerful. Aim to be concise and speak in plain language that athletes will understand—avoid jargon. Frame your comments in relation to their presentation (the specific injury rather than the condition broadly/theoretically). Inspire them to be confident that you will be able to assist them back to participation, even if that may be some time away (see also Chapter 3).

After providing your advice, notice how the athlete absorbs or interprets your message. This may influence how effective the shared treatment plan will be. If you notice they seem to have reservations, give them a chance to share their thoughts. "Am I sensing some reservations about ...? Is there something I can clarify further? I really want to hear your thoughts."

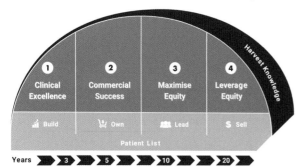

**The Health Practitioner's Journey**™

**Figure 7.2** The arc of the clinician's journey. The model is based on a private practice setting where the clinician is able to develop a practice and potentially sell their equity. The principles that underpin a successful private clinical practice apply equally to those aspiring to serve in the public system or work with non-governmental organisations.
Source: Image reproduced from Mike Kenihan, *The Health Practitioner's Journey*

**TABLE 7.1** Eight steps to providing your patients with a quality experience for every consultation

| Step | Brief description |
|---|---|
| 1. Prepare | Make sure you are ready, that the consulting room is clean and you have read the intake/referral notes. |
| 2. Build rapport with the patient | Show genuine interest, listen intently and empathetically, and use non-verbal cues to make the patient comfortable. |
| 3. Analyse the patient's need | Why is the patient here?<br>How did they find you?<br>What concerns do they have?<br>What is their expectation of treatment? (don't assume that you know) |
| 4. Develop a solution | Is the patient's expectation realistic?<br>Involve the patient in treatment planning (see Chapter 4).<br>Remember, a good referral can be as productive as a treatment from you. |
| 5. Explain the benefits of treatment | Many clinicians fail to sell the benefits of the treatment plan—they assume the patient will be motivated. Treatment takes time and can be costly: explain that this is worth it—be specific. |
| 6. Demonstrate the value (if you can change a patient's symptoms during one visit) | If you can provide immediate relief (e.g. manual therapy, taping), be sure to reassess the patient after applying the treatment. This can apply to some injections as well (e.g. with local anaesthetic).<br>Provide extra information (e.g. websites) to help with education, a powerful part of treatment (see Chapter 25). |
| 7. Offer a brief summary | Recount what you have discussed, observed and provided (treatment).<br>Detail your instructions—what should the patient do at home? Detail the intensity, as patients are often inclined to do more than asked! |
| 8. Provide a caring close | Clarify your expectations (yours and the patient's).<br>Remind them of what you think the problem is and how you plan to assist them.<br>Be clear on next steps (e.g. next appointment).<br>Ensure you provide a caring farewell. |

Consider also how you use supplementary material. This may be existing material from your practice, digital links including commercial exercise platforms, or old-school drawings that can still resonate with some patients.

To promote successful outcomes, work closely with the athlete (see also Chapters 2, 3 and 4). Provide them with specific opportunities to share what they understand about the condition and what they think they should and will do.

Being part of the multidisciplinary team means you will generally have immediate access to your professional colleagues. They are powerful allies to help you assist the athlete but they can teach you a great deal too. Athletes at all levels will expect others in the team to be involved in their treatment, recovery and performance.

## GOAL SETTING AND TIME MANAGEMENT

There is always more to do than there is time in the day. Should you volunteer or spend time reading? How is your work–life balance? Being proactive means thinking about what's important to you and setting goals, then assessing whether you have met those goals. The business term "key

performance indicators (KPIs)" has gained a foothold in common parlance. KPIs are quantifiable indicators of progress towards an intended goal. What will you set as your KPIs? How will you find the time to work on them?

## Goal setting

University health-related training usually doesn't help much with setting goals. I recommend using the well-known SMART objectives to ensure that your goals are:

- Specific
- Measurable
- Achievable
- Realistic
- Timely.

My book, *The Health Practitioner's Journey*, provides great detail regarding goal setting but there is one key factor involved in setting goals: a study into goal setting conducted by Dr Gail Matthews, a psychology professor at the Dominican University of California, provides clear evidence that those who write down their goals accomplish significantly more than those who do not write them down.[2]

## Developing KPIs

Here's a practical example of KPI development. Your goal might be to learn more about treating spinal conditions. You need to be able to evaluate whether you have learned more about such conditions. To do this, your KPIs should direct your performance. Make sure you set KPIs that are binary: that is, you achieve them or you do not. Your KPIs might be to:

- identify and attend a course where the topic is being presented within the next quarter
- read two relevant articles in the next month and review/ discuss them with someone more experienced than you.

## Time management

I will remind you of the very widely recognised "quadrants" of time management. They have been associated with former US President Dwight Eisenhower, which indicates they have enduring value. Stephen Covey certainly amplified the concept as it is a core element (Habit 3) in *The 7 Habits of Highly Effective People.* One way of categorising tasks (and then acting on them) is to create a 2 × 2 matrix (Fig. 7.3) and then place tasks into the four quadrants. Clinicians who find themselves too often in quadrant 1 may not be spending enough time in quadrant 2. The vicious cycle is that the more you are battling crises in quadrant 1, the less time you have to address preventive measures in quadrant 2. Quadrant 2 items need to be scheduled and attended to— even when they are challenged by items in quadrant 3.

| Quadrant 1. Urgent and important | Quadrant 2. Not urgent and important |
|---|---|
| • Crises<br>• Pressing problems<br>• Deadlines | • Planning<br>• Relationship building (professional and personal)<br>• Crisis prevention<br>• Preparation |
| Quadrant 3. Urgent and not important | Quadrant 4. Not urgent and not important |
| • Interruptions<br>• Some phone calls, meetings, urgent emails | • Doomscrolling<br>• Procrastination<br>• Some emails |

**Figure 7.3** The four quadrants of time management. The challenge is to do the important work of quadrant 2 when the urgent items pull you strongly to quadrants 1 and 3.

## BUILDING REFERRALS: RELATIONSHIP MARKETING

The idea of building relationships with referrers is known as relationship marketing and at first this may seem intimidating. When presenting this idea to practitioners I often receive the reply, "I haven't been trained in marketing." This may be true, although some health courses focus heavily on marketing because they realise that most of those who graduate will move into private practice and will need to know how to build a practice or business.

During your professional life you will constantly build relationships and most clinicians have very precious lifelong professional friendships. Developing referrer relationships is like nurturing friendships. There is mutual respect and admiration. Your patients will be delighted with you when you refer them to an expert who can solve their issue.

Essential behaviours that help with relationship building include:

- be professional in everything you say and do and how you present yourself
- attend totally to the task at hand so that the patient feels the personalisation of your service
- be engaged and not distracted
- listen attentively and with empathy. If your patient feels that you truly understand what they may be going through, they will align more readily with the recovery or treatment plan.

## OTHER SKILLS THAT MAKE YOU A BETTER CLINICIAN

Here I outline four other skills you might consider developing. The stars of the clinical community I have worked with over 30 years have all been excellent listeners, great with people, able to prevent and resolve conflict, as well as having tremendous communication skills. These skills are summarised in Table 7.2 later in this section.

## Listening is underrated

Reflect on the five levels of listening below. How well do you listen? If you aren't already an empathetic listener, focus on improving your listening skills so that you reach this level.

- *Ignoring:* The lowest level of listening is ignoring—not listening at all!
- *Pretend listening:* This form of listening is often employed by parents when their 2-year-old is talking incessantly on learning to talk. You are there but not eagerly engaged with the content.
- *Selective listening:* During selective listening you pay attention to the speaker as long as they are talking about things you like or agree with.
- *Attentive listening:* Attentive listening occurs when you carefully listen to the other person, but, while they are

speaking, you are deciding whether you agree or disagree, often determining when they are about to stop talking.

- *Empathetic listening:* This is the fifth and highest level of listening. The empathetic listener is aware of, and tries hard to appreciate, the speaker's feelings and emotions, as well as the words they are using. This means not only listening to what the speaker is saying but also trying to get behind the words–to hear what they are *not* saying. Try to develop your listening to this level.

## Read the room and stay in your lane

The expression "reading the room" is not uncommon but many people don't read it very well. If you keenly observe the behaviour of others, it will help you to see opportunities and improve how you connect with other team members.

"Staying in your lane" can be wise, knowing when you are not the expert. I am aware of scenarios where surgeons have regaled the details of post-ACL injury rehabilitation when surrounded by physiotherapists with vast experience; similarly, it doesn't pay for a sports physician who has assisted at surgery to extoll inexpert opinions on surgical management of complex fractures. Of course, multidisciplinary spaces are great for discussion, learning and contributing novel ideas from a different viewpoint, but the tone of the conversation is critical. "I've been wondering ..." can be an appropriate opening for a respectfully challenging opinion. Bombastically launching a polemic on how another clinician should do things differently is never a good idea.

## Solve problems and resolve conflict

You know people who seem to be able to make the world a better place and you know others who some would describe as being "hard work", or words to that effect. I'm not judging here and everyone has reasons for their behaviour. In the clinical sports setting you find all types–of course. But I didn't have any courses on interpersonal relations, conflict resolution or organisational behaviour (the clinic level) when I was learning to be a physiotherapist. Before long, I was leading a physiotherapy department and then all the disciplines in our group sports practice.

What I learned through experience–and subsequently from courses, reading and listening to podcasts–is that listening (again!) is a key element in conflict resolution. Above, I mentioned empathetic listening in the context of the patient consultation but here I am referring to listening to find out what the conflict is about. Is there tension between a physiotherapist and a strength and conditioning coach over the late-stage management of an injured player who is soon to return to sport? Is there disagreement among managing physicians and team physiotherapists about how

long a football player with an anterior tibial stress fracture needs to be on crutches? Stephen Covey's Habit 5–"Seek first to understand, then to be understood"–provides a good foundation for the wise clinician. If you remember this, your colleagues will see you as a sensible, positive influence.

Another area of conflict can be rosters. Who does the unpopular shifts? Who jumps in to cover for a colleague when they have a real emergency? My advice is the obvious–but difficult: to earn a reputation of being a team player. This doesn't mean you allow yourself to be taken advantage of but you demonstrate that you are unselfish– that you appreciate the communal good.

If you are in a formal or informal leadership position and you find yourself losing sleep over interpersonal conflict issues, I suggest taking a conflict resolution course that others in your community can vouch for.

## Get media and communication training

You might wonder how media training makes you a better clinician. What's the core material in media training? It's how to share clear messages so that others can understand them. If you learn how to speak in front of a camera or microphone, you will explain things better to your patients. If you learn to make a pitch in 30 seconds for television, you will be able to explain a patient's tendinopathy clearly during a consult.

Expanding from traditional media to social media, skills such as writing blogs, creating graphics, and recording and editing videos and podcasts enable you to create customised patient education materials should you desire. The importance of patient education in clinical practice is outlined in Chapter 15.

When you first graduate as a clinician, it's probably wise to focus on your clinical skills–and clinical skills need attention for your entire career. After a few years in clinical practice, however, many clinicians feel the urge to contribute to the community in additional ways. How to set yourself up to do that is shown in Table 7.2 and discussed below.

## TAKE CONTROL OF YOUR CAREER

You need to be the chief executive officer (CEO) of your career rather than hoping that you'll be swept in a favourable direction. Expert clinicians have all had terrific mentors, worked hard to refine their skills and made time to volunteer strategically. Here I provide some more background on six ways to move your career forward. This builds on the previous section, which focused on how to be a top-class clinician. In this section, I assume you are one of them!

**TABLE 7.2**  How to be your best clinician and develop your career

| In the clinical setting: how to become better at diagnosing and treating patients | How to progress your career as you gain experience |
|---|---|
| • Gain as much experience as possible: "put yourself out there" and take opportunities<br><br>• Network widely and ask questions<br><br>• Sit in with others during their consultations and ask questions<br><br>• Volunteer and ask questions (event coverage)<br><br>• Learn from other professions and disciplines in the clinical team<br><br>• "Be present" (a term introduced by Eckhart Tolle) to learn and grow by experiencing the moment | • Consider specialised hospital rotations to upskill if you are a sport and exercise physician (e.g. sports cardiology)<br><br>• Attend courses<br><br>• Prioritise purposeful professional development<br><br>• Volunteer to edit podcasts, support the clinic social media, make educational videos for patients or be part of patient engagement or student education events<br><br>• Learn a language or other skills (such as coding skills if you are working with data/data analytics, or podcast editing skills)<br><br>• Get involved in research: volunteer to do work such as literature searches, data collection or knowledge translation activities |

## Find a career sponsor, mentors and clinical advisor

The words "mentor" and "advisor" are widely used, but "sponsor" is perhaps a lesser-used term. Although the labels are not as important as the roles, I connect the labels and roles below. These categories aren't water-tight containers though so the question to ask yourself is: Am I covered across the domains of sponsor, mentors and clinical advisor?

### Career sponsor

If you speak to the leaders in our field, they will all tell you of at least one person who provided them with a very powerful "big-picture" opportunity. Note that I wrote "opportunity" not just advice.

Sponsors may choose to open doors if they think you are ready (Fig. 7.4). You need to have skills to do what's on the other side of the door. This is where performance matters—just as in sport. If you do well, the sponsor may look to create further opportunities for you. Some junior clinicians think that a fellowship director will automatically play a sponsor role, but in a large facility the fellowship director will have numerous trainees per year. There are a limited number of major opportunities (roles with teams and major games) so there is competition for the plum jobs.

### Mentors

You can have wonderful mentors who provide career advice but who may not have the gravitas of a sponsor. I deliberately use the plural, "mentors", as you may have at least one mentor in your work with a sporting team, a different academic mentor if you are in research and another mentor in a multidisciplinary clinical setting. If any

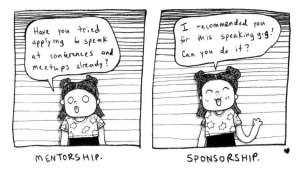

**Figure 7.4**  As a junior clinician you will often receive advice to find a mentor, but the concept of finding a sponsor is rarely discussed. There are very important differences, as illustrated here.
REPRODUCED WITH PERMISSION FROM CATT SMALL

of these mentors plays a sponsor role from time to time, that's a bonus. That potential switch in roles illustrates why roles are more important than labels.

### Clinical advisor

If you are working in a healthcare practice or a sporting team with a senior clinician, you'll notice that there are experts who are always fully booked and who give lectures or conduct courses. These people can provide great tips in the immediate office setting—when you are with a patient or when you ask them about a patient after a consultation. "My patient, a heptathlete, has had midfoot pain for a few weeks now. I'm worried about a navicular stress injury but I wasn't completely sure where to palpate as I haven't seen one before. I palpated the dorsal talus and the proximal navicular and there was no difference from the other side."

This opening can lead to you being shown precisely where the injury occurs and the expert reminding you to consider the diagnosis of relative energy deficiency in sport (REDs).

## Observe experts

One stereotype of a busy clinician has them in a white coat seeing one patient at a time. Many clinicians practice in group settings so it's possible for you to observe a colleague in action. If you have a gap in your appointment list and a colleague is seeing a patient, it may help you to ask to sit in. Patients generally appreciate that clinicians are trying to improve and will see their clinician as an expert when they have a professional colleague who wants to learn from them. (Of course, you can reverse roles with your colleagues at other times!)

If you are a junior clinician (e.g. resident/fellow), you may have a formal mentor you can observe working with a wide range of patients. Another way to hone your practice is to ask to spend time with a clinician who has a specialised focus. For example, they might treat many patients with headaches or who present with back pain. This type of learning is easy to arrange in practices in larger centres. If this isn't the case for you, try to arrange a few days with such a mentor away from your hometown. You may be pleasantly surprised how willing experienced clinicians are to make time for such teaching.

## Be purposeful about personal and professional development

Reading (or listening to) at least 2–4 relevant articles per month helps you keep growing in your clinical practice. Listening to podcasts is a very popular and very effective method of learning. Our field is particularly rich in quality podcasts and most of them are free. Share these products with your colleagues and discuss what you each learned. Try to spend at least 5–6 hours per month in such purposeful learning.

## Attend courses with a view to the future

Completing courses is part of professional development, but I want to separate the process of attending the occasional course from the ongoing commitment to professional development. In your early years as a clinician, you will get opportunities to attend courses to expand your skill base. The practice you work in may also offer courses for its clinicians. I recommend that you undertake general courses rather than those with a narrow focus.

A good example would be to undertake a shoulder course or a workshop on dealing with difficult people or how to set up an injury prevention surveillance program. Set your focus on problems and conditions that commonly present in your practice. Courses that develop your skills with such everyday problems should be your focus at this stage.

## Volunteer

Making yourself available to volunteer—strategically—at various stages of your career enables you to gain skills that make you attractive for paid employment. It is a way of avoiding the vicious cycle: you can't get hired for a job because you have no experience, and because you can't get a job you can't get experience.

In your early career, volunteering at a local sporting club or to support clinicians who provide event coverage will help your learning and build your reputation for knowing about a sport. You will learn to treat athletes and see clinical reasoning play out in real time. (Does the player need to come off? Can they return to play after this assessment?) You will hone your manual skills and your exercise prescription and progression, without the pressure that comes at higher levels. It can help build your patient list over time too. Because you are passionate about sport and your vocation, you will also gain the sense of satisfaction that comes from helping people and belonging in your community.

At later stages in your career your volunteering may take different forms. You may be part of larger, more prestigious event coverage, you may serve on important committees for your professional body, organise continuing education events or give time to worthy academic journals by way of peer-review or social media contributions. In this way you are benefitting—learning more about a sport, connecting with people who can make you a better clinician or who can potentially advance your career (sponsors).

## Learn another language

Depending on the sporting environment and the athletes in the team, it may be useful to learn another language. As anyone who has tried to learn a language as an adult knows, there is no substitute for immersion. Can you work in another country? If you are a clinician who speaks more than one language, think about whether you can bring this asset to your clinical work.

## CHOOSE AN EMPOWERED WORKPLACE

As an excellent clinician you will have choices as to where to work. Remember that the best salary doesn't always come with factors that can greatly influence your quality of life, such as location, colleagues, support staff, the non-financial benefits of work (e.g. formal and informal continuing education) and freedom to arrange your own schedule. As a clinic leader, I aimed to create an "empowered work environment"—a place where all staff (not just the clinicians) had all they needed to grow and develop.

Empowered workplaces:

- give you access to key personnel who can mentor you and assist you to become more efficient in how you work
- offer world-class colleagues from whom you can obtain informal second opinions, learn from over coffee or refer challenging patients to
- have challenging and interesting patients and a good selection of athletes who visit the practice
- offer opportunities for learning and growth
- provide the flexibility in your work to allow you to also work with sporting teams
- have up-to-date equipment for testing and treatment
- give you a level of independence to explore how you can improve and grow.

## Intrinsic factors you need to develop and exhibit

There are two sides to the excellence coin: you also need to bring your best self to the clinic every day. In the health professions we are used to the concept of specialisation; it may be formal specialisation such as a sports designation or others such as cardiac or neuro. If you think of the prominent leaders in the field, their specialisation may be in areas that are not formally accredited by the profession: for example, sports injury prevention, tendinopathy, shoulder injuries, dance/rugby injuries, Parasport. In business, specialisation is also referred to as differentiation (a marketing term) or value proposition. In short, it's why a patient may choose you rather than a colleague who is undifferentiated, as it were.

As you develop your career, what are you going to do to differentiate yourself? Leading clinicians follow a common pattern: they undertake strategic volunteering, have mentors, do additional formal/informal study to gain greater insight, undertake research in the area, and proactively pursue focused education while all the time being clinically active—seeing patients in their area of specialisation so that they keep getting better. The virtuous circle is obvious: by being better you get referred the more challenging cases and you learn more. You might attend focused conferences or be invited to contribute, and this makes you better again. You have a high-quality network of colleagues you can consult with immediately. This is great for your patients—if anyone can help them, you can.

Box 7.1 details tips based on one very successful team physician's career (so far).

---

**BOX 7.1** One "pathway" as a team sports physician

Dr Laura Lallenec (Fig. 7.5), a sport and exercise physician (Fellow of the Australasian College of Sport and Exercise Medicine), shares her journey and pathway to being engaged with team sport for international and Australian professional sport.

Dr Lallenec's tips include:

- When working as a junior doctor in the hospital system, choose specific rotations to assist you to develop knowledge and skills that will help you when you enter the sports and exercise medicine training program. In Dr Lallenec's case, that meant rotations in orthopaedics, emergency medicine, plastics, rehabilitation, ENT and maxillofacial.
- Find mentors and develop supportive peer networks.
- Broaden your clinical experience by seeing a variety of sports medicine presentations including both in elite and recreational athletes.

Dr Lallenec progressed her career by:

- taking opportunities to travel with teams, both domestically and internationally
- covering local sport events and building her experience base to enable her to work at larger events
- accepting opportunities when the chance presented itself to develop her communication, presentation and media skills, as well as taking opportunities to learn about governance in sport
- talking to colleagues ahead of her on the training pathway to learn from their path and developing her own personal sports medicine pathway.
- covering local events and building up to bigger events where there was more risk when more experienced people were there to assist and teach her
- accepting media opportunities when the chance arrived, and learning about governance in sport and developing supportive networks.

A

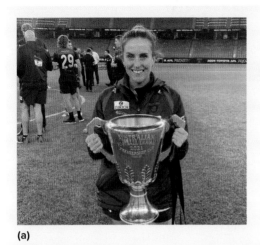

(a)

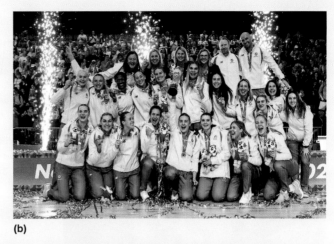

(b)

**Figure 7.5** (a) Dr Lallenec holding the 2021 Australian Football League premiership cup. Melbourne Football Club supporters hope they don't have to wait 57 years to win the cup again. (b) Dr Lallenec with the Australian Diamonds world champion netball team
IMAGES COURTESY OF LAURA LALLENEC

## COMMON CONCERNS

In any career there will be specific problems and challenges to navigate.

### Income

Aiming to be a sport and exercise clinician doesn't come with salary guarantees. Although some clinicians work in one practice and receive a proportion of the fees they bill (fee-for-service model), many have a variety of income streams. They might work in several practices, and/or be paid to work at a school, academy or club. They may have other roles in private or public medicine or work part-time in an academic setting.

As with any financial transaction, absence of information is a major disadvantage so get advice when you are considering signing on for work. The employer does reference checks on you—have you researched the history of your potential employer? Are staff satisfied? Is there rapid turnover? Have you spoken to staff who have left? The setting may be a wonderful launching pad for better options or it might be a terrible place to work. Ask trusted colleagues about specific salary details. The first offer you get isn't necessarily the one you should accept.

Factors other than remuneration can be crucial, particularly in the first phase of your career. Are there opportunities to learn from colleagues in the clinical setting? Is there a professional development program? Will

you get opportunities to attend professional development events? Is there ongoing research in the environment?

### Taking opportunities

If you want to grow, you need to show initiative. You need to put time into the task of becoming a better clinician. Attend events, conferences and forums where you find the tribe you want to be with. Look at events at the periphery of your interests to be sure that interest is peripheral and you aren't missing something great. For example, if vestibular rehabilitation is of interest because you see post-concussion patients, but you don't think you want to be a full-time vestibular clinician, attend a relevant event to see whether there is more to the field than you appreciate.

### Roadblocks

Glass ceilings, sexism, racism, ageism (towards youth as well as older people) and ableism are all too real, sadly. Be diplomatic where appropriate and try to discover what avenues are open to you to achieve the change you see is needed. Sometimes crashing boldly through the roadblock may be needed—but crashes do come with scrapes, at a minimum.

In this chapter I have deliberately focused on a setting where many clinicians work: the outpatient office. But our field comes with a wide range of job options including in the military, specialised sports institutions and public health systems (Box 7.2).

## BOX 7.2  Are you exploring the full range of career options?

There are many options to consider when seeking career opportunities in health and sport/physical activity/rehabilitation.

### The military

The modern military needs highly skilled professionals to assist with matters of health, wellness, physical fitness and injury prevention (Fig. 7.6). Joining the military will often assist you to gain qualifications and further education. Chapter 36 of *Clinical Sports Medicine 6e: Managing Injuries* focuses on injuries among military personnel.

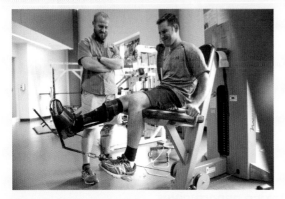

**Figure 7.6**  The large military hospital complex at Fort Sam Houston, near San Antonio, Texas, contributes to the service of more than 36,000 active duty servicemen and women
COURTESY OF TECH. SGT. VERNON YOUNG, JR

### Sports academies/sports institutes/college sport

Many countries have formal sports academies or institutes that employ sport and exercise clinicians (Fig. 7.7). In many cases the term "academy" is used when the athletes are junior or youth. Institutes have no age connotations and are often national or regional.

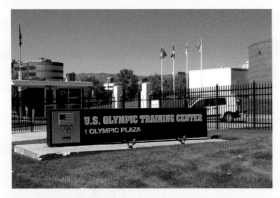

**Figure 7.7**  The US Olympic Training Center in Colorado Springs, Colorado
COURTESY OF DR DANIEL FRIEDMAN

In the US, college sport is the dominant sport setting between high-school level sport and professional sport.

Academy work can provide experience in business and management skills, in addition to the clinical training that comes with the role. This experience can be invaluable in the private sector or in a sporting organisation. Most clinical disciplines (e.g. physiotherapy, medicine, soft-tissue therapy, psychology, nutrition) are represented in sports academies and they often provide the clinical staff for national and other sports teams. Sports academies also help develop policies and position papers and staff often provide advice to government and sporting bodies.

### Public health systems

In health systems such as the National Health Service (NHS) in the UK there are many healthcare practitioner opportunities. Positions for specialist physiotherapists, emergency medicine practitioners, psychologists and others are available. There is also the opportunity to work with larger organised sporting events that involve both athlete and spectator/general public care when working in the public healthcare system (Fig. 7.8).

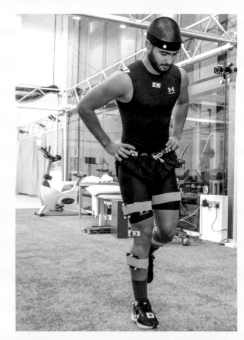

**Figure 7.8**  The Aspetar Orthopaedic and Sports Medicine Hospital in Doha, Qatar, is an example of a large employer of sports health professionals and administrators. It provides a public health service but its scope is restricted to the gamut of sports medicine (using that term very widely and inclusively).
COURTESY OF THE ASPETAR ORTHOPAEDIC AND SPORTS MEDICINE HOSPITAL, DOHA, QATAR. COURTESY OF ANIS MAHER KASSIM. @ANIS.MAHER.KASSEM15

## KEY POINTS

- The successful sport and exercise clinician should possess a varied set of skills related to their clinical practice and interpersonal interactions. Personal qualities like humility, eagerness, thoughtfulness and attentiveness are worth cultivating.

- Clear, honest communication in the clinical setting can help to build trust. Avoid over-promising and setting unrealistic expectations.

- Active listening is a cornerstone of delivering good quality healthcare. It is also a key component of resolving conflict.

- Mentorship is an important part of career development. You may also benefit from having a career sponsor and clinical advisor.

- Depending on the context in which you work, it may be worthwhile developing a number of other skills, including learning additional languages, acquiring media training, and learning to resolve conflict.

- Working as part of a multidisciplinary team requires humility, attentiveness and good communication skills. Practise within your abilities and approach clinicians from other domains with curiosity.

- Workplace satisfaction and success involve a combination of extrinsic factors (like having an empowered workplace) and intrinsic factors (including enthusiasm, trustworthiness and time management).

- Developing your career is an active process. Seek and seize opportunities, ask to learn from others, network widely and put yourself in a place to acquire new experiences and knowledge.

## REFERENCES

References for this chapter can be found at www.mhprofessional.com/CSM6e

## ADDITIONAL CONTENT

 Scan here to access additional resources for this topic and more provided by the authors

PART B

# Clinical sciences

## CHAPTER 8

# Acute injuries

with **PAUL BLAZEY and NICOL VAN DYK**

*It's almost like … mourning, you actually mourn the loss of like the gymnast you were or the athlete you were. And it sort of feels like you're never gonna get back to that level … [it's] devastating. It's very frustrating. Like, mentally, you're ready to go, but you know, your body doesn't allow it anymore.*

RENÉ COURNOYER, OLYMPIC ALL-AROUND GYMNAST (AND PHYSIOTHERAPIST) AFTER A SEVERE ACUTE KNEE INJURY, INTERVIEWED BY FELLOW ATHLETE BRIAN WALLACK

## CHAPTER OUTLINE

| | |
|---|---|
| Mechanisms of acute injury | Muscle |
| Pathophysiology and initial management | Tendon |
| Bone | Fascia |
| Joint | Bursa |
| Hyaline cartilage | Nerve |
| Fibrocartilage | Fat pad |
| Ligament | Skin |

## LEARNING OBJECTIVES

By the end of this chapter you should be able to:

- identify the various ways in which sport-related injuries can be classified
- discuss the factors that influence an athlete's risk of injury
- describe what is happing at the cellular level after soft-tissue injury and how that informs acute management principles of soft-tissue injuries
- summarise the features of injuries specific to individual tissue types (e.g. muscle, tendon, ligament, bone, skin)
- discuss treatment and return-to-sport strategies for injuries across tissue types
- recognise the signs or symptoms of an injury that indicate the need for urgent medical attention.

This chapter aims to build on your prior knowledge of anatomy and physiology by detailing the fundamental pathologies in our field: muscle strains, ligament sprains, fractures and other everyday sports injuries. Classifying items helps make them easier to understand and discuss. We could classify injuries by body part or by sport, but the most fundamental division is into "acute" and "overuse" injuries (Table 8.1), based on the mechanism of injury and the speed of symptom onset.

An acute injury occurs during a single, identifiable traumatic event—when the force applied to a tissue generates stresses and/or strains that are greater than the tissue can withstand. This results in a sprain, strain, fracture and/or dislocation of a specific body tissue.

Tissue failure generates macroscopic damage and the rapid onset of pain, dysfunction and impairment of the affected area. Neglecting or improperly treating acute injuries can lead to long-term health consequences. A comprehensive approach to managing these injuries is essential to minimise the risk of recurrent or chronic problems (described with overuse injuries in Chapter 9).

## MECHANISMS OF ACUTE INJURY

Acute sports injuries occur for a variety of reasons, including direct impact (e.g. blunt trauma from a tackle); indirect impact (e.g. twisting and landing on a surface); overuse (Chapter 9); muscle imbalance or poor technique; falls or slips; and shear forces (e.g. skin abrasions from rubbing along rough surfaces). All of these mechanisms can be distilled into whether the forces exerted on the tissues are related to an extrinsic or intrinsic load.

**TABLE 8.1**   Classification of sporting injuries into "acute" and "overuse"

| Site | Acute injuries | Overuse injuries |
| --- | --- | --- |
| Bone | Fracture (including growth plate)<br>Periosteal contusion | Stress injury (including stress reaction and stress fracture)<br>Osteitis, periostitis<br>Apophysitis, enthesopathy<br>Osteophyte/bone spur |
| Joint | Dislocation<br>Subluxation | Synovitis<br>Osteoarthritis/osteoarthrosis<br>Instability |
| Hyaline cartilage | Chondral/osteochondral injury | Chondropathy (e.g. softening, fibrillation, fissuring, chondromalacia) |
| Fibrocartilage | Acute tear (including meniscal, labral and intra-articular and inter-vertebral discs)<br>Intervertebral disc herniation | Degenerative tear (including meniscal, labral and intra-articular and intervertebral discs)<br>Intervertebral disc herniation |
| Ligament | Sprain/tear (grades I–III) | Chronic ligament rupture (e.g. ankle instability) |
| Muscle | Strain/tear<br>Exercise-induced muscle soreness<br>Contusion<br>Acute compartment syndrome<br>Cramp<br>Myositis ossificans | Chronic compartment syndrome<br>Focal tissue thickening/fibrosis |
| Tendon | Tear (partial or complete) | Tendinopathy (as an umbrella term that includes paratenonitis, tenosynovitis, tendinosis and tendinitis) |
| Fascia | Tear (partial or complete) | Fasciitis (e.g. plantar fasciitis); some clinicians prefer the term "fasciopathy" |
| Bursa | Traumatic or "acute" bursitis | Bursitis/bursosis |
| Nerve | Neuropraxia | Entrapment<br>Minor nerve injury/irritation<br>Adverse neural dynamics |
| Fat pad | Bruise/contusion | Impingement/irritation |
| Skin | Laceration<br>Abrasion<br>Puncture wound | Blister<br>Callus |

**B**

**TABLE 8.2**   Examples of non-modifiable and modifiable injury risk factors

| Non-modifiable risk factors | Modifiable risk factors |
|---|---|
| Age | Body composition |
| Sex | Physical fitness to compete (strength, flexibility, etc.) |
| Individual injury history | Skill level (technical experience) |
| Anatomy (i.e. genetics, which may be assessed by family history) | Training load |
| | Playing environment (e.g. surface) |
| | Equipment (e.g. helmet, shoes) |
| | Biomechanics (e.g. riding position in cycling, foot strike pattern in running) |
| | Rules of the sport |

Extrinsic loads come from outside the body, such as from a direct blow or collision with an external object. Intrinsic loads come from inside the body, such as from muscle contractile forces, and arise in relation to specific joint and tissue biomechanics. You should consider whether acute injuries have either a primarily extrinsic or intrinsic cause. This allows you to design ways that may prevent or mitigate the risk of acute injuries (or re-injury).

Table 9.1 (in Chapter 9) outlines many of the differences between extrinsic and intrinsic factors that may alter forces acting upon the body. To summarise, extrinsically generated forces can be modified by altering equipment (e.g. new helmet designs in American football), the playing surface or the rules of the sport (e.g. new tackle height rules in rugby union). Intrinsically generated forces require changes in an athlete's characteristics and capabilities (e.g. muscle strength, endurance and flexibility, motor control, joint range, biomechanics, proprioception). All acute injuries result in intrinsic changes and therefore, regardless of the cause (intrinsic or extrinsic structure overload), an individual athlete's characteristics and capabilities need to be considered and where possible improved to facilitate their return to participation and prevent re-injury.

## Modifiable versus non-modifiable factors

When a force is applied to a tissue, the nature of the force being applied (such as the direction, magnitude and rate of loading) and the mechanical properties of the tissue in the direction of loading determine whether the tissue fails.

The mechanical properties of an athlete's soft tissues are determined by a combination of innate (non-modifiable) factors, whereas the magnitude of load applied is the result of environmental (modifiable) factors. Modifiable factors can dictate whether a load is safe or injurious by either increasing or decreasing genetically endowed tissue strength. Modifiable injury risk factors can lead to acute or chronic injury.

Although there is some overlap between intrinsic and extrinsic loading, they are distinct. Table 8.2 lists some potential non-modifiable and modifiable injury risk factors. Chapter 17 focuses on what can be done to address modifiable injury risk factors.

An example of the relationship between intrinsic/extrinsic loads and modifiable/non-modifiable factors is shown in Table 8.3. The balance between loads and risk factors is further discussed in Chapter 9.

Regardless of how or why an injury is sustained, there is some consistency in how the body reacts to an acute injury.

## PATHOPHYSIOLOGY AND INITIAL MANAGEMENT

Acute injury initiates a common sequence of preliminary processes, irrespective of the specific tissue injured. Haematoma formation from damaged blood vessels gives way to an acute inflammatory response involving fluid exudation and phagocytosis. Fluid exudation contributes to oedema formation (i.e. swelling) and the delivery of white blood cells to the injured site, while phagocytosis aids in the removal of damaged tissue and cellular debris.

**TABLE 8.3**   Example demonstrating the relationship between intrinsic and extrinsic load considerations for an American football quarterback and their relationship to modifiable or non-modifiable risk factors

| | Intrinsic | Extrinsic |
|---|---|---|
| **Modifiable** | Reactive muscle strength/power, flexibility, proprioception and other factors all affect the ability to absorb a tackle during game play | Changes to the design of helmets to mitigate the forces acting on the body during a tackle |
| **Non-modifiable** | The player's genetic tissue capacity or their previous injury history, which may have reduced their ability to withstand a heavy tackle to a specific area of the body | Players colliding in a dynamic team sport such as American football |

Swelling occurring within a joint is referred to as an effusion and usually takes place slowly over the course of 12-24 hours. More rapidly occurring joint swelling (e.g. within the first 2-3 hours after injury) indicates that the effusion contains blood (i.e. haemarthrosis) and that an intra-articular structure has been damaged (as often occurs post ACL injury).

The acute inflammatory response to injury stimulates nociceptors to activate pain pathways. Pain is the body's way of protecting the injured site from further damage and leads to muscle inhibition and functional limitation. Muscle inhibition is also affected by swelling. Reactive muscle spasm serves as an additional protective mechanism to reduce the potential of further injury, but also contributes to pain.

The acute inflammatory phase protects the damaged tissue from further injury, prepares the injured site for repair and stimulates the recruitment and activation of reparative cells. The inflammatory phase is generally thought to persist for 48-72 hours; however, the duration within a particular individual can vary, and can be influenced by the tissue damaged, the severity of the damage, and early management. Signs of persistent acute inflammation include ongoing pain at rest and/or night, prolonged (>30 minutes) morning pain and stiffness, and ongoing swelling that changes in volume according to recent activity.

Early management of acute injuries traditionally focused on Protection, Rest, Ice, Compression and Elevation (PRICE).[1] However, due to the benefits of maintaining physical activity a new acronym was coined in the early 2010s to encourage Protection, Optimal Loading, Ice, Compression, Elevation (POLICE) of the body part or area injured.[2]

More recently, the use of cryotherapy and routine use of anti-inflammatory medications have been questioned. This has resulted in suggestions for a new protocol that focuses on Protection, Elevation, Avoid anti-inflammatory medication, Compression, Education, and Load, Optimism, Vascularisation, Exercise (PEACE & LOVE).[3] For the detailed management of acute injuries, see Chapter 24.

Both POLICE and PEACE & LOVE identify tissue load as an important aim of acute injury management, as this can help take advantage of the responsiveness of musculoskeletal tissues to mechanical stimuli. Progressive functional loading stimulates connective tissue synthesis and counteracts the loss of muscle mass due to immobilisation. Reducing muscle loss can enable faster return to participation (and ultimately performance). "Optimal" loading promotes healing, but without causing further damage.

## BONE

Acute bone injuries include fractures and contusions. Bone stress injuries are addressed in Chapter 9.

## Fracture

There is a large safety factor between the forces bone is exposed to during athletic activities and the forces required to generate a fracture. In the absence of bone pathology causing generalised or localised fragility, large forces are required to fracture a bone. Such forces can result from direct trauma, such as a blow, or indirect trauma, such as an awkward fall or twisting motion.

### Classification

Traumatic fractures can be classified as either closed (simple) or open (compound). The skin is intact over the fracture site in closed fractures, whereas in open fractures skin integrity is lost, often due to penetration from within by the fractured bone. The presence of a skin wound in open fractures that is continuous with the fracture site enables pathogens to enter and contribute to bone infection. Thus individuals with an open fracture should be treated with prophylactic antibiotic therapy.

Within the dichotomy of open and closed fractures, fractures can be further classified according to their fracture pattern (Fig. 8.1), the location in terms of both the affected bone and the location within that bone, the amount and type of displacement of the fractured ends of the bone, and/ or the specific name of the fracture. For instance, a Colles' fracture refers to a fracture of the distal radius with dorsal (posterior) and radial displacement of the distal fracture segment, whereas a Smith's fracture refers to a fracture of the distal radius, but with ventral (anterior) displacement of the distal segment.

> **PRACTICE PEARL**
>
> The immature skeleton presents some unique fractures because of its lower mineralisation and the presence of unfused secondary ossification centres with interposed growth plates.

The lower mineralisation of the immature skeleton makes it more flexible than the adult skeleton and, consequently, susceptible to buckling.

When sufficient bending force is applied to an immature bone the cortex on the concave side buckles, while the cortex on the opposite side cracks open due to tensile forces. The resultant greenstick fracture is named according to how a green (i.e. fresh) stick buckles and cracks when bent. When the injurious force causes axial compressive loading of an immature bone as opposed to bending, the result can be a torus or buckle fracture characterised by buckling and bulging of the cortex on all sides.

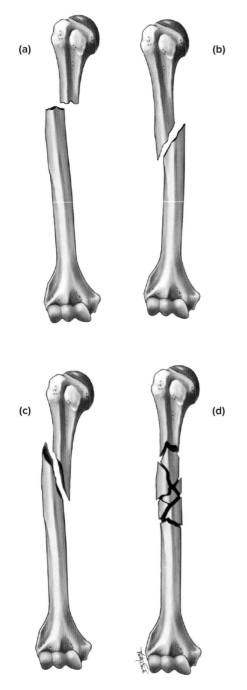

in the young skeleton. They serve to develop bony prominences, such as tubercles and epicondyles, upon which tendons and ligaments attach. With an appropriate tensile pull from a tendon or ligament, a secondary ossification centre can be pulled away from the rest of the bone at its growth plate, resulting in the development of an avulsion fracture. Avulsion fractures can also occur in the adult skeleton when extreme tensile forces at the insertion site of a tendon or ligament pull off a portion of bone.

## Management

The primary aim of fracture management is to enable the fracture to heal in the most anatomical position possible so that the mechanical function of the bone can be restored. If the fracture is displaced, it should be reduced to realign the bone fragments back to their anatomical position. A fracture that heals in an abnormal position (i.e. malunited fracture) can lead to the long-term development of secondary complications, such as osteoarthritis. Fracture reduction is typically extremely painful and resisted by muscle spasm. Thus, it is usually performed under a short-acting anaesthetic, sedative or nerve block, and with muscle relaxants. Once the fragments are reduced, the fracture needs to be held in place to permit fracture gap bridging.

The appropriate method of stabilisation depends on the nature of the fracture. Stable fractures may be managed with a simple sling, cast or fracture brace, whereas more rigid stabilisation is required for unstable fractures. Rigid stabilisation may consist of open reduction and internal fixation, in which the fracture site is opened surgically, reduced and fixed using metal plates, rods, screws, pins and/or wires. Open reduction and internal fixation has the advantage of allowing earlier introduction of forces across the fracture site. However, the trade-offs include:

- potential hardware loosening, failure and irritation
- opening the fracture site to the possibility of infection
- too rigid stabilisation of the fracture, leading to insufficient fragment micromotion and atrophic non-union
- peri-implant fracture resulting from regional osteoporosis due to stress shielding.

**Figure 8.1** Types of fracture: (a) transverse, (b) oblique, (c) spiral, (d) comminuted

It is necessary to assess and monitor all fractures whether managed surgically or not for other possible complications. Infection and malunion post-surgery have already been mentioned. Potential acute complications from any fracture include acute compartment syndrome (discussed later in the chapter), associated injuries (e.g. nerve, vessel), deep venous thrombosis/pulmonary embolism, and delayed or non-union.

Growth plate fractures in children and adolescents present a particular problem. The most common growth plate fracture is an avulsion fracture. Unfused secondary ossification centres represent an area of relative weakness

Soft-tissue injury, such as ligament or muscle damage, is often associated with a fracture, and may cause more long-term problems than the fracture itself. Thus, it is important to address any concomitant soft-tissue injury.

### Delayed or non-unions

Delayed or non-united fractures lead to persistent pain and disability, and can be caused by several factors, including:

- excessive or insufficient fracture site stabilisation
- the presence of a complicated fracture type (e.g. open or highly comminuted fracture)
- insufficient or disrupted blood supply (e.g. due to normal regional anatomy or the presence of comorbid conditions such as diabetes)
- lifestyle factors (e.g. smoking, excessive alcohol intake and poor nutrition).

Management options for delayed or non-united fractures include non-surgical treatments, such as low-intensity pulsed ultrasound and electromagnetic therapies, as well as surgical treatments, such as bone graft or bone graft substitute, internal fixation and/or external fixation. Researchers are striving to provide effective biological compounds and small molecule pharmaceuticals that promote fracture healing. Specific fractures that are common in athletes are discussed in various chapters in *Clinical Sports Medicine 6e: Managing Injuries.*

## Periosteal contusion

The periosteum is a dense, fibrous tissue that is firmly attached to the outer surface of bones and is richly vascularised and highly innervated. At subcutaneous skeletal sites (such as the medial surface of the tibia and iliac crest), the periosteum is susceptible to acute trauma from a direct blow with an external object, such as a ball, stick, opponent or playing surface.

The blow damages periosteal blood vessels and causes sub-periosteal haematoma, also known as a periosteal contusion. The confined space beneath the periosteum limits the spread of the haematoma, occasionally leading to the development of a palpable lump. As the raised periosteum is inflamed and under tension, the region is often particularly tender to palpation and painful on contraction of the muscles that attach to the injured region.

A periosteal contusion at the iliac crest, often referred to as a "hip pointer" injury, can be extremely painful because of involvement of the cluneal nerve which runs along the iliac crest. Management of periosteal contusions focuses on minimising the extent of the haematoma using conventional first aid approaches (as discussed under "pathophysiology

and initial management" above) followed by a gradual return to activity. Protective equipment (such as shin guards and padding) should be considered for future prevention.

## JOINT

Acute trauma in the sporting context can occur due to high velocity contact with an external object (e.g. a collision between players) or low-velocity contact between a player and an external object such as the playing surface. This can result in injuries such as joint dislocation and subluxation.

### Dislocation and subluxation

Joint stability depends on the interaction between the passive, active and neural subsystems. Muscles and tendons combine to form the active subsystem, which is controlled by the neural subsystem, to provide dynamic joint stability. When the force applied to a joint exceeds the capabilities of the active subsystem or when the active and/or neural subsystems are compromised, loads are transferred to the passive subsystem. The passive subsystem consists of non-contractile connective tissues, which includes the bony anatomy, joint capsule, ligaments and fibrocartilage joint structures (e.g. labrum, volar plates, menisci).

Excessive load placed on the passive subsystem can cause the bones forming a joint to abnormally translate or luxate relative to one another. When the bones are forced to completely separate so that the articulating surfaces are no longer in contact, it is referred to as dislocation (Fig. 8.2a). Subluxation (partial dislocation) refers to when the bones shift relative to one another, but the articulating surfaces remain partially in contact (Fig. 8.2b).

Luxation of a joint invariably results in damage to passive subsystem structures such as fibrocartilage and ligaments,

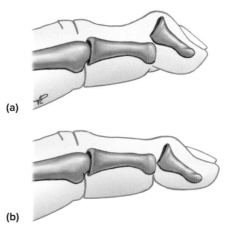

(a)

(b)

**Figure 8.2** Acute finger joint injury: (a) dislocation, (b) subluxation

with synovial joint surfaces (bone and hyaline cartilage) also at risk. The structures damaged and the extent of the damage depend on the direction and magnitude of the luxation force and the inherent stability of the joint created by the passive subsystem.

The hip joint is inherently stable because the large ball-shaped femoral head is well encased in a reciprocating socket-shaped acetabulum, and the bones are supported by a strong joint capsule that is reinforced by robust ligaments. Thus, considerably more force is required to luxate the hip joint compared with a less stable joint, such as the shoulder. The shoulder lacks inherent stability because the large humeral head outsizes the small, shallow glenoid fossa, and the joint possesses a thin, loose capsule that is minimally supported by ligaments. The heightened force required to luxate inherently stable joints (such as the hip, elbow, ankle and subtalar joints) means that subluxation or dislocation of these joints is more likely to be associated with damage beyond that to the joint capsule and ligaments, including fractures and damage to cartilage, vessels and nerves.

A dislocated joint is readily identifiable by gross deformity with complete loss of joint function. The individual presents in intense pain and often has the afflicted limb cradled or held to keep it immobile. Following a neurovascular screen to assess for nerve and blood vessel damage, the dislocated joint should be reduced as quickly as possible. In most cases, this can be performed by applying gradual and controlled distraction of the joint while simultaneously moving the joint through a passive range of motion. When distraction is unable to overcome the opposing muscle spasm and the joint does not readily reduce, use of an injected muscle relaxant or general anaesthetic may be required.

After reduction, ensure that dislocated joints are radiographed in case there is an accompanying fracture. The joint should be protected to allow the joint capsule and ligaments to heal. Early protected mobilisation is encouraged to promote functional healing, and training of the active and neural subsystems should commence as early as possible and progress to functional activities.

In some joints (e.g. the shoulder) and in some patients, active and neural subsystem training may be insufficient to prevent re-dislocation or chronic subluxation. In those cases, the patient benefits from surgical reconstruction of the damaged capsule and ligaments.

# HYALINE CARTILAGE
## Chondral and osteochondral injuries

Hyaline or articular cartilage lines the articular surface of bone regions forming synovial joints. It provides a smooth, lubricated surface allowing for low-friction gliding and possesses unique viscoelastic properties that facilitate the absorption and distribution of loads to the underlying subchondral bone. In fulfilling these roles, hyaline cartilage is principally exposed to compressive loads.

### Classification

Acute joint subluxation or dislocation (discussed above) and acute ligament sprain or rupture (discussed later) can lead to locally high compressive forces and the superimposition of shearing forces due to excessive joint translation. The net result can be development of an acute chondral (cartilage) (Figs 8.3a and b) or osteochondral injury (Fig. 8.3c), with the latter involving both the articular cartilage and underlying (subchondral) bone.

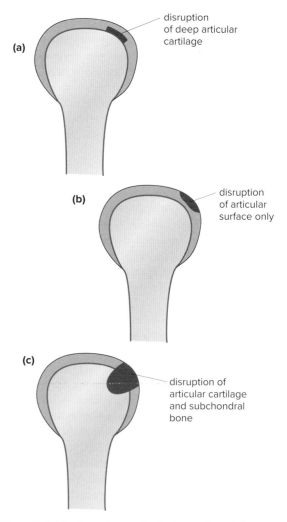

**Figure 8.3** The three types of articular cartilage injury

Articular cartilage is radiolucent and therefore most chondral injuries are not visible on conventional radiology. As a result, these injuries have historically been underdiagnosed. With the advent of magnetic resonance imaging (MRI) and direct visualisation via arthroscopy, it has become clear that chondral injuries are far more common than previously realised.

Common sites for chondral and osteochondral injuries are the femoral condyles, the superior articular surface of the talus and the capitellum of the humerus. The patella chondral surface is another common site for chondral injuries. It can be damaged acutely in a patellar dislocation but is also vulnerable to repetitive trauma resulting in patellofemoral pain.

## PRACTICE PEARL

Maintain a high index of suspicion for chondral involvement if an apparently "simple joint sprain" remains painful and swollen for longer than expected, despite the presence of normal radiography.

Chondral injuries can contribute to the development of premature osteoarthritis. Articular cartilage has limited regenerative and repair capacity due to its avascular nature. As larger lesions or defects have lower probability of healing, classification systems have been developed to quantify the severity of chondral damage and guide prognosis.

Chondral lesion severity is determined by the depth the injury extends towards the underlying bone and the areal size of cartilage affected, whereas osteochondral lesion severity is determined by the continuity of the overlying cartilage and stability of the lesion. Scales generally extend from 0 (normal) to 4 (exposed bone for chondral injuries; fragment displacement for osteochondral lesions), with higher scores indicating greater damage and a worse prognosis.

### Management

Chondral and osteochondral injuries in young active individuals represent a therapeutic challenge. The goal of treatment is to restore the structural integrity and function of the affected surface so that it can withstand the significant stresses associated with athletic endeavours. The hope is to permit a return to participation while minimising cartilage degeneration and the need for early arthroplasty (joint replacement).

Treatment options for chondral injuries range from longstanding techniques such as chondroplasty to smooth loose edges of damaged cartilage, and arthroscopic washout to remove debris to contemporary techniques aimed at stimulating cartilage repair or restoration. Reparative techniques include bone marrow stimulation techniques such as abrasion arthroplasty, drilling and microfracture, whereas restorative approaches include autologous osteochondral mosaicplasty, osteochondral allograft transplantation, and chondrocyte and mesenchymal stem cell-based therapies wherein cells are implanted into the cartilage lesion under a periosteal or collagen-membrane cover.

Treatment choice depends on the size of the chondral or osteochondral lesion, with great debate continuing as to the most effective approach. Ultimately, return to sport depends on a range of factors, including the athlete's age, the duration of symptoms, the level of play, repair tissue morphology, lesion size, type and location, and the number of surgeries and concomitant procedures.[4]

## FIBROCARTILAGE

### Acute tear

Fibrocartilage consists of a mixture of fibrous and cartilaginous tissue in varying proportions, which provide it with both toughness and elasticity. Fibrocartilage forms a range of structures in different joints with varying functions, but roles generally include enhancing joint stability, contributing to shock absorption and distribution, and promoting joint lubrication. Fibrocartilage structures include the knee menisci, the glenoid and acetabular labra, the triangular fibrocartilage complex at the radiocarpal joint, volar plates of the digits, and articular discs within the acromioclavicular and sternoclavicular joints.

Given the predominantly mechanical roles of fibrocartilage structures in enhancing joint congruency and distributing stresses, it is not surprising that they are at risk of acute injury when excessive forces are introduced. The knee menisci are at risk when the athlete rotates on a flexed and loaded knee, whereas a fall onto an outstretched hand can acutely injure the triangular fibrocartilage complex at the radiocarpal joint.

Joint fibrocartilage structures can be injured in isolation; however, simultaneous injury with associated joint structures (e.g. ligaments and joint capsule) is common due to their close anatomical and mechanical relationships. For example, it is common for a knee meniscus and the ACL to be simultaneously injured as they share a common mechanism of injury (i.e. rotating on a flexed and loaded knee). Similarly, shoulder dislocation often damages the anterior glenoid labrum as well as the glenohumeral ligaments and joint capsule due to their anatomical connections.

B

Signs and symptoms of acute fibrocartilage injury are region- and injury- specific, but generally include pain and swelling in the affected joint combined with joint clicking, catching or locking. These latter symptoms are often delayed in their presentation, occurring once the initial acute symptoms have subsided and the athlete is again using the joint "normally". Joint clicking, catching or locking can contribute to reflex muscle inhibition and the sensation of the joint "giving way" during load bearing.

Management of acute fibrocartilage injuries depends on the type, size and location of damage (e.g. meniscal or labral tear). Management options are both exercise-based (conservative) and surgical; surgical options including repair, removal and replacement of the damaged fibrocartilaginous structure. Surgery has traditionally been reserved for individuals who have failed to respond to conservative management. In certain settings, randomised clinical trials support surgery as first-line management for fibrocartilage injuries (Chapter 26).

## Intervertebral disc herniation

Herniation of the nucleus pulposus in athletes most commonly occurs secondary to damage accumulation within the disc in response to repetitive flexion and/or rotational loading. Thus, the vast majority of disc herniations are overuse injuries, despite the onset of symptoms often occurring relatively spontaneously and in response to an apparently trivial loading event.

However, it is possible to acutely prolapse or herniate an otherwise healthy intervertebral disc with sufficiently high compressive force. This can occur during contact sports when the spine is axially loaded while in a flexed position, such as when driven into the ground when being tackled. The disc may protrude or herniate radially beyond the usual margins of the annulus fibrosus or herniate through the vertebral body endplate into the vertebral body to form a Schmorl's node.

Intervertebral disc herniation varies in scale and may progress as shown in Figure 8.4. It can be asymptomatic, with a large body of MRI evidence demonstrating its presence in asymptomatic individuals. In those who do experience severe and immediate pain, management will depend on the presence of red flag symptoms (e.g. bladder or bowel dysfunction, saddle anaesthesia) or severe radicular pain. Chapter 15 in *Managing Injuries* provides more detail to help guide the nuanced decision making that occurs following intervertebral disc injuries.

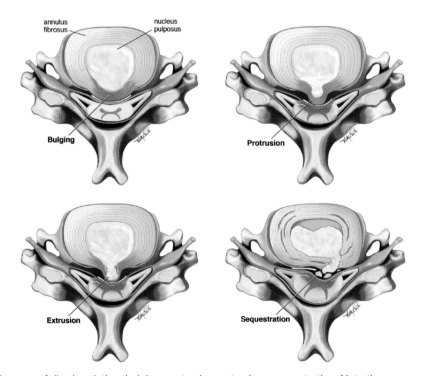

**Figure 8.4** Four degrees of disc herniation: bulging, protrusion, extrusion, sequestration. Note the progressively greater damage (red) of the annulus fibrosus from bulging through to sequestration. Extrusion and sequestration may cause pressure on the exiting nerve root (purple) and sequestration has indented the spinal cord in this image. Remember that symptoms do not always mirror the physical appearance.

## LIGAMENT

### Sprain/tear

Ligaments typically span joints to connect articulating bones, and present as either discrete extra-articular structures or thickenings of the joint capsule. Their structure—tightly packed bundles of collagen arranged almost in parallel along the longitudinal axis of the ligament—is designed to resist tensile loads.

Ligaments function to provide passive stability and guide what directions of motion are available at a joint. When force is applied to a joint that attempts to move the bones in a direction they are not designed to move, passive tension rises in ligaments on the side of the joint being opened. When the load is sufficient, and dynamic joint stabilisation afforded by the active and neural subsystems is insufficient, collagen fibres within the ligaments begin to yield, resulting in an acute ligament injury (commonly referred to as a sprain).

Ligament sprains range in severity from mild injuries involving tearing of only a few fibres to complete tears of the ligament where ligament continuity and its stabilising role are completely lost. Based on the number of fibres torn and the subsequent degree of joint instability, ligament sprains are classified into three grades, each representing an increase in injury severity (Table 8.4).

Management of acute ligament sprains is summarised in Figure 8.5. Initial management consists of first aid techniques to minimise bleeding and swelling (Chapter 17). For grade I and II sprains, subsequent treatment aims to promote tissue healing, prevent joint stiffness, protect against further damage and strengthen muscle to provide dynamic joint stability.

Return to sport usually takes place prior to tissue-level healing being complete, with healing of collagen in a partial ligament tear taking several months.[5,6] Earlier return to sport is facilitated by the use of bracing or taping to help protect against re-injury.

Rehabilitation (especially neuromuscular training) should continue in some form following return to sport as injury risk is heightened, and individuals often have ongoing objective mechanical laxity and subjective instability. For instance, one-third of individuals report ongoing pain and subjective instability one year following acute ankle sprain, and up to one-third report at least one re-sprain within a period of 3 years.[7]

The treatment of a grade III sprain may be either conservative or surgical. For example, the torn medial collateral ligament of the knee and the torn lateral ligament of the ankle may be treated conservatively with full or partial immobilisation. Alternatively, the two ends of a torn ligament can be reattached surgically and the joint then fully or partially immobilised for approximately 6 weeks.

During the past few decades, there have been mounting efforts to develop tissue engineering strategies that encourage ligament regeneration (as opposed to repair) so that the final product matches that of native ligament. Strategies have included the use of growth factors, cell-based therapies, gene transfer and therapy, and artificial scaffolding materials.[8] These approaches have not been proven to be clinically useful as this edition of *Clinical Sports Medicine* goes to press (mid-2024).

## MUSCLE

> **PATIENT VOICE** A wet kitchen towel
>
> Kevin De Bruyne (Manchester City midfielder) suffered a recurrence of his hamstring injury in 2023. He said that it was important that he recovered completely. His hamstrings could have torn at any time. They were like a wet kitchen towel.

Muscle injuries account for up to half of all sport-related injuries at the elite level. They result from either intrinsic or extrinsic causes, with the former contributing to muscle strains/tears and the latter resulting in contusions or modifying the environment and predisposing muscles to an injurious load.

### Strain/tear

A muscle is strained or torn when excessive tensile forces generated by the muscle—often when the muscle is in a stretched position—cause muscle fibres to detach from their connective tissues (e.g. the muscle aponeurosis, tendon or fascia). Muscles consist of a hierarchy of active contractile elements and passive non-contractile connective tissue. The actin and myosin machinery responsible for producing active contractile forces form myofibrils which are housed in elongated, rod-shaped cells known as muscle fibres.

The cell membrane of the muscle fibre (i.e. sarcolemma) attaches to a basal membrane surrounded by a connective tissue sheath called the endomysium. Groups of muscle fibres bundle together to form fascicles encased in a connective tissue sheath known as the perimysium. The fascicles in turn combine to form the muscle which is surrounded by a final dense sheath of connective tissue called the epimysium.

During normal muscle contraction, actin and myosin form cross-bridges to generate force, which is transmitted both via the surrounding connective tissue and directly to an attached tendon and, subsequently, the skeleton to produce motion. High-load activities (e.g. repeated eccentric contractions) can cause muscle damage without breaking

**TABLE 8.4**    Ligament sprains: (a) grade I, (b) grade II, (c) grade III

| Grade | Pathology | Clinical findings | |
|-------|-----------|-------------------|---|
| I | Some disruption of collagen fibres | • Local tenderness<br>• Minimal swelling<br>• Normal range and end feel on ligament stress test, but test may be painful<br>• Little functional deficit | |
| II | Considerable disruption of a proportion of collagen fibres | • Significant tenderness<br>• There can be considerable swelling which may involve the whole joint (effusion)<br>• Greater than normal ligament laxity on stress tests; ligament has a definite end feel<br>• Moderate functional deficit | |
| III | Complete disruption of all collagen fibres | • There may be an audible "pop" at the time of injury<br>• Often immediately painful, but may become pain-free a short time after the injury; pain and effusion return thereafter<br>• Can be considerable rapid swelling due to bleeding into the joint (haemarthrosis)<br>• Significantly increased joint play on ligament stress test with no discernible end point<br>• Significant functional deficit | |

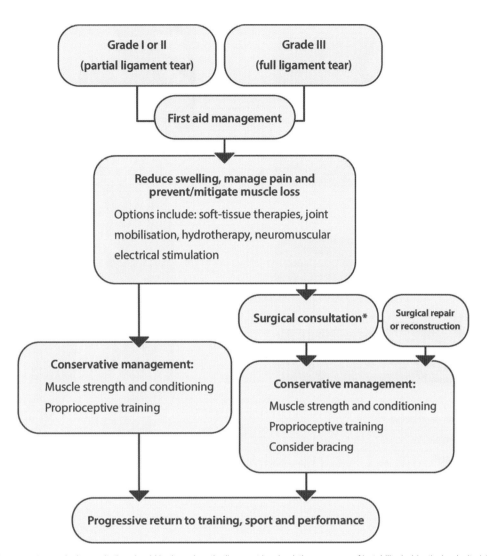

**Figure 8.5** Management of acute ligament sprains

*The decision to request a surgical consultation should be based on the ligament involved, the presence of instability (subjective) or laxity (objective), and shared decisions made between the athlete, coach and medical team.

the contractile or non-contractile elements. This results in the muscle getting stronger and being more resistant to future high-load activities (known as the "repeated bout" effect). Often these events will be associated with delayed-onset muscle soreness but will not prevent an athlete from continuing to participate in their sport.

Muscle strains most commonly occur within the hamstring, quadriceps and calf muscle groups, as these muscles are exposed to the highest amounts of total tension. Total tension is the sum of active tension generated by muscle fibre contractile forces and passive tension due to stretch on the connective tissue components. Active tension can be high in the hamstring, quadriceps and calf muscles as these muscles often have to contract eccentrically, generating large forces as they do so. Passive tension is also often high in these muscle groups as they are biarthrodial (cross two joints) and are often required to contract while on passive stretch over more than one joint. The microscopic process of muscle repair is depicted in Figure 8.6.

Hamstring, quadriceps and calf muscle tears commonly occur at or near the musculotendinous junction, which appears as an area of relative weakness in skeletally mature individuals. The traditional view of the muscle-tendon unit involved a relatively distinct separation between the muscle belly and the free tendon at the end via which active contractile forces are transmitted to the bone. However, advanced imaging and anatomical dissection studies have

**Injury**

**Day 7**

**Day 30**

**Month 3**

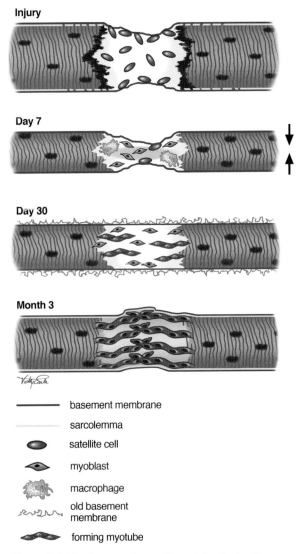

basement membrane

sarcolemma

satellite cell

myoblast

macrophage

old basement
membrane

forming myotube

**Figure 8.6** Healing muscle myofibre at day 0, day 7,
day 30 and 3 months after injury. Note this example applies
to injuries where the basement membrane remains intact.
Source: Adapted from Mackey, A.L., Kjaer, M. The breaking and
making of healthy adult human skeletal muscle in vivo. *Skeletal Muscle*
2017;7(24).

clearly shown that tendinous structures extend deeply into
the muscle belly and that some muscles also have isolated
central tendinous structures within the muscle belly
themselves.

Depending on the severity of the injury, the insertion
between muscle fibre and the connective tissue (fascia,
intramuscular tendon—more accurately called the
"aponeurosis") is torn off, to a varying degree.[9] Figure 8.7
demonstrates a common site of hamstring muscle injury
along the muscle-tendon (intramuscular tendon) junction.

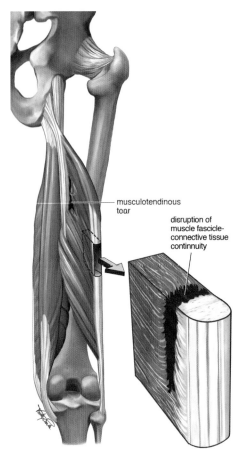

musculotendinous
tear

disruption of
muscle fascicle-
connective tissue
continnuity

**Figure 8.7** Hamstring muscle tear at the site of the
intramuscular tendon

At the muscle fibre level, a strain may include rupture
of the muscle cell membrane and the basal membrane
to which the membrane attaches. Figure 8.6 illustrates a
healing muscle myofibre where the basement membrane
has remained intact and demonstrates the subsequent
sarcolemma. Healing often continues beyond the 30 days
when players traditionally have returned to sport.

**PRACTICE PEARL**

Muscle healing processes continue long after we see
clinical resolution (often up to months beyond the initial
injury); thus, continued and thoughtful active loading
is vital to ensure that the muscle regains strength and
adapts to the loads required for sport.

Damage may also occur within blood vessels contained
within the connective tissue sheaths. The net result can
be pain on active contraction and passive stretch of the

muscle, and some loss of strength due to a disruption of the functional muscle–tendon interface.[10] Strength loss might additionally be caused by pain inhibition, decreased range of motion due to muscle spasm, and loss of function.

## Grading muscle injuries

To guide prognosis, muscle strains were historically graded using a three-tier system, with increasing grade suggesting a greater severity of injury requiring longer recovery.[11] This system has been considered too imprecise to explain the variations seen in muscle injuries, leading to the development of several new classification systems, the most prominent of which is the British Athletics Muscle Injury Classification (BAMIC) system—see Table 8.5.[12] BAMIC has been recommended as the best classification system for grading hamstring injuries.[13]

The BAMIC system takes account of both the degree of the strain and the location. There are six categories, with an "extensive" category added between moderate tears (the old grade II) and complete ruptures (the old grade III).

Perhaps the most significant addition was to acknowledge grade 0a/0b injuries. Grades 0a and 0b reflect clinicians' experience of athletes presenting with a clinical syndrome of muscle abnormality, but without imaging evidence of pathology. Grade 0a often has the clinical hallmarks present in any of grades 1–3 (i.e. sudden-onset pain), but players may make a fast return to sport (often within several days), although they remain at high risk of a recurrence of pain. Grade 0b was added to acknowledge the significant impact that delayed-onset muscle soreness can have on performance. No definitive aetiology of grade 0 injuries has yet been established, but you should carefully monitor players who have suffered a grade 0a injury. Consider having those athletes perform additional rehabilitation exercises (e.g. enhanced neuromuscular warm-up prior to training/playing).

> ### PRACTICE PEARL
>
> Players who have suffered sudden-onset muscle injury but show no visible injury on diagnostic scans can be classed as having suffered a grade 0 injury. These players may be at risk of recurrence and therefore greater adherence to neuromuscular warm-up programs for the subsequent 2 weeks is recommended.

We encourage clinicians working without access to diagnostic imaging such as ultrasound or MRI to continue using the traditional three-grade classification. In this instance, you should maintain awareness of the potential for greater variation in the level of muscle injury than can be assigned using clinical testing alone, and especially in athletes who do not progress as expected (or have recurrent injuries) you should consider the possibility that the athlete has suffered injury to the intramuscular tendon.

## Prognosis

Grading systems provide an indication of the severity or extent of muscle damage; however, the variable recovery time for individuals with similarly graded injuries suggests that other factors influence prognosis. With advances in

**TABLE 8.5** Muscle injury classification

| Traditional classification[11]<br>*Clinical diagnosis—severity only* | British Athletics Muscle Injury Classification (BAMIC)[12]<br>*Radiographic diagnosis—severity and location* | |
|---|---|---|
| **Grade 1** Mild<br>Strain affects a limited number of muscle fibres. There is no decrease in strength and there is full active and passive range of motion. Pain and tenderness are often delayed until the day after the injury. | **Severity**<br>**0a** Focal neuromuscular injury with normal MRI<br>**0b** Generalised muscle soreness (delayed-onset muscle soreness) with normal MRI<br>**1** Small injuries (tears) | **Location**<br>**a** Myofascial injury<br>**b** Intramuscular, usually at the musculotendinous junction<br>**c** Extends into tendon |
| **Grade 2** Moderate<br>Strain affects approximately half of the muscle fibres. Acute and moderately severe pain is accompanied by swelling and a small loss of muscle strength. | **2** Moderate injuries (tears)<br>**3** Extensive tears | |
| **Grade 3** Severe<br>A complete rupture of the muscle. The tendon may be separated from the muscle belly or the muscle belly may be torn in two parts. Swelling, pain and a complete loss of function characterise the grade 3 strain. | **4** Complete tears | |

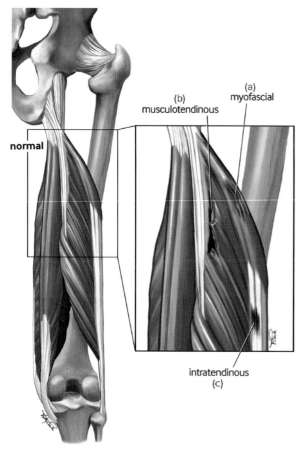

**Figure 8.8** Letter classification based on the anatomical site of muscle injury within the BAMIC system: (a) myofascial, (b) musculotendinous, (c) intratendinous

MRI and ultrasonography, it is now possible to also classify or categorise injuries in terms of their anatomical location and the type of tissue involved (Fig. 8.8).

The role of imaging in predicting recovery time from muscle strains remains unclear.[14] However, there is increasing recognition of the benefits of combining clinical and radiological findings, as reflected by the updates to the muscle injury classification system. Classification systems have yet to be convincingly validated,[15] but may represent a new era in understanding and establishing prognosis for muscle strains.

Common to the new grading systems is recognition that strains involving tendinous components of the muscle have a worse prognosis. It is well established that muscle strains involving concomitant damage to the free tendon (e.g. proximal hamstring tendon) require a longer recovery time than strains isolated to the musculoskeletal junction. However, damage within or adjacent to the intramuscular tendon may explain why some individuals with historically labelled "muscle belly strains" have a slower than expected recovery.

The presence of intramuscular tendinous structures means that musculotendinous junctions occur throughout a greater length of a muscle and that muscle belly strains still represent an injury occurring at one or more of these junctions.

As tendinous structures have a slower healing rate than muscle tissue, a muscle strain that also involves damage to intramuscular tendinous structures has the potential to slow healing and delay return to sport.[15] One study showed that strains of the biceps femoris muscle with and without central tendon disruption had median recovery times of 72 and 21 days, respectively.[16]

### Managing acute muscle strain injury

The goal when managing an acute muscle strain is for the athlete to return to activity at the prior level of performance with minimal risk for re-injury. This requires the underlying pathology, and the changes that it introduces (i.e. pain, swelling, weakness, reduced range of motion), to be addressed. It also requires causative risk factors to be addressed, with a previous muscle injury being the single largest risk factor for a future strain.

Acute management of muscle strains focuses on education, restoring neuromuscular control at slow speeds and preventing excessive scar formation while mobilising/loading the injured muscle groups as early as possible without excessive lengthening. Recommended early techniques include the application of the principles outlined in POLICE or PEACE & LOVE. As part of this, athletes are encouraged to mobilise the affected area using pain limits as guidance (e.g. tolerance up to 5 on a numerical pain scale), while avoiding aggressive stretching techniques and any fast or explosive movements.[17]

Subsequent management allows for increased exercise intensity, the initiation of moderate and eventually heavy eccentric resistance training and finally neuromuscular training at faster speed and larger amplitudes. The final stage of recovery prior to return to sport progresses to high-speed neuromuscular training and eccentric resistance training in a lengthened position in preparation for return to sport.[18]

In the context of strain injuries, the high risk of re-injury is a clinical problem. A recurrent strain injury occurs often in the early phase post return to sport and at the same location as the first strain injury in the majority of the cases (Fig. 8.9).[19] High re-injury rates suggest that tissues involved in a strain injury (i.e. the interface between muscle fibres and the connective tissue) cannot withstand the high forces they are exposed to during sprinting or jumping. The consequence is a new injury. High tissue turnover continues even months after athletes return to sport,[20] indicating that the repair of the injured tissues is not completed at the time of return to sport. Therefore, continuing strengthening

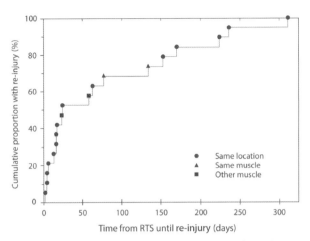

**Figure 8.9** Graph showing the site and speed of muscle re-injury in male athletes who re-injured following their return to sport (RTS); the median time to re-injury was 19 days
Source: Wangensteen A, Tol JL, Witvrouw E, et al. Hamstring reinjuries occur at the same location and early after return to sport: a descriptive study of MRI-confirmed reinjuries. *Am J Sports Med* 2016;44(8):2112–21.

exercises of the injured muscle groups may help to minimise the risk of re-injury after return to sport.

Recent studies have also shown that after strain injuries muscle shows pathological signs as loss of muscle mass, fatty infiltration and loss of contractile elements within muscle fibres.[21] In addition, a strain injury may result in an area where muscle fibres are not actively contracting, and the intramuscular tendon is altered in both structure and function even years after the injury.[22] All of these pathological characteristics appear irreversible. It is therefore vital for an athletic career to maintain focused strengthening of the injured muscle and its agonists.

## Exercise-induced muscle soreness

Exercise-induced muscle soreness is a common complaint during or immediately following vigorous unaccustomed exercise. Muscle soreness that develops 24–48 hours after unaccustomed high-intensity activity is known as delayed-onset muscle soreness. Delayed-onset muscle soreness appears to be more severe after activities that involve eccentric muscle contractions; that is, when muscle contracts while simultaneously lengthening. Activities that involve both high muscle forces and eccentric muscle contractions, such as skiing and downhill running, are a common cause of delayed-onset muscle soreness in untrained individuals.

The exact cause of acute exercise-induced muscle soreness and delayed-onset muscle soreness is unclear. Although debate about the mechanism of muscle soreness is ongoing in the literature, the general consensus is that the soreness is caused by microtrauma to muscle cells and connective tissue. Microtrauma is followed by a local inflammatory process within the extracellular space, which sensitises nerve endings via mechanical, chemical or thermal stimulation.[23-25]

### Signs and symptoms

Exercise-induced muscle soreness is often accompanied by muscle stiffness, aches and mild cramping. Symptoms can persist for several hours post-exercise before resolving.[24] Delayed-onset muscle soreness is characterised by tenderness on palpation and a sense of stiffness with physical activity. Soreness can peak around 48 hours after exercise. Resolution of symptoms can take up to 10 days.[23] Soreness can vary from mild discomfort to incapacitating pain; this is largely dependent on the intensity and volume of training, as well as the actual inducing event.

Importantly, delayed-onset muscle soreness may be associated with muscle strength deficits, which may affect physical performance. Strength deficits associated with delayed-onset muscle soreness are typically greatest between 24 and 48 hours after activity.[26-27] A reduction in muscle power and reduced joint range of motion may also affect an athlete's performance. Local muscle swelling and intracellular proteins in the blood are also common signs.[23, 26-28] Exercise-induced muscle soreness and delayed-onset muscle soreness are often associated with elevated levels of creatine kinase in the blood. However, given the self-limiting nature of acute muscle soreness and delayed-onset muscle soreness, blood tests are rarely warranted, and the clinical interpretation of such tests is unclear.[28]

### Management

Management strategies in the treatment of delayed-onset muscle soreness focus on encouraging healing and recovery of the inflamed and damaged muscle tissue. Intense exercise during the symptomatic period can potentially cause more microtrauma and muscle injury, particularly as strength, power and coordination of movement are compromised. Therefore, during the symptomatic period, training and competition performance should be modified accordingly.

Common modalities used to treat exercise-induced muscle soreness and delayed-onset muscle soreness include massage, cryotherapy, stretching and active recovery.

### Prevention of exercise-induced muscle soreness and delayed-onset muscle soreness

Prevention of exercise-induced muscle soreness should be centred on a properly planned training program, which adequately addresses strength, power, endurance and quality of movement. Adequate periods of training and conditioning are needed before individuals participate in strenuous activity, to ensure that the exercise-induced muscle soreness is minimised and more serious injuries are prevented.

Delayed-onset muscle soreness occurs less in those who train regularly, although even trained individuals may become sore after an unaccustomed exercise bout. There is little evidence to support the use of static stretching to prevent acute muscle soreness and delayed-onset muscle soreness.[24] Variable results have been shown with preventive approaches such as the use of vitamins C and E and protein supplements.[29] Understanding an athlete's current training volume—including exercise intensity, duration, current rate of progression and recovery—will provide a context for understanding and preventing future episodes of muscle soreness.

## Contusion

Muscle contusion is the term for a muscle bruise and refers to bleeding and subsequent haematoma formation within the muscle and its surrounding connective tissue sheaths. Contusions occur when a muscle is compressed against underlying bone by a blunt, external force. The force can result from a direct blow or collision with an external object, such as an opposing player, teammate or piece of equipment. Thus, contusions are common in contact sports and sports involving the use of rapidly moving, hard objects (e.g. sticks and balls).

The most common site for muscle contusion is the quadriceps, with contusions at this site being referred to as a "corked thigh", "charley horse" or "dead leg". Other common sites for contusion include the calf and gluteal muscles; however, a contusion can occur in any muscle exposed to a blunt compressive force. Muscle compression causes muscle fibre damage and rupture of microvessels. The released blood clots to form a haematoma that initiates an acute inflammatory reaction aimed at removing the haematoma and damaged tissue and initiating a repair response. The haematoma may form either within (i.e. intramuscular) or between (i.e. intermuscular) the fascial coverings of the muscle.

Intramuscular contusions affect function more as pressure rises within the fascial compartment, reducing blood flow. They are generally more painful and more restrictive because muscle contraction results in further rises in compartment pressure and stimulation of nociceptors. In contrast, intermuscular contusions are generally less painful as the fascial sheath is damaged, which allows the haematoma to spread to relieve compartment pressure. Intermuscular haematomas are generally more evident externally as the blood is able to travel distally due to gravity and into the subcutaneous tissues, resulting in a visible bruise.

Initial management of a muscle contusion involves ruling out an acute compartment syndrome (discussed later), controlling bleeding to reduce secondary injury (i.e. muscle fibre hypoxia) and protecting the injured site from further injury. Techniques include compression and ice with the muscle placed in a pain-free stretched position to help stop the bleeding and reduce muscle spasm. Applying heat, drinking alcohol and vigorous massage are all likely to increase blood flow and/or cause a re-bleed; these should be avoided in the acute and subacute stages.

As this book goes to press, trials of tranexamic acid are underway.[30] This antifibrinolytic drug is used to suppress bleeding in major orthopaedic surgery (e.g. joint replacement) and nosebleeds. Some clinicians are using tranexamic acid off-label for contusion to reduce inflammation, accelerate recovery and reduce the incidence of myositis ossificans (see below). The studies that are underway will provide results in the late 2020s.

Subsequent management focuses on restoring muscle function via progressive stretching and strengthening. The use of protective equipment in the form of force dissipating and dispersing padding should be considered to prevent re-injury on return to participation. However, the reduction in injury risk gained by using protective equipment will need to be weighed against any associated reduction in athlete mobility and performance.

## Myositis ossificans

Myositis ossificans is a form of heterotrophic ossification and refers to the formation of bone within a muscle. It is an infrequent complication of a contusion injury wherein bone-forming osteoblasts invade the haematoma and begin to lay down bone. The cause remains unknown; however, risk factors include severe contusions that limit joint range of motion (e.g. thigh contusions that limit knee flexion to <45°), repeat contusion injury and inappropriate initial management that causes a re-bleed.

Myositis ossificans should be suspected in muscle contusions that do not resolve in the expected time. Signs and symptoms include initial improvements in range and pain followed by subsequent deterioration and ongoing or reappearance of inflammatory symptoms (i.e. resting, morning and night pain). The bone grows 2–4 weeks after injury at which time an area of calcification may be visible on radiographs (Fig. 8.10a) or ultrasound (Fig. 8.10b), and a firm lump may be felt. Once active bone formation ceases, the area of calcification gets slowly reabsorbed. As myositis ossificans is self-limiting, management is typically conservative and consists of anti-inflammatory approaches and non-painful stretching and strengthening.

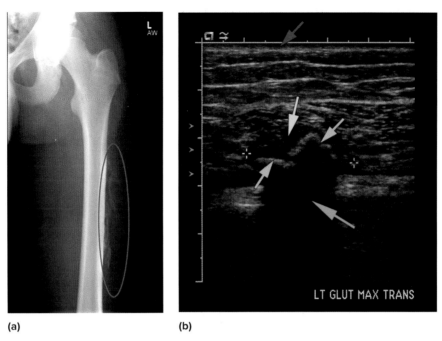

(a)                                    (b)

**Figure 8.10** Myositis ossificans: (a) radiographic appearance, (b) ultrasound appearance. Yellow arrow points to haematoma within the gluteal muscle; blue arrows point to calcium within the gluteal muscle; green arrow points to acoustic shadowing associated with calcification; red arrow points to skin and then subcutaneous fat. Below that are layers of gluteal muscles.

## Acute compartment syndrome

Muscles in the extremities are surrounded by a strong, thick connective tissue called fascia. The fascia serves as an attachment site for muscle, aids in force transmission and forms non-distensible compartments that facilitate muscle-pump-mediated venous return. Injuries such as a bone fracture or contusion that lead to swelling or bleeding into one of the fascial compartments (usually the flexor compartment of the forearm or anterior compartment of the lower leg) can result in the development of acute compartment syndrome.

Acute compartment syndrome occurs when interstitial pressure within a compartment exceeds perfusion pressure, leading to the onset of ischaemia and, ultimately, cellular anoxia and death. It is characterised by pain that is out of proportion to the inciting injury, pain on passive stretch and at rest, paraesthesia and pulselessness (although the latter is a late finding as the interstitial pressure needs to be high enough to occlude arterial flow).

Acute compartment syndrome represents a medical emergency that may require urgent fasciotomy (i.e. release of the fascia surrounding the muscle compartment) in order to prevent permanent, irreversible damage.[31] Hence, referral to an orthopaedic emergency specialist is recommended.

## Cramp

Muscle cramps are sudden, painful, involuntary contractions characterised by repetitive firing of motor unit action potentials. When they occur during or immediately after exercise in healthy individuals with no underlying metabolic, neurological or endocrine pathology, they are referred to as "exercise-associated muscle cramps" ("cramps" in the rest of this chapter).[32] Cramps are usually temporary (lasting 1–2 minutes) but often incapacitating and tend to recur if activity at the same exercise intensity level is continued without an adequate recovery period. The most common sites of cramps are the calf and foot muscles, followed by the hamstring and quadriceps muscle groups.

Previously, cramps were thought to be due to dehydration and/or electrolyte depletion, but this hypothesis has not been supported. As cramps most commonly occur towards the end of, or after, fatiguing exercise or following a rapid increase in exercise intensity, fatigue is a contributing factor. Cramps probably result from abnormal neuromuscular control at the spinal level in response to fatiguing exercise— specifically increased excitatory (accelerator) and decreased inhibitory (brake) afferent inputs to motor neurons during fatigue.[32] This results in sustained motor neuron activity (accelerator to the floor) and a cramp-inducing

85

discharge. The most recent update to this theory involves a variety of intrinsic and extrinsic factors (such as pain, stress and inadequate conditioning) converging to create circumstances under which altered neuromuscular control and thus exercise-associated muscle cramps are possible.[10]

Immediate treatment of cramp aims to reduce motor neuron activity, with the most popular and effective technique being cessation of the current activity and passive stretching. Passive stretching increases the Golgi tendon organ's inhibitory activity to reduce muscle electromyographic activity within 10–20 seconds and provide symptomatic relief. Ideally, passive tension should be maintained to the affected muscle for up to 20 minutes or until fasciculation ceases.[33] If the cramps were particularly intense or prolonged, icing while the muscle is on stretch may be considered to offset any potential delayed-onset muscle soreness resulting from microscopic muscle fibre damage. Other potential methods of reducing motor neuron activity during cramps include electrical stimulation of tendon afferents and antagonist contraction to induce reciprocal inhibition.

Our incomplete knowledge of the aetiology of cramps has limited the development of preventive strategies. Fluid and electrolyte replacement has not been shown to be beneficial, consistent with the now debunked dehydration-electrolyte imbalance theory. In contrast, strategies aimed at modulating fatigability and altering neuromuscular control may be beneficial.[10]

Fatigability may be modified by improving generalised conditioning and endurance, and ensuring and maintaining adequate carbohydrate reserves. Neuromuscular control may be targeted by performing plyometric and eccentric exercises, which may elicit changes in muscle spindle and Golgi tendon organ firing to enhance the efficiency and sensitivity of reflexive and descending pathways used for neuromuscular control. Given the likely multi-factorial nature of cramps, a thorough investigation of all potential inciting factors should be conducted and an individualised prevention strategy developed.

## TENDON

Tendons connect muscle to bone and function to transmit the muscle contractile forces necessary for motion. They consist of collagen fibres that are more tightly packed and arranged in parallel than in ligaments, which endow tendons with the consummate ability to resist tensile loading.

### Tear/rupture

The tensile strength of tendons is so great that acute tear or rupture of a normal, healthy tendon is relatively rare, with forces more likely to cause an avulsion fracture or failure at the musculotendinous junction (i.e. muscle strain). The pathology (tendon rupture) is usually asymptomatic such that the tendon failure appears to occur without warning. As the presence of pathology increases with age, tendon ruptures most frequently occur in middle-aged to older athletes.

The two most commonly ruptured tendons are the Achilles and supraspinatus tendons, with ruptures involving either a portion (partial rupture) or the full thickness (complete rupture) of the respective tendon (Fig. 8.11). Partial ruptures are characterised by the sudden onset of pain, localised tenderness, and a loss of tendon function that is inversely related to the size of the tear. In contrast, complete ruptures are associated with total loss of tendon function and acute pain, but the pain often settles quickly due to concomitant damage of nociceptor afferents.

Diagnosis of tendon ruptures can be confirmed using imaging, with ultrasonography and MRI both useful at distinguishing between partial and complete rupture. Partial tendon ruptures may be managed conservatively using progressive rehabilitation; however, complete ruptures may be treated by surgical repair to restore tendon continuity and function, followed by rehabilitation, or treated by rehabilitation alone. The risk of complications, speed of recovery and ability to return to performance outcomes are all likely to impact shared decision making on surgery versus conservative management in athletes post Achilles rupture.

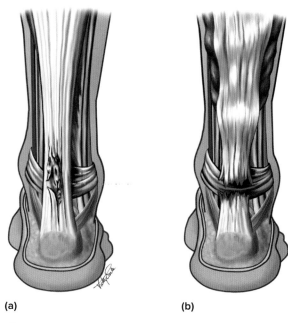

**(a)**                    **(b)**

**Figure 8.11** Tendon rupture: (a) partial, (b) complete

## FASCIA

### Tear/rupture

Fascia is a dense, regular connective tissue consisting of closely packed bundles of collagen fibres. It divides muscles into compartments and forms specific force-transmitting structures, such as the iliotibial band and plantar fascia. Most injuries to fascia are associated with overuse, with prominent conditions being iliotibial band syndrome and plantar fasciopathy (both considered in detail in *Managing Injuries*). Acute sprain or rupture of fascia is rare but has been reported. Plantar fascia ruptures are rare in asymptomatic individuals—usually patients present with a history of fasciopathy managed via corticosteroid.[34]

## BURSA

### Traumatic bursitis

Bursae are small, synovial membrane-lined sacs filled with an inner layer of viscous fluid. They are frequently found between bone and overlying connective tissues (such as tendon, muscle and skin) where they function to provide cushioning and facilitate movement by reducing friction.

Most injuries to bursae are associated with overuse (Chapter 9), but occasionally a direct fall onto a bursa may result in acute traumatic bursitis due to bleeding into the bursa. The management of acute haemorrhagic bursitis involves the application of ice and compression. Aspiration may be considered if the condition does not resolve, but corticosteroid injection is rarely indicated.

Aseptic bursitis is usually a time-limited condition but if an athlete presents with a fever and has a painful bursitis which feels hot and looks red, suspect septic bursitis, a relative medical emergency. Diagnosis will be through aspiration of the bursal fluid, and treatment will probably require oral or IV antibiotics. In extreme cases, bursectomy may be required.

## NERVE

Peripheral nerve injuries can broadly be divided into three categories: neuropraxia, axonotmesis and neurotmesis (Fig. 8.12). Neurotmesis is unusual in athletes. Neurotmesis, or severance of all neural layers, represents permanent damage and requires surgery if sensation and functional capacity are to be restored. In contrast, both axonotmesis and neuropraxia indicate temporary damage to the nerve.

Axonotmesis injury involves damage to the axon and its myelin sheath. Patients with an axonotmesis injury will present with pain, muscle wasting and complete motor, sensory and sympathetic neural function loss. However, as the epineurium and perineurium layers of the nerve remain

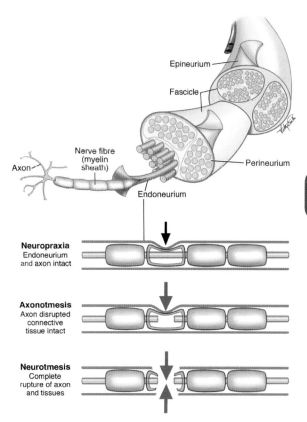

**Figure 8.12** Anatomy of a peripheral nerve, combined with Seddon's classification of nerve injuries into three categories: neuropraxia, axonotmesis and neurotmesis

intact, regeneration is possible. Axonotmesis injuries usually end in a complete recovery but take significantly longer than a neuropraxic injury.

### Neuropraxia

Neuropraxia is the most common form of nerve injury in athletes. Athletes usually present with pain, numbness, muscle weakness and proprioceptive deficits but importantly no muscle wasting. Injury most often occurs due to compression, traction or friction which may all lead to localised ischaemia (within the nervi nervorum), inflammation, oedema and/or fibrosis. A temporary functional block in nerve conduction can occur due to the loss of nerve myelin around the site of the injury.[35]

Specific nerves are susceptible to compression or friction injury because of their subcutaneous location, including the ulnar nerve at the elbow and the common peroneal nerve at the neck of the fibula. Similarly, some nerves are vulnerable to being co-injured with other tissues, such as axillary nerve injury during shoulder dislocation and radial nerve injury with humeral shaft fracture.

The most common example of traction causing an acute nerve injury in athletes is a "stinger" or "burner". A stinger or burner results from an overstretching injury to the brachial plexus. Neural fibres are elastic but have a finite stretching capacity. Exceeding the nerve's capacity to stretch can, for instance, occur when the head is forcibly bent away from the shoulder while the shoulder is simultaneously depressed. This may also occur when an athlete is driven into the playing surface during a high-contact sport, such as ice hockey, rugby, wrestling and various football codes.

Symptoms are a stinging or burning sensation that spreads from the shoulder to the hand, which may be associated with numbness in the sensory distribution of the involved nerves. The paraesthesia is often temporary, disappearing in minutes and usually within hours. In cases that do not resolve within several weeks, electromyography and nerve conduction studies may be considered to determine the extent of nerve damage.

## FAT PAD

### Bruise/contusion

Fat pads consist of closely packed adipose cells surrounded by fibrous septa, which commonly divide the fat pad into separate compartments. The function of fat pads is not well established and may vary according to anatomical location. However, they appear to have roles in cushioning and facilitating joint lubrication. It is in their cushioning role that fat pads are susceptible to acute compression injury. In particular, the calcaneal fat pad under the heel and the infrapatellar fat pad located behind the patellar tendon can be acutely injured. The plantar fat pad can be injured during landing onto the heel from a height, while the infrapatellar fat pad can be injured by landing on the knees or pinching the fat pad between the femoral condyles, proximal tibia and inferior pole of the patella during knee hyperextension. The infrapatellar fat pad is also often acutely injured when creating portals during knee arthroscopic surgery.

Fat pads are well vascularised and innervated. The blood supply contributes to haematoma formation (contusion) in response to acute injury, but also enables fat pad injuries to readily heal. The rich innervation of fat pads means that they can be a significant source of pain, with the infrapatellar fat pad being reported to be the most pain-evoking structure in the knee.[36]

The integrity and function of the calcaneal fat pad may be compromised if its organised compartments are disrupted; however, this is rare, with compression injuries sufficient to fracture the calcaneus not damaging the fibrous septa.[36]

Management of fat pad injuries, beyond acute care techniques, includes externally padding using heel cups or knee pads and using tape to limit radial expansion of the calcaneal fat pad or unload the infrapatellar fat pad. These injuries can take considerable time to heal.

## SKIN

Acute skin injuries are common in athletes, particularly those competing in contact sports and cycling. Open wounds may be caused by a scraping (abrasion), cutting (laceration) or piercing (puncture) force. Possible damage to underlying structures, such as tendons, muscles, blood vessels and nerves, should always be considered. The principles of treatment of all open wounds are shown in Table 8.6.

**TABLE 8.6**   Principles of treatment of all open wounds

| Principle | Details |
| --- | --- |
| 1. Stop any associated bleeding | Apply a pressure bandage directly to the injured part and elevate it. If the wound is open and clean, bring the wound edges together using adhesive strips or sutures. A contaminated wound should not be closed. |
| 2. Prevent infection | Remove all dirt and contamination by simple irrigation. Extensively wash and scrub with antiseptic solution as required as soon as possible. If the wound is severely contaminated, prophylactic antibiotic therapy should be commenced (e.g. flucloxacillin, 500 mg orally four times a day). If anaerobic organisms are suspected (e.g. wound inflicted by a bite), add an antibiotic such as metronidazole (400 mg orally three times a day). |
| 3. Immobilisation (where needed) | This applies when the wound is over a constantly moving part (e.g. the anterior aspect of the knee). Certain lacerations, such as pretibial lacerations, require particular care and strict immobilisation to encourage healing. |
| 4. Check tetanus status | All contaminated wounds, especially penetrating wounds, have the potential to become infected with *Clostridium tetani*. Tetanus immunisation consists of a course of 3 injections over 6 months given during childhood. Further tetanus toxoid boosters should be given at 5–10-year intervals. In the case of a possible contaminated wound, a booster should be given if none has been administered within the previous 5 years. |

## KEY POINTS

- Injuries can be classified in several ways, including by body region (upper versus lower limb), tissue type (ligament, tendon, muscle) and mechanism of injury (acute versus chronic).

- Recognising the intrinsic and extrinsic factors that contribute to injury can help focus injury prevention efforts.

- The standard of acute care for soft-tissue injuries has evolved over time, based on our understanding of the inflammatory process. Recent models question the use of ice or anti-inflammatory medications in the early stages of healing and prioritise early mobilisation.

- Fractures represent a broad range of bone injuries, from simple to compound, which can be treated with simple casting or bracing or may require surgical intervention with implanted hardware.

- Dislocation or subluxation can occur at joints when the passive and/or active stabilisers are disrupted. After a neurovascular screen, reduction should occur as soon as possible, and post-reduction imaging should be done to rule out associated injuries.

- Chondral injuries may be sustained secondary to serious ligament injuries, dislocations and subluxations. These are particularly painful injuries that tend not to heal well. Imaging may be necessary to confirm the presence of a chondral injury.

- Fibrocartilage injuries, including those to the labrum, intervertebral discs and menisci, can occur secondary to other nearby capsular or ligament injuries. Treatment depends on a number of factors including the location and severity of injury and associated dysfunction.

- Ligament injuries should be managed initially with usual soft-tissue injury principles. Lower grade ligament injuries can be treated conservatively, while surgery may be an option for full ligament ruptures.

- Muscle strains can be classified using different grading scales, depending on the availability of medical imaging. Whether or not there is tendon involvement in a muscle strain contributes to the overall prognosis. Athletes with muscle strain injuries are at high risk of re-injury after returning to sport.

- Exercise-induced muscle soreness, often referred to as delayed-onset muscle soreness, is a very common but poorly understood phenomenon. Well-designed training programs are the best prevention strategy.

- Acute injuries can occur at other soft-tissue sites, including fat pads, bursae, fascia, nerves and skin. Treatment varies by tissue type, location and severity of injury.

## REFERENCES

References for this chapter can be found at www.mhprofessional.com/CSM6e

## ADDITIONAL CONTENT

Scan here to access additional resources for this topic and more provided by the authors

## CHAPTER 9

# Overuse injuries

with PAUL BLAZEY, ROBERT-JAN DE VOS and STUART WARDEN

*The injury was super-upsetting, but you have to realize that it's real, that you have to give up your race, and that you'll get better.*

DES LINDON (2018 WOMEN'S BOSTON MARATHON WINNER)

## CHAPTER OUTLINE

Have we made progress with the challenges of overuse injuries?
Bone stress injuries: nomenclature and pathophysiology
Bone stress injuries: management principles
Other bone-related overuse injuries
Articular cartilage
Joint
Ligament
Muscle
Tendon
Tendon management principles
Bursa
Other tendon pathologies
Nerve
Skin
But it's not that simple

## LEARNING OBJECTIVES

By the end of this chapter you should be able to:

- summarise sport-related overuse injuries according to the affected tissue type
- list intrinsic and extrinsic risk factors for overuse injuries
- describe the pathophysiology of common overuse injuries
- discuss some common and emerging approaches to treat overuse injuries.

Overuse injuries such as tendinopathies and bone stress injuries continue to affect large numbers of people—from recreational athletes to world champions in many different sports. In the first edition of *Clinical Sports Medicine* (1993), we wrote that overuse sports injuries posed three distinct challenges to the clinician: (1) accurate diagnosis, (2) understanding why the injury occurred and (3) management.

Some 30 years later, athletes are more likely to receive an accurate diagnosis. Clinicians have better understanding of sport injuries and imaging advances have revolutionised our field.

## HAVE WE MADE PROGRESS WITH THE CHALLENGES OF OVERUSE INJURIES?

Does the "why" remain a challenge? Perhaps less so than it used to. Clinicians better understand the effects of load on tissue than they did. Clinicians and athletes have greater access to data, including the loads athletes place on their bodies (see Chapter 15). These data have been available in the professional club setting for decades but the advances in wearable technologies mean access to training data is essentially universal now.

Beyond load, clinicians are now aware of a wider range of antecedents to overuse injuries than their 1990s counterparts were: for example, inadequate nutrition (relative energy deficiency in sport, REDs) contributes to overuse injuries—this condition was not named until the 2010s. The causes of overuse injuries are still divided into extrinsic factors such as training surfaces, equipment or environmental conditions, and intrinsic factors such as age, gender and muscle weakness (Fig. 9.1).

In this chapter we illustrate how bone, joint, muscle and tendon adapt—or fail to adapt—to physical activity/exercise/sport. There are wonderful accurate and detailed books on each of the major overuse injuries (e.g. bone stress injuries, tendinopathy). Here, we share the principles of management of overuse injuries, while detailed treatment of specific overuse injuries is covered in *Clinical Sports Medicine 6e: Managing Injuries*.

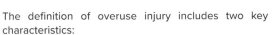

**PRACTICE PEARL**

The definition of overuse injury includes two key characteristics:

1. a gradual onset of injury
2. underlying pathogenesis that includes repetitive microtrauma to the tissues—there is no single identifiable event.[1, 2]

**Training errors:**
Change in load volume, intensity, etc. with inadequate recovery

**Surfaces:**
Hard, soft, cambered, uneven

**Equipment (including shoes):**
Inappropriate, worn out

**Environment:**
Hot, humid, cold, polluted

**(a)**

**Malalignment:**
At the foot, leg, hip (e.g. genu valgum)
Leg length discrepancy

**Muscle:**
Strength imbalances or muscle tightness

**Sex, size, body composition:**
Can contribute to injury risk

**Other:**
Genetic susceptibility, endocrine/metabolic conditions (see also Chapter 22)

**(b)**

**Figure 9.1** Risk factors for overuse injury: use the clinical encounter to try to identify (a) extrinsic risk factors and (b) intrinsic risk factors.

## BONE STRESS INJURIES: NOMENCLATURE AND PATHOPHYSIOLOGY

The term "stress fracture" refers to the structural failure of bone in response to repetitive mechanical load.

### The bone strain/stress continuum

The term "bone stress injury" (BSI in many papers, but we use the full term here) is common in publications, podcasts and videos. It is an umbrella term that includes both the pre-stress fracture condition known as stress reaction and stress fracture. It is critical to appreciate the pathology continuum from bone strain (no pain) to stress reaction (pain, but no visible fracture) to complete stress fracture (Fig. 9.2). Bone strain is a normal response of bone that has undergone loading and is remodelling (adapting)—the athlete has no pain. Box 9.1 defines these terms.

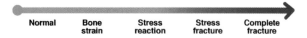

| Normal | Bone strain | Stress reaction | Stress fracture | Complete fracture |

**Figure 9.2** The bone strain/stress continuum. Note that the term "bone stress injury" refers to two stages in that continuum: stress reaction and stress fracture. The athlete with bone strain has no pain and is not "injured". The green to red transition reflects the extent of structural change/damage based on MRI.

---

**BOX 9.1** Bone stress injury definitions

- *Bone strain:* there are signs of excessive load leading to accelerated bone turnover on imaging, but the athlete does not yet feel pain.
- *Stress reaction:* bone stress injury is severe enough to cause local bone pain, which is aggravated by sporting activities. Athletes often report tenderness on palpation at the affected area and there may also be swelling.
- *Stress fracture:* a break that can be seen on medical imaging. Typically athletes can localise the pain, and weight-bearing through the affected limb provokes pain.

---

To form a mental picture of the bone stress continuum, imagine 100 army recruits training by marching on a concrete surface in low-quality boots:

- After a few days, many will have bones that are not coping with the load, but they won't feel bone pain yet. Some of them would have abnormal magnetic resonance imaging (MRI) scans (i.e. the definition of bone strain).
- After a few weeks, some will have pain (e.g. metatarsal pain) and MRI will reflect the bone beginning to fail. If these recruits have normal radiographs, they will be given the diagnosis of stress reaction. They have (1) pain, (2) MRI features of bony pathology, but (3) no fracture line.
- If the training program continues unchanged, some of these recruits will develop radiographic features of a fracture on their metatarsal bones (and perhaps at other lower limb sites). Once a fracture is evident on radiographs or computed tomography (CT) scans, they have a stress fracture.

Table 9.1 summarises the relationship between pain and imaging appearance at different stages of the continuum.

Stress fractures account for approximately 20% of bone stress injuries.[3] When radiographed, stress fractures appear as a sclerotic (hard, white) line at trabecular bone-rich sites (e.g. the calcaneus; Box 9.2) or later as lines (gaps, cracks) at sites rich in cortical bone (e.g. the shaft of long bones such as the 5th metatarsal; Box 9.2). The remaining 80% of bone stress injuries are stress reactions, evident by altered signal intensity within the marrow, endosteum and/or periosteum on MRI.

In the lower leg, there is debate as to whether medial leg pain (commonly referred to as medial tibial stress syndrome or the lay term "shin splints") is a bone stress injury. In athletes with medial tibial stress syndrome, MRI can reveal periosteal tissue changes consistent with a low-grade bone stress injury, but they typically have more diffuse pain than is typical of the usual bone stress injury.

**TABLE 9.1** Symptoms and imaging appearance at different stages of the bone stress continuum

| Diagnosis (using MRI as the gold standard) | Does the patient have localised pain? | Is pathology evident on radiography? | Is pathology evident on CT scan? | Is pathology evident on MRI (gold standard)? |
|---|---|---|---|---|
| Bone strain (stress response) | No | No | No | Yes |
| Stress reaction | Yes | Uncommon (often need repeated radiographs to assess for periosteal reaction) | Sometimes (often need repeated scans) | Yes |
| Stress fracture | Yes | May be (depending on the site of injury, may see cortical lucency) | Yes | Yes |

**BOX 9.2** Making sense of the different radiological appearances of bone stress injury

Stress fractures manifest in different ways in different locations:

- Stress fractures in cortical bone appear as either periosteal new bone (Fig. 9.3a) or a crack (radiolucent line) (Fig. 9.3b).

- Stress fractures in trabecular bone (such as the calcaneus) appear whiter (more radiopaque) than normal trabecular bone. This greater whiteness is due to sclerosis (hardening) of trabeculae that have collapsed (i.e. stress fracture) (Fig. 9.3c).

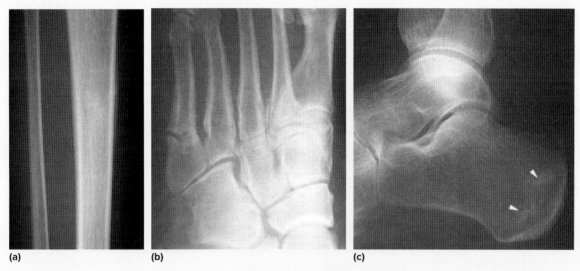

(a)                    (b)                    (c)

**Figure 9.3** Stress reactions and stress fractures on radiography. (a) Stress reactions can manifest as periosteal new bone formation. (b) Stress fractures are demonstrated in cortical bone as a focal line of radio-opacity/sclerosis. (c) Stress fractures are demonstrated in trabecular bone as a sclerotic line, as shown in the calcaneus (arrowheads).

MRI is particularly useful at identifying features associated with a stress reaction. Areas of periosteal and bone oedema (accelerated bone remodelling) appear even though there are no features of fracture (i.e. crack in cortical bone) (Fig. 9.4a). If a stress fracture is present, MRI will reveal a fracture line within the area of bone oedema (Fig 9.4b). Dual-energy CT is proving useful in detecting bone marrow oedema (Fig. 9.4c).

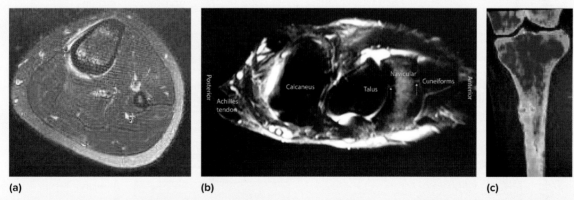

(a)                    (b)                    (c)

**Figure 9.4** MRI and CT appearances along the bone continuum. (a) Stress reaction: the patient had activity-related bone pain and a normal radiograph. Note the increased periosteal and bone marrow signal in the tibia, which reflects periostitis/bone marrow oedema. There was no MRI fracture line. (b) Stress fracture: MRI fluid-sensitive sequence showing subtle low-signal fracture lines (arrows) at both the proximal navicular (articulation with talus) and the distal navicular (articulation with the cuneiforms). (c) Stress reaction: coronal image using dual-energy CT showing bone marrow oedema (green) and no fracture line oedema.

Tissue biopsy of patients with medial tibial stress syndrome has revealed normal bone remodelling—not the elevated remodelling associated with a bone stress injury[4] (see "Pathophysiology" below). Therefore, whether to classify medial tibial stress syndrome as a very early part of the bone stress injury continuum is debatable.

---

**PRACTICE PEARL**

Bone stress injuries are presented here as a continuum, but it is possible for a patient to present with a stress fracture that is not preceded by a stress reaction.

---

## Bone remodelling and bone stress injuries

Bone stress injuries result from an imbalance between the removal and formation of bone following repetitive loading. Synchronised bone removal and formation at the same location is known as remodelling. Figure 9.5 depicts how bone responds to load either positively (bone strain resulting in positive remodelling, which may include changes to bone geometry or material properties) or negatively (e.g. bone removal exceeds bone formation, resulting in symptoms such as pain and the diagnosis of a bone stress injury).

Microdamage is a normal response to load. It helps dissipate energy and stimulates local remodelling. During this remodelling, bone-resorbing osteoclasts remove the damaged tissue before bone-forming osteoblasts fill the resorbed space with new bone. Targeted remodelling preserves (or enhances) a bone's mechanical properties and enables bone to adapt over time. The physiology underpinning this remodelling is known as mechanotransduction—the cellular process that controls remodelling (Chapter 24).

The healthy skeleton can increase the speed of remodelling in response to increased microdamage (e.g. during an increase in the frequency of heavy bouts of

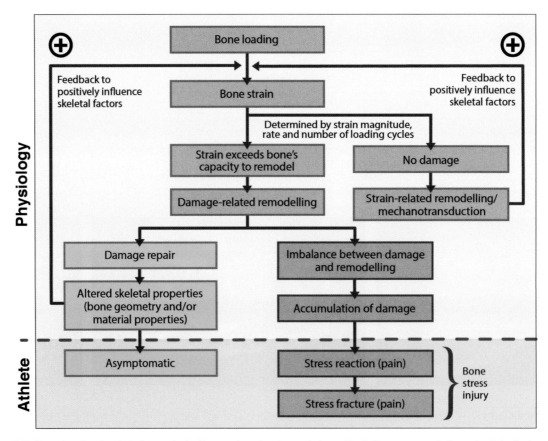

**Figure 9.5** Bone loading leads to bone strain (the engineering term, deformation). Bone responds in a physiological manner (mechanotransduction leads to normal remodelling, a positive feedback loop) or it begins to fail. If repair can match the accelerated rate of bone turnover (microdamage), bone remains intact—promoting stronger bone. When the load simulates excessive turnover for too long, damage accumulates. The clinical pictures associated with these bony states are below the dotted line (asymptomatic or bone stress injury).

exercise that include activities like running or jumping). Thus, changes in loading can generally be tolerated. However, remodelling can produce a positive feedback loop that drives further damage under certain conditions (e.g. when training is progressed too rapidly).

Remodelling takes about 4 weeks to remove damage and 3 months to fill the void. As bone resorption precedes formation in remodelling, an increase in active remodelling temporarily reduces local bone mass and energy-absorbing capacity. This can heighten damage and lead to "microcracks", which can extend and/or coalesce, and ultimately turn into a stress fracture.

## Epidemiology of bone stress injuries

Bone stress injuries occur in active individuals.[5] Between one- to two-thirds of runners have a history of a first stress fracture (index injury) and the 2-year recurrence rate is about 10–12% in cross-country and track and field athletes.[6]

Bone stress incidence varies by both sex and type of physical activity. Females have more than twice the rate of stress fractures compared with males. The higher incidence in female athletes may be partially explained by the association of stress fractures with low energy availability, a condition more prevalent in active females than males.[7] Bone stress incidence is greatest in those participating in sports where leanness is desirable (e.g. distance running and gymnastics) and sports involving high-magnitude repetitive loads (e.g. basketball and track).

Stress fractures predominantly occur at weight-bearing sites, with the most common sites being the tibia, metatarsals and fibula. However, they also occur in response to repetitive muscular loading at non-weight-bearing sites—think of rib stress fractures in rowers and humeral stress fractures in adolescent baseball pitchers.[8] Figure 9.6 depicts a list of common stress fracture locations and the sports/activities associated with their occurrence.

> **PRACTICE PEARL**
>
> Bone stress injuries can occur in virtually any bone exposed to sufficient novel loading and need to be considered in the differential diagnosis of all presenting overuse injuries.

| Site of stress fracture | Associated sport/activity |
|---|---|
| Coracoid process of scapula | Trapshooting |
| Scapula | Running with hand weights |
| Humerus | Throwing; racquet sports |
| Olecranon | Throwing; pitching |
| Ulna | Racquet sports (esp. tennis); gymnastics; volleyball; swimming; softball; wheelchair sports |
| Ribs—1st | Throwing; pitching |
| Ribs—2nd–10th | Rowing; kayaking |
| Pars interarticularis | Gymnastics; ballet; cricket fast bowling; volleyball; springboard diving |
| Pubic ramus* | Distance running; ballet |
| Femur—neck | Distance running; jumping; ballet |
| Femur—shaft | Distance running |
| Patella | Running; hurdling |
| Tibia—plateau | Running |
| Tibia—shaft | Running; ballet |
| Fibula | Running; aerobics; race-walking; ballet |
| Medial malleolus* | Running; basketball |
| Calcaneus | Long-distance military marching |
| Talus | Pole vaulting |
| Navicular | Sprinting; middle-distance running; hurdling; long jump; triple jump; football |
| Metatarsal—general | Running; ballet; marching |
| Metatarsal—2nd base | Ballet |
| Metatarsal—5th | Tennis; ballet |
| Sesamoid bone—foot | Running; ballet; basketball; skating |

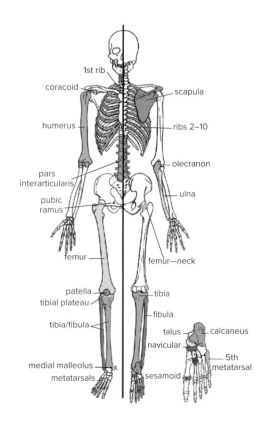

**Figure 9.6** Stress fracture location and associated sport/activity

## Load and bone health

The cause of bone stress injuries is multifactorial and contributing factors vary. A history of previous bone stress injury is one of the strongest risk factors for future bone stress injury—associated with a 5-fold[9] increase in risk. Risk factors for bone stress injuries can be grouped into:

- factors that may increase the load applied to a bone
- factors modifying the ability of a bone to resist and/or respond to damage (Fig. 9.7).

### Factors that load bone

The load applied to bone is the sum of external and internal forces. External forces have received a lot of attention as they can be measured using force plates, accelerometers and pressure-sensing insoles. It was once believed that higher magnitudes and rates of external forces around the time of initial ground contact during running activities were correlated with higher bone stress injury risk, but this is being challenged (Chapter 12).

Scientists and clinicians now recognise that internal tissue loads should also be considered because they are greater than those indicated by external measures due to the pull of a muscle on structures around it. Laboratory-based musculoskeletal modelling reveals that muscle loads, and consequently bone loads, reach their peak nearer midstance of the running gait cycle, not near initial contact.[10, 11]

Muscle-generated loads are introduced at a slower rate than those experienced with the impact peak, but their magnitude is much greater. It is the magnitude of bone load

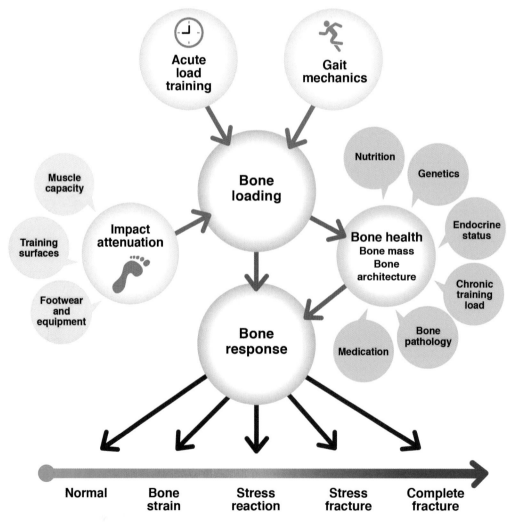

**Figure 9.7** How various load-related (blue) factors interact with bone health (pink) to influence the bone response

(as opposed to the rate of bone loading) that appears most relevant to bone fatigue.[12] At this stage, there is no clinically applicable means of estimating internal bone forces.

The role of muscle-generated internal forces in bone stress/strain begs the question as to whether strong muscles cause bone stress injuries or protect against them. On the one hand, muscle generates the highest bone loads and contributes to microdamage which can extend to bone stress injury. On the other hand, muscle activity can dampen landing forces—think of the quadriceps cushioning the landing force that affects the knee. Fatigue increases the load bone sees[13, 14] and lower muscle size and strength is a risk factor for bone stress injury.[15-18]

## Biomechanical factors

Faulty biomechanics can contribute to stress fracture risk because abnormal motion increases forces at a specific site. Excessive hip external rotation,[19] leg-length discrepancy,[20] and both pes planus[21] and pes cavus[22]—all "static" measures—increase the risk of an athlete having a stress fracture. Kinematic variables—greater peak hip adduction, excessive knee internal rotation and peak rearfoot eversion in the frontal plane during running,[23-25] less knee flexion in the sagittal plane—have also been associated with stress fractures.[26]

## Training factors

Increases in frequency and volume of loading and an athlete's usual workload are central to developing bone stress injuries. In military populations who suddenly launch into full training, pain appears as early as 3 weeks and injury incidence peaks 8 weeks after the unaccustomed activity began.[27]

Historically, considerations regarding workload have focused on training volume (e.g. weekly running distance). This led to the "maximum 10% rule" to guide weekly increases in training volume. However, there is much individual variability with respect to tolerance to changes in training loads[28] and it is unlikely that a single "rule" can be uniformly applied to eliminate running-related bone stress injuries[29] or any other type of complex tissue-loading behaviour (see also Chapter 15).

Training workloads should be individualised since two runners may have identical training loads but different injury patterns. A runner's risk of injury relates to the complex interaction between rapid changes in workload and their biomechanics, physiology, musculoskeletal qualities (including anatomy), energy availability and psychology.

There has also been a shift away from focusing on training volume/distance to incorporating metrics of intensity (e.g. speed) and perceived effort.[30] Running at faster speeds increases bone stresses and strains. Bone can less readily tolerate increases in bone stress and strain than it can tolerate an increase in the number of loading cycles. For loads relevant to running, it has been estimated a 10% increase in tissue stress or strain results in halving the number of loading cycles before fatigue failure.[12] Thus, rapid increases in training intensity, despite maintenance of training volume, heighten bone stress injury risk.

## Playing surface

Playing surface has historically been considered a contributor to bone stress injury risk. Competing on harder surfaces (such as asphalt/bitumen) was thought to increase loading compared with softer surfaces (such as grass, rubber and sand) but the interaction between playing surface and injury risk is complex. Athletes alter their leg stiffness when running on surfaces of differing compliance, apparently to maintain a constant vertical excursion of their centre of mass.[31] Athletes also subconsciously accommodate their leg "stiffness" when running on harder surfaces. However, loading rates do increase when running on surfaces that are less compliant.[32] Ultimately, what may be important with bone stress injuries is whether there has been a recent change in running surface.

## Shoes and inserts

The role of shoes and inserts (orthotics and insoles) on bone loading and ultimately stress fracture risk is a topic of ongoing debate. Shoes and inserts act as filters that theoretically attenuate ground impact forces. They have the potential to influence motion of the foot and ankle, and the subsequent mechanics proximally in the kinetic chain. Interestingly, a recent case series suggested an association between the wearing of "supershoes" containing a carbon fibre plate and navicular bone stress injuries in runners.[33] The impact of supershoes on bone loading and injury risk is being investigated. See Chapter 13 for further discussion of how shoes may affect biomechanics and subsequently different types of injury risk.

### *Factors modifying the ability of bone to resist and/or respond to damage*

Three modifiable factors may affect bone's ability to resist loading:

- physical activity history: a longer history of physical activity protects against bone stress injury[34-38]
- energy availability: see Box 9.3 and Figures 9.8 and 9.9
- calcium and vitamin D status: both are essential for bone health, but adequate loading is also essential for bone.

**BOX 9.3**   Relative energy deficiency in sport

Low energy availability results from insufficient dietary intake to meet exercise energy expenditure. It can result from low dietary energy intake (whether inadvertent, intentional or psychopathological) and/or excessive exercise energy expenditure. When sustained over medium to long periods of time, low energy availability can affect hormone function in athletes of both sexes and lead to problems associated with REDs[7] (discussed in *Clinical Sports Medicine, 5e: The Medicine of Exercise*). Figure 9.8 summarises the effects of low energy availability on different aspects of an athlete's health.

Female athletes have a greater risk of bone stress injury.[43] This appears to be related to sex differences such as lower total bone mass, but may also be related to sociocultural factors that put pressure on females

(and some males) to maintain a low body weight leading to lower energy intake and subsequently low energy availability.

It is increasingly recognised that low energy availability leading to REDs can impact both the development and prognosis of a bone stress injury. The new REDs Clinical Assessment Tool, Version 2 can help detect REDs and grade its severity and risk (Fig. 9.9).

IOC consensus statement on REDs

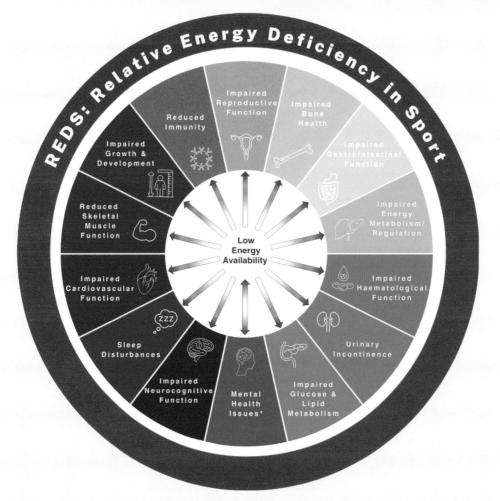

**Figure 9.8** Effects of sustained low energy availability on different aspects of health

Source: Mountjoy M, Ackerman KE, Bailey DM, et al. 2023 International Olympic Committee's (IOC) consensus statement on relative energy deficiency in sport (REDs). *Br J Sports Med* 2023;57(17):1073–98. © 2023 BMJ Publishing Group Ltd & British Association of Sport and Exercise Medicine. All rights reserved.

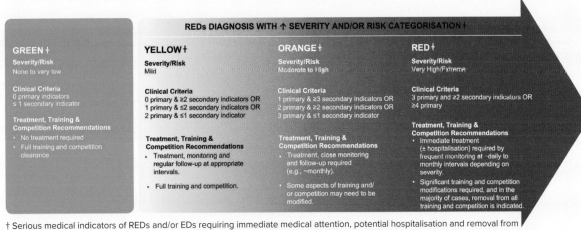

REDs DIAGNOSIS WITH ↑ SEVERITY AND/OR RISK CATEGORISATION †

**GREEN †**

Severity/Risk
None to very low

Clinical Criteria
0 primary indicators
≤ 1 secondary indicator

Treatment, Training &
Competition Recommendations
• No treatment required
• Full training and competition clearance

**YELLOW †**

Severity/Risk
Mild

Clinical Criteria
0 primary & ≥2 secondary indicators OR
1 primary & ≤2 secondary indicators OR
2 primary & ≤1 secondary indicator

Treatment, Training &
Competition Recommendations
• Treatment, monitoring and regular follow-up at appropriate intervals.
• Full training and competition.

**ORANGE †**

Severity/Risk
Moderate to High

Clinical Criteria
1 primary & ≥3 secondary indicators OR
2 primary & ≥2 secondary indicators OR
3 primary & ≤1 secondary indicator

Treatment, Training &
Competition Recommendations
• Treatment, close monitoring and follow-up required (e.g., ~monthly).
• Some aspects of training and/ or competition may need to be modified.

**RED †**

Severity/Risk
Very High/Extreme

Clinical Criteria
3 primary and ≥2 secondary indicators OR
≥4 primary

Treatment, Training &
Competition Recommendations
• Immediate treatment (± hospitalisation) required by frequent monitoring at ~daily to monthly intervals depending on severity.
• Significant training and competition modifications required, and in the majority of cases, removal from all training and competition is indicated.

B

† Serious medical indicators of REDs and/or EDs requiring immediate medical attention, potential hospitalisation and removal from training and competition, include: ≤75% median BMI for age and sex; electrolyte disturbances; ECG abnormalities (e.g. prolonged QTc interval or severe bradycardia [adult: HR ≤30 bpm; adolescent: HR ≤45 bpm]); severe hypotension: ≤90/45 mmHg; orthostatic intolerance (adult and adolescent a supine to standing systolic BP drop >20 mmHg and a diastolic drop >10 mmHg); failure of outpatient ED treatment program; acute medical complications of malnutrition; any condition that inhibits medical treatment and monitoring while training and/or competing.

**Figure 9.9** REDs Clinical Assessment Tool, Version 2
Source: Mountjoy M, Ackerman KE, Bailey DM, et al. 2023 International Olympic Committee's (IOC) consensus statement on relative energy deficiency in sport (REDs). *Br J Sports Med* 2023;57(17):1073–98. © 2023 BMJ Publishing Group Ltd & British Association of Sport and Exercise Medicine. All rights reserved.

Consuming more calcium and vitamin D alone will not support effective bone health or healing.[39,40] In a large randomised trial, female Navy recruits who had suboptimal baseline daily calcium intake and took daily calcium and vitamin D supplements had 20% fewer stress fractures than their control counterparts during basic training.[41] Athletes should have sufficient calcium and vitamin D intake to meet or exceed the current recommended dietary allowance of 1000–1300 mg and 600 IU (for individuals aged 14–50 years), respectively.[42] Note that food sources provide calcium more effectively than do supplements.

## Diagnosis of bone stress injuries

History taking and physical examination are the foundation stones for diagnosis. Imaging may be used to confirm a suspected diagnosis and support decisions on management of the injury. Suspicion of a bone stress injury is increased in the presence of prominent risk factors, such as participation in an "at-risk" activity (e.g. distance running or ballet dancing), symptoms presenting at a skeletal site known to be loaded during the athlete's activities, recent changes in activity levels, a history of previous stress fracture and/or the presence of indicators suggestive of REDs.

The patient with a bone stress injury reports activity-related pain. The features and nature of pain can vary greatly between individuals and depending on the location of the injury. An athlete may initially describe that their pain started as a mild ache occurring after a specific amount of exercise. It may also have developed during or immediately after loading. The athlete may report pain the day after training when they initially passed off the post-training pain as typical soreness.

On physical examination the most obvious feature is localised bony tenderness. Certain bones (such as the tibia, fibula and metatarsals) are easy to palpate. Direct palpation is not possible at deeper sites (such as the femur and pars interarticularis of the spine); you can diagnose injury at these sites with specific bone-loading tests, such as hopping[44] and the fulcrum test for the femoral shaft.[45] These tests have limited sensitivity and specificity—you will need to apply reasoning to decide whether the patient should be investigated further or not. Therapeutic ultrasound and vibrating tuning forks are *not* useful in diagnosing bone pathology.[46]

### Imaging and grading severity of bone stress injuries

MRI is the modality of choice when investigating bone pain because of its high contrast resolution, lack of ionising radiation and combined high sensitivity and specificity. Plain radiographs have a role because of their low cost and wide availability; however, they should not be used to look for pars stress fractures because of the high dose of truncal radiation. If an athlete has had a recent onset of pain,

**TABLE 9.2**   The Fredericson MRI bone stress injury classification system adapted to include updated nomenclature and potential differences in prognosis at different severities of bone stress injury

| New nomenclature | | Historical nomenclature | Potential prognosis |
|---|---|---|---|
| **Grade 0** | Normal | Normal | Normal |
| **Grade 1** | Periosteal oedema | Stress reaction | Variable time period to recovery but prognosis is that the athlete may begin impact activities again within 8 weeks[48] |
| **Grade 2** | Marrow oedema (visible on MRI T2-weighted images) | | |
| **Grade 3** | Marrow oedema (visible on MRI T1- and T2-weighted images) | | |
| **Grade 4a** | Intracortical signal changes (multiple focal areas) | | |
| **Grade 4b** | Linear region of intracortical signal change | Stress fracture | Indicates worse prognosis, likely to take at least 9–10 weeks before return to impact activities posslbly longer |

radiographs are very unlikely to be of use as bone changes lag weeks behind.

CT involves high exposure to ionising radiation and lacks sensitivity but may be used if you feel that visualising a fracture line may affect treatment (e.g. with a femoral neck stress fracture). CT can also be considered in cases with high concern for injury, including the tarsal navicular (sometimes missed on MRI), that have clinical concern for non-union, or to evaluate an athlete for avascular necrosis. Dual-energy CT shows promise in visualising the bone marrow oedema/trabecular microfracture seen with bone stress injury.[47] Radionuclide bone scan uses extremely high ionising radiation, relegating recommendations for its use to situations where other methods of diagnosis are unavailable.

**PRACTICE PEARL**

MRI is the preferred imaging technique for diagnosing bone stress injuries due to its greater specificity and sensitivity at all stages of the bone strain/stress continuum.

The ability of MRI and other imaging modalities to predict when an athlete will return to sport is a subject of controversy. Certainly, there are high-risk anatomical areas (e.g. the femoral neck, anterior mid-tibial diaphysis and tarsal navicular) in which delayed return to sport can be expected.[6] Imaging findings of bone healing tend to lag behind clinical healing. Imaging should be considered as part of the decision matrix, strongly supported by clinical findings.

Dr Michael Fredericson's MRI classification system was published in 1995 and was primarily directed at tibial injuries;[48] other systems have since been proposed.[49] The most significant finding on imaging is a T1-weighted low-signal discrete cortical line (Fredericson 4b), often indicating a prolonged return to sport. This suggests an abbreviated classification system of bone marrow oedema (periosteal, cortical and medullary) as one stage, and the identification of a cortical line as the other. Table 9.2 demonstrates how the Fredericson classification can support clinical decision making, but the imaging information has to be considered alongside the anatomical site of the injury.[50]

## Why are some stress fractures low risk and others high risk?

Stress fractures can be classified into low or high risk according to their location. The "risk" refers to the natural history of these injuries and the chances of a poor outcome. For example, most patients who have a fibular stress fracture recover well if they stop loading their leg. In contrast, many promising athletic careers have been curtailed by a stress fracture of the navicular bone. Figure 9.10 details which stress fractures are considered low and high risk.

In Chapter 12 we outline that tension and compression forces act on bone. Compression forces help bone to heal, whereas tension forces pull the healing ends of a fracture apart. Low-risk stress fractures predominantly occur on the compression side of a bone's bending axis and have a favourable natural history in that recovery occurs with a low incidence of complications and without the need for aggressive intervention (such as surgery and/or prolonged

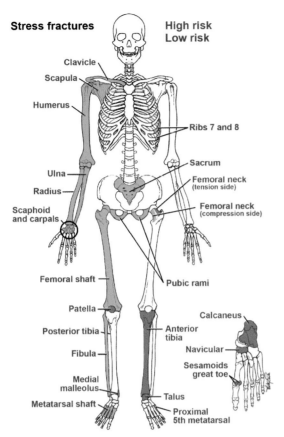

**Stress fractures**

High risk
Low risk

Clavicle

Scapula

Humerus

Ribs 7 and 8

Ulna

Sacrum

Radius

Femoral neck
(tension side)

Scaphoid
and carpals

Femoral neck
(compression side)

Femoral shaft

Pubic rami

Patella

Calcaneus

Posterior tibia

Anterior
tibia

Fibula

Navicular

Sesamoids
great toe

Medial
malleolus

Talus

Metatarsal shaft

Proximal
5th metatarsal

**Figure 9.10** High- and low-risk stress fractures. Note all high-risk sites are located in the lower limbs and feet.

modified weight-bearing). In contrast, high-risk stress fractures often occur on the tension side of a bone's bending axis and present treatment challenges demanding specific attention because they are prone to delayed or non-union and/or are at high risk for progression to complete fracture.

One particularly good example of how the site of a stress fracture influences management is at the femoral neck where compression-side fractures are often treated conservatively, whereas tension-side stress fractures would leave an athlete at risk of requiring surgery. Figure 9.11 depicts compression and tension at different surfaces of two bones.

## Healing of bone stress injuries

We close this section on bone pathophysiology by underscoring that healing (part of the natural history of bone stress injuries) must be assessed clinically by the absence of local tenderness and functionally by the ability to perform without pain. It is not useful to attempt to monitor healing with radiographs, CT or MRI.[51] CT scan appearances of healing stress fractures can be deceptive as in some cases the fracture is still visible well after clinical healing has occurred.[51] Figure 9.12 shows the relationship between imaging appearance and the various stages of bone stress.

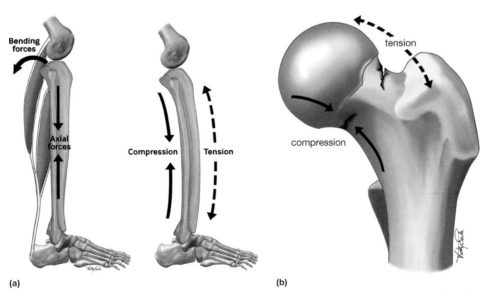

Bending
forces

Axial
forces

Compression    Tension

(a)

tension

compression

(b)

**Figure 9.11** The concept of compression and tension is fundamental to understanding why the precise location of a bone stress injury bone stress injury affects its prognosis. (a) Tibial stress fractures on the tension side (anterior tibial cortex) have a much greater risk of non-union and complete fracture than stress fractures on the compression side (medial tibial cortex). (b) Image of the neck of the femur: weight-bearing tends to "open" the tension side (prevent healing).

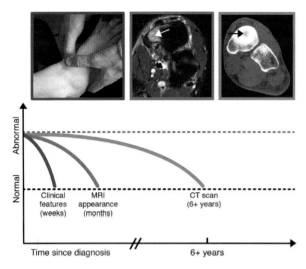

Figure 9.12 Stress fracture healing. Timeline for recovery in clinical features, appearance on MRI and appearance on CT scan. Note imaging findings resolve much later than clinical union occurs.

## BONE STRESS INJURIES: MANAGEMENT PRINCIPLES

*Clinical Sports Medicine 6e: Managing Injuries* deals with common bone stress injuries and their specific management. Here we outline some common principles relevant to low- and high-risk stress fractures.

### Low-risk bone stress injuries

The cornerstone of low-risk bone stress injury management is a period of modified activity followed by a gradual return to physical activity/sport and exercise.

#### First things first: reduce load

An axiom of bone stress injury management is that the athlete must become pain-free during and after activities of daily living before they return to function. Cushioned shoes and/or insoles may help dissipate impact forces during daily living for athletes with a rearfoot or leg bone stress injury, whereas athletes whose midfoot or forefoot is injured may consider wearing a stiff-soled shoe to reduce bending forces and symptoms. The athlete should minimise walking and if they demonstrate an antalgic gait, they should use an aid (e.g. an elbow crutch). If pain persists despite these interventions, a brief period (days) of reduced weight-bearing in a walking boot may prove useful.

> **PRACTICE PEARL**
>
> While recovering from a bone stress injury, the athlete should not tolerate any pain during or after activity. If pain occurs, activities should be reduced further until the athlete is pain-free.

Early in rehabilitation, athletes may continue to notice pain at rest around the fracture site, but this should disappear within 2–3 days of limiting activity. When activities resume, the athlete should be pain-free around the fractured bone both during the activity and for 24 hours afterwards. If the athlete experiences pain, the intensity of the loading should be reduced or removed until their pain has settled. Athletes may ask you about non-steroidal anti-inflammatory drugs (NSAIDs) or other analgesics; discourage use of these medications as they can mask pain and may impede bone repair.[52]

To prepare the athlete for a return to running and to prevent deconditioning, they should begin rehabilitation immediately. Options for rehabilitation while an athlete is still unable to fully weight-bear through the affected bone include using the antigravity treadmill or pool running to maintain running specific benefits. Athletes may also be able to undertake other types of cross-training to maintain aerobic fitness depending on the severity and site of the bone stress injury. You should prescribe strength and conditioning programs to support areas surrounding or adjacent to the injury prior to the return-to-running stage.

Athletes should not attempt to restart running until they are able to walk pain-free, perform a single-leg hop pain free and with good form. Athletes should also be declared medically fit to resume exercise; for instance, they should be cleared of any underlying concerns that may further impact their bone health.

#### Return to running in four stages

Once the athlete is completely pain-free walking and during other normal activities for 5 consecutive days, they can begin to progressively add back running-related loads. For distance-running athletes this can be divided into four stages:

- *Stage 1* introduces loading in 30-minute sessions separated by rest days. Sessions consist of increasing durations of running at a steady pace ("steady" is based on the rate of perceived exertion or heart rate) and decreasing durations of walking. This may be best achieved in a controlled environment such as on the treadmill.

- *Stage 2* may include a small increase in pace but focuses on increasing the frequency or length of running. This includes a return to consecutive days of running followed by recovery days.
- *Stage 3* focuses on increasing the intensity so that the athlete begins to return to their prior running speeds. Intensity is best measured using an internal load measure such as heart rate.
- *Stage 4* involves individualised running until there is a complete return to desired running activities. This can mean changing pace and terrain, and adding significant amounts of climbing or descending if running on trails, etc.

Table 9.3 provides an example of taking an athlete through the four stages and includes suggested criteria for progressing between stages. The primary criterion for progressing within or between stages is pain experienced at the bone stress injury site. If the athlete experiences pain during or after a session, they should stop the session and return to the previous level at which they were pain-free (e.g. 1-min run, followed by 2-min walk repeated 10 times). Patients with lower-grade bone stress injuries may progress more quickly through a graduated loading program. Program duration should be based on the known clinical time course for recovery as a minimum, but the patient's program should be individualised.

### Antigravity treadmill training

Athletes who have access to an antigravity treadmill may exchange or supplement a usual return to run program with running in a reduced bodyweight environment (Box 9.4).

### Can running gait retraining prevent bone stress injury recurrence?

Several gait retraining techniques have been suggested by runners, coaches and clinicians to limit running-related injuries (including stress fractures). As discussed earlier, ground reaction forces (our current best way to measure running-related forces) are not highly correlated with internal tissue stress. Gait retraining doesn't eliminate the role of force, but it can shift forces away from tissues with lower tolerance to load. It may still be worth considering as a short- to medium-term measure with athletes who wish to return to running as soon as possible.

Some methods to support gait retraining include:

- *Using accelerometer-based biofeedback:* this can be used to reduce the magnitude and rate of loading.[56] An athlete can use on-screen real-time feedback with instructions to find a way to land that reduces the impact peaks of each foot strike (often with verbal feedback to "land quietly").

- *Increasing stride rate:* this aims to increase the athlete's number of steps per min over a specific distance. This reduces their stride length, affecting several kinematic variables around the point of contact.[57] Although the total load will remain the same (the forces absorbed by bone and other tissues will just be spread over a greater number of foot strikes), the peaks of each individual loading cycle (foot strike) will be reduced.[58]

  Athletes tend to self-select their own favoured stride rate based on their individual anatomy and physiology, so changes should be individualised and aim to increase their stride rate by no more than 10% in total. This increase should be trained incrementally (e.g. an athlete who runs at 150 steps per min should aim to go no higher than 165 and may initially increase to 155 for a period before attempting 160 etc.). Athletes asked to increase immediately by 10% often run faster without reducing stride length, increasing bone loads and perhaps even increasing their risk of injury.

- *Modifying foot strike:* prevailing dogma suggests that athletes should be encouraged to adopt a forefoot strike. While this may be advantageous for performance at sprint and middle-distance events, it is often less successful for the half-marathon or longer due to fatigue in the plantar flexors (fatigue can also cause changes mid-event).[59] The majority of runners adopt a foot-strike pattern that feels best for them and both elite and recreational runners tend to run with either mid- or rear-foot strike in longer distance events.[60,61]

  However, runners with specific stress fractures may be asked to adopt an alternative foot-strike pattern (either temporarily or long term). For instance, a runner with a metatarsal stress fracture may find it beneficial to move from a forefoot to a mid- or rear-foot strike. Each case should be evaluated individually and discussed with the athlete based on their condition.

- *Switching shoes:* not a gait retraining intervention in itself, but switching shoes can influence the ease with which an athlete can attempt to change associated variables. For instance, wearing a shoe with a lower heel-to-toe drop and lower overall stack height can support an athlete to adopt a more mid- or forefoot strike. Therefore, this may be considered as an adjunct intervention for those undergoing gait retraining.

### Caveat emptor—buyer beware!

Gait retraining efficacy is variable as running patterns (i.e. motor control) are engrained over long periods of time, making short-term bouts of retraining ineffective for anything beyond symptom relief.

**TABLE 9.3**   An example of a four-stage program to return to running after bone stress injury

| Stage 1 | Initial loading, going from walking to running | Progression criteria |
|---|---|---|
| | Athlete should be able to tolerate weight-bearing in walking. Focus is on increasing the amount of running vs walking. Starting point will be dictated by the athlete, the severity of their injury and their previous capacity. | Pain-free completion of each run session |
| | Running frequency should be no more than every 48 hrs to allow the athlete to monitor 24-hr response to running loads. | 30 mins of running with no or less than 10% walking |
| | Begin run:walk ratio below the athlete's pain threshold, for instance 1-min run, 3-mins walk and repeat × 7. Slowly increase the ratio of running to walking as the athlete's symptoms allow. Keep all stage 1 activities to 30 mins maximum. | Maintain strength and conditioning program |
| | Often runners may be asked to complete each session pain-free *twice* before progressing to the next cycle of run:walk. | |

| Week 1 | Week 2 | Week 3 |
|---|---|---|
| Day 1 Run 1 min, walk 4 mins (× 6) | Day 8 Rest | Day 15 Run 5 mins, walk 1 min (× 5) |
| Day 2 Rest | Day 9 Run 2 mins, walk 1 min (× 10) | Day 16 Rest or cross-training |
| Day 3 Run 1 min, walk 3 mins (× 7) | Day 10 Rest or cross-training | Day 17 Run 6 mins, walk 1 min (× 4) |
| Day 4 Rest | Day 11 Run 2 mins, walk 1 min (× 7) | Day 18 Rest or cross-training |
| Day 5 Run 1 min, walk 2 mins (× 10) | Day 12 Rest or cross-training | Day 19 Run 7 mins, walk 1 min (× 4) |
| Day 6 Rest | Day 13 Run 4 mins, walk 1 min (× 6) | Day 20 Rest or cross-training |
| Day 7 Run 1 min, walk 1 min (× 15) | Day 14 Rest or cross-training | Day 21 Run 9 mins, walk 1 min (× 3) |

Run intensity should stay at 5/10. Alternatively, if the athlete uses heart rate to measure training intensity, they can be advised to stay at the low end of heart-rate zone 2 (5-zone model).

| Stage 2 | Increasing exposure to distance OR frequency | Progression criteria |
|---|---|---|
| | Athlete can now run 30 mins pain-free. | Pain-free completion of each run session |
| | **Progressions should focus on increasing the amount of time OR frequency** that the athlete is able to tolerate running. For example: | Maintain strength and conditioning program |

| Week 1 | Week 2 |
|---|---|
| Day 1 Run 30 mins | Day 8 Run 30 mins |
| Day 2 Run 30 mins | Day 9 Rest or cross-training |
| Day 3 Rest or cross-training | Day 10 Run 30 mins |
| Day 4 Run 30 mins | Day 11 Run 30 mins |
| Day 5 Run 30 mins | Day 12 Rest or cross-training |
| Day 6 Rest or cross-training | Day 13 Run 30 mins |
| Day 7 Run 30 mins | Day 14 Run 30 mins |

Run intensity should stay at a 5–6/10. If the athlete uses heart rate, they can be advised to stay in heart-rate zone 2 (5-zone model).

| Stage 3 | Reducing recovery time and testing intensity tolerance | Progression criteria |
|---|---|---|
| | Athlete is running >80% of their pre-injury frequency OR over 1 hr of steady-paced (zones 2–3) running without symptoms. | Pain-free completion of each run session |
| | To improve tolerance for faster running, add strides, drills or bounds for short distances before or following a run. | Limb symmetry index back to less than 5% deviation |
| | Run intensity can increase to 8/10 for short periods. If the athlete uses heart rate, they can reach zone 4 (5-zone model). | Maintain strength and conditioning program |

| Stage 4 | Return to performance | Progression criteria |
|---|---|---|
| | Athlete progresses different training variables depending on their goals. Variables include speed, distance, frequency, elevation gain/loss, work on technical surfaces. | Progressions based on performance rather than rehabilitation goals |
| | | Athlete bone health should be monitored. |

**BOX 9.4** How to prescribe return to running on an antigravity treadmill

The antigravity treadmill (Fig. 9.13) was a product of NASA research[53] and was first used by professional sports teams around 2008. An antigravity treadmill includes an air-filled pressure-controlled chamber that surrounds the lower half of the body from the waist down. Pressure in the chamber is modulated to unweight the runner in 1% increments so that they are running with between 100% and 20% body weight.

Demonstration of antigravity treadmill

When available, an antigravity treadmill may replace overground running and permit a faster return to running (due to the reduction in recovery time required between sessions), as well as enabling the athlete to run at higher intensities earlier during recovery. Many athletes prefer this to pool-based running, a traditional method to maintain fitness in a low-impact environment.[54] Pool running remains relevant for those without the resources to access an antigravity treadmill.

Running with a lesser body weight (i.e. using a harness) reduces the metabolic and cardiac cost of running.[55] To keep athletes working at a level consistent with their cardiovascular fitness, you can consider having them run at higher speeds or at an incline. Table 9.4 provides speed conversions for different body-weight support percentages with an athlete's corresponding overground speed.

Runners with a low-risk bone stress injury can start antigravity treadmill training once they are pain-free during walking and activities of daily living. A typical starting point is to run 2–3 times per week, performing 30-min sessions consisting of five 1-min repeats at between 50% and 70% body weight with 4–5 mins walking between repeats. You can try to increase the run: walk ratio and the body-weight percentage by 5–10% each week. Over 5–6 weeks (depending on the athlete's tolerance), the number of sessions can increase to 3 times per week between 90% and 100% body weight and to 5 repeats of 5 mins running. If the athlete is able to successfully (pain-free) perform this final session, you can discuss the resumption of overground running with an equally gradual progression back to their previous level of frequency, distance and intensity.

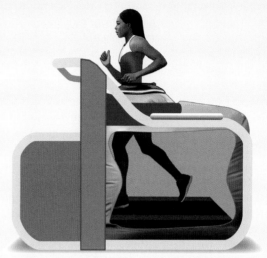

**Figure 9.13** A patient training on an antigravity treadmill

**TABLE 9.4**   Speed conversions to maintain cardiovascular fitness when using an antigravity treadmill

| Treadmill support | Corresponding speed |
| --- | --- |
| 50% bodyweight | 24.1 km/hr (2:30 min/km) |
| 60% bodyweight | 22.4 km/hr (2:41 min/km) |
| 70% bodyweight | 22.0 km/hr (2:43 min/km) |
| 80% bodyweight | 19.6 km/hr (3:04 min/km) |
| 90% bodyweight | 17.7 km/hr (3:24 min/km) |

Source: Based on Kline JR, Raab S, Coast J et al. Conversion table for running on lower body positive pressure treadmills. *J Strength Cond Res* 2015;29(3):854–62.

The current guidelines for progression using antigravity treadmill running come from literature reviews: we have relatively little evidence available to titrate these guidelines to individuals or different types of bone stress injury. Belt placement (either above or below the iliac crest height) when in the antigravity harness can also affect the accuracy of the body weight percentage reading. Try to ensure consistency between sessions and base all progressions on the athlete's symptoms.

Interventions require sustained practice on the part of the athlete with regular feedback from the practitioner in charge of supporting this adaptation. Moving forces from one area to another also risks overloading musculoskeletal structures that were previously under less stress, therefore making any transition to new stride rates, length or foot-strike patterns a risk for secondary injuries in the short- to medium-term (e.g. Achilles tendinopathy following a switch to a forefoot strike).

However, athletes with repeated stress fractures (and other injuries) may consider gait retraining. To support the ability of tissues to adjust to new forces, the athlete can also undergo a pre-conditioning program to improve their ability to tolerate new loads.

*Running program design*

If an athlete increases their training load too rapidly or frequently relative to their usual activities, they can upset the balance between bone microdamage formation and its removal. Unfortunately, there is no algorithm for how much an individual can modify their training program before their risk of bone stress injury starts to accelerate.

To advise an athlete returning from a stress fracture it is important that you obtain as much information as you can about their pre-injury training regimen. This includes information on changes in any feature that may have altered the load, including training intensity, duration, frequency, type, surface, technique and shoes. In addition, recovering athletes should be encouraged to maintain a training diary containing these data to not only track their training progress, but also to provide reliable data regarding their training program for future reference.

Encourage periodised training. Chapter 15 discusses using data to monitor athlete health and wellbeing and may provide additional information if you are looking to support athletes who need to track important training variables over time.

Following the diagnosis of a stress fracture, we recommend scheduling an appointment with the athlete to help them understand their injury and discuss how to stay fit while recovering. This appointment can also be used to support shared decision making about the athlete's injury management and how they can prevent future injuries (often including lifestyle or training changes). Box 9.5 covers three common questions athletes will ask following a bone stress injury.

## High-risk bone stress injuries

Most textbooks don't include a section on treatment of high-risk stress fractures and for good reason: each stress fracture in this category demands different treatment. For example, first-line treatment for a navicular stress fracture is prescription of a non-weight-bearing boot. Traumatic scaphoid fractures are best managed with screw fixation—randomised trials have proven that surgery is associated with faster recovery than cast immobilisation.

There is both an unspoken and a spoken pressure to consider surgery, particularly in the elite athlete. There is currently no evidence that surgery speeds return to sport in stress fractures other than stress fracture in the Jones position (proximal 5th metatarsal). Despite this, some in our field have great faith in surgery. They argue—correctly—that absence of evidence (no studies) is not absence of effectiveness. Treatment of individual high-risk stress fractures is described in the relevant sections of *Managing Injuries.*

Table 9.5 lists several high-risk stress fractures and the sports with which they are most commonly associated.[62]

What is common across high-risk stress fractures is that you should look for an underlying contributing cause such as energy insufficiency (which has numerous causes), endocrine disorder (such as abnormal thyroid function) or secondary to osteoporosis. Try to find the cause—don't assume the stress fracture is purely mechanical (even though it may be).

We close this discussion of the foundations of bone stress injury management with Box 9.6, which examines whether athletes can find marginal gains in their management of bone stress injuries.

**TABLE 9.5**   High-risk stress fractures and the sports with which they are most commonly associated

| Site of stress fracture | % | Common sports |
| --- | --- | --- |
| Pars interarticularis | <1 | Cricket fast bowling, high jump, gymnastics |
| Femoral neck | <5 | Running, endurance athletes |
| Patella | <1 | Running, basketball, gymnastics |
| Anterior tibia | 0.8–7 | Basketball, gymnastics |
| Medial malleolus | 0.6–4.1 | Running, track and field, basketball, gymnastics |
| Talus | Rare | Running, pole vaulting, basketball, gymnastics |
| Navicular | 14–25 | Track and field, football, basketball |
| Proximal 5th metatarsal | <1 | Football, basketball |
| Sesamoid | Rare | Dance, gymnastics, racquet sports |

Source: Adapted from McInnis KC, Ramey LN. High-risk stress fractures: diagnosis and management. *PM&R* 2016;8(3 Suppl):113–24.

**BOX 9.5** Discussing risk factors for a bone stress injury with the athlete

### Why did this happen to me?

The athlete will want to know why they got the injury (i.e. what are the risk factors from your perspective). These injuries are usually multifactorial and the discussion may touch on several of the following topics:

- *Age:* hormonal changes as we age make us more susceptible to lower bone mineral density so older athletes (>30) may have a higher risk.
- *Family history:* low bone mineral density may have a genetic component so athletes who have a family history of osteoporosis/osteopenia may be more susceptible.
- *General health:* other conditions that can lead to reduced bone density include coeliac disease, thyroid disorders, inflammatory bowel disease, kidney or liver disease, cancer, multiple myeloma and rheumatoid arthritis.
- *Medications:* certain medications can lead to reduced bone mineral density, including steroids (medical or non-medical use), autoimmune medications and medications that affect digestion.
- *Previous history of stress fractures:* a very important predictor of stress fracture; how was the previous fracture managed?
- *Load or factors that alter tissue stress:* a detailed activity history is important. Many athletes have data they can share (e.g. through training platforms like Strava, Garmin or TrainingPeaks). Discuss recent changes in activity frequency, duration and intensity, changes in playing surface or equipment (e.g. shoes) and ask about participation in physical activity beyond running.
- *Leanness and nutritional status:* low body mass index is a risk factor associated with inadequate nutrition. Maintain a high index of suspicion regarding athletes who participate in weight-dependent or "leanness" sports. Note that a body mass index of <19 is mentioned in some studies, but that is a statistical cut-off whereas risk of injury associated with leanness is a continuum and will be similar at a range of BMIs in real life. Low BMI may be relative to the athlete's previous history, so discussing their weight history may be key, even if they are currently within the normal or healthy weight range.
- *REDs:* linked to leanness and nutritional status, REDs is perhaps the most critical risk factor in otherwise young healthy adults. Explore a detailed dietary history to evaluate deficits in energy intake and/or eating disorders. Inexperienced clinicians focus on calcium and vitamin D intake but overall nutrition influences risk of injury far more than calcium intake alone. In endurance sports, adequate carbohydrate intake is key to recovery and to avoid periods of energy deficit. Management of REDs is ideally done in a multidisciplinary team setting (taking athlete agency and preference into account of course).
- *Detailed menstrual history:* often linked as a symptom of REDs, assess age of menarche and how menstrual status has varied over time with training and/or nutrition changes. You may also need to ask about the nature of menstruation (e.g. whether periods are light, short) and particularly whether this has changed recently, as this may indicate a change in hormone production.

### Did biomechanical factors contribute?

Biomechanics alone can lead to stress fractures in otherwise healthy adult athletes. Athletes naturally push their bodies to extreme lengths to go faster, longer, harder than their competition. Changes in training are a risk factor but repetitive biomechanical overload of specific structures can also lead to bone stress injuries. Assess the athlete's:

- history of overuse injuries (which may give additional pointers for where musculoskeletal structures are being overloaded)
- static posture and alignment
- gait, using recent videos of the athlete running
- unilateral dominance (i.e. movement asymmetry)
- hip, knee and foot mechanics during non-painful activities such as walking or single-leg squats
- shoe wear pattern.

Depending on the individual and preliminary examination findings, initial biomechanical interventions may address suspected deficits. Interventions may include muscle strength, endurance and motor-control training to address muscle length and/or joint mobility. Key areas to consider include motor control; endurance and strength at the hip, knee and ankle; core stability; and strength of the intrinsic and extrinsic muscles of the foot. Activities may need to be modified to be pain-free, and performed non- or partial weight-bearing.

### How can I maintain my fitness?

Maintaining physical conditioning during recovery is important for a seamless return to activity, as the athlete's pathology permits. If the athlete has hormonal changes (such as low testosterone in males), it may be best to counsel against endurance activities and instead focus on anabolic (bone-building) activities, including heavy resistance training (depending on the fracture site).

If the injury precludes heavy loading in one limb (e.g. a calcaneal stress fracture), the athlete may be able to focus on upper limb or contralateral limb training. The focus should be on maintaining a positive energy balance, but general conditioning activities should be introduced early.

For low-risk stress fractures, activities such as cycling, swimming, deep-water running and antigravity treadmill training should be encouraged early on. The latter two may be most specific in running athletes as they more closely reproduce the neuromuscular recruitment patterns involved in running. Deep-water running can be introduced as long as the athlete is pain-free during and after sessions, progressing towards antigravity treadmill training, which increases the load on bones in the lower limb.

**B**

We estimate that hundreds of millions of dollars have been spent in the search for an electrotherapy or pharmaceutical treatment to accelerate the repair of bone stress injuries. However, there is no convincing evidence to support the use of any such treatment at present.

### Electrotherapy

Preclinical and preliminary clinical support exists for using low-intensity pulsed ultrasonography in managing bone stress injuries, but a pilot randomised trial did not find a benefit to recovery from low-risk tibial, metatarsal and fibular bone stress injuries.[63] Despite this lack of high-level evidence of efficacy, low-intensity pulsed ultrasound therapy is used in clinical management of bone stress injuries.

Similarly, in a randomised controlled study of tibial bone stress injuries, capacitively coupled electric field therapy did not induce faster healing across all injuries, although higher grade injuries healed faster with this treatment.[64] The application of pulsed electromagnetic fields is not fully established in clinical routine.[65]

No high-level studies have been performed to evaluate the efficacy of extracorporeal shockwave therapy, but resolution of non-union with this approach in delayed union of stress fractures has been documented in a number of case series.[66–68]

### Pharmaceuticals

A number of pharmaceutical agents may help bone stress injuries to heal, yet they are unlikely to receive regulatory approval due the difficulty in establishing their efficacy in clinical trials. Thus, their use will likely remain off-label. The two agents with the most promise are parathyroid hormone and anti-sclerostin antibody therapy.

Parathyroid hormone, when administered intermittently, promotes osteoblastogenesis and osteoblast survival, which promote bone gain.[69–70] Because the protein sclerostin reduces osteoblastic bone formation, anti-sclerostin antibody promotes osteoblast proliferation and function.[71,72] So these two agents achieve osteoblast activity but via different cell communication pathways. Both accelerate fracture healing in preclinical models, but whether the same fracture healing benefits carry over to humans with bone stress injuries remains unknown. Further research is required before recommending either treatment.

## OTHER OVERUSE CONDITIONS OF BONE

### Osteitis

Osteitis (impaction trauma or primary inflammation of bone) and periostitis (abnormal histological appearance of periosteal collagen) are overuse injuries. Although traditionally they may have been seen as separate from bone stress injuries, we encourage you to think of them as low-risk injuries on the bone stress continuum. Both conditions result from chronic repetitive loading in the absence of time to functionally adapt (or where there are underlying reasons why adaptation is slow to occur).[73]

The most common examples include osteitis pubis, which occurs in the pubic bones of the pelvis and is characterised by deep-seated pain and tenderness of the symphysis pubis. It was historically diagnosed using radionuclide bone scan but now MRI is used and shows bone marrow oedema. However, the imaging appearance does not correlate well with clinical findings. The current thinking is that this condition may be a form of apophysitis. It is discussed more fully in Chapter 18 of *Managing Injuries*.

### Periostitis

Periostitis, most often at the medial tibial border, was traditionally regarded as inflammation of the periosteal layer of bone ("shin splints" or medial tibial stress syndrome). In this condition, tenderness along the medial border of the tibia at the interface between the muscles and their bony attachments corresponds with an area of increased MRI signal in the periosteal tissue and sometimes in the bone marrow. Clinically, the symptoms often differ from those of a tibial bone stress injury by the breadth of the tenderness (bone stress injuries are often more pinpoint), but it can be difficult to differentiate periostitis from a bone stress injury without further investigation.[73]

Many clinicians believe that periostitis is a form of bone stress injury and manage it accordingly. It is discussed more fully in Chapter 27 of *Managing Injuries*.

### Apophysitis

Bony injury caused by overuse may occur at the attachment of the strong, large tendons to areas where bone is developing rapidly (i.e. during adolescence). This condition is known as apophysitis and the most common examples are Osgood-Schlatter disease (attachment of the patellar tendon to the tibial tuberosity) and Sever's disease (attachment of the Achilles tendon to the calcaneus). Apophysitis is considered to be a mixture of both bone and tendon overload. Management of apophysitis is detailed in Chapter 32 of *Managing Injuries*.

## ARTICULAR CARTILAGE

Overuse injury can affect the articular cartilage lining of joints. Changes range from microscopic inflammatory changes to softening, fibrillation, fissuring and ultimately gross visible changes. In younger people, this pathology can arise at the patella (patellofemoral pain), but it is important to note that patellofemoral pain can occur in the presence of normal joint surfaces. This very common condition is discussed in Chapter 24 of *Managing Injuries*.

## JOINT

Inflammatory changes in joints associated with overuse are classified as synovitis or capsulitis. Examples include the sinus tarsi syndrome of the subtalar joint[74] and synovitis of the hip joint.

Impingement syndromes occur when a bony abnormality, either congenital or acquired, causes two bony surfaces to impinge on each other (e.g. femoroacetabular impingement syndrome at the hip, or posterior impingement at the ankle), or impinge on a structure passing between them (e.g. supraspinatus tendon at the shoulder) causing damage to that structure. Treatment requires either modification of the athlete's biomechanics to relieve the impingement or removal of the structural abnormality (e.g. surgery).

In patients with femoroacetabular impingement syndrome, surgery for cam-type impingement may be successful,[75] whereas shoulder surgery (sub-acromial decompression) has failed to demonstrate long-term efficacy.[76] As overall results are still mixed and physiotherapy provides benefit and does not negatively impact patients who progress to surgery, it may be considered as the first-line option in many cases.[77]

## LIGAMENT

Overuse injuries of ligaments are uncommon but may occur as a result of excessive load. Injuries to the ulnar collateral ligament of the elbow in baseball pitchers are the most common ligamentous overuse injury.[78] Management of this condition is discussed in Chapter 10 of *Managing Injuries*.

## MUSCLE

Athletes with overuse muscle conditions may present with several conditions, including myofascial pain and chronic exertional compartment syndrome.

### Myofascial pain

The clinical phenomenon of muscle tenderness is, dare we say it, universal but scientists don't agree on the pathology.

### *The trigger point model*

The myofascial trigger point theory was pioneered by Travell and Simons more than 30 years ago.[79] The theory has had widespread acceptance until recent times. Trigger points are classified as either active or latent, with only active trigger points being symptomatic. Active trigger points are thought to be tender to palpation, generate a local twitch response on stimulation and create a predictable pattern of referred pain on compression.

The term "myofascial pain syndrome" is commonly used to describe the clinical signs thought to represent active trigger points. As per Travell's original description, this is characterised by:

1. localised areas of deep muscle tenderness or hyperirritability, referred to as trigger points—palpable taut bands within the muscle associated with muscle inhibition, intolerance to stretch as well as autonomic symptoms such as vasoconstriction or dilation
2. a predictable, discrete reference zone of deep aching pain that is worsened by palpation of the trigger point. This may be located in the immediate region of or remote from the trigger point.

Dommerholt expanded on Travell's theory, postulating a role for excessive release of acetylcholine from dysfunctional neuromuscular endplates, causing taut bands and subsequent muscle ischaemia. This muscle ischaemia was thought to precipitate an energy crisis in the muscle, causing the release of pro-inflammatory molecules, thereby activating nociceptive neurons.[80] Newer theories subject to research include the principle of neurogenic inflammation leading to sensitisation of innervated muscle,[81] secondary allodynia secondary to irritation of deeper structures such as ligament or bone (central sensitisation),[82] descending inhibitory pain modulation[83] and diffuse noxious inhibitory control.[84]

Despite the abundance of hypothesised theories regarding the pathophysiology of myofascial trigger points, their existence is not widely accepted in the medical literature. Furthermore, much of the research to date is limited by significant methodological flaws.[81] Consequently, despite many years of research endeavour, the diagnosis, treatment and pathophysiological mechanisms underlying localised palpatory muscle pain remain an area of vigorous debate.[81, 85] Despite this, the lack of definitive anatomical or biochemical evidence has not prevented the concept of trigger points from achieving popularity among sports and musculoskeletal medicine clinicians.

A diagnosis of trigger points causing pain must only be made following the appropriate exclusion of alternative diagnoses. Failure to respond to appropriate treatment should necessitate a review of the diagnosis.

Fluctuations in pain over the course of a day or longer periods are typical of trigger points and suggestive that acute tissue trauma is not involved. Fluctuations usually follow particular events, such as lying on a particular side in bed, or computer-based work. This is quite distinct from the diurnal variation seen in inflammatory conditions. While the pain of trigger points has a different temporal pattern to that of tissue trauma, it is important to note that trigger points are often secondary to, and therefore frequently coexist with, acute tissue trauma.

The spatial distribution of pain also differs between trigger points and localised tissue trauma. Travell describes predictable referred pain patterns attributed to myofascial trigger points,[86] derived from the injection of hypertonic saline into muscle. As referred pain tends to be poorly localised, patients often indicate the location of referred pain with a wave of the hand. Direct stimulation of tissue nociceptors, in contrast, as may occur with a ligament rupture, typically results in more precisely located pain, able to be indicated with a pointed finger.

While Travell described palpable taut bands in muscle as a diagnostic feature of trigger points,[86] several controlled studies have found this to be unreliable and therefore not recommended.[87-90]

In contrast, the identification of localised muscle tenderness based on patient feedback has shown acceptable inter-examiner reliability,[91] presumably by removing the subjective phenomenon of palpatory pareidolia. Thus, on the basis of existing research, clinical identification of trigger points should be based primarily on localisation of maximally tender points within muscle. Consideration also may be given to the reproduction of any referred pain patterns.

Treatment of myofascial pain and trigger points is discussed in Chapter 24.

## Chronic exertional compartment syndrome

Chronic exertional compartment syndrome refers to the intermittent and reversible pathological elevation of compartment pressures following exertion.[92] The condition usually affects the lower legs but may also occur in the forearms in tennis, rock climbing and weightlifting.[93] Chronic extertional compartment syndrome is listed here as a muscle injury but is not itself a muscular disorder. Intra-compartmental pressure is likely the source and multiple tissues are affected, including the nerves and vascular supply.

The muscles of the lower leg are divided into a number of compartments by fascial sheaths, which are relatively inelastic thickenings of collagenous tissue. Exercise raises the intracompartmental pressure and may cause a muscle to swell and fluid to accumulate in the interstitial spaces. The tight fascia prevent expansion. This impairs the blood supply and causes pain with exertion. Compression of neurological structures may also contribute to the clinical presentation. Muscle hypertrophy may precipitate chronic exertional compartment syndrome.

The main symptom is pain that commences during activity and ceases with rest. This differs from other overuse injuries such as tendinopathies, where pain may be present with initial exercise, then diminish as the affected area warms up, only to return when activity stops. The role of imaging in diagnosis is unclear.[94]

The gold standard for diagnosis has always been measurement of compartment pressures at rest and during pain-provoking exercise. In recent years, various authors have expressed reservations regarding the reliability and validity of these tests.[95-97]

> **PRACTICE PEARL**
>
> Chronic exertional compartment syndrome in the lower limb should initially be managed with an intensive gait-retraining intervention before considering fasciotomy.

Results of conservative treatment by gait retraining and treatment with BoNT-A (Botox) injections are promising. Specifically, gait retraining may be considered a treatment of choice in military personnel, as in this population fasciotomy appears to be less effective than in athletes.[98]

Fasciotomy is the preferred operative treatment for both lower-extremity and upper-extremity chronic exertional compartment syndrome. Good results have been reported after open, single-incision, minimally invasive, percutaneous, endoscopic and ultrasound-guided techniques. Nerve damage, haematoma and wound issues are the most common complications. Improved surgical outcomes are seen in younger patients and those who undergo fasciotomies of all compartments. Worse outcomes are seen in those with lower compartment pressure, military personnel, older individuals and adults with a longer duration of symptoms.[99]

## TENDON

Up until the early 1990s, tendon injuries received relatively little attention compared with acute injuries but the advent of ultrasound and then MRI helped clinical research to flourish. The major risk factors for overuse tendon injury include being overweight or obese, systemic disorders (e.g. diabetes mellitus, hyperlipidaemia), inflammatory conditions and connective tissue disorders (e.g. hypermobility syndrome or Ehlers-Danlos syndrome) (see also Chapter 22). In this chapter we focus on the extrinsic risks associated with sports. Sports often place high, repetitive loads on tendons, which are slow to adapt and thus susceptible to cumulative microdamage with increasing tissue pathology over time.

## Tendon overuse injury (tendinopathy)

Tendons are primarily responsible for transferring forces from muscle to bone, as well as storing and releasing energy to reduce the work required by the muscle during "elastic" activities such as running or throwing. These repetitive activities can injure tendon.

In lower limb tendons with overuse-related tendinopathy, such as the Achilles, histopathological findings collected during surgical debridement reveal:[100, 101]

* the loss of a well-organised hierarchical collagen structure
* changes in tenocyte morphology (e.g. more numerous tenocytes with rounded nuclei, or a relative absence of tenocytes indicative of more advanced pathology)
* excessive interfibrillar proteoglycans (also called matrix or ground substance)
* more prominent blood vessels—these are believed to be newly generated (i.e. often referred to as neovascularisation).

These anatomical changes—found at surgery in patients whose symptoms had been present for at least 3 months— are illustrated in Figure 9.14. Normal and pathological specimens are shown in Table 9.6.

### Theories of how tendons fail (with overuse)

Unlike bone, where the pathogenesis of stress injury has been well characterised, the process by which tendons fail is not crystal clear. There are numerous explanations and all have an absence of proof for some of the proposed steps (Table 9.7).[102] The main mystery is the association between structural abnormality (morphology) and symptoms (pain, perhaps swelling, crepitus). Regarding overuse tendinopathy, experts agree that the disease process (e.g. changes in structure detectable by biochemical and imaging methods) precedes the onset of symptoms.[103]

### The continuum model

The continuum model of tendon pathology, often referred to as the Cook–Purdam model after its authors, was

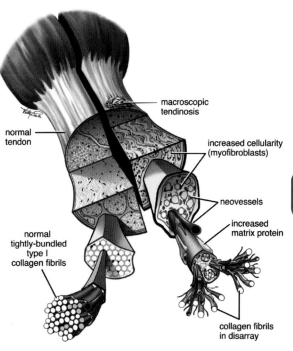

**Figure 9.14** Tendinosis: the contrasting features of normal tendon (left side) and tendinosis (right side). Characteristic features at this macroscopic level are the collagen fibres of different sizes in disarray, abnormal cell numbers (decreased and increased), abnormally prominent blood vessels and an increase in matrix proteins.

designed to blend clinical knowledge and laboratory-based research to aid in treatment decisions for different presentations of tendinopathy.[113] The model outlined three stages: (1) reactive tendinopathy, (2) tendon disrepair and (3) degenerative tendinopathy. The authors proposed an initial non-inflammatory proliferative response in tendon cells and non-collagenous matrix due to tendon overload. Further stages involve collagen disorganisation, neovascularisation and apoptosis of tendon cells. Therefore, the model draws on all of the theories presented in Table 9.7.

Many clinicians find the continuum model useful, but as with all models, it has limitations. Labelling a tendon as reactive suggests it passes through a different state before clinical tendinosis (speaking at the structural/pathology level, not the clinical level). However, there is no agreement on the histopathological/biochemical features of such a phase. The model suggests that an "optimally loaded" tendon can return to a structurally "normal" state but this is a sticking point—tendons with tendinosis rarely (if ever) return to their pre-tendinopathic state with full "healthy" type 1 collagen based on biopsy analysis (few of these in humans) or on imaging.[114]

111

**TABLE 9.6**   Differences in normal and pathological tendon specimens observed using different types of light microscopy (the specimens were obtained from patients undergoing surgery for tendon pain)

| Tendon element | Normal appearance (or early tendinosis, Fig. 9.15g) | Pathological changes observed in end-stage tendinopathy |
| --- | --- | --- |
| Cells—tenocytes (specialised fibroblasts) | 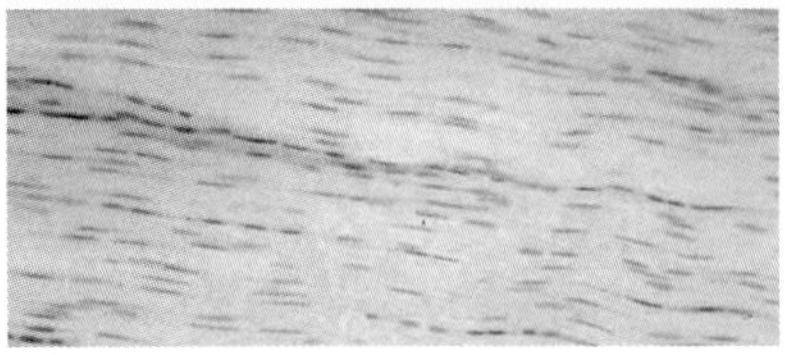 <br>**Figure 9.15(a)**  Spindle-shaped tenocyte nuclei. The cell nuclei cluster in longitudinal chains. In your mind's eye, see cell cytoplasm around each nucleus and link those cells in a network (H&E stained tendon) | 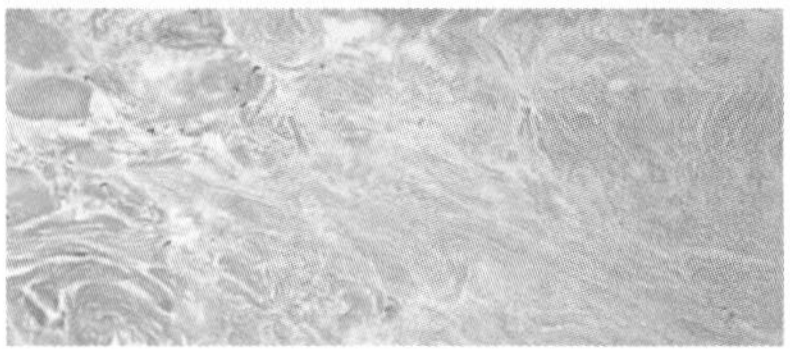 <br>**Figure 9.15(b)**  Cell nuclei clusters are no longer visible, likely as a result of apoptosis. Before this late stage, cell nuclei can become rounded and more prolific than in normal tendon (not shown here) (H&E stained tendon) |
| Collagen | 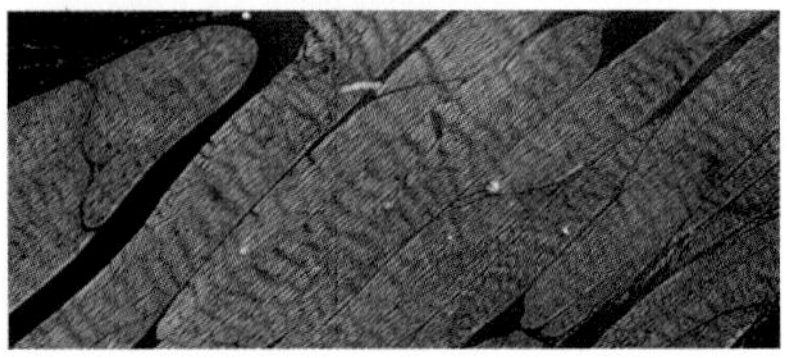 <br>**Figure 9.15(c)**  Collagen (all the golden tissue) has a linear arrangement, is tightly bundled and has a characteristic crimp and reflectivity when viewed with the polarised light microscope. The collagen is predominantly type 1. | 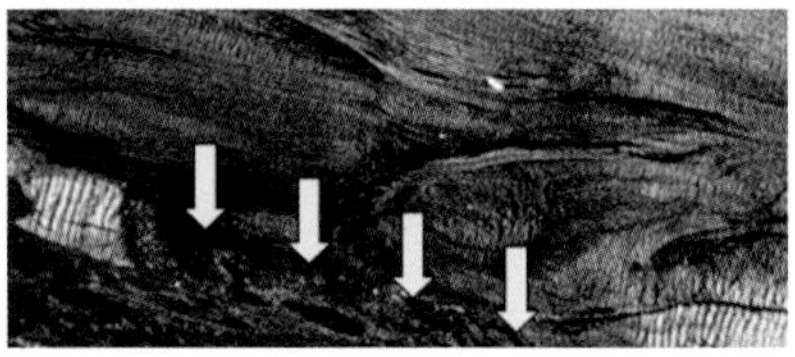 <br>**Figure 9.15(d)**  This specimen came from a patient with painful patellar tendinopathy. The arrows point to frank gaps in a collagen fibril. Note also the loss of golden reflectivity above and below that fibril—absent collagen. (Polarised light microscopy as in c.) |
| Vessels | 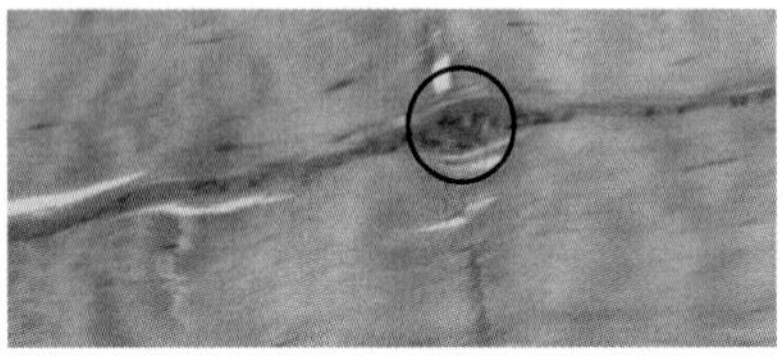 <br>**Figure 9.15(e)**  Vessels (circled) are rarely seen under light microscopy. Nerves run alongside vessels but cannot be seen without special stains. | 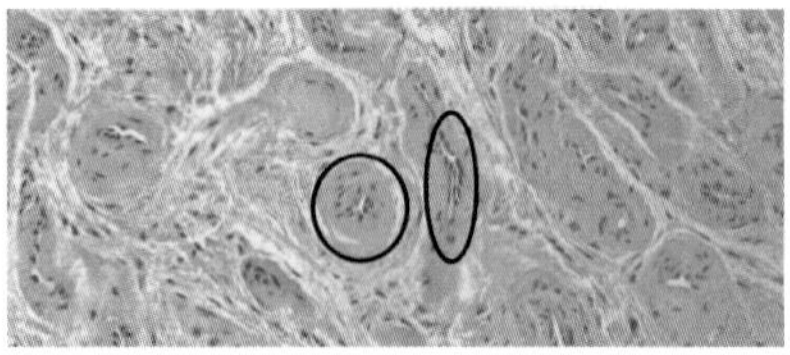 <br>**Figure 9.15(f)**  Abnormally prominent nerves and vessels. The small black dots are tendon cell nuclei; the abnormal vessels are visible (circle and oval). |
| Ground substance/ matrix proteins | 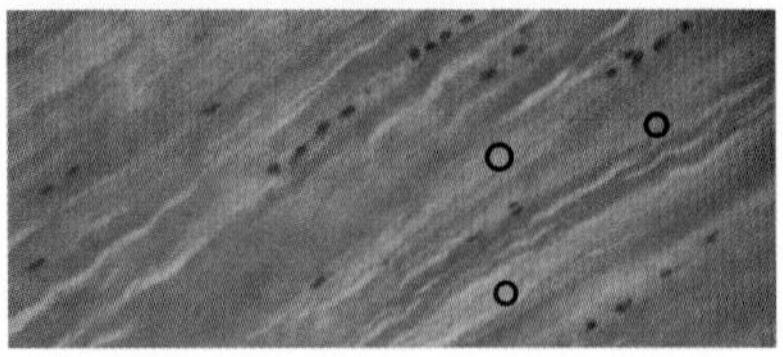 <br>**Figure 9.15(g)**  Early tendinosis: plump round tenocytes (abnormal), collagen bundles separated (not bundled) with pale-blue ground substance (abnormal proteoglycans, circles). | 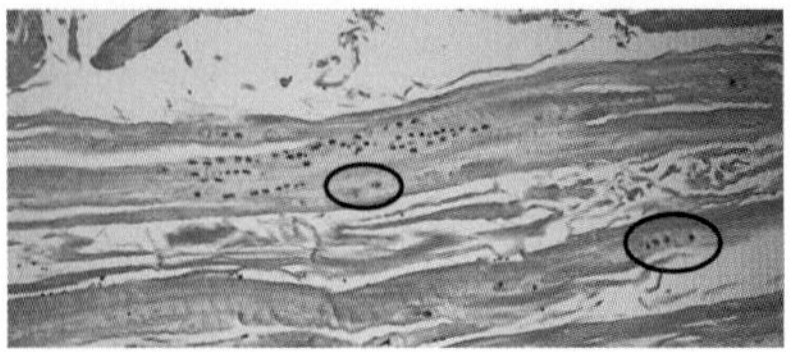 <br>**Figure 9.15(h)**  Severe tendinosis: very rounded cells (circled); pools of ground substance (blue); frayed, fragmented collagen fibrils. |

**TABLE 9.7**    Some of the theories that aim to explain the pathogenesis of overuse tendinopathy

| Name | Theory |
|---|---|
| Mechanical theory[104–106] | The mechanical theory proposes that collagen breakdown or separation in tendons is induced by excessive mechanical stimulation, caused by repetitive tensile strain or compression. This mechanical stimulation is also thought to be a harmful trigger for tendon cells. An inadequate repair can eventually result in progressive tenocyte apoptosis. This theory highlights the importance of the interplay between tendon cells and their mechanical environment in the development of tendinopathy. |
| Inflammation theory[107–109] | The inflammatory theory implies that the emergence of pathological alterations in the tendon is due to inflammatory mechanisms. This inflammation may be triggered by mechanical stimulation. Recent research has verified the existence of inflammatory mediators in patients with tendinopathy. |
| Hypoxia theory[110] | According to the hypoxia theory, degenerative tendon changes are associated with oxidative stress due to mechanical overload. Matrix metalloproteinases are activated, causing collagen breakdown. Increased oxygen free radicals have been implicated in apoptotic pathways. Tendon cells become more rounded with features of a cartilage phenotype and eventually undergo apoptosis. |
| Neurovascular theory[111,112] | The neurovascular theory is based on the observation that tendinopathy is associated with vascular and neural tissue ingrowth into the tendon. Several neurotransmitters (e.g. glutamate, calcitonin gene-related peptide [CGRP] and substance P) have been identified as a potential mediator of adaptive responses of tendons to mechanical overloading and to initiation of pain. |

The model emphasises that when tendons with an area of tendinosis are loaded appropriately, they can return to a "silent and well-performing tendon" state (the patient is asymptomatic in the presence of structural tendinosis).

Figure 9.16 is the result of our synthesising several contemporary papers on tendon pathology.[102, 114, 115] Our aim is to support athletes and clinicians to understand the pathology and what happens when we are rehabilitating a tendon with tendinosis.

## Clinical presentation of tendinopathy

Athletes often report gradual onset of dull but occasionally sharp pain around a tendon. Pain will linger following exercise, is often worse in the morning (especially following more intense exercise or physical activity the preceding day) and may persist over several days before settling with relative rest. Athletes may report a pain that is "manageable" and disappears following appropriate warm-up.

Patients with overuse tendinopathy often provide three cardinal clues to the clinician:

1. They localise the pain—they point with one or two fingers to a small area around the tendon.
2. They note that the pain is aggravated by activities that load the tendon (running, jumping).
3. They say the pain disappears or significantly reduces following warm up—they can function after warming up only to have more pain the next day (often presenting as morning stiffness).

## Diagnosing tendinopathy

The tendons most commonly injured are:

- in the upper limbs, the rotator cuff tendons and the common extensor tendon at the elbow (i.e. "tennis elbow")
- in the lower limbs, the gluteal, proximal hamstring, patellar, Achilles, tibialis posterior and peroneal tendons.

Athletes reporting pain in any of these regions and who have symptoms consistent with the three cardinal clues should be considered as highly like to have a tendinopathy.

Palpation is not useful for monitoring changes in tendon pathology but it can help to clinically isolate tendon problems and support a suspected diagnosis;[116] for instance, pain specific to the inferior pole of the patellar tendon may be consistent with patellar tendinopathy. However, palpation tests alone are often sensitive but non-specific, thus pain on palpation at the inferior pole of the patella does not rule out conditions related to the infrapatellar fat pad, or the pre patellar bursa.

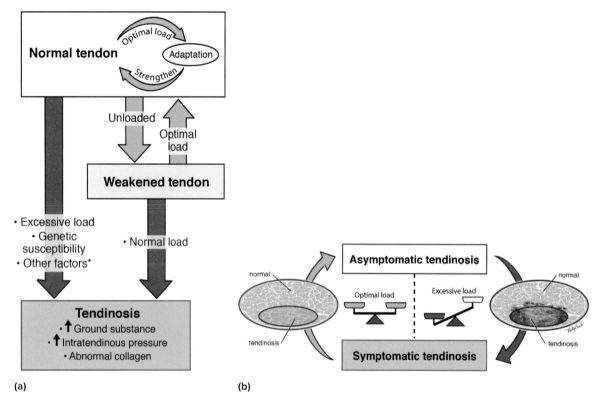

(a)                                    (b)

**Figure 9.16** Tendon symptoms and tendon pathology. (a) How tendinosis develops. In athletes, the most common cause of tendinosis is the athlete exceeding the tendon's capacity through chronic repetitive loading. Genetic susceptibility refers to an individual's genetic makeup (remembering that risk of tendon disorder is polygenetic) and relates to genes that have been linked to the development of tendon-related disorders. Other factors (*) include risks such as smoking, inflammatory conditions, metabolic diseases (e.g. hypercholesterolaemia) and medications. Note that unloading tendon can also lead to symptoms (usually pain). Athletes may unload if they take a complete break at the end of a season or with another injury/surgery. Consistent training promotes a virtuous cycle (to the right of the "normal tendon" box). (b) Cross-sectional view of a tendon with tendinosis, demonstrating the importance of maintaining load in an optimal range to keep athletes asymptomatic. The area of tendinosis remains consistent but becomes asymptomatic with balanced load.

In the lower limbs, tendon loading tests such as the hop test, heel-rise test (Achilles tendon) or single-leg stance (gluteal tendons) are used to support diagnosis. Provocation of pain increases the likelihood or suspicion of a tendon-related condition, but as with palpation, these tests have mixed success in the specificity of their findings. Diagnostic imaging is often not required in cases of suspected tendinopathy, but for cases that do not resolve with appropriate conservative rehabilitation, ultrasound or MRI may be considered to confirm and also rule out concomitant conditions. Therefore, diagnosis is often made using a combination of the patient's history, palpation tests and loading tests.[117] Individual tests for each tendon are discussed in the respective sections of *Managing Injuries*.

If the athlete participates in a sport that does not include running or jumping and they report tendon pain, maintain a healthy dose of suspicion about the diagnosis. For example, cyclists often describe Achilles tendon pain which turns out to be tenosynovitis or paratenonitis (swelling in the sheath around the tendon) rather than tendinopathy and should therefore be diagnosed and managed differently.

Before we discuss the principles of tendon rehabilitation, remember that medications can cause tendon harm (Box 9.7).

**BOX 9.7** Medications and tendon-related disorders: which cause harm and which cure?

Table 9.8 lists medications that may contribute to an athlete developing tendinopathy or suffering a tendon rupture. The effects of the medication may be apparent within days, but can also take months to affect a tendon.

### Fluoroquinolones

Fluoroquinolones are the drug most commonly associated with tendon injury (including tendon rupture). Flouroquinolones are used to treat bacterial infections. There are at least three pathways by which fluoroquinolones could affect tendon health—they may:

- impair the function of tenocyte cell cycle regulatory proteins to cause cell arrest[118]
- produce reactive oxygen species that damages tenocyte DNA and thus apoptotis (cell death)[119]
- upregulate tendon matrix metalloproteinases (MMP-2) which degrade collagen type 1.[120]

Risk is higher when these are used alongside corticosteroids.[121]

### Glucocorticoids

Glucocorticoids (see also Chapter 24) have a strong anti-inflammatory action and are used to treat a range of musculoskeletal and systemic conditions that may coexist in an athlete (e.g. asthma). They may be given as a vapour for asthma, or orally/intravenously for systemic disorders. With respect to tendons, both oral and injected glucocorticoids inhibit normal tenocyte proliferation.[122,123] Oral and local glucocorticosteroid medication has been associated with Achilles tendon rupture.[124,125]

### Statins

Statins (HMG-CoA reductase inhibitors) are lipid-lowering medications used for people at high risk of cardiovascular disease. In the clinical sport setting, two groups use statins: the small group of elite athletes with a genetic predisposition to high cholesterol, and recreational athletes who are among the 20–30% of the general population taking statins.

Some studies show that people who take statins have a greater rate of tendon disorders than population norms but data are inconsistent. Note that high cholesterol itself is a cause of tendon pathology. Statins can potentially compromise tendons by limiting the (needed) cholesterol content of cell membranes (leading to apoptosis). Statins also limit tenocyte migration[126–129] (an essential part of mechanotransduction/tissue repair).

### Aromatase inhibitors

Aromatase inhibitors are commonly used to treat hormone receptor-positive breast cancer, particularly in postmenopausal women. They reduce the level of circulating oestrogen by blocking the activity of the enzyme aromatase, which converts androgens into oestrogens.

The use of aromatase inhibitors may be associated with an increased risk of tendon-related disorders.[130,131] However, the evidence is not entirely consistent, and at present there is no causal link. As oestrogen helps maintain collagen synthesis and tendon integrity, a drug that lowers oestrogen has the potential to harm tendon.

### Others

"Anabolic steroids increase the risk of tendon ruptures" has been an accepted wisdom in sports medicine and athletic circles for more than 30 years. Case reports suggest the supraphysiological, steroid-induced growth of muscles generates forces that exceed tendon capacity, leading to injury.

**TABLE 9.8**  Medications associated with tendinopathy and tendon rupture

|  | Drug class | Example |
|---|---|---|
| **Associated with tendon-related disorders** | Fluoroquinolones | Ciprofloxacin, ofloxacin, levofloxacin, pefloxacin |
|  | Glucocorticoids | Prednisolone, dexamethasone, betamethasone, hydrocortisone |
| **Likely associated with tendon-related disorders** | Statins | Simvastatin, atorvastatin |
|  | Aromatase inhibitors | Letrozole, anastrozole |
| **Potentially associated with tendon-related disorders** | Retinoids | Isotretinoin |
|  | Metalloproteinase inhibitors | Prinomastat, ilomastat |
|  | Anabolic steroids | Testosterone |
|  | Antiretroviral drugs | Abacavir, tenofovir |

*continues*

A 2017 cross-sectional study reported an abnormally high rate of tendon rupture among athletes who used anabolic-androgenic steroids.[132] However, there are those who feel the jury is still out.[133,134]

### Patients with tendon pain or rupture who use one of these medications

Tendon pain or rupture is a serious side effect of certain medication. In 2008, the Food and Drug administration (FDA) published a black box warning for fluoroquinolone-induced tendon disorders. Black box is the strongest possible warning issued by the FDA.[135] With respect to tendons, you might consider advising individuals to avoid medications that are associated with harm or to consider alternative medications.[136]

If you suspect a drug-induced tendon-related disorder, you should discuss this with the athlete and support them to understand the multifactorial onset of the disorder. It is unlikely to directly affect the basic treatment principles of tendinopathy, as it is currently unknown whether this subgroup of drug-induced tendon-related disorders respond differently to treatment.

If there is a clear association between the medication and onset of tendon-related disorder, the medication may be stopped if the clinical picture allows. Another consideration might be to change to another medication within the same class (e.g. from atorvastatin to simvastatin).[129] These considerations should always be taken with the athlete's general health in mind.

## TENDON MANAGEMENT PRINCIPLES

There is no such thing as a generic tendon overuse injury: all athletes with a tendinopathy will have differing levels of pain and irritability. Therefore, we provide a principle-based set of recommendations for managing a "simple" tendinopathy. There is no consideration for concurrent bursopathy or other conditions commonly found in addition to tendinopathy, such as with greater trochanteric pain syndrome.[137]

We acknowledge that much of what we recommend is based on evidence for managing lower limb tendinopathy. The greater need for dexterity and lower loads (reduced need to support body weight) may mean we need to treat upper limb tendons differently, but at present the principles that follow apply to all tendons.

Figure 9.17 provides an overview of the process for rehabilitation of tendinopathies.[138] Previously the steps

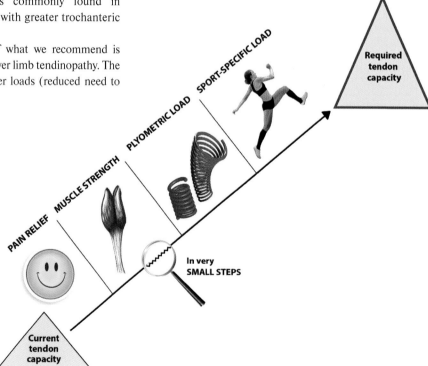

**Figure 9.17** Overview of tendon rehabilitation

were divided into four distinct categories but often elements of each phase (muscle strength, plyometric load and sport-specific load) occur concurrently.

## Pain relief

Tendons that have areas of tendinosis can be both symptomatic and asymptomatic (Figure 9.16b), and researchers remain uncertain about the primary drivers of pain in a tendon. However, Dr Ann Cools describes an "irritable" shoulder tendon (a reactive tendon using the continuum model) as: (1) being painful at rest, (2) referring pain down the arm and (3) affecting the patient's sleep. Difficulty with sleep is also a common feature of gluteal tendinopathy but less so with other lower limb tendinopathies.

When a patient first presents with tendon pain, the pain tends not to settle at rest and is worse upon waking. Athletes often report sharp, quite intense pain. Later, after pain has been present for 4 weeks or more, they report a dull ache or nagging pain.

To assess capacity and support effective rehabilitation, first consider pain relief. Highly irritable tendons may require a short period of rest from loads that involve shear/friction, compression or tensile forces (Fig. 9.18). Therefore, you should consider prescribing activities that avoid such loads.

This does not often require total rest from activities. True tendinopathies often respond well to alternative activities such as cycling, which involves a much greater need for isometric muscle activation in the calves, reduced need for eccentric (braking loads) from the quadriceps and less eccentric (stability) requirements at the glutes. Insertional tendinopathies such as proximal hamstring or insertional Achilles tendinopathy may simply require activities to take place through a reduced range of motion, avoiding compressive/friction by reducing approximation with the calcaneum bone. Isometric contractions held for up to 45 seconds can help alleviate tendon pain[139,140] in 7–10 days in patients with mild tendinopathy (shorter duration symptoms, first or second episode of tendon pain), but can take up to 6–8 weeks in more challenging cases.

## Assess current and desired capacity

As the stress-shielding response postulates, tendons (and the cells within) need load to maintain their tensile capacity. Rest reduces immediate pain but doesn't allow an athlete to return to their previous level of activity. Therefore, it is important to also assess current and desired capacity.

Sports-related tendinopathy is most often the result of an imbalance between the athlete's current (or at least recent pre-injury) capacity and their desired capacity to perform in their sport.

Figure 9.19 demonstrates how load—in this example, training load—and tissue capacity interact. The example of exceeding one's current tissue capacity could be applied to many overuse conditions, and the factors that make up daily load are complex. For a more in-depth consideration of load, including measurement of load, see Chapter 15.

Athletes have differing requirements for capacity. For instance, a track and field sprinter will require extremely high amounts of strength and power from their calf and Achilles, thus the focus may be on assessing their ability to calf raise with added resistance (most often using weights). However, a marathon runner requires high amounts of endurance, and therefore their ability to push body weight multiple times (i.e. a focus on the number of "quality" reps they can achieve) may be the focus of capacity testing. Often, assessing capacity requires a mixture of strength and endurance.

If the athlete can tolerate it, you can also assess their plyometric capacity, but this should be done with caution for those with highly irritable "symptomatic" tendons. A single-leg-hop test, where the athlete hops on one leg for 30 seconds, can tell you much about their ability to store and release load. It can also tell you valuable information such as:

- whether the athlete is using compensatory movements to avoid loading a painful tendon (e.g. athletes with patellar tendinopathy will avoid knee flexion and jump with a "stiff" leg)
- if the athlete has additional areas of weakness that may be contributing to reduced movement efficiency or

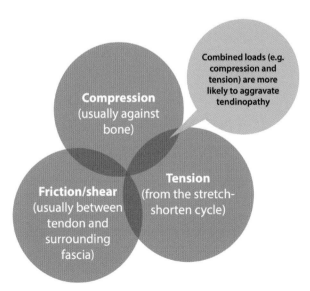

**Figure 9.18** Clinical experience suggests that tendinopathy-related pain is often aggravated by one of three types of load, or a combination of them.

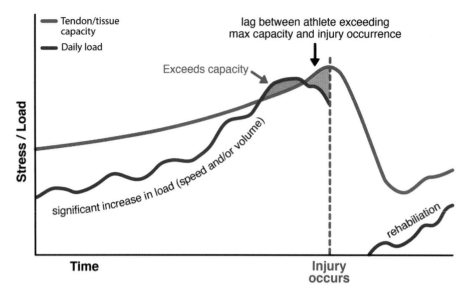

**Figure 9.19** The relationship between load (in this case, increased training load) and tissue capacity. Note there is often a delay between an athlete exceeding their tissue capacity and the onset of injury (true for both bone and tendon overuse injuries). This is simplified for illustrative purposes.

weakness and an increased burden on the tendon (e.g. the Trendelenburg sign during the stance phase of the hop, or an inability to produce enough height with the hop)

- whether the athlete stays on the ground or appears to "stick" rather than "spring" from the floor (ground contact time; can be measured with many widely available wearable devices); if so, they are likely lacking capacity to store and release energy from one of their lower limb tendons (note: this can also indicate shutdown due to other pathologies such as a bone stress injury so always keep differential diagnoses in mind).

Once you have an idea of the athlete's current capacity (e.g. they can do 8 single-leg standing calf raises and 12 single-leg seated raises at a tempo of 2 seconds up, 2 seconds down), you can determine how to raise the ceiling of their capacity using a combination of strength, endurance and, when appropriate, plyometric exercises. The goal should be to raise capacity in all three areas regardless of the athlete's sport-specific demands, as they are likely to require a combination of all three once they restart sport-specific training.

### Raising an athlete's capacity through progressive loading

There is no magic type of muscle contraction that best supports recovery from tendinopathy. Eccentrics and isometrics have both had their time in the limelight, but neither has been shown to be superior to isotonic

(concentric–eccentric muscle contractions) when tested in isolation.[141-144] The "correct" exercise is the one that you know the athlete is ready for because you have assessed them, and you know it will support them to progress towards their functional goal.

Progressive loading can occur through many mechanisms, but should be made specific to the athlete's goals. This often requires manipulation of the weight lifted, the time that the respective tendon is placed under tension or the speed of the movement performed. Progressions can incorporate a mixture of these elements to achieve the desired outcomes. It is important to perform exercises as single-limb exercises so that you can be confident the region being treated is being loaded; however, both the affected and unaffected limbs should be trained in order to take advantage of the cross-education effect.[145, 146]

Traditionally this step started with slow, heavy loading using appropriate resistance equipment for the tendon in question. Research has provided progressive loading scales based on the amount of tendon-specific load that goes through both the patellar and Achilles tendons with different exercises.[147, 148] This allows you to select a starting point based on the athlete's reaction to certain exercise and progress or regress their exercises according to the amount of pain they experience both immediately performing the exercise and within the 24-hour period afterwards.

*Managing Injuries* provides detailed recommendations for specific tendons based on the available data for progressing and regressing loads. Where data are not available, you should use your clinical reasoning to assess which exercises are most likely to place additional loads through a tendon, remembering that tendons are exposed to greater loads during fast-and-heavy loading exercises.

Tendons may require approximately 48 hours to remodel and this fits with leading clinicians' experience; very irritated/irritable tendons may respond better with some down time between exercise bouts.

> **PRACTICE PEARL**
>
> Building strength and power in the rehabilitation period is key to successful return to sport. And the athlete should continue to do strength and power exercises to prevent recurrence or further episodes of reactive tendinopathy.

## How to use the numerical pain rating scale

Tendon rehabilitation is not without pain—explicitly, even patients who are on a very successful rehabilitation journey will report pain at some time during their exercise program. What is "acceptable" pain to the patient and the clinician should be discussed between them. The patient outlines their pain level and the clinician makes suggestions as to whether that level is acceptable from their experience or there is too much pain. The "correct" answer reveals itself the next day. This illustrates shared decision making (Chapter 4) regarding how hard to push certain exercises. This management style also vivifies patient (self) education as an important part of treatment (Chapter 25).

Studies (primarily in the lower limb) have outlined a pain-monitoring approach to guide which exercises are acceptable at a specific stage of rehabilitation.[149-151] Figure 9.20 illustrates the numerical pain rating scale as a "traffic light" system to indicate what pain may be acceptable during rehabilitation with a tendinopathy.

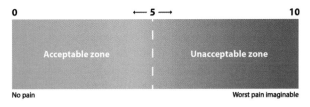

**Figure 9.20** The pain-monitoring model numerical pain rating scale. Pain is allowed to reach 5 on the scale during activity. Pain after activity is allowed to reach 5 on the scale. Pain the morning after the activity should not exceed 5 on the scale. Pain and stiffness should not increase from week to week.

## Addressing the kinetic chain

As tendinopathies often result from repetitive overload, it is reasonable to believe that deficits in the kinetic chain may cause or exacerbate tendinopathy. It is difficult to study this in the real world due to the complex interplay of muscle actions that produce human movement, but if athletes have deficits in their antigravity muscles such as the calf (especially soleus), quadriceps and gluteal muscles, this needs to be addressed. Hamstrings are clearly addressed as a priority in hamstring tendinopathy.

In the upper limbs, the transfer of forces across the kinetic chain often happens over an even greater number of connective tissues. For instance, a force generated from pushing off the ground to hit a backhand in tennis will transfer forces all the way from the toes and feet through the lower limbs, core, scapula, shoulder, elbow and eventually to the wrist and hand (the contact point with the racket). Theoretically, weakness across any one of these regions can have a knock-on effect for surrounding or even distal tendons. This is discussed in greater detail in Chapters 12 and 13.

Exercise should be continued until there is "good" strength in the affected musculotendinous unit and the agonists in the kinetic chain that are relevant to the athlete's sport-specific movements. What constitutes "good" will depend on the athlete's previous capacity and the demands of their sport. For example, although being able to lift 1.5–2x body weight in deadlift may be relevant to athletes playing football (requirement for repeated sprints), athletes performing long-distance events such as marathon running may be able to aim for slightly lower values. If normative strength values exist for a sport, we encourage you to use these as potential reference values to aim for.

## Plyometrics exercises

Once the athlete has demonstrated no "reactivity" to strength training and is progressing well, the tendon can be loaded with plyometric exercises. Plyometric exercises involve a rapid transition from the eccentric (energy storage) phase to the concentric (energy release) phase. This places a high amount of load on the tendon as shorter ground contact times reduce the ability of the muscle to absorb load, requiring a greater elastic contribution from tendon. This simulates forces that often occur during sports where a rapid change of direction, high speed sprint or jumping and push off are required.

Initially, exercises can focus solely on the eccentric loading component (e.g. stepping off a box and landing from a small height without a subsequent movement places demands on the Achilles and patella tendons to absorb greater forces, without the need to then elastically recoil into a [concentric] jump). If these are well tolerated, progressing the intensity of the eccentric phase (e.g. bigger box height) or adding the concentric phase by asking the patient to focus on "quickly leaving the floor once they land" can begin.

As these exercises place high loads on the tendon, they are best completed only 2–3 times a week. Plyometric exercises need to be controlled in terms of numbers and/or time, started at a low level and gradually increased.

### Return to sport

Once the athlete's tendon can tolerate plyometric loads, functional activity-specific exercises can be introduced in a clinical setting. These can replace the plyometric loads in many cases and initially there should be a minimum of 48 hours between training sessions that involve increasing amounts of running, jumping or throwing. Once the tendon tolerates training across a high number of functional activities, the athlete can return to a controlled training environment and from there to a graduated return to competition.

The increased availability of data from wearable technology does offer insights into an athlete's previous capacity or their desired capacity to perform sport-specific movements and allow you to tailor the rehabilitation. For instance, running itself is a plyometric exercise and therefore using an athlete's previous running volumes (including the amounts performed at higher intensity) can support return-to-sport decisions.

### Can we apply these principles to upper limb tendinopathies?

The principles outlined have been well studied in the lower limb, especially the patellar and Achilles tendons. Although consensus suggests that the upper limb can be treated in a similar fashion, note the substantial difference between plyometric loads (with body weight) acting on the lower limb and those acting on the upper limb (often without body weight).

We encourage you to follow the same principles for managing tendinopathy regardless of the area of the body, but reinforce that upper limb tendinopathies may require a greater focus on kinetic chain deficits to help balance the load applied and the athlete's capacity.

### Medications

Although certain medications may induce tendon-related disorders (Box 9.7), Box 9.8 highlights that medications have also been used to treat tendons clinically with considerable uncertainty regarding their efficacy.

## OTHER TENDON PATHOLOGIES

Although the most-used clinical label for tendon overuse injuries is tendinopathy (e.g. Achilles tendinopathy), the conditions of paratenonitis, partial tear and enthesopathy also need consideration.

### Paratenonitis

Paratenonitis, peritendinitis, tenosynovitis (single layer of areolar tissue covering the tendon) and tenovaginitis (double-layered tendon sheath) all relate to overuse disorders of the connective tissue that surrounds a tendon. This occurs where the tendon rubs over a bony prominence and/or where repeated movement directly irritates the paratenon. Uncommonly, it can coexist with partial tears and tendinopathy, but is most often a differential diagnosis for an athlete presenting with pain in the Achilles region.

Unlike tendinopathy, which requires a progressive loading program to return to sport, pain from the paratenon—often with accompanying swelling (caused by a fibrinous exudate that fills the tendon sheath)—requires rest from aggravating activities to allow the problem to settle before the initiation of progressive loading. Classically, there will be a palpable crepitus over the region affected that can also be heard when using a stethoscope.

Treatments for respective paratenon injuries revolve around methods to reduce the inflammation and are discussed in *Managing Injuries*.

### Partial tears

The term "partial tear" should be reserved for a macroscopically evident subcutaneous partial tear of a tendon, an uncommon acute (not overuse) injury, at least in the Achilles and patellar tendon (Chapter 3). In our experience a partial tear usually occurs in a patient with underlying tendinopathy, either subclinical or symptomatic. The distinction between tendon degeneration and partial tear on imaging is difficult; there are no definite signs that allow a clear distinction and diagnosis is reliant on radiologist expertise.

Unless a patient experiences acute-onset pain, a partial tear diagnosed on a scan should be treated the same as regular tendinopathy. Patients should be reassured that their prognosis for recovery from a degenerative partial tear is the same as for anyone who has been diagnosed with tendinopathy.

### Enthesopathy

Entheses are bony insertion sites of tendons and ligaments. Enthesopathies most often occur at the bone–tendon

## BOX 9.8 Medication to treat tendinopathy

Commonly used medical treatments include corticosteroid injections, platelet-rich plasma, high-volume injections (often saline), prolotherapy (dextrose injections) and glyceryl trinitrate (GTN) patches.

### Corticosteroids

Glucocorticoids (commonly given as a corticosteroid injection when used to treat tendons) impair tenocyte production and can be linked to tendon injury, so their use as treatment is discouraged. The use of corticosteroid injections directly into tendons is contraindicated, while the use of corticosteroid injections "around" tendons (e.g. under ultrasound control) remains debated. There are still conflicting results in some studies.[152,153]

Based on evidence synthesis, guidelines and clinical experience, there is no compelling evidence to encourage clinicians to use corticosteroid injections to help athletes gain superior mid- or long-term outcomes. There is no doubt that corticosteroids can provide superior short-term pain relief from tendinopathy-related pain compared with placebo injection. We appreciate that experienced clinicians may discuss corticosteriods as a potential treatment to provide short-term pain relief when the athlete has a very important short-term goal. Such shared decision making should also include a discussion with the athlete about the risk of tendon rupture.

### Platelet-rich plasma

Autologous platelet-rich plasma has been proposed to produce greater inflammation and fibrotic response of tendons leading to improved recovery. However, although widely used by clinicians with good anecdotal evidence, platelet-rich plasma has no benefits over placebo in multiple well-conducted trials for treating Achilles, patella, elbow and shoulder tendinopathies.[154–157]

### High-volume injections

Saline injected at high volumes has primarily been proposed as a method to reduce neovascularisation associated with Achilles tendinopathy. While evidence for efficacy is mixed, a high-quality clinical trial demonstrated no added effect of high-volume injections over placebo.[158]

### Prolotherapy

Prolotherapy injects small amounts of an irritant solution (usually dextrose) into tendon that is symptomatic. This is done multiple times and is hypothesised to stimulate the growth of normal cells/tissues in the affected areas.

The most recent evidence demonstrates that, when compared with placebo, prolotherapy has no significant added benefits,[159] and when added to physiotherapy has no added benefit over the physiotherapy alone.[160] Therefore, prolotherapy for tendon pain is not recommended.

### Glyceryl trinitrate

There is currently a mismatch between the quality of evidence (fairly robust) and clinicians' prescribing (fairly limited) glyceryl trinitrate to treat tendinopathy.[161] Evidence synthesised from 10 RCTs suggest that it can be an effective treatment alongside exercise prescription. If you imagine various treatments (glyceryl trinitrate, corticosteroid, platelet-rich plasma etc.) to be contestants in a blind audition, then glyceryl trinitrate should be much more acclaimed than corticosteroid or platelet-rich plasma. Our impression of clinical practice is that the latter treatments are much more widely used.

The reason for this mismatch in evidence versus usage could include marketing, financial incentives and the fact that glyceryl trinitrate is a patch rather than a pill. Our advice is to consider the evidence and consider a trial in your own practice. There are clinicians who use glyceryl trinitrate consistently with what they consider good effect. The commonly discussed side effect is headache (as with medications that affect blood flow) and for some patients this is a deal-breaker. Some clinicians titrate the dose and keep it below the level associated with headaches. There is a zone for many patients where the dose of glyceryl trinitrate is therapeutic and they do not suffer headaches.

### Others

The list of other drugs that have been trialled to treat tendinopathy is long. Polidocanol, autologous blood, skin-derived fibroblasts/stem cells, aprotinin, aprotinin polysulfated glycosaminoglycan, botulinum toxin and sodium hyaluronate have all been trialled and largely discontinued. None of these treatments is supported by research evidence. Refer to the *Clinical Sports Medicine* website where we cover future updates and clinical breakthroughs.

---

junction. All tendons undergoing high amounts of load (mechanical stress) can develop an enthesopathy. The most common areas affected include the supraspinatus, gluteal and Achilles tendons.

Enthesitis is also a hallmark sign of spondyloarthropathy.[162] If you suspect an insertional tendon issue, you are encouraged to screen for other common comorbidities or symptoms such as skin conditions (e.g. psoriasis), bowel complaints (colitis or Crohn's), eye issues (acute anterior uveitis, causing blurred vision), dactylitis (swelling of the fingers or toes) and early-morning stiffness. The acronym SCREEND'EM is discussed in Chapter 22. It may be difficult to differentiate between tendinopathy and enthesopathy without imaging.

If left untreated, there will be loss of fibrillar structure caused by local oedema and mineralisation.[163] This can progress to include calcification and/or ossification. There is no consistent evidence that calcification or ossification leads to a worse prognosis; they are simply a common feature associated with tendinopathy.

Enthesopathies are similar to tendinopathies in that they are primarily degenerative in nature, so treatment principles are broadly similar.

## BURSA

The human body contains many bursae situated usually between bony surfaces and overlying tendons. Their role is to facilitate movement of the tendon over the bony surface. All bursae are susceptible to injury. Typically, these are overuse injuries resulting from excessive shearing and/or compressive forces.[164, 165]

Overuse injuries in bursae are quite common, particularly at the subacromial bursa,[166] the greater trochanteric bursa,[143] the bursa deep to the iliotibial band at the knee[165, 167] and the retrocalcaneal bursa separating the Achilles tendon from the calcaneus.[168] Overuse pathologies affecting bursae commonly couple with other local pathologies such as tendinopathies and impingement syndromes.[169, 170]

Symptoms include localised pain and swelling and typically increase with activity. Conservative approaches to treatment are often trialled first. Treatment involves removal of irritating loads, reduction of inflammation and a progressive to return to pain-free activity. Specific treatments include ice, electrical stimulation, iontophoresis and gentle stretching. Once initial inflammation subsides, a stretching and strengthening program for the surrounding tissues and muscles can commence. NSAIDs are widely prescribed for these conditions, and corticosteroid injections, often guided by ultrasound, are considered where conservative approaches have failed.

## NERVE

Nerve entrapment syndromes occur in athletes as a result of swelling in the surrounding soft tissues or anatomical abnormalities. These may affect the suprascapular nerve, the posterior interosseous, the ulnar and median nerves in the forearm, the obturator nerve in the groin, the posterior tibial nerve at the tarsal tunnel on the medial aspect of the ankle and, most commonly, the interdigital nerves, especially between the third and fourth toes, a condition known as Morton neuroma. This is not a true neuroma but rather a nerve compression. These nerve entrapments occasionally require surgical decompression.

Chronic mild irritation of a nerve may result in damage manifested by an increase in neural mechanosensitivity. This may be the primary cause of the symptoms or may contribute to symptoms. This concept is discussed more fully in Chapters 10 and 11.

## SKIN

The skin's integrity is constantly challenged by athletic activity, weather conditions and pathogenic organisms.

### Pressure injuries

Pressure injuries (also known as pressure wounds) are a serious skin condition. There is a great deal of information about pressure injuries in the general population and the hospital setting; the following high-value resource focuses on Para athletes:

Pressure injuries in Para athletes

Pressure injuries are particularly prevalent in athletes who have had a spinal cord injury and now have altered sensation below the level of the injury. The ischial tuberosities are the site of most lesions. These injuries can be devastating (Fig. 9.21).

We recommend that a multidisciplinary team of clinicians contribute to the athlete's care. In keeping with quality clinical care principles, the athlete should be at the centre of the team's focus—and support staff and coaches should be included in management.

### Blisters

The skin of many athletes is subjected to friction-related forces, compounded by perspiration.[137, 138] Exposure to shearing and compressive forces can lead to mechanical separation of the epidermal cell layers. Hydrostatic pressure causes further separation and allows plasma-like fluid or sweat into the space to form a blister.[171] The repair process starts 24 hours post incident and blisters generally heal in approximately 5 days.[171] Blisters may occur at any site of friction with an external source, such as shoes or sporting equipment.

Blisters are common in marathon runners, rowers, race walkers, triathletes, hikers and military personnel. Foot blisters are painful and can have an impact on sporting

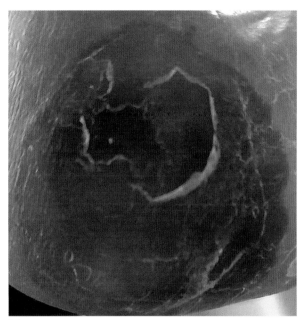

**(a)**

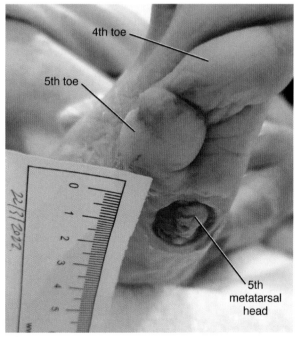

4th toe

5th toe

5th
metatarsal
head

**(b)**

**Figure 9.21** Examples of skin lesion illustrated in the Australian Institute of Sport Pressure Injuries guideline (see QR code for details on diagnosis, management and documentation). (a) Suspected deep-tissue injury, which may recover if the cause is removed. (b) Stage 4 pressure injury with extension into deep layers showing muscle, bone and tendon. Stage 4 injuries have healing times of months to years, if they heal at all.

IMAGES COURTESY OF JAN RICE

performance. Sock type, ethnicity, previous hiking or military experience and certain orthopaedic foot conditions predict the development of foot blisters in the military population.[172]

Foot blisters can be prevented by wearing-in new shoes, wearing socks and smearing petroleum jelly over the sock at sites of friction. Strategies to prevent blisters also serve to prevent callus. Symptomatic callus can be pared down with a scalpel blade, taking care not to lacerate the normal skin.

At the first sign of a blister, the aggravating source should be removed and adhesive tape applied over the blistered area or blister pads applied. Blister pads prevent blisters by acting as a barrier between skin and shoe.

Treatment of blisters involves prevention of infection with antiseptics and protection with sticking plaster. Fluid-filled blisters may be punctured and drained.

## Skin infections

Almost any cutaneous infection can afflict athletes. However, their activities place them at higher risk of developing and subsequently transmitting their skin ailment to competitors. Athletes acquire infections as a result of their interactions with other athletes and with the environment in which they compete. An athlete's skin is often macerated from sweating which promotes most common infections in sports include bacterial, fungal and viral infections, but parasites can also afflict the athlete.[173]

### *Dermatitis*

An athlete's skin can suffer repeated exposure to trauma, heat, moisture and numerous allergens and chemicals. These factors may combine with other unique and less well-defined genetically predisposing factors in their skin to cause both allergic dermatitis and irritant contact dermatitis. As with other cases of contact dermatitis, these eruptions present on a spectrum from acute to subacute to chronic. Recognising the unique environmental irritants and allergens encountered by athletes is paramount to facilitate appropriate therapy and prevention.[174]

### *Skin cancer*

Skin cancers are not true overuse injuries, but perhaps can be described as "overexposure". Nevertheless, athletes are particularly venerable as many sports involve prolonged exposure to sun during training and games.

The incidence of melanoma and non-melanoma skin cancers is increasing worldwide. Ultraviolet light exposure is the most important risk factor for cutaneous melanoma and non-melanoma skin cancers. Non-melanoma skin cancer includes basal cell carcinoma and squamous cell carcinoma. Constitutive skin colour and genetic factors, as well as immunological factors, play a role in the development of skin cancers. Ultraviolet light also causes sunburn and photoaging damage to the skin. Studies in athletic populations have found that certain sports are associated with increased risk of skin cancers.[175]

Athletes should avoid excessive exposure to ultraviolet light and particularly avoid sunburn.

## BUT IT'S NOT THAT SIMPLE

Although it is important to have a good understanding of the conditions outlined in this chapter and Chapter 8 on acute injuries, three important additional components are necessary for successful management of athletes with sporting injuries.

### Pain

The pain the athlete feels at a particular site may not necessarily be emanating from that site. It is essential to understand pain, which is the topic of Chapters 10 and 11.

### Red flags

There are many medical conditions whose presentation may mimic a sporting injury. While some of these conditions are relatively rare, it is nevertheless important to keep them in mind. If the clinical pattern does not seem to fit the obvious diagnosis, think of the conditions that may masquerade as sporting injuries. These are described in Chapter 22.

## The kinetic chain

We have already touched on the importance of the body acting in synergy to produce movements when looking at tendinopathy. Every athletic activity involves coordinated movements of joints and limbs. The sequencing of the links is known as the kinetic chain.[176] Studies of sporting biomechanics in part look to find the most efficient way to transfer force and energy to produce a specific movement.

Injuries or maladaptations in some areas of the kinetic chain can cause problems not only locally but also distally, as distal links must compensate for the lack of force and energy delivered through the more proximal links. This phenomenon, known as catch-up, is inefficient and poses a risk to the distal links because it may cause more load or stress than a specific—often smaller—link can handle. These changes may result in anatomical or biomechanical situations that increase injury risk, perpetuate injury patterns or decrease performance. For example, a tennis player with stiffness of the lumbar spine may overload the rotator cuff muscles while serving as they try to generate their maximum force. This may result in a tear (acute) or repetitive (overuse) injury at the rotator cuff muscle-tendon unit.

Deficits in the kinetic chain must be identified and corrected as part of the treatment and rehabilitation process. We will return to the theme of the kinetic chain in the following chapters.

## KEY POINTS

- Our knowledge of overuse injuries has been greatly expanded by advances in research, knowledge translation and medical imaging. At the same time, there is a great deal of misinformation related to overuse sports injuries.

- The risk of sustaining an overuse injury is determined by external factors including training load and internal risk factors including metabolic disorders and genetic variants.

- Bone stress injuries in the skeletally mature athlete include pubic bone stress and medial tibial stress syndrome. In skeletally immature athletes, training overload may result in injury to the apophyses (apophysitis).

- Synovitis, capsulitis and impingement syndromes are common overuse injuries at the joints.

- Overuse injuries of the ligaments are generally uncommon, but baseball pitchers are at risk of overuse injury to the ulnar collateral ligament of the elbow.

- Myofascial trigger points are thought to be tender, taught bands of soft tissue. There is significant debate about trigger points: what they are, whether they can be imaged and how to treat them.

- Chronic exertional compartment syndrome is most common in the lower leg but can occur in the forearm. It results from stiff fascia restricting the space available for exercising muscle to expand. Neurovascular structures are at risk due to high intracompartmental pressure.

- Our understanding of tendon response to overload has been greatly improved by advances in research and medical imaging. Using microscopy, we can visualise the structural differences in healthy and overloaded tendons (with tendinosis).

- Tendon overuse injuries are distinct from acute tendon injuries like partial and complete tears.

- Bursae throughout the body are at risk of overuse injury due to shearing and/or compressive forces. Treatment often begins with load modification, a progressive return to activity and a comprehensive exercise rehabilitation program.

- Swelling or anatomical abnormality may predispose an athlete to secondary nerve entrapment.

- Skin is susceptible to overuse injuries like blisters and overexposure conditions like dermatitis or skin cancers.

## REFERENCES

References for this chapter can be found at www.mhprofessional.com/CSM6e

## ADDITIONAL CONTENT

 Scan here to access additional resources for this topic and more provided by the authors

# How does pain work? Using contemporary neuroscience to understand pain, performance and recovery

**with G. LORIMER MOSELEY**

*Taking a neuroscience-informed approach to pain, performance and rehab, totally fits with high performance principles. I've seen athletes who were close to stepping away from the sport, engage with an education-based approach and return faster and stronger. Even more importantly, they were way more informed about how to optimise their preparation and recovery moving forward.*

**DR DARREN BURGESS, 2024 (PERFORMANCE DIRECTOR)**

## CHAPTER OUTLINE

What is pain?
What is nociception?
The "fit for purpose/play/performance" model
Always a nanostep ahead: our internal models, predictions and corrections
The brain is different in those with persistent pain
Treating someone in pain: a complex system requires a comprehensive approach

## LEARNING OBJECTIVES

By the end of this chapter you should be able to:

- describe the complex and variable relationship between tissue damage and pain
- distinguish between the concepts of nociception and pain
- explain our evolving understanding of central and peripheral sensitisation
- consider cognitive, sensory and motor processing issues when developing an intervention for an athlete with persistent pain
- educate an athlete on how pain works
- identify clinical signs and symptoms that may indicate increased sensitisation in an athlete.

Even the simplest organisms can protect themselves from threatening stimuli by altering their path of movement away from the source of the threat.[1] As evolution has honed us into ever more sophisticated creatures, we have also refined this fundamental capacity to protect ourselves from threat. Perhaps our most sophisticated protective strategy is pain.

## WHAT IS PAIN?

Almost everyone experiences pain. Those who do not experience pain are at a distinct disadvantage in life and are likely to die young without living fast.

Pain is an unpleasant sensory and emotional *experience* that is felt in the body and motivates us to do something to escape it. These two characteristics of pain—its unpleasantness and its bodily location—appear to be inseparable dimensions of a unified experience.[2] They are what makes pain such an effective protective feeling (although it is not our only protective feeling).[3]

Pain alerts us to tissue damage or the threat thereof. Pain makes us seek care. Pain stops us competing, keeps us seeking a cure, compels us to prioritise pain relief above almost everything else. That's the rub: pain changes our behaviour. This is a critical consideration when we think about pain within the context of performance: pain and performance have different objectives—they will always be in competition.

That is the key to really understanding pain: it is as simple and as difficult as this—if the brain concludes that a body part is in danger and needs protecting and that volitional behaviour is required, then the brain will make that body part hurt.[4]

There is a critical caveat here. This convention to ascribe pain to the brain is flawed, because a brain, on its own, almost certainly would not and probably could not produce pain. There has been some criticism of this position.[5] The caveat is this: to attribute it all to the brain is simplistic and denies the role of physiological mechanisms that extend beyond the brain.

Yet, as much as we know now, networks of brain cells (neuronal and non-neuronal) are the most obvious "last step" and the emergence of consciousness (and therefore pain) is likely to be most closely related to the activation patterns of these neuroimmune networks.

With that rather perplexing caveat out of the way, let's consider what is good about this concept of pain. This concept of pain integrates a vast body of basic, applied and clinical research. It differs greatly from conventional theories, which have changed little since the 17th century when Rene Descartes was ridiculed for suggesting that we were not made from 4 bodily humors.[6]

> **PRACTICE PEARL**
>
> Pain is not a measure of tissue damage: it's an indicator of the brain's conviction that certain tissue needs protection.

To better understand pain as a protective output of the brain, not as a marker of tissue damage, consider several contrasts between the two models (Table 10.1).

## WHAT IS NOCICEPTION?

Nociception is not pain. Nociception refers to detecting, transmitting and processing noxious stimuli. A noxious stimulus is one that is potentially or actually damaging. The neurons that detect noxious stimuli and transmit a nociceptive message to the spinal cord are known as primary nociceptors, or just nociceptors ("danger or difference receptors").

In reality, activity in nociceptors is always associated with activity in other afferent neurons—mechanoreceptors and thermoreceptors most obviously. This is because when we talk about nociceptors, we usually mean "high-threshold

**TABLE 10.1**   Contrasts between pain as a protective output of the brain and pain as a marker of tissue damage

| Pain is in consciousness | Damage is in the body |
|---|---|
| One can't be in pain and not know about it | One can be severely damaged and not know about it |
| No brain, no pain | No body, no damage |
| Pain is affected by what else is at stake | Damage is not |
| Pain is affected by who is in the area | Damage is not |
| Pain is affected by beliefs | Damage is not (well, not directly) |
| Pain can occur in a body part that does not exist | Damage cannot |
| Pain can occur in a body part that is not damaged | Damage can occur in a body part that is not painful |
| Pain can occur without activation of primary nociceptors (see below) | Damage cannot (excepting local anaesthetic or pre-injury nociceptor death) |

neurons", which means that in order to activate them, the intensity of the stimulus needs to be approaching that which is damaging to the tissue in which the neuron resides. Remarkably, when that tissue is damaged, the sensitivity of nociceptors increases so as to remain a viable protective mechanism (see later in the chapter).

Nociceptors are thinner than other peripheral neurons and many of them are not myelinated at their distal endings. Sometimes, all unmyelinated or thinly myelinated neurons are classed as nociceptors, but many of them have very low thresholds, disconnecting them from a role in detecting potentially dangerous events. It is easier to think about nociceptors according to their role in protection and therefore to class a neuron as a nociceptor if it (1) does not have a specialised receptor on its distal end and (2) has a high threshold for activation.

Nociceptors fall into two classes:

- C fibres (unmyelinated, slow-conducting neurons)
- Aδ fibres (myelinated, slow-conducting neurons).

According to our criteria, all nociceptors are C or Aδ neurons, but not all C and Aδ neurons are nociceptors.[7]

Nociceptors are located in almost all body tissues with the notable exception of the brain.

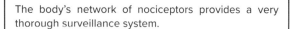

> ### PRACTICE PEARL
>
> The body's network of nociceptors provides a very thorough surveillance system.

Of course, the surveillance function of the peripheral nervous system is much more comprehensive than nociceptors alone, it's just that nociceptors are always surveying the anatomical landscape for dangerous events. These events fall into one or more of three categories: thermal, chemical or mechanical. Thus, nociceptors have specialised receptors in their cell walls that are cold-sensitive, hot-sensitive, chemosensitive or mechanosensitive.

Humans have low-threshold neurons that are solely interested in one modality or another, such as thermosensitive Aβ fibres, which inform brainstem areas of even tiny fluctuations in tissue temperature—fluctuations that are well within a safe operating range.

In contrast, nociceptors are most often bimodal or multimodal. That is, they are responsive to thermal and mechanical input, or to thermal, mechanical and chemical input. These nociceptors, which are situated in the tissues of the body, are known as primary nociceptors.[8,9] That primary nociceptors are multimodal and only project as far as the spinal cord clearly shows that the nociceptive system,

per se, is not able to transmit information specific to each modality. That is, the nociceptive system does not tell the brain that something is dangerously hot or dangerously cold, or dangerously squashed. It most definitely can't tell the brain that something is painful.

Rather, the nociceptive system has the apparently simple task of telling the brain that something is "potentially dangerous". It is the non-nociceptive inputs (including non-somatosensory cues[10]) that provide critical information about the nature of the danger.

The polymodal characteristic also means that if a stimulus is both dangerously hot and dangerously squashing, it evokes quicker firing of primary nociceptors, which effectively tells the spinal cord that something is "doubly dangerous". To consider a clinical example: if a primary nociceptor is activated by heating of the skin to 42°C, the addition of a mechanical input to the hot input will increase the firing of nociceptors to a greater extent than either would alone.

Primary nociceptors terminate in the dorsal (or sensory) horn of the spinal cord. The dorsal horn is grey matter. It consists almost entirely of interneurons (neurons that connect to other neurons in the area).

The grey matter of the spinal cord (the dorsal horn and the ventral [or motor] horn) is similar in structure to the grey matter in the brain—neuroimmune networks offering an extraordinary capacity for processing of incoming sensory information and modulating outgoing motor commands. Neurons that emerge from the dorsal horn and carry nociceptive data to the brain are known as secondary or spinal nociceptors (see below).

> ### PRACTICE PEARL
>
> Primary nociceptive input is open to modulation at the spinal "processing station". Therefore, other peripheral input and descending input from the brain can both decrease the likelihood of the brain receiving nociceptive signals.

The processing role of the dorsal horn is one reason we can, for example, "rub it better" or use TENS to provide pain relief. In fact, TENS was born from Melzack and Wall's famous gate control theory of 1965[11] and is thought to reduce the likelihood of activating spinal nociceptors by flooding the dorsal horn with non-nociceptive input from the skin.

The other way the spinal processing station can be modulated is by descending input from the brain, and it is this descending input that arguably represents a more important and potent modulatory influence.[12]

## Sensitisation of primary nociceptors

Primary nociceptors become sensitised in the presence of inflammation. This means that they are subsequently activated at a lower threshold than is ordinarily required. In the presence of tissue injury, the mix of molecules released is collectively referred to as "inflammatory soup". The exact ingredients of any particular soup will vary, depending on the particular situation/injury/context/chemical stimuli and, critically, person.

Figure 10.1 depicts typical inflammation-mediated sensitisation of primary nociceptors. This "peripheral sensitisation" is exactly that—nociceptors become responsive to stimuli that are not normally evocative. One example

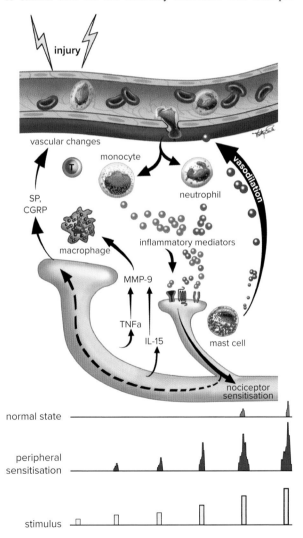

**Figure 10.1** A simplified illustration of the connection between nerve terminals and vasculature. The green (normal) and red (sensitised) bars depict nociceptor responses to test stimuli (yellow bars). When there is peripheral sensitisation (red bars), even tiny stimuli evoke responses.

is sunburn: sunburnt skin is painful in a shower of 40°C because nociceptors are sensitised sufficiently to be activated by a thermal stimulus 4–5°C cooler than would normally be required.

> **PRACTICE PEARL**
>
> That peripherally sensitised tissues are heat-sensitive is a very important clinical phenomenon because spinal nociceptor sensitisation does not result in heat sensitivity.

If you have concluded that there is a peripheral problem and can heat the culprit tissues to 42°C, you can confirm the conclusion, or question it, by determining whether the tissues are more sensitive in the presence of thermal stimuli that normally do not activate nociceptors (see also Fig. 10.2).

Another aspect of sunburn, reddening of the skin, is an important aspect of peripheral sensitisation. Reddening of the skin is a sign of neurogenic inflammation, also known as peptidergic inflammation because it is mediated by nociceptors releasing peptides into the tissue.

Peptidergic inflammation occurs when nociceptors are activated. Impulses transmit along every branch of the nociceptor. If an impulse transmits in the opposite-to-usual direction and arrives at another terminal branch, it causes the release of peptides. These peptides (CGRP and substance P) are inflammatory and cause vasodilation.[7]

This mechanism is responsible for the flare around a skin wound or scratch. Peptidergic inflammation is an important mechanism if the nociceptor is being activated proximally—for example, in the dorsal root ganglion or spinal cord—because it means that the tissues become inflamed as a consequence of action potentials being propagated elsewhere (in this situation, peptidergic inflammation is not being driven by activation of nociceptors within the sensitised tissue).

## Central sensitisation version 1.0: altered response profiles in the dorsal horn

If nociceptive networks in the dorsal horn are repeatedly active, they become sensitised—their activation threshold reduces such that a smaller stimulus is required to evoke the same response as it did previously, or the same stimulus evokes a bigger response than it did previously. The response may well be activation of spinal nociceptors.

The notion of central sensitisation has changed substantially since it was first documented in 1983,[13] but the early idea (version 1.0) remains dominant and warrants describing. The landmark paper[13] describes animal experiments demonstrating that, in the presence of peripheral nerve injury, the stimulus required to activate

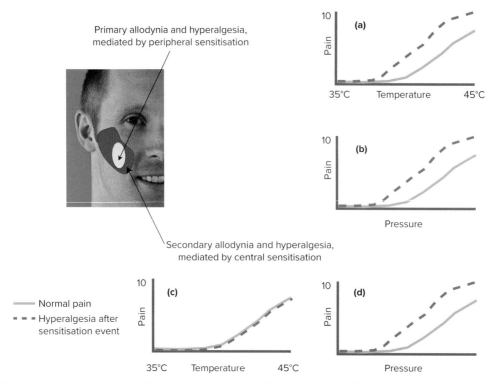

**Figure 10.2** Peripheral and central sensitisation. A change in sensitivity to stimuli delivered to the skin in an area of inflammation (white circle), in which inflammatory soup sensitises nociceptors (peripheral sensitisation), and in the surrounding area (grey) in which changes inside the central nervous system cause the effect. Graphs represent the effect of peripheral sensitisation on pain evoked by increasing (a) temperature or (b) pressure and the effect of central sensitisation on pain evoked by increasing (c) temperature or (d) pressure.

a response in a spinal nociceptor reduces over time. The spinal nociceptor seems to become *sensitised*. Because this sensitivity occurs in the central nervous system, it was termed central sensitisation.[14] (There are numerous reviews of this original paper.[12, 15, 16])

### Central sensitisation version 2.0: altered response profiles in the nociceptive system

Since that landmark work of the 1980s, our understanding of how the dorsal horn works has transformed and similar processes of sensitisation have been observed at numerous levels within the central nervous system. These discoveries prompted Woolf to update his definition of central sensitisation to include sensitivity at one or more locations across the entire nociceptive system (see Box 10.1).[17]

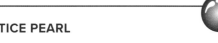

**PRACTICE PEARL**

Central sensitisation manifests as *mechanical sensitivity* beyond the area of injury and peripheral sensitisation.

**BOX 10.1** Key definitions

- *Peripheral sensitisation:* a physiological process. Increased sensitivity of primary nociceptors, caused by tissue damage or inflammation and mediated by a cascade of events that occur inside the primary nociceptors themselves.
- *Central sensitisation version 1.0:* a physiological process. Altered stimulus-response profiles in neuron-to-neuron synapses in the dorsal horn such that the activation threshold of the post-synaptic neuron is reduced.
- *Central sensitisation updated version 2.0:* a physiological process. Altered stimulus-response profiles such that the activation threshold of the post-synaptic neuron is reduced, occurring in one or more locations within the nociceptive system (spinal cord or brain).

## Clinical manifestations of peripheral and central sensitisation

Peripheral sensitisation results in sensitivity to somatosensory stimuli applied in the area of tissue damage or inflammation. There are two manifestations:

- *allodynia*, which reflects pain in response to stimuli that are normally not painful
- *hyperalgesia*, which reflects more intense pain to stimuli that are normally painful.

When these clinical signs are confined to the local area and attributed to local injury or inflammation, they are known as primary allodynia and primary hyperalgesia. In peripheral sensitisation, primary allodynia and primary hyperalgesia will be observed for mechanical, heat and chemical stimuli.

When the sensitivity extends beyond the area of tissue injury or inflammation, they are known as secondary allodynia and secondary hyperalgesia. In central sensitisation, secondary allodynia and hyperalgesia are much more marked for mechanical stimuli than for heat and chemical stimuli.

## Pain system hypersensitivity

Recent progress in biological sciences has revealed that there are many more locations within the brain and body at which sensitivity to somatosensory stimuli can be mediated. These changes are not limited to the nociceptive system but include a wide range of processes involved in pain more broadly—processes that relate to factors across biological, psychological and social domains.

Through more than a decade of consumer-focused research (e.g. talking to patients), we have gained great insight into how we can capture these complex processes that contribute to and underpin persistent pain, in terms and labels that can be readily understood and used to promote evidence-based care and better outcomes.[18-23]

One concept to emerge from this is the term "pain system" to describe the diverse range of processes and bodily systems that can be involved in pain. Patients, the general public and clinicians immediately resonate with this idea, find it intuitive and report the notion that pain involves an entire system helps explain their experiences. Patients have extended this idea of a pain system to suggest that this clinical state in which we experience pain in response to a wide range of normally not-painful stimuli from across biopsychosocial domains as "pain system hypersensitivity" (Box 10.2).[21-22]

> **BOX 10.2** A note on the terms "central sensitisation" and "pain system hypersensitivity"
>
> Many people with persistent pain have reduced pain thresholds to mechanical stimuli in the area of their pain. This sensitivity may extend beyond the painful area, or across half or all of their body.
>
> While peripheral sensitisation can explain local sensitivity, the most obvious biological substrate for wider sensitivity is the central nervous system. Central sensitisation is the proposed physiological process by which sensitivity to mechanical stimuli occurs across the body.[17]
>
> Critically, peripheral and central sensitisation are physiological mechanisms, not clinical states. Pain system hypersensitivity is a patient-generated term to describe a clinical state of sensitivity to stimuli. It is mechanism-agnostic insofar as it accommodates sensitisation processes anywhere within the wider pain system. It is mechanism-considerate insofar as it attributes sensitivity to biological mechanisms, not to a psychological or moral flaw or insufficiency in the person in pain. This is a critical consideration because many patients with persistent pain feel invalidated or blamed by usually very well-meaning health professionals.

## THE "FIT FOR PURPOSE/PLAY/PERFORMANCE" MODEL

The last 30 years of research into chronic pain and performance have revealed important new targets for treatment. A number of research groups have explored cognitive-, sensory- and motor-processing abnormalities in people with chronic pain,[23-38] developing and testing new interventions to correct them[39-47] and, if they work, running clinical trials to assess whether they can change pain and function.[48,49]

Clinically, this work has been integrated into complex, multimodal treatment approaches that are grounded in enabling, empowering pain education and both brain and body-targeted interventions.

An example of a complex care package is the RESOLVE intervention, a standardised progressive treatment program for chronic back pain.[48] It is based on the "fit for purpose" model, whereby chronic musculoskeletal pain has been conceptualised by Professor Ben Wand of Notre Dame University as an information-processing problem with three broad intervention targets (pillars):

1. understand that the body is fit for purpose
2. refine the neural networks that represent the body and the space around it so that the body feels fit for purpose
3. ensure that the body is fit for purpose.[50]

131

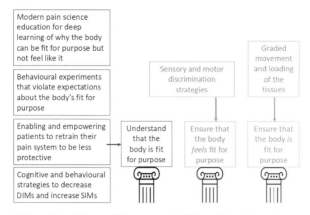

DIM: credible evidence of "danger in me"; SIM: credible evidence of "safety in me"

**Figure 10.3** The three pillars of the "fit for purpose" model
Source: Moseley G, Butler D. *The Explain Pain Handbook: Protectometer.* Adelaide: Noigroup, 2015.

The most important mechanism by which the intervention seems to work is a shift in how the person in pain conceptualises the problem.[51]

This is consistent with a growing number of studies, from clinical trials to clinical audits,[52] which point to the powerful role of changing understanding of the problem in facilitating recovery from chronic pain. Our paper in *Journal of Pain*[22] outlines pain education delivery and learning frameworks.

When working with recreational and elite performers, the "fit for purpose" model (Fig. 10.3) can easily be adapted to a "fit for play" or "fit for performance" model:

1. the literature on the first pillar of promoting understanding of the problem is growing rapidly (see above)
2. aspects of the second pillar of refining neural networks are covered in many articles[53-56]
3. the principles of the third pillar of ensuring the body is fit for play/performance are already well understood and applied across the sport and performance sectors.

The power of the "fit for play/performance" model is that it:

1. is grounded in and guided by reconceptualisation of the problem through a range of educational strategies, behavioural experiments and intentional learning activities
2. integrates brain and body training all the way to returning to full performance.

The practical application of these ideas is covered in Chapter 11.

## ALWAYS A NANO STEP AHEAD: OUR INTERNAL MODELS, PREDICTIONS AND CORRECTIONS

The pain chapter in the 5th edition of this book described a way of thinking about how the brain works. That model was drawn from several fields and focused on neuroimmune networks, or "neurotags". According to that model, pain emerges from the brain as a result of a complex hierarchical process by which these neurotags influence each other.

In practical terms, this process represents the constant evaluation of threats to body tissue and whether an experience is required to motivate protective action. It is true to say that this model is neurocentric[5] insofar as pain does not emerge from the brain or, in fact, from a nervous system sitting in isolation from the rest of our body. How our biology produces consciousness—a manifestation of "the unified human"—is thus far beyond comprehension.

We might concede this neurocentricity but accept that to conceptualise it in this way is faithful to much of our understanding and is very clinically applicable. Thus, you are encouraged to revisit the pain chapter in the 5th edition or refer to references that describe action and modulation neurotags and the principles that govern them.[55, 57-59]

The last 15 years have seen growing support for the notion that the brain does not produce outputs (e.g. feelings, motor commands) in *response* to what is happening, but rather in *anticipation* of what will happen next. Therefore, brain outputs are predictions based on a best guess or inference.[60] Some predictive processing theories propose that predictions reflect our internal models of things (Fig. 10.4).

Neurotags provide a biological substrate that represents these internal models; as such, our internal models reflect the constant competition and collaboration of neurotags. Indeed, the earliest presentation of the neurotag model[9] clearly stipulated that in any given pain experience, we can be sure that the neurotags that produce pain are being activated, but we cannot be sure that the painful tissue is actually under threat—that nociceptors are active. That is, pain occurs because neurotags are activated and this provides evidence that the organism has concluded that protective action is required to safeguard against the very next moment.

### The very next moment

Neurotag and predictive processing theories can be difficult to grasp. Understanding them as a single combined model is likely to be even more difficult. Feedback from numerous professional development courses has highlighted the usefulness of walking through the process of pain with tissue injury or threat, and the resolution of pain as tissues recover, from a predictive processing perspective.

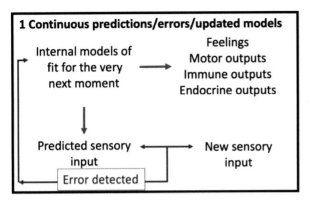

**Figure 10.4** Predictions reflect our internal models of things

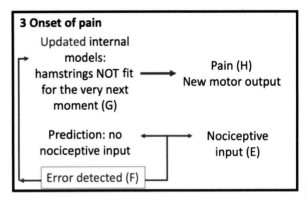

**Figure 10.6** The onset of pain

**B**

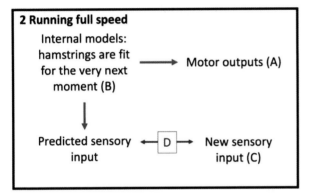

**Figure 10.5** Running at full speed

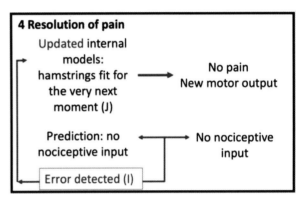

**Figure 10.7** Resolution of pain

### *The onset of pain*

Imagine an athlete running at full speed. Take a moment to ponder on the remarkable complexity of this act—to produce optimal torques at multiple joints with precise temporal and spatial patterns. We can conceptualise that these motor outputs (Fig. 10.5) are produced by neurotags.

These neurotags are influenced by a wide range of other neurotags that represent the size, weight, location and alignment of the body, the strength and length of muscles, the surroundings, and the surface on which the athlete runs. These neurotags can be considered the neuroimmune substrate of this athlete's internal models of things. The internal models of the body will be consistent with hamstrings that are fit for the very next moment (B in Fig. 10.5). The athlete may not have any particular feeling in their body.

Now take a moment to contemplate the amount of sensory data that will be generated by the various tissues of the legs (for example). According to predictive processing theory, there is no possibility for the dorsal horn of the spinal cord to process this information and send to the brain a real-time, precise and comprehensive account of what is happening in the legs. Instead, the dorsal horn is thought to compare what sensory data are predicted to arrive in the very next moment with what sensory data actually arrive. During performance, these predictions and new sensory data are well-matched and the internal models regarding fitness for the task remain unchanged (D in Fig. 10.5).

Now imagine that the mechanical load on the hamstring muscle approaches or exceeds that tissue's tolerance. This activates the nociceptors. Now the sensory data arriving at the dorsal horn (E in Fig. 10.6) do not match the prediction. An error message is generated (F in Fig. 10.6) and the internal models (neurotags) concerning whether the leg is fit for purpose are quickly updated: the hamstring is *not* fit for the very next moment (G in Fig. 10.6). Immediately the system adjusts motor output and produces a *feeling* that will alert the athlete to this situation (H in Fig. 10.6). They immediately back off, perhaps clutch their leg and collapse to the ground, *because of pain.*

A wide range of cues can influence the neurotags that represent the internal models of how fit for purpose the body is: the athlete may have heard a pop; the trainer explains that it looks bad on the replay; the athlete had a previous injury on the other leg or a previous injury at that exact site.

133

### Inflammation increases the safety buffer by transforming the internal models of the body

Inflammation rapidly changes the activation thresholds of nociceptors. This is a spectacularly effective protective strategy.

Consider it from the perspective of neurotags, internal models and predictive processing. Inflammation causes nociceptors to be activated with very little mechanical load on the tissues. As long as the sensitivity of the nociceptors is *increasing,* there is a constant mismatch between the predicted sensory input and the actual sensory input. At each mismatch event, the internal models of the hamstring's fitness for purpose are updated towards being *less fit for purpose.*

Remember, according to the theories above, these internal models are held by neurotags. A day after injury, when the sensitivity of the nociceptors may well have reached its peak, the internal models will suggest that the hamstring is not even fit to walk. As a result, should the athlete attempt to walk, they will experience pain at the injury site.

Resolution of pain reflects updating the internal models of how fit for purpose the body is for the very next moment (Fig. 10.7).

Now consider the gradual reduction in pain as the tissues heal and remodel, until full mechanical characteristics and skill are returned. Every progression of loading on the hamstring provides an opportunity to update the internal models by producing errors between the predicted sensory input and the actual sensory input (I in Fig. 10.7).

This time, however, the internal models are updating towards the hamstring being *more* fit for purpose (J in Fig. 10.7). Progressive loading of the tissues allows for progressive updating of the internal models of the hamstring, right up to being fit for purpose for full competition/play.

### When rehabilitation doesn't go according to plan

If we consider the neurotag and predictive processing theories discussed here, we can be sure that persistent feelings in the body reflect slow updating of the internal models of the body's fitness for purpose. But we cannot be sure that it reflects the slowed return of the tissues themselves to pre-injury characteristics, because these feelings reflect predictions generated by internal models. Here, your clinical reasoning is critical because you must decide where to target your interventions.

Table 10.2 presents things to consider when making this decision for *anyone* with persistent pain. Weekend warriors, elite athletes and non-athletes have a great deal in common—their pain is a multifactorial output that reflects whether or not their body is considered, within the complex network of neurotags, to be fit for purpose. When working with athletes for whom return to play is slow, it is surprising that so much focus is placed on the tissue that hurts, even when all available evidence suggests it is on track.

### Why don't internal models update when the sensory data don't match the prediction?

This question gets to the challenge, and opportunity, of working with athletes/performers for whom return to sport has been slow. According to the theories discussed here, whether an error is detected between a prediction and incoming sensory data depends on the relative weighting of each.

**TABLE 10.2**  Things to consider for tissue properties and internal models

| Tissue properties | Internal models/neurotags |
|---|---|
| Tissue healing is consistent within individuals: what is the healing history of this individual? | Internal models of the body are affected by the sensitivity of the pain system: is there evidence of secondary allodynia or hyperalgesia? |
| Tissue healing is consistent between individuals: what is the usual healing time for this type and degree of injury? | Internal models can be very different between individuals: is this variability being considered? |
| Tissue properties can be visualised using scans: is there any evidence that healing or remodelling has not occurred? | Internal models can be explored through careful questioning: what does the athlete think this part of their body looks like? Could they draw it? What treatment or investigations do they think they need and why? |
| Tissue healing is affected by medications and loading progression: is there any reason to expect tissue healing to be hampered? | Internal models are affected by anything associated with danger or safety to the body: what other danger cues are present in this athlete's life? |
| Tissue strength is assessed by strength tests: is performance on non-functional tests disrupted? | Internal models are affected by training or play-related characteristics other than loading: is the pain affected by location, context, weather, who's around, coach, stakes (e.g. contract pending)? |

Considering the principles that govern how neurotags work,[54, 55, 59] the influence of a neurotag (or the weighting of its output) is associated with its neuronal mass (the number of neurons involved), precision and synaptic efficacy.[58] Applying these principles to this question leads to the hypothesis that the error will not be detected if the prediction is very heavily weighted or the incoming sensory data are not very heavily weighted, or both.

Therefore, according to this way of thinking, strong internal models may well overpower incoming sensory data such that the error is never detected. In such cases, a movement that does not generate the predicted sensory data associated with danger may still result in pain, which actually strengthens the internal model that the body is not fit for that purpose.

Consider Figure 10.8. The internal models suggest that the hamstring is not fit for the very next moment (G in Fig. 10.8). Pain is produced (H in Fig. 10.8) and a prediction of sensory data including nociception is generated (K in Fig. 10.8). The incoming sensory data do not include nociception, but the error is not detected (L in Fig. 10.8). As a result, the model is not updated. In fact, the model is strengthened and pain persists.

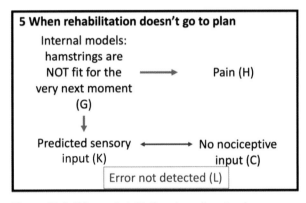

**Figure 10.8** When rehabilitation doesn't go to plan

### What is the solution to this problem?

This line of thinking points to two strategies:

- *increase the influence of incoming sensory data:* this is possible by training the precision of sensory input via, for example, tactile discrimination training[44]
- *decrease the influence of internal models:* this provides the greater opportunity because our internal models are based on many modifiable variables (Table 10.2).

The practical tips in Chapter 11 can all be viewed through the neurotag/predictive processing and biopsychosocial lens.

Hopefully you can now appreciate why Descartes' idea that we have pain receptors in the tissues and that pain signals are transmitted to the brain[6] is as inadequate as it is popular. While its simplicity may be seductive, the ever-increasing body of evidence suggests it simply does not hold up.

If we accept the true complexity of pain as evidenced by the huge amount of experimental and clinical literature[9] and conceptualise pain as being the output of neurotags that represent whether the body is fit for the very next moment, then we must also accept that activity in primary nociceptors is not sufficient for pain.

In fact, when we recognise the potential of strong internal models that the body is not fit for purpose/play/performance to outweigh incoming sensory data, then activity in primary nociceptors is not necessary for pain. These ideas put renewed emphasis on robust clinical reasoning, astute use of scans and clinical tests, sound knowledge of tissue healing properties and load progression/management.

Charles Darwin suggested that young scientists should write down the results that do not support their current beliefs because they are the results that are most forgettable.[61] As clinicians we should do the same.[62]

With regard to pain, this might mean taking note:

- when the same mechanical input flares a condition one day and not the next
- when pain is worse in competition or in build-up than it is in training
- when strength, endurance, control and flexibility are exemplary but the athlete still "tweaks" a hamstring or feels tightness running at 90% effort
- when a 20-second manual therapy technique increases hip range of motion by 25°
- when pain and tightness do not resolve alongside tissue healing and strengthening
- when scans and tests are clear but symptoms persist.

## THE BRAIN IS DIFFERENT IN THOSE WITH PERSISTENT PAIN

It is commonly held that, in much the same way that spinal nociceptors adapt to become more sensitive, so do brain cells that underpin pain.[63-66] That is, the more the pain neurotags are active, the better they get at being active. This manifests in more and more advanced hyperalgesia and allodynia, extended across modalities and exhibiting "overgeneralisation".

Overgeneralisation refers to the phenomenon in which pain begins to be evoked by more innocuous stimuli, in different contexts and under different circumstances.[67-69]

TABLE 10.3  Clinical patterns of increased sensitivity to peripheral stimuli and possible underlying mechanisms

| Clinical manifestation | Possible underlying cause |
| --- | --- |
| Mechanical allodynia: mechanical stimuli that do not normally evoke pain now do | Peripheral sensitisation, pain system hypersensitivity |
| Thermal allodynia: the heat pain threshold is decreased | Peripheral sensitisation |
| Hyperalgesia: normally painful stimuli are now more painful | Peripheral sensitisation, pain system hypersensitivity |
| Primary hyperalgesia (in the painful area) | Peripheral sensitisation |
| Secondary hyperalgesia (beyond the painful area) | Pain system hypersensitivity |

Spreading pain, unpredictable pain and pain less and less related to tissue state and activity are cardinal signs of these cortical changes.

The full mechanisms and manifestations of pain system sensitivity are not fully understood. The complexity of pain and the adaptability of the nervous system should prompt the modern clinician to think well beyond the tissues when dealing with anyone in pain. Indeed, common changes in the sensitivity of the nociception/pain system can be mediated at various levels of the neuraxis (Table 10.3).

An important implication of the disrupted sensory-motor processing now widely documented in people with persistent pain[26] is that it suggests the neurotags representing the characteristics of the body and those associated with movement become less precise. This disruption may underlie feelings (other than pain) that are consistent with the body not being fit for purpose.

It is beyond the scope of this chapter to delve deeply into this, but it is covered in an account by Wand and colleagues.[50] This disruption in neurotags representing the body and its movement is targeted in the second pillar of the "fit for purpose/play/performance" model (Fig. 10.3).

## TREATING SOMEONE IN PAIN: A COMPLEX SYSTEM REQUIRES A COMPREHENSIVE APPROACH

This chapter is not designed to provide a comprehensive guide to treating athletes in pain. Instead, it provides an account of pain that can underpin the assessment and management of pain, whatever your "clinical toolbox". Perhaps the key take-home message here is that you need to consider whether (1) the patient understands that the body is fit for purpose (i.e. the internal models of the body), (2) the body otherwise *feels* fit for purpose and (3) the body is *in fact* fit for purpose.

A contemporary approach to rehabilitation of the athlete in pain places great weight on understanding how pain works, how the body can feel broken or vulnerable when it is not, how many factors influence pain and how there are many ways to reduce the sensitivity of the pain system. These concepts are covered in detail elsewhere.[18, 20] Clinical care must integrate the complexity, context, expectations and resources of the individual. Practical application of the theories and principles presented here is covered in Chapter 11.

## KEY POINTS

- Pain is not a direct indication of tissue damage in the body, but rather the brain's conviction about protecting its tissues. Pain and tissue damage are distinct concepts.

- Pain is a complex biological, cognitive and psychological experience. Nociception refers to the nervous system's handling of noxious stimuli. Pain and nociception are distinct concepts.

- Sensitisation occurs when neurons respond to stimuli that would normally not evoke a response. Our understanding of sensitisation in relation to pain has evolved in recent decades.

- Allodynia is experiencing pain in response to stimuli that are not normally painful. Hyperalgesia is a more intense than expected pain in response to a normally painful stimulus.

- The experience of pain is mediated by many structures throughout the brain and body. The pain system crosses biological, psychological and social domains.

- Researchers and clinicians are beginning to develop interventions for people with persistent pain that consider cognitive-, sensory- and motor-processing abnormalities.
- Changing the way people understand chronic pain is a powerful point of intervention.
- There are physical changes to the brain in people with persistent pain. Spreading pain, unpredictable pain and pain less and less related to tissue state and activity are cardinal signs of cortical changes.
- There are clinical clues that should alert you to a possibility of pain system hypersensitivity in the athlete with whom you're working. Treatment should be individualised accordingly.

## REFERENCES

References for this chapter can be found at www.mhprofessional.com/CSM6e

## ADDITIONAL CONTENT

Scan here to access additional resources for this topic and more provided by the authors

**B**

## CHAPTER 11

# Managing pain

with **KAL FRIED** and **DANIEL FRIEDMAN**

*Understanding pain biology changes the way people think about pain, reduces its threat value and improves their management of it.*

DAVID BUTLER AND LORIMER MOSELEY (IN *EXPLAIN PAIN*)

## CHAPTER OUTLINE

The pain spectrum

Contextualising pain for the individual

Neuropathic pain or neuropathic "contribution" to pain?

Somatic and radicular referred pain

Rethinking models of care: biomedical versus biopsychosocial

Managing acute and subacute pain

Managing persistent pain

Other treatment tools

Bringing it all together

## LEARNING OBJECTIVES

By the end of this chapter you should be able to:

- explain the evolution of how we understand what causes a person's pain
- adopt a biopsychosocial approach to managing pain by practicing patient-centred care that examines how multiple domains of a patient's life can contribute to their experience of pain
- reframe the value you place on unnecessary medical imaging, pain medication and surgical intervention for pain
- discuss pain with patients using accurate, appropriate and sensitive language
- present evidence-based treatment options for the management of persistent pain
- implement an exercise rehabilitation plan that integrates the principles of biopsychosocial care.

In Chapter 10, we explored fundamental neurobiological principles that untangle what can be described as the "circuitry" of pain. Pain is a protective response. If it is accepted that this is a powerfully influential component of pain rather than just an inconvenient by-product, we can change the pain = nociception narrative and improve patient outcomes.

The significance of this extends further because pain is only one of an array of centrally modulated biological processes that align with the brain's discernment of the need for protection. These processes include excessive inflammation, muscle spasm and somatoform disorganisation, as well as complex autonomic nervous system and immune system changes (Fig. 11.1).[1]

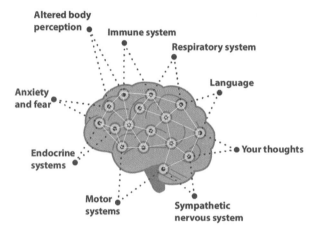

**Figure 11.1** Protective "circuitry" comprises extensive neural pathways that involve multiple systems
ADAPTED WITH PERMISSION FROM THE EXPLAIN PAIN HANDBOOK (MOSELEY, BUTLER, 2015) NOIGROUP PUBLICATIONS.

There is a tendency towards teaching and implementing a linear construct: A leads to B, which can be managed with C. This might work reasonably well for some health conditions, such as using antibiotics to treat a bacterial infection, but health is rarely linear. Acceptance of the broad and dynamic spectrum of manifestations that commonly defy our attempts to pigeon-hole them is a more realistic and potentially more helpful way of conceptualising a variety of health issues.

This is especially evident when it comes to pain. We need to move beyond a linear biomedical model that unhelpfully conceptualises pain as being reliably reflective of physical tissue damage towards a biopsychosocial (BPS) model of management that aligns tightly with contemporary understanding of pain neurobiology.

## THE PAIN SPECTRUM

Physical injuries and degenerative changes are certainly significant, but they are not directly painful. Injuries and illnesses produce electrical signalling (nociception) with pain generated and modulated centrally based on a myriad of other simultaneous and ongoing contributors. These include information provided by clinicians and others that form beliefs and expectations, external stressors, fatigue and a broad variety of contextual factors.

This is why at one end of the pain spectrum it is common to observe severe physical injury or degenerative changes with no pain, while at the other end severe pain is experienced with no changes discovered—and there is a great diversity of presentations in between these two extremes (Clinical case 11.1).

> **PRACTICE PEARL**
>
> Nociceptive contribution to pain is neither sufficient on its own nor necessary for pain to be experienced.

That nociception on its own is insufficient for pain is depicted well at one end of another spectrum when survival is an overriding contextual factor. There are two examples of individuals who were compelled to amputate their own trapped arm to save their life.[2,3] Both individuals were astonished to find that the experience of cutting through soft tissues and nerves and breaking bone was nowhere near as painful as they had anticipated. At the other end of this spectrum is the well-recognised "phantom limb" pain phenomenon where there is no nociception, but pain is still experienced.

As another example of the importance of context, consider injuries suffered in a sporting context versus those in a "perception of injustice" context in an occupational setting. In the former, severe injuries generally result in recovery and return to sport, often within a shorter than anticipated time frame. By contrast in the latter, an event, with or without an objective injury, may result in lifelong pain and even inter-generational, maladaptive pain sequelae.[4] If physical damage was linearly responsible for pain, this wide variability in outcomes doesn't make any sense.

Practical clinical considerations are abundant. Avoid pushing patients further down the maladaptive end of the spectrum. This may happen inadvertently when you invalidate their pain by using judgmental terminology such as "non-organic pain" or "abnormal illness behaviour" when it doesn't fit standardised concepts and resists standard interventions.[5]

> **PRACTICE PEARL**
>
> Protective biological processes are powerful. They are not linear constructs but are variable and dynamic, and often unrelated to tissue change or severity of injury.

## CLINICAL CASE 11.1 A tale of two nails

Two brief case reports involving construction injuries demonstrate the phenomenon of expectation beautifully:

- In the first report, a builder jumped onto a large nail, which pierced his boot at the toe (Fig. 11.2a). He was rushed to hospital and treated with strong pain medication, as he found even the slightest movement to be incredibly painful. However, when the boot was cut

away, they discovered that the nail had actually passed between his toes rather than impaling his foot.[6, 7]

- In the second report, a construction worker was operating a nail gun when it discharged unexpectedly. He was unaware that he had been injured. A radiograph (Fig. 11.2b) was taken 6 days later when he attended his dentist with a toothache.

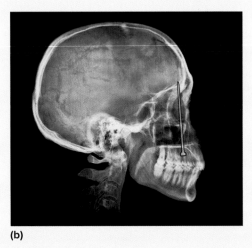

**(a)**                                              **(b)**

**Figure 11.2** (a) This nail pierced the patient's boot, passing between the toes; the patient was in severe pain. (b) This nail in the head caused no pain for 6 days and was then perceived as a toothache.

(A) ADAPTED FROM ISTOCK/DHEO TEGAR PRATAMA, (B) ADPATED FROM ISTOCK/DABOOST

## CONTEXTUALISING PAIN FOR THE INDIVIDUAL

### A "cause" or "contribution"?

Pain is not caused by a single noxious stimulus, but rather is the result of a variety of simultaneous physical, psychological and social contributions that are always in play simultaneously. The experience of identical noxious stimuli can be profoundly influenced by seemingly simple sensory cues.

In an Australian study (Fig. 11.3), participants consistently rated the sensation of touching the same −20°C rod to be more painful when shown a red visual cue representing heat and the potential for more tissue damage than when shown a blue visual cue representing cold and less potential for tissue damage.[8]

Like visual cues, auditory cues can also influence our experiences. Individuals with persistent, maladaptive pain often ascribe high significance to various noises emanating from body tissues when describing both acute injury events and ongoing musculoskeletal concerns.

In a similar, more recent study that explored sound association with perceived feelings of back pain and stiffness, researchers found that providing auditory input in synchrony to forces applied to the spine modulated individuals' prediction accuracy of forces without altering actual back stiffness.[9] Rather than being a marker of the biomechanical characteristics of one's back, this suggests that feeling stiff can be thought of as a "multisensory perceptual inference" that, like pain, aims to protect.

The extrapolation of researched phenomena in relation to understanding pain as a protective construct that is always influenced by a great many idiosyncratic factors is fundamental to optimal management of pain and pain-related disability (Fig. 11.4).[10]

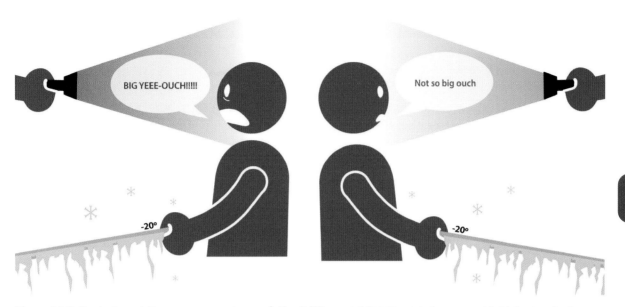

**Figure 11.3** Context can influence our experience of stimuli. When participants were shown a red light, the touch of a −20°C metal rod to the hand was rated as more painful than when participants were shown a blue light.
Source: Adapted from Moseley L, Arnoud A. The context of a noxious stimulus affects the pain it evokes. *Pain* 2007;133(1–3):64–71.

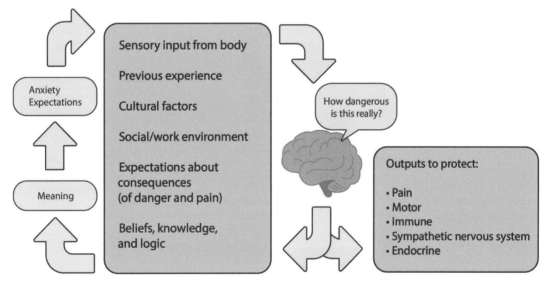

SNS, sympathetic nervous system

**Figure 11.4** Reconceptualising pain according to modern pain science
Source: Adapted from Moseley I. Reconceptualising pain according to modern pain science. *Phys Ther Rev* 2007;12:169–78

## Pain sensitisation

If the brain consciously or subconsciously processes that there is a potential or actual threat, and there are no other (e.g. survival) priorities, pain will be experienced.

The persistence of pain then invites a wide variety of maladaptive processes and complications.

After an injury, a period of increased sensitivity is an adaptation that reduces the risk of a secondary injury

---

**BOX 11.1** The twin peaks model

The twin peaks model (Fig. 11.5) metaphorically illustrates pain sensitisation as a change in our peak protective buffer.[13] We have an innate physical tissue tolerance level that alters with time and after certain injuries. There is a buffer region that protects this tissue tolerance level, usually by producing pain before the tissue fails, but again, many other biopsychosocial factors influence whether pain is experienced and to what level. When pain persists, this buffer increases and can become very large.

Some people can't even tolerate the feeling of clothes on their skin (allodynia). Their protective buffer is a long way from their tissue tolerance level. In these cases, pain from standard activities and physical harm to tissues are unrelated. Understanding this is the basis for a graded exposure rehabilitation program (discussed later in this chapter).

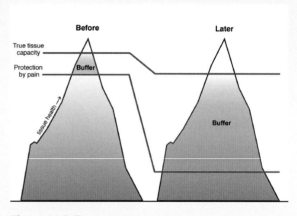

**Figure 11.5** The twin peaks model

---

and provides an opportunity for tissue to heal. However, when pain persists for any reason, sensitisation is virtually inevitable as the brain develops a heightened awareness of the painful region. This means it takes less or even no contribution from physical structures for an amplified pain response (Box 11.1), and responses to interventions targeting these structures become increasingly erratic.[11]

In the clinical setting, sensitisation can manifest overtly as hyperpathia. Hyperpathia is an abnormally painful reaction to a stimulus, especially a repetitive stimulus. It includes hyperalgesia, allodynia, hyperaesthesia and dysaesthesia (Box 11.2). Individuals may find it difficult to identify and localise the stimulus, and may experience a delay in sensation, radiating sensation and/or aftersensation. The pain is constant and easily aggravated. It is objectively resistant to even potent analgesia and may contribute to sleep disturbance, which feeds into the perpetuating cycle.

---

**BOX 11.2** Common presentations of hyperpathia

- *Hyperalgesia:* increased pain from a stimulus that would be expected to provoke less pain, such as slightly more firm clinical palpation.
- *Allodynia:* pain due to a stimulus that does not normally provoke pain, such as light touch.
- *Hyperaesthesia:* increased sensory sensitivity (i.e. heightened sensation of touch, smell, sight).
- *Dysaesthesia:* abnormal, unpleasant sensation in response to touch.

---

These symptoms and signs can be difficult to assess clinically. They have mainly been reported using methods such as qualitative sensory testing, which can be impractical due to cost and time restraints, as well as light touch testing (e.g. with von Frey filaments) and two-point discrimination testing, but these have questionable reliability and rely on the assumption that there are established normative data (which do not exist).

Be vigilant for any features of sensitisation and signs of hyperpathia and contextualise your findings within the bigger clinical picture.[12] Consider sensitisation as having a spectrum of manifestations, rather than rigidly relying on current consensus derived definitions, which can be problematic given the broad spectrum and dynamically changeable nature of maladaptive pain responses. For example, signs of hyperpathia or autonomic dysfunction may not be apparent on the day of presentation but if a patient is asked, they will often respond that they have been present at other times.

## Autonomic dysfunction

A detailed discussion of the many biological system processes that influence pain-related presentations is beyond the scope of this chapter. However, autonomic nervous system involvement merits highlighting as an example of how profound maladaptive processes can be in certain individuals.

The sympathetic nervous system is inherently involved in pain experiences and links to all other systems. Its general involvement can be understood via the "fight or flight" response in relation to an immediate threat, such

---

**BOX 11.3** Budapest diagnostic criteria for CRPS

1. Continuing pain that is disproportionate to any inciting event.
2. Must report at least one symptom in three of the following four categories:
   - *Sensory:* reports of hyperaesthesia and/or allodynia
   - *Vasomotor:* reports of temperature asymmetry and/or skin colour changes and/or skin colour asymmetry
   - *Sudomotor/oedema:* reports of oedema and/or sweating changes and/or sweating asymmetry
   - *Motor/trophic:* reports of decreased range of motion and/or motor dysfunction (weakness, tremor, dystonia) and/or trophic changes (hair, nail, skin).

3. Must display at least one sign at the time of evaluation in two or more of the following categories:
   - *Sensory:* evidence of hyperalgesia (to pinprick) and/or allodynia (to light touch and/or deep somatic pressure and/or joint movement)
   - *Vasomotor:* evidence of temperature asymmetry and/or skin colour changes and/or asymmetry
   - *Sudomotor/oedema:* evidence of oedema and/or sweating changes and/or sweating asymmetry
   - *Motor/trophic:* evidence of decreased range of motion and/or motor dysfunction (weakness, tremor, dystonia) and/or trophic changes (hair, nail, skin).

4. There is no other diagnosis that better explains the signs and symptoms.

---

as being faced by an aggressive beast. The physical effects that a sudden, frightful sensory stimulus have on heart and respiratory responses, pupillary dilation, sweating, sphincter action among others are well recognised and commonly experienced.

But what if the beast stays with you? What if the ongoing threat from the beast is encouraged by the persisting pain, as well as a multitude of idiosyncratic sociological, psychological and contextual factors including what is thought to be causing the problem, focusing on physical factors, either alone or in an unbalanced way. The sympathetic nervous system's response to the ever-present beast persists and this response and its manifestations become increasingly disordered.

How the sympathetic nervous system responds is best conceptualised via a spectrum, with what is currently described as complex regional pain syndrome (CRPS) situated at the severe end of this spectrum.

CRPS is essentially a visible pain-related manifestation. It is a markedly aberrant response to tissue injury, but there is no evident injury in approximately 10% of cases. Multifactorial pathophysiology is being studied extensively, with the literature presenting varying interpretations including noting the roles of disordered neurogenic inflammation, central reorganisation, maladaptive neuroplasticity, autonomic dysregulation and nociceptive sensitisation.[14, 15] Consensus-derived Budapest criteria are currently widely used as an aid in diagnosis of the two types of CRPS (Box 11.3).[16]

- CRPS-1: a nerve lesion cannot be objectively identified
- CRPS-2: a nerve lesion can be identified.

CRPS management approaches involving various oral pharmaceuticals, intravenous infusions and other interventions have demonstrated limited value and validity.[17-19] Conservative measures endorsed as key first-line treatment options include education, graded motor imagery such as mirror therapy, tactile discrimination training and graded exercise exposure.[20]

Clinical case 11.2 probably depicts a manifestation of a maladaptive response that includes subtle, migratory autonomic dysregulation that does not fit into any standard box. In contrast, Clinical case 11.3 illustrates the dynamic and variable potential of a maladaptive response that would easily fit the criteria for CRPS when present sporadically, but not at other times.

## Expectation responses: placebos and nocebos

A discussion of individual pain contextualisation would be incomplete without considering expectation responses. Top-down psychobiological modulations influenced by expectations include responses to placebos and nocebos (Box 11.4).[21, 22]

Placebo and nocebo construct responses are embedded in the very fabric of therapeutic relationships and are a manifestation of the rituals that characterise clinical practice. Placebo and nocebo could be considered redundant terms if neurobiology fundamentals were to be considered more broadly.[23, 24]

It is important to keep this in mind for many reasons, including so that problems associated with the common habit of drawing direct cause-and-effect relationships between various interventions and outcomes in clinical

## CLINICAL CASE 11.2  A swollen foot 1

A 12-year-old girl presented to her family doctor with spontaneous foot pain. An MRI (Fig. 11.6) revealed bone and soft-tissue oedema which were considered to be stress injuries, so she was advised to rest. Her pain persisted and despite rest, further imaging revealed worsening oedema. After review from multiple medical specialists, she was advised to further rest and off-load her lower limb. The pain persisted for more than 2 years. On repeated clinical assessments, she had no clinical signs externally (e.g. swelling, skin changes). There were no externally visible CRPS-type changes, including hyperpathia. There was very little tenderness at all. Further investigations and specialist reviews did not reveal or suggest anything different.

A follow-up MRI was performed in a phase in which the girl was improving clinically. The "migratory" local oedema persisted and was similar to what is seen in CRPS despite no external evidence of this being the case. From a biopsychosocial perspective, there were recognisable potential contributors to a maladaptive pain process. She struggled with a re-adaptive program but improved overall with an interdisciplinary approach, pain education and a graduated progression to regular activity.

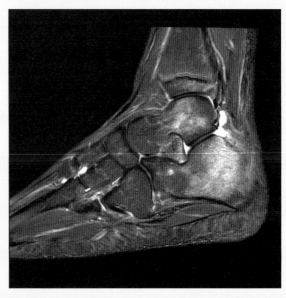

**Figure 11.6** MRI showing significant bone and soft-tissue oedema

### BOX 11.4  Placebos and nocebos

- *Placebos:* inert treatments, such as pills that do not include any pharmacological ingredients. The placebo effect is a beneficial outcome attributable to the expectation response to the context in which the treatment is delivered, rather than to the specific actions of the treatment itself.
- *Nocebos:* inert treatments with a negative outcome, such as the aggravation of symptoms.

practice can be acknowledged properly. Given what we now know about expectation responses in relation to pain interventions including surgery, contemporary perceptions of "improvements" afterwards shouldn't be deemed as having a direct causal relationship.[25-28]

Some of the fascinating research in this area includes 'open label placebo' in irritable bowel syndrome and low back pain. In these trials, placebo responses were explained and the participants knew they weren't receiving active treatments, yet a similar number of unblinded to blinded participants still had significantly positive responses.[29, 30]

Research also indicates that there is a placebo hierarchy (Fig. 11.8). Certain coloured or capsuled medications work better than white tablets. Placebo injections and infusions produce greater levels of responses than placebo oral medications.[31, 32] Sham/placebo surgery may produce an even greater response.

Similar to medications, an increasing number of surgeries targeting pain have been exposed as not having the direct effects we once thought. In sham surgery comparison trials, those who received surgery and those who simply believed they received surgery had comparable results.[28, 33-37] That surgery for pain may only be indirectly effective via expectation responses is problematic for many reasons, including contextual vulnerability, significant harm potential and because it is the gold standard by which many diagnostic and management pathways are retrospectively validated.

The placebo's dark side is the nocebo response. Importantly, this seems to have more profound consequences in a negative direction than placebo has in a positive direction. Unlike placebo analgesia, nocebo hyperalgesia is resistant to extinction, and it can spread socially. Watching another person experience nocebo hyperalgesia from a treatment can lead the observer to experience nocebo hyperalgesia when they receive the treatment.[38, 39]

Again, there is wide-ranging relevance to everyday clinical interactions. For example, reframing the way pharmacy side effect information is provided can affect the

## CLINICAL CASE 11.3  A swollen foot 2

A woman in her early 20s presented with intermittent, severe foot pain when running, but not on every run. On three consecutive reviews, there were no apparent clinical signs of concern. However, she persistently described florid, transient foot changes when experiencing the pain.

During a subsequent review, the woman presented a photo of her foot (Fig. 11.7), which appeared swollen and erythematous—an extreme case of CRPS, but which only occurred sporadically and transiently, and never when being reviewed in the clinic. The woman underwent extensive investigations for other causes of this phenomenon, such as peripheral vascular pathology, but no other aetiology was found.

From a biopsychosocial perspective, it is important to note that the woman discovered running for weight loss after being teased when younger for being obese and was desperate to maintain this activity. She responded very well to a re-adaptive program that included learning the neurobiological basis for her maladaptive pain response, graded but confident "I am doing no harm" activity re-exposure and a short course of low-dose amitriptyline targeting her maladaptive neural response.

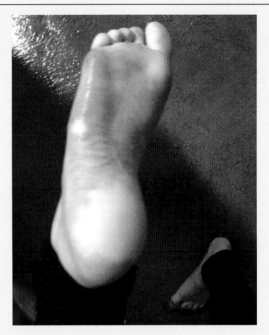

**Figure 11.7** Florid skin changes

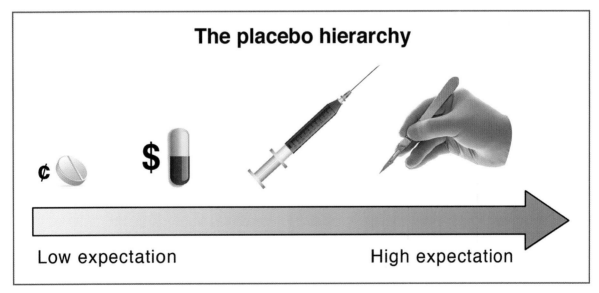

**Figure 11.8** The placebo hierarchy. Patients impose their expectations on the effect of treatments. White tablets come with the lowest expectations of success. Different colour medications come with different placebo effects (e.g. red = stimulating, blue = tranquilising). Price contributes to expectation. Placebo surgery produces the strongest response of the treatments depicted in this hierarchy.

ARTWORK BY VICKY EARLE. PHOTO CONTRIBUTOR: KRAN77/123RF, ISTOCK/CONTRAIL1

incidence of those side effects.[40] This can be extrapolated to understanding the potential major impact of phrases such as "You have bone-on-bone arthritis" or "Your pain is due to your slipped disc ... have a look at this model I have on my desk ..."[41]

## NEUROPATHIC PAIN OR NEUROPATHIC "CONTRIBUTION" TO PAIN?

Neuropathic contribution to pain is best conceptualised similarly to nociceptive contribution to pain, but the nociceptive component is directly from neural tissue. Although a neural lesion or disease is necessary by definition, it is not sufficient to generate what is commonly described in a linear way as neuropathic pain.[42]

Neuropathic processes can be central or peripheral, and include various mononeuritis and polyneuritis, as well as other neuropathic conditions that are usually managed by neurologists. From a clinical sports and exercise medicine perspective there can be objective trauma to neural structures, but the situation is commonly non-objective and, as such, careful judgment is required. An example of this is in relation to spinal imaging where canal stenosis and cord compression of varying severity are seen commonly in asymptomatic people as a well-adapted change.[43, 44]

There are abundant clinical descriptors such as "burning", "tingling" or "pins and needles" which are commonly considered to be diagnostically suggestive of neuropathic contribution, but these can be offered when there is no objective evidence of neural involvement and so the pain spectrum cautions discussed previously remain applicable.

## SOMATIC AND RADICULAR REFERRED PAIN

Similar considerations apply to other commonly used pain descriptors, such as somatic and radicular referred pain.

### Somatic pain

Somatic pain is a highly variable clinical manifestation that can be conceptualised by considering central imprecision as the brain attempts to localise pain in response to ambiguous input from various deeper structures including joints and intervertebral discs.[45] Somatic referred pain can be manifest by myofascial trigger points or fibromyalgia (Fig. 11.9).

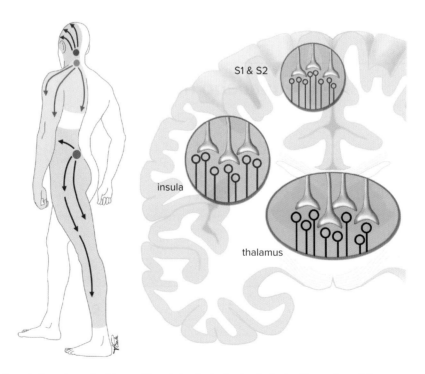

**Figure 11.9** Somatic pain is an important type of input-dominated pain. As in the illustration of the person on the left side of the figure, pain can be referred in non-radicular patterns such as within a limb or quadrant. Nociceptive signals converge in higher centres, e.g. thalamus, insula, and primary (S1) and secondary (S2) somatosensory areas.

The validity data concerning popular treatments for fibromyalgia are not robust and a practical problem is the variability in how the condition is interpreted, informed and most importantly understood by patients.[46] Diagnostic and prognostic beliefs of this nature, which are ultimately based on fragile evidence, commonly become entrenched and can inadvertently contribute to "over-protection" based maladaptive processes.

## Radicular pain

Radicular pain is taught as being pain associated with nerve root compression or irritation. Neuropathic descriptors apply in a dermatomal distribution, but again there is high variability in clinical presentations and interpretations (Fig. 11.10).[47]

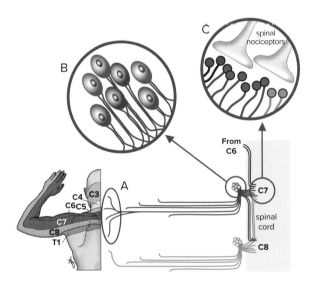

**Figure 11.10** Radicular pain runs in well-characterised narrow bands according to which nerve root is affected. The left panel shows the dermatomal distribution of the neck region. The image also explains mechanisms that can underpin radicular pain—convergence of multiple incoming nociceptors. Note that radicular pain within the peripheral supply of a single spinal segment can occur via convergence of multiple branches of single nociceptors (A). Radicular pain can also occur via nociceptors within the dorsal root ganglion of that peripheral nerve (B). Pain can occur within the adjacent spinal nerve root territory via convergence within the dorsal horn, where projections from levels above (C6) or below (C8) can terminate alongside those from the spinal segment concerned (C).

Objectively concordant, dermatomal reduced sensation and/or myotomal weakness can accompany or occur without radicular pain and then the term "radiculopathy" is applied. Once again, radicular pain and radiculopathy

are seen when an objective compressive lesion is absent and, in this situation, localised inflammation is a possible factor.

> **PRACTICE PEARL**
>
> Always maintain clinical perspective based on fundamental pain biology principles, and re-frame existing definitions. Terms such as "nociceptive/neuropathic pain" suggest a reliable linear relationship and are better considered as "nociceptive/neuropathic contribution to pain" along with many other simultaneous contributions including context, beliefs and expectations.

## RETHINKING MODELS OF CARE: BIOMEDICAL VERSUS BIOPSYCHOSOCIAL

There is growing recognition of the low value associated with an intrinsically flawed biomedical model approach to musculoskeletal care. It relies on an absent linear relationship between musculoskeletal structural damage, pain and interventional outcomes.[48]

The biomedical model assumes that when a person presents for assessment of their pain or disability, not only can the exact pathoanatomical cause be located through examination and imaging, but directed treatment such as medication or surgery will fix the pain and correct the problem.

In sports and exercise medicine, accurate structural diagnosis is often impossible. Many "abnormal" imaging findings may be considered normal age-related changes that can also be found in asymptomatic individuals.[49-59] Injudicious use of imaging, in attempts to isolate a cause and/or rule out red flags, is contributing to alarming levels of ballooning healthcare costs, as well as preventable downstream clinical harms.[60]

Rapid advances in imaging technology and pharmacology have not helped the disturbing increases in the number of patients who report persistent pain.[61,62] An opioid epidemic and widespread use (and misuse) of non-steroidal anti-inflammatories have taught us that while effective in appropriate clinical situations, they come with real and impactful side effects. Patients sold magic bullet interventions for pain—such as arthroscopic surgery for non-traumatic meniscal tears or knee osteoarthritis,[63-65] SLAP tears[66] and subacromial impingement[67]—take the risk of potential harms inherent in these procedures that have now been exposed to be no more effective than a placebo intervention.[68]

## A biopsychosocial approach is not the sum of its parts

As a clinician, you are first taught to rule out red flags, and then advised to screen for yellow ones. Yellow flags, now widely recognised as psychosocial factors that influence a person's health and pain trajectory, were introduced in the late 1990s in New Zealand as part of a framework designed to help primary healthcare clinicians screen for factors contributing to long-term disability in patients with low back pain.[69]

Yellow flags worth exploring with patients include their beliefs, anxieties, self-efficacy and fear-avoidance behaviours. By attempting to understand a person's (mis)conceptions about their pain and expectations of their condition and treatment options, you can begin to identify the many contributions to the person's experience.

While it sounds good in practice, the addition of psychosocial considerations to a biomedical approach does not result in a biopsychosocial model of care. This is a misconception of what the model represents. Engel introduced the BPS model in 1977 to challenge the dominant, reductionist biomedical model, which he described as a model that "leaves no room within its framework for the social, psychological, and behavioural dimensions of illness".[70]

Updates to this definition led to the shared understanding of the BPS model as we know it today, in alignment with fundamental pain neurobiology. It is a model that "focuses on both disease and illness, with illness being viewed as *the complex interaction of biological, psychological, and social factors* ... The distinction between disease and illness is analogous to the distinction that can be made between nociception and pain ..."[71, 72] To aid your understanding of the difference in clinical thinking between the older biomedical model and the more contemporary BPS model, see Table 11.1.

To advance our current practice and improve patient outcomes, clinicians must accept the complex, dynamically fluctuating and interactive nature of this model (Fig. 11.11).[73] The acceptance is the pivotal factor. In the clinic or on the field it may only be possible to identify the overtly recognisable factors. Many other factors do and will always fly under the radar, but they are still present and influential. This is one reason why screening is useful but will never predict all maladaptive pain outcomes.[74]

## Adopting a biopsychosocial approach

One of the fundamental objectives of explaining pain is to shift conceptualisation of pain from that of a marker of tissue damage or pathology to that of a warning signal of the perceived need to protect. An interconnected BPS model reflects pain biology, where complex and dynamic contributions from biological, psychological and psychological domains are all relevant. In other words, when it comes to pain, *everything* matters.

**TABLE 11.1**   Comparison of the biomedical and biopsychosocial perspectives

| Biomedical perspective | Biopsychosocial perspective |
|---|---|
| Involves a search for a cause or causes | Recognises complex interactive contributions from biological (including neurobiological), psychological and sociological domains |
| Strongly focuses on anatomical and mechanical factors, i.e. start with tissue pathology and work backwards | Strongly acknowledges interactions between brain and body, i.e. highlights top-down considerations |
| Focuses on disease or pathology | Focuses more on health |
| Focuses on and informs the need for physical healing ± fixing discovered damage | Focuses on and informs regarding bioplasticity and the extraordinary capacity for adaptation |
| Patient management is often passive and disempowering | Patient management is active, including a high focus on self-management techniques |
| Curative therapies attempted sequentially with increasing risk (e.g. manipulations, injections, surgery ...) | Therapies are rehabilitative/interdisciplinary/re-adaptive |
| Higher perceived harmfulness of physical activity | Lower perceived harmfulness of physical activity |
| Tendency to neglect the significant contextual factors, beliefs and expectation (i.e. placebo/nocebo construct) responses | Implicitly recognises the powerful role of context, beliefs and expectations |
| Research is aimed more at cellular, molecular and genetic levels, with some engagement with neuroscience | Research is aimed more at psychological contributions, with increasing engagement with neuroscience |
| May fail to recognise preventive medicine | Recognises psychological contributing factors as precursors to injury/disease |

Source: Adapted with permission from Explain Pain Supercharged (Moseley, Butler, 2017) Noigroup Publications.

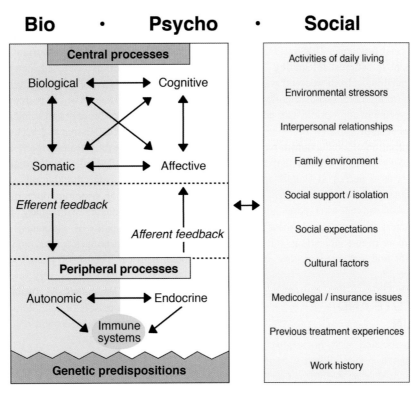

# Bio • Psycho • Social

**Figure 11.11** A biopsychosocial model is not simply the addition of psychosocial considerations to a biomedical model. It also isn't achieved by separating the biopsychosocial into the biological, psychological and sociological, or considering these as primary or secondary factors. Rather, it is a non-linear, dynamic and multidirectionally interactive relationship.
Source: Gatchel RJ. Comorbidity of chronic mental and physical health disorders: The biopsychosocial perspective. *Am Psychol* 2004;59:792–805.

> **PRACTICE PEARL**
>
> To optimally manage pain, we must appreciate how a wide biopsychosocial array of cues affects the brain's evaluation of the need to protect tissue.

You can explore a patient's existing knowledge and behavioural and physical patterns as it relates to their pain. While a focused and classical pain history (e.g. SOCRATES) is essential, you should question a patient's beliefs about their pain and the impact it is having on their mood, wellbeing, ability to work or study, be physically active and engage in relationships, among other important and relevant aspects we recognise throughout the clinical encounter.

By listening to a patient's existing pain and movement beliefs, you can begin to understand and acknowledge the thoughts, emotions and stressors that underlie their potentially problematic conceptual framework. Screening and matching approaches using questionnaires may be helpful for identifying important psychosocial factors and stratifying risk, but do not rely on these as a sole substitute for discussing psychosocial factors with patients.

A patient's apprehension and guarding when performing different movements during clinical examination may also give clues about their pain beliefs and self-efficacy. These protective movement patterns are important to address in rehabilitation (discussed later in this chapter).

## Graded exercise rehabilitation is a core component of the biopsychosocial approach

Fundamental sports and exercise medicine emphasises "doing the basics well". This translates to providing appropriate perspective, reassurance and graded exercise rehabilitation.

Graded exercise is highly recommended for pain management and regional musculoskeletal pain conditions, regardless of severity of degenerative change.[75] Exercise is commonly conceptualised as physical rehabilitation only, but exercise also helps mitigate endogenous pain (Chapter 24), improves cognition and enhances capacity for plasticity.[76,77]

Essential management also includes facilitating return to sport or work, as well as social and community re-connection (i.e. normal function). This results in broad biopsychosocial re-adaptive benefits. Integrating "context" management for all individuals, from weekend warriors to those injured at work, within a biopsychosocial framework, together with careful, recipient-appropriate pain education, is a synergistic, high-value approach.[78]

Resisting the prioritisation of a reductionist, biomedical model of care in this way does not mean that attention to the physical factors is neglected. It should mean that you can support better and safer re-adaptive recovery outcomes. It should also mean that when potentially unsafe interventions and surgery are performed, these are not only undertaken for more robust indications, but that the chances of meaningful and sustained positive outcomes afterwards are enhanced.[79]

## MANAGING ACUTE AND SUBACUTE PAIN

Acute injuries are associated with nociceptive sensory contribution from injured tissues. When a hamstring is torn or a bone is fractured, sensory information from the periphery that has stimulated a nociceptor is sent onwards along the sensory pathway. Nociceptors may respond to different thresholds of thermal, mechanical or chemical stimuli, and encode the noxious stimuli into an electrical message that is transduced at different speeds, depending on the type of nociceptor.

In acute states, pain associated with nociceptive contribution is generally considered to be more closely linked with injury and is an important element of the repair process. However, as discussed, non-linear considerations remain applicable in everyday management. One example is severe pain experienced when spraining an ankle. This pain response can vary broadly and diminish quickly for many. The patient can be pain-free at 2 weeks post-injury, but their ankle may not be fully healed for 6 weeks. In fact, the tissue may never be "fully healed" to its original state.

You should avoid thinking of pain presentations in absolute terms of symptom duration or even as always having proportionality with injury. Pain associated with patellar tendinopathy is intimately linked with patellar tendon load and implies a nociceptive contribution, even though pain can persist for years.[80] First-time episodes of acute low back pain can be very severe without objective evidence of an associated significant structural change.[81] There is always a reason for pain. Remember that even in an acute event, pain is the end point of a complex system that aims to protect (Fig. 11.12).

**PRACTICE PEARL**

When managing acute injuries, aim to support the best physical outcome. Also, quite separately, aim to prevent or at least not inadvertently to contribute to persistent pain.

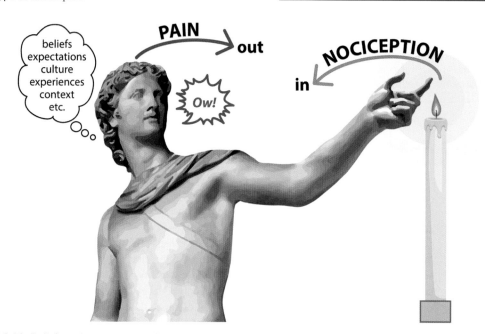

**Figure 11.12** Beliefs and expectations play an important role in how nociceptive inputs are perceived

## Sticks and stones can break bones and words can hurt you too

Consider the important potential long-term influence of how you deliver your clinical opinion in this acute and subacute phase.[82-85] Diagnoses are commonly speculative and inconsistent among clinicians. They are not always as objectively apparent as a fractured bone.

The way even this objective diagnosis is discussed, as seen in Figure 11.13, combined with the idiosyncratic personality and contextual factors in play, combine to be a powerfully influential force in the experienced pain, the degree of inflammation, sympathetic responses and other protective manifestations. Inadvertent clinical contribution to this possible "perfect storm" can profoundly affect recovery outcomes and potentially tissue healing itself.[84, 86]

Acute and subacute back pain presentations are well-recognised to be particularly problematic in this regard. Guidelines firmly recommend that routine scanning be avoided if red flag concerns are absent,[87-89] yet it is not the scan that causes the downstream problems but the way the diagnostic findings are interpreted and communicated. We can apply this rationale to most musculoskeletal findings.

## Injury versus "pain event"

Observing normal, age-related degenerative findings on imaging highlights why differentiating between objectively traumatic physical injury and what may be best described as a "pain event" is so important. Too often, non-objective injuries are speculated based on imaging, or degenerative changes are upgraded in status and assumed to have been created by the recent pain event, regardless of the low mechanical force associated with that activity.

Clinicians must appreciate the commonality of such changes and desist from the over-pathologising that creates downstream harms and associated costs. Instead, when faced with common age-related changes, look to provide broader perspective, explain and reassure. This is applicable at all levels of activity, from an occupational setting to high-performance sport.[90]

A standard biomedical model of care diagnosis following onset of pain commonly focuses on the clinically suspected and/or investigation-evident structural change. A practical change that could be made here is highlighting the pain itself as the diagnosis, with potential physical contribution based on clinical and imaging findings. This is part of the thinking behind the widespread adoption of regional pain labels, such as shoulder-related pain or lateral hip pain. For example:

- Replace "The diagnosis is rotator cuff tendinopathy and subacromial bursitis" with "The diagnosis is a painful shoulder with (potential contribution from) clinical ± investigational features of rotator cuff tendinopathy and subacromial bursitis."

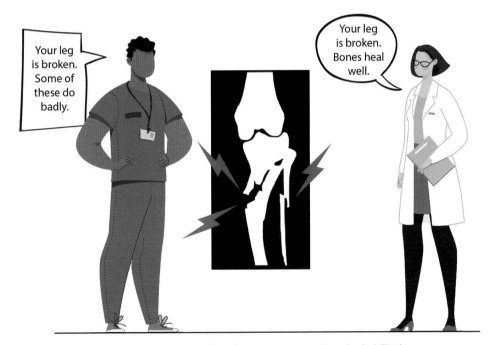

**Figure 11.13** How you convey the diagnosis can profoundly impact prognosis and rehabilitation success
ARTWORK BY VICKY EARLE. PHOTO CONTRIBUTOR: CHARACTERVECTORART/123RF

- Replace "Knee pain secondary to chondral wear" with "Knee pain with (potential contribution from) MRI findings of chondral wear".
- Replace words that convey undue "danger" messages about normal age- or activity-related changes, so instead of "degenerative meniscal tear" or "osteoarthritic wear and tear" use "meniscal change" or "age-related cartilage changes".

Various other investigation findings that commonly exist as well-adapted changes in asymptomatic people should be qualified as such in reporting, and when explaining the imaging and report to patients, rather than speculating that they are the "cause" of pain (Fig. 11.14).[91, 92]

| 2  INCIDENT & WORKERS INJURY DETAILS |
| --- |

What is your injury/condition, and which parts of your body are affected?

3 SLIPPED DISCS IN LOWER SPINE

I REPORTED INCIDENT BUT DIDN'T KNOW I HAD CRUSHED DISC TILL I HAD MRI.

**Figure 11.14** Two unfortunately typical comments on work injury claim forms—both were associated with a persistent, maladaptive pain outcome

---

**PRACTICE PEARL**

When considering a pathoanatomical or structural diagnostic label, ask yourself two pivotal questions:

1. Is the diagnostic label also commonly seen as a well-adapted asymptomatic change?
2. Is pain in the region of interest also experienced by people with no discoverable physical changes?

---

## MANAGING PERSISTENT PAIN

Persistent (chronic) pain is a consensus-derived definition of pain lasting longer than 3 months.[93] This well-intentioned definition inadvertently encourages a linear approach for the first 3 months of therapy to focus on physical targets—a potentially flawed approach that remains difficult to discourage even after the 3-month mark has passed.

---

**PRACTICE PEARL**

The longer pain persists, the less aligned it becomes with nociceptive contribution from tissues and the more sensitisation and other maladaptive processes become influential.

---

A foundation requirement for an optimal re-adaptive recovery is an appropriate level of pain literacy, for clinician and patient alike.[94] There is compelling evidence that by having an optimal understanding of pain, and empowering patients through pain education, we can help improve outcomes synergistically with well-structured, graded exercise rehabilitation. When pain persists, and especially when it is aggravated by physical activity, the assimilation of pain education becomes even more important.[76, 95-97]

Another practical conundrum is that distractions incurred from well-intentioned but disempowering, low-value and low-validity interventions can detract from optimal plasticity-based re-adaptive recoveries. Contentious interventions, prominently including surgery, are commonly proposed because of "failed conservative management". This is highly problematic and may eventually attract serious "informed consent" considerations if the conservative management was not optimally applied and particularly if it lacked contemporary model of care guidance and appropriate pain education.[98]

### What does optimal contemporary "conservative" pain management look like?

Exercise rehabilitation is safe and effective in the management of persistent musculoskeletal pain. There is a growing body of evidence to support combining exercise rehabilitation with a biopsychosocial approach—in programs that provide recipient-appropriate pain education and facilitate confidence in patients that not only is it safe to move, but that this is needed for a re-adaptive recovery (see Table 11.2).[97, 99-102]

Therapeutic exercise rehabilitation intrinsically challenges the threat response to pain and is a pivotal ingredient in the re-conceptualisation of the pain that might accompany movement (Fig. 11.15). In other words, "motion is lotion". For those who do not respond to exercise rehabilitation alone, central pain processes and affective aspects of pain have a better chance of responding differently

**TABLE 11.2**   Upgrading your approach to pain management

| Common approach to pain management | Contemporary, integrated approach to pain management |
|---|---|
| • Focus on and communicate the need for caution<br>• Protect with more activity avoidance and rest<br>• Search further for a physical or pathoanatomical "cause"; refer on because of "failed conservative care" | • Be vigilant for red flag concerns, but maintain full perspective of changes on imaging<br>• Reframe the problem by prioritising the neurobiology and a BPS model of care, which supports the overall benefit of pain during exercise<br>• Frequently reassure the patient that it is safe to move/pace up despite their symptoms<br>• Lower exercise dosage and change type, then gradually build up again<br>• Emphasise developing and restoring movement confidence and quality of movements |

**B**

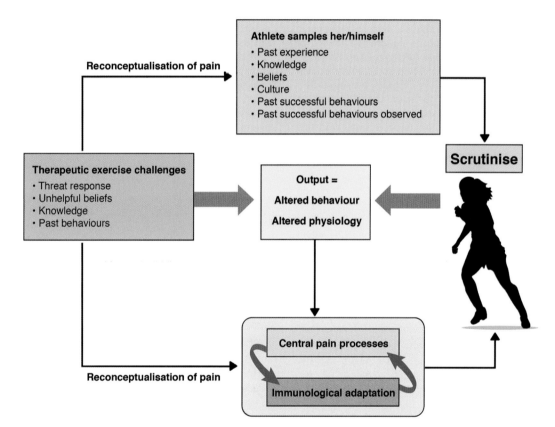

**Figure 11.15** Exercise rehabilitation challenges the threat response to pain and aids the process of reconceptualisation to advance recovery

when pain is conceptualised as non-threatening and unaligned with physical harm (Clinical case 11.4).[97, 103–105]

## Pain education

The aim of pain education is to subdue protective symptom severity via a broader science-based explanation of how the unpleasant sensations are being experienced. But ultimately, it is not the education that is of utmost importance for optimal adaptive recovery, it is the learning. This is best achieved by a management program that implements practical neuroplastic physical and psychological practices with a focus on the process rather than the outcome. A suitable sporting analogy for this is "play the next ball and don't think about the scoreboard".

## CLINICAL CASE 11.4  The man with the bow legs and sore knees

A man in his mid-50s presented after years of bilateral knee pain and repeated arthroscopic surgery on both knees. On examination, both knees were varus aligned and had clinical features of degeneration. He had significant knee effusions and wasted and inhibited quadriceps.

For many years, clinicians had communicated perceptions of non-adaptable damage (e.g. wear and tear, bone on bone), caution and required protection. He attempted exercise programs several times but was repeatedly deterred by his knee pain. He was eventually advised by multiple clinicians that his only option was to have bilateral knee replacements.

Unsatisfied with his prognosis and apprehensive to have knee replacements, he sought the advice of another sport and exercise clinician. This clinician focused on broader pain education and challenged him to a progressive strengthening program, framing it as a "nothing to lose" scenario: if he "failed" the strengthening program, he would find himself where he started, facing the prospect of bilateral knee replacements. And this way, at least he could feel satisfied that he had exhausted

all options if he did end up back on the operating table. He now had a licence to undertake a strengthening program, regardless of pain, before opting for surgery.

This no-lose approach resonated and he pushed through a graduated but vigorous exercise rehabilitation program over the next 6 months. During this period, his ability to control his quadriceps and adjacent muscles improved, his effusions slowly disappeared and his pain improved markedly. His regular reviews became increasingly infrequent as his pain settled and he was able to maintain his improved knee function. When he presented for review 3 years later, this time for elbow pain experienced when playing his weekly tennis match, he still had minimal disturbance from his well-adapted but degenerative knees.

This all-too familiar story is an example of the importance of the clinician understanding contemporary pain neurobiology, patient education and communication, and graded exercise therapy. Advising patients that they simply need to "get stronger" or "lose weight" misses the pivotal ingredient of re-framing pain and beginning the re-adaptation process.

---

Prominent barriers to learning (i.e. the deep integration of pain knowledge) include:

- deeply entrenched reductionist linear concepts about pain causation held by patients and well-intentioned clinicians alike
- the common prioritisation of a biomedical model of care and inconsistent/poor application of an authentic biopsychosocial model of care
- an abundance of fear-inducing and "snake oil" information via widespread misconception augmented by various media, "Dr Google" and a health industry trained narrowly and financially incentivised to "fix" rather than "empower"
- interventions that are interpreted as having a direct cause-and-effect relationship, but lessen in perceived effectiveness with the passage of time and repetition, and encourage escalation in harm risks
- confusing pain syndrome diagnoses and prognostic information with information provided based almost entirely on observations with a dearth of objective data in support; these then develop a life of their own and become the patient's unhelpful, maladaptive reality
- mixed message pain management that often alludes to a biopsychosocial model but implements waves of low-value and low-validity investigations and interventions; this is done simultaneously with curiously little appreciation of

the self-defeating conundrum intrinsic to this approach for the many whose pain persists or recurs.[106]

Despite ardent efforts, clinicians are regularly deflated by the "You are telling me it's in my head and I'm imagining it" reaction. It is therefore not surprising that even though pain education effectiveness data are promising, there is great heterogeneity in process and outcomes, especially when it is education implementation that is being assessed not recipient understanding and deep integration.[95, 107–109]

In 2022, the University of South Australia Pain Revolution group analysed the effectiveness of pain education messaging for people who had been challenged by persistent pain and then recovered. The researchers started with 11 statements capturing target concepts (Fig. 11.16)[110] and were able to refine them to 4 key learning statements (see Box 11.5).[111]

### BOX 11.5  Key learning statements (essential pain facts)

1. Pain protects us and promotes healing.
2. Persistent pain overprotects us and prevents recovery.
3. Many factors contribute to pain.
4. There are things you can do to reduce pain.

## The Target Concepts of Pain Revolution

Target concepts are gateways to new knowledge, activities, retraining overprotective systems and freedom. They are not always easy to grasp, but when you do, you will be well on your way to your own personal pain revolution. Ask your health professional about any of these concepts.

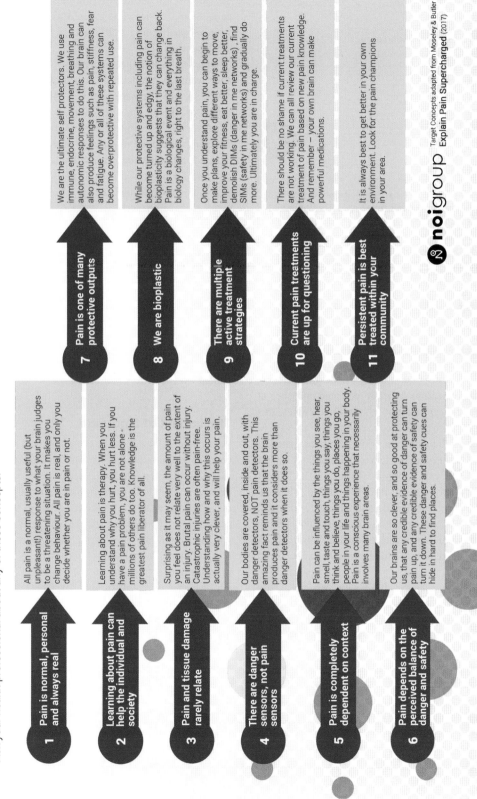

**1 Pain is normal, personal and always real**

All pain is a normal, usually useful (but unpleasant!) response to what your brain judges to be a threatening situation. It makes you change behaviour. All pain is real, and only you decide whether you are in pain or not.

**2 Learning about pain can help the individual and society**

Learning about pain is therapy. When you understand why you hurt, you hurt less. If you have a pain problem, you are not alone - millions of others do too. Knowledge is the greatest pain liberator of all.

**3 Pain and tissue damage rarely relate**

Surprising as it may seem, the amount of pain you feel does not relate very well to the extent of an injury. Brutal pain can occur without injury. Catastrophic injuries are often pain-free. Understanding how and why this occurs is actually very clever, and will help your pain.

**4 There are danger sensors, not pain sensors**

Our bodies are covered, inside and out, with danger detectors, NOT pain detectors. This amazing fact reminds us that the brain produces pain and it considers more than danger detectors when it does so.

**5 Pain is completely dependent on context**

Pain can be influenced by the things you see, hear, smell, taste and touch, things you say, things you think and believe, things you do, places you go, people in your life and things happening in your body. Pain is a conscious experience that necessarily involves many brain areas.

**6 Pain depends on the perceived balance of danger and safety**

Our brains are so clever, and so good at protecting us, that any credible evidence of danger can turn pain up, and any credible evidence of safety can turn it down. These danger and safety cues can hide in hard to find places.

**7 Pain is one of many protective outputs**

We are the ultimate self protectors. We use immune, endocrine, movement, breathing and autonomic responses to do this. Our brain can also produce feelings such as pain, stiffness, fear and fatigue. Any or all of these systems can become overprotective with repeated use.

**8 We are bioplastic**

While our protective systems including pain can become turned up and edgy, the notion of bioplasticity suggests that they can change back. Pain is a biological event and everything in biology changes, right to the last breath.

**9 There are multiple active treatment strategies**

Once you understand pain, you can begin to make plans, explore different ways to move, improve your fitness, eat better, sleep better, demolish DIMs (danger in me networks), find SIMs (safety in me networks) and gradually do more. Ultimately you are in charge.

**10 Current pain treatments are up for questioning**

There should be no shame if current treatments are not working. We can all review our current treatment of pain based on new pain knowledge. And remember – your own brain can make powerful medications.

**11 Persistent pain is best treated within your community**

It is always best to get better in your own environment. Look for the pain champions in your area.

noigroup — Target Concepts adapted from Explain Pain Supercharged (2017)

B

**Figure 11.16** The target concepts of Pain Revolution: see QR code for more details
Source: Adapted with permission from Moseley & Butler, Explain Pain Supercharged, 2017.

Pain Revolution group

## PRACTICE PEARL

Just because there are barriers to taking a biopsychosocial approach and implementing optimal pain management, it doesn't mean you should avoid it altogether. Always provide your patients with information about their treatment options and the opportunity to be empowered in their recovery.

Regardless of the barriers, and the effect these barriers have on research and clinical interactions, it is not difficult to argue philosophically that those who attend for your clinical assessment and management should be informed optimally according to best available data and science. Given the powerful neurobiologically mediated influence of context, beliefs and expectations in overall outcomes, this becomes an even more pivotal requirement.

This approach fundamentally differentiates science-based practices from pseudo-science and charlatanism. It is often argued that expert opinion based on the "art of medicine" should be respected. If there is an art to clinical practice, it is in the individualised implementation of a biopsychosocial model of care; it is not the implementation of potentially harmful management based on observations that are not aligned with fundamental science and contemporary data.

It is also not unusual for those with persistent pain who have exhausted all interventional options to be advised, "You'll have to learn to live with your pain". Yes, this can be appropriate and helpful for some individuals, but it is a concerning observation that patients in this situation regularly retain an either surprisingly poor or suboptimal understanding of fundamental pain biology and biopsychosocial considerations. They rarely prioritise this perspective.

Re-thinking and re-engaging with a re-adaptive, plasticity-oriented approach can indeed mean that recovery is back on

the table.[112] All those suffering persistent musculoskeletal pain should at least be offered an optimally delivered, science-based and safe "escape hatch" opportunity (Patient voice 11.1).

Practically, it is useful to have an array of resources and resource modalities at hand when adding pain education to management.[112] This provides external validation of the material being provided and allows for idiosyncratic learning factors. Virtual reality programs are being developed to assist in this regard.[113, 114] These will help educationally but could also add value with active re-training programs, especially for patients with high levels of movement fear avoidance.

Pain Revolution group resources

For further discussion about the role of education in patient care, refer to Chapter 25.

## The impact of language

As a clinician, think about the number of times you have heard a patient state negative beliefs derived from others (e.g. "The doctor told me I would never [insert activity] again ..."). Even if that patient may have had a lower chance of returning to their preferred activity, these clinician-delivered predictions create sizeable roadblocks for the patient to reframe and begin their journey of positive re-adaptation. Patients too often arrive at consults with indelible quotes that anchor and reinforce their pain beliefs and fear of movement. In contrast, recovery occurs loudly in those who complete the sentence, "The doctor told me I would never [insert activity] again but I didn't believe that and now ..."

Experiencing persistent pain inherently challenges a patient's resilience and self-efficacy, making them more vulnerable to the words of the clinician. And even if well-intentioned, a clinician's language is almost never neutral. The same words that have the potential to heal also have the potential to harm.[118-120] Table 11.3 lists some examples of ways to communicate with patients.

**PATIENT VOICE 11.1** Finding the "escape hatch"

A 47-year-old female police officer with a persistent pain condition was in the audience at a Pain Revolution outreach event in Tasmania, Australia, in 2019. She had been a police officer for more than 20 years and participated in ironwoman races and ultra-marathons. After having a brain haemorrhage, followed by an accident where she was hit by a motor vehicle, she experienced persistent pain long after her injuries had healed.

She received standard pain management, including various pharmaceuticals of considerable doses that only resulted in minor perceived benefit. Her experience of persistent pain spiralled into multiple years of medications, procedures and depression:

"You follow the doctor's advice, but your discomfort grows. You go back to the doctor, and get a scan done. The results are a bit inconclusive, so you reach out to some other health providers ... but nothing helps. So you move on to cortisone injections, opioid medications, even nerve blocks. Before you know it, you are seeing a surgeon and you are having surgery done. The pain doesn't go away ... the pain is moving and growing ... You stop going to work and social events ... Your world becomes smaller and scarier ... You turn to your doctor desperately asking to find what's wrong and make it stop. And they can't. And you have no answers and no belief."

She became curious about pain and read, watched and listened to every resource she could find, notably from Pain Revolution and Pain Australia. Until she discovered what was wrong—nothing.

"I no longer had physical injuries. My body had healed. My pain was very real, but it didn't relate to damage in my body ... My brain had developed an opinion that I was in danger, and it was sending me warning messages in the form of pain.

Normally these messages are a good thing ... but in some cases, the brain gets overprotective and it can keep sending these messages even when we don't need them any more ... This was the first breakthrough moment in my recovery, where I understood that the pain I was feeling, that was very real, was no longer related to damage in my body."

She began a re-adaptive program with a local Pain Revolution "pain coach":

"I had spent a lot of time practising pain. Just as you can train your brain to wind up the pain ... you can consciously train the brain to wind it back ... I made a conscious and deliberate decision to change my approach to pain, from passive to active. I stopped seeing my body as broken and dysfunctional, and I become grateful for this amazing organ that was trying way too hard to protect me."

A year later, her pain had reduced significantly, enabling her to come off medication completely and return to work. She went on to participate in the next Pain Revolution outreach as a cyclist, completing 800 km.

Further details of this fascinating re-adaptive recovery story are available in her TEDx talk, "A new way to think about pain"[115] and Chapter 1 of *Why Does it Still Hurt?* by Dr Paul Biegler.[116]

This isn't an isolated, unusual outcome: other similar "escape hatch" recoveries are described in various media, including Dr Biegler's book and *Pain Heroes* by Alison Sim.[117]

**TABLE 11.3**   The impact of language

| The bad (and based on real quotes) | The not-so-good (what is commonly stated) | The good (and evidence-based) |
|---|---|---|
| "You're a builder, aren't you? . . . Well then, you're screwed." "Every bend or twist at the waist that you can avoid is a victory." | "Your back is degenerated and your pain is because of a disc bulge/prolapse/slip/malalignment/instability." | "There is no evidence of anything nasty; degenerative change is seen commonly in people with no pain and we know it to be highly adaptable." |
| "With each passing moment, you may be doing further damage to your S1 nerve root." "... disc prolapse at T7/8 ... surgery needed due to risk of paraplegia ..." | "Your nerve is damaged/compressed and you have neuropathic pain. This can be difficult to manage and may need intervention/surgery." | "There is likely signalling contribution to pain from the nerve but even this is adaptable because we often also see it in people with no pain." |
| "There is significant knee wear and I certainly don't think the arthroscopy will be the definitive procedure. You will need a joint replacement in the future." | "You have a torn meniscus and wear and tear in your knee which can only get worse with time." | "The best evidence supports exercise (and weight loss) as the best re-adaptive treatment for knee pain, regardless of the grade of joint and cartilage wear." |

# OTHER TREATMENT TOOLS

Maladaptive processes can start early and be exceedingly resistant to standard treatments. There is a foundational need to facilitate a neuroplastic basis for recovery according to the overarching principles discussed above. Once this is appreciated and implemented, the chance for other interventions to have a direct or indirect "circuit breaker" effect is enhanced.

## Medications: options and problems

Medication options include the following:

- "simple" analgesia (e.g. paracetamol [acetaminophen])
- anti-inflammatory medications: non-steroidal anti-inflammatory medication (e.g. ibuprofen, naproxen, celecoxib) and steroids (e.g. oral prednisolone)
- opiates/opioids (synthetic) (e.g. oxycodone, morphine, fentanyl)
- "anti-neuropathics": antidepressants/anticonvulsants
- others: this long list includes local anaesthetics, benzodiazepines, muscle relaxants, cannabinoids, clonidine, ketamine and capsaicin.

These treatment options are also discussed in Chapter 24, exploring their application to different musculoskeletal injuries.

> **PRACTICE PEARL**
>
> Medications can be important in managing acute and persistent pain. At all stages, you should prepare for and discuss future medication reduction management plans.

Opiates and opioids can have opioid-focused activity with higher risks of dependence and respiratory depression; this includes codeine, morphine, oxycodone, hydromorphone and fentanyl. Medications that combine opioid and non-opioid activity have lesser (but not absent) risk of respiratory depression and dependence as tolerance develops more slowly; this includes tramadol, buprenorphine, tapentadol and methadone. The prescribing clinician must appreciate the important nuances of opiates/opioids in acute pain and in persistent, non-cancer pain. Contemporary guidelines reflect these concerns and should be adhered to tightly.[121, 122]

Anti-neuropathic medications emanate from antidepressant and anticonvulsant origins. Antidepressants that are used are tricyclics (amitriptyline and nortriptyline) and serotonin noradrenaline reuptake inhibitors (duloxetine and venlafaxine). Anticonvulsants that are used are gabapentin, pregabalin, valproate, carbamazepine and topiramate.[123]

Both antidepressants and anticonvulsants have been investigated in relation to neuropathic pain with questionably extrapolated use in pain sensitisation. Antidepressant medication action is thought to be through mediation of the modulatory descending inhibitory pathway and the analgesic benefit is thought to be independent of antidepressant action. Amitriptyline has a "number needed to treat" of 4 to achieve 30% perceived pain reduction and there are a wide range of potential adverse effects largely due to its anticholinergic action.[124]

Anticonvulsant medication action is thought to be via effects on synaptic calcium channels. Pregabalin has a number needed to treat of 6 to achieve 30% perceived pain reduction in central neuropathic pain, with once again a wide range of potential adverse effects.[125]

Relevant to all pain medication is expectation response, as discussed above. This is another reason for the firm recommendation of judicious use and close monitoring.[126-128] A further major concern relevant to both new medications and interventions is that uptake and marketing commonly fuel expectations and develop far in advance of appropriate level validation. A good example is the most recent upsurge in popularity of medicinal cannabis. Position statements are often presented "after the horse has bolted", which is a repeated pathway that has significant clinical and fiscal ramifications.[129-131]

> **PRACTICE PEARL**
>
> Always start at the lowest dose possible. Monitor perceived benefits and adverse effects closely.

> **PRACTICE PEARL**
>
> Rationalise and/or cease medications if there are adverse effects or cognitive impairment. Cognitive impairment limits a patient's ability to use re-adaptive techniques.

## Interventional pain management

The range of interventions available for pain management is extensive and far exceeds the scope of this chapter. There is ample literature for both believers and sceptics of this approach, yet higher level analyses generally urge caution, and if support is offered it is generally trepidatious and highly qualified.

There appears to be a common misconception in the application of many interventions that treating nociception

**TABLE 11.4**   The three stages of graded motor imagery

| Stage | Activity | Explanation |
| --- | --- | --- |
| 1. Left/right discrimination | Quick judgments of left or right images, usually using flashcards | Individuals with persistent pain can lose the ability to distinguish between their left and right sides when viewing images of painful body parts. Before they can progress to successfully visualise painful body parts moving in specific ways, they need to be able to discriminate between their left and right. |
| 2. Explicit motor imagery | Rehearsing imagined movements | Mirror neurons are neurons that modulate their activity both when an individual executes a specific movement, observes the same or similar movement performed by another individual, or visualises the movement themselves. Explicit motor imagery enables an individual to visualise executing movements that have been causing pain, starting with smaller components of the movement pattern and building up from there. |
| 3. Mirror therapy | Using a mirror box to create the illusion of therapeutic movement | When an individual places their pain-free limb in front of a mirror and hides their painful limb within the mirror box, they can "trick" their brain into believing the reflection is their painful limb. This activates motor neurons and helps reduce the perceived pain sensitivity of the affected limb through pain-free movement of the limb being reflected. |

is the same as treating pain,[132] which is fundamentally incorrect. Beware of "catch-22" considerations inherent in approaches that prioritise directing sequential interventions to physical targets.[133]

## Graded motor imagery

Graded motor imagery is a sequential process that aims to facilitate sensory cortical reorganisation. It is used in the management of persistent pain and has specific application in phantom limb pain and complex regional pain syndrome.[134] The three stages of graded motor imagery (Table 11.4 and Fig. 11.17) are designed to optimise sensory-motor processing and gradually engage the cortical motor networks without triggering the protective pain response.

## Manual therapy/acupuncture/dry needling/transcutaneous electrical nerve stimulation

Touch and electrical stimulation have theoretical nociceptive modulating effects that can provide benefits

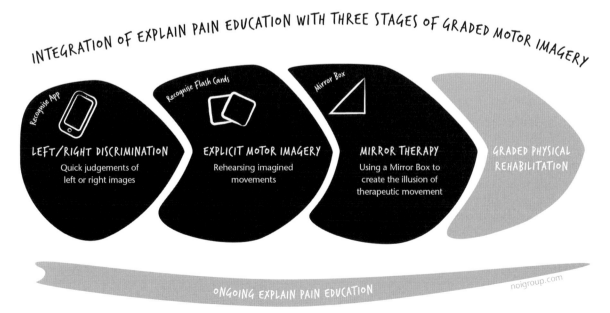

**Figure 11.17** The three stages of graded motor imagery
Source: Reproduced with permission from Noigroup Publications, noigroup.com

for many individuals. They are best used as part of a wider re-adaptive program. However, clinician statements regarding manual therapy such as "putting your spine back in place" are not only grossly inaccurate but also unhelpful from a pain biology perspective.

Similar to many other pain treatments, the direct effectiveness of dry needling treatments and transcutaneous electrical nerve stimulation (TENS) is tenuous.[135,136] Perceived responses are commonly partial and short term, with susceptibility to contextually vulnerable expectation responses.

To learn more about manual therapy and dry needling in the management of sporting injuries, see Chapter 24.

### PRACTICE PEARL

Long-term dependence on passive therapy is counterproductive and is best discouraged.

## Psychological treatment approaches

In a biopsychosocial approach, awareness of psychological influencing factors is pivotal in recognising risk of a maladaptive outcome in the acute pain phase. Subsequent to this, psychological management is implicitly required in persistent pain management. Pain education and some formal psychological treatment programs are often referred to as "talk therapies"; other programs are described as mind–body therapies.

### Meditation and mindfulness

Meditation and mindfulness are closely linked and are helpful in winding down heightened, maladaptive processes. Meditation sessions involve three key components: ritual, focus and management of intrusive thoughts. Mindfulness can be conceptualised as the integration of these components in everyday activities and interactions.[137]

### Cognitive behavioural therapy

Cognitive behavioural therapy aims to facilitate awareness of inaccurate or negative thinking so that challenging situations can be viewed more clearly, and patients can respond to them in a more effective way.[138]

### Acceptance and commitment therapy

Acceptance and commitment therapy focuses on helping patients apply mindfulness and acceptance skills to their responses to uncontrollable influences and commit to behave more consistently with constructive values. There is specific relevance here to "perception of injustice" and compensable contexts, both associated with increased risk of maladaptive, persistent pain outcomes.[139]

### Eye movement desensitisation and reprocessing

Eye movement desensitisation and reprocessing is a psychotherapy treatment program that facilitates the accessing and processing of traumatic memories and other adverse life experiences, aiming to bring these to an adaptive resolution. During therapy, patients attend to emotionally disturbing material in brief sequential doses while simultaneously focusing on an external stimulus.

Therapist-directed lateral eye movements are the most commonly used external stimulus, but a variety of other stimuli including hand-tapping and audio stimulation are also used. These new associations are thought to result in complete information reprocessing, new learning, elimination of emotional distress and development of cognitive insights. There is much relevance for persistent pain conditions with current data showing promising crossover benefits.[140]

## Nutrition and other lifestyle factors

Optimising nutrition and other lifestyle factors are mentioned here last, but these are certainly not the least important management considerations. General stress, lack of sleep (no longer a badge of honour[141]), sedentary behaviour, smoking and poor diet among other troublesome lifestyle behaviours are recognised to heighten and perpetuate pain.[142]

In recent years research has uncovered more about the link between nutritional neurobiology and sensitisation in people with persistent pain.[143] Diet-induced neuroinflammation caused by pro-inflammatory ultra-processed foods and high consumption of sugar has been proposed as a potent contributor to pain outcomes. Inversely, wholefoods and antioxidant-rich plates (think Mediterranean diet) show an inverse relationship with systemic inflammation and may alleviate persistent musculoskeletal pain via their positive effects on gut microbiome and other mechanisms.[144-148]

In sports and exercise medicine, there has been a seismic shift in thinking about the classical "wear and tear" mechanical paradigm of osteoarthritis to a more complex inflammatory systems model that recognises the role of the immune system as well as biomechanics.[149] Losing even 10% of body weight can significantly reduce pain and function in those with knee osteoarthritis, probably due to both reduced mechanical load and the anti-inflammatory effects of the loss of adipose tissue itself.[150,151]

There is a growing body of research exploring how when and what we eat affects pain,[152] with particular focus on dietary polyphenols.[153] Blueberries have been touted for their anti-inflammatory effects and benefits in symptomatic knee osteoarthritis.[154] Similarly, omega-3 fatty acids in the form of fish oil have been found to have equivalent effects in reducing arthritic spinal pain as some non-steroidal anti-inflammatories.[155]

But as simple as it may seem to ask patients to eat more "[insert superfood here]", isolating individual foods or components of foods that yield positive and significant research findings perhaps loses sight of the bigger picture. Just like pain, nutrition is far from linear.

### PRACTICE PEARL

Consider the evaluation of diet as a routine part of the work-up for persistent pain, alongside other lifestyle factors such as sleep and physical activity.

## BRINGING IT ALL TOGETHER

In managing pain, the most helpful approach to breaking pain's vicious cycle, or preventing it from occurring in the first place, is to consider the wide biopsychosocial array of cues that affect the brain's evaluation of the need to protect tissue. Understanding that pain is, by definition, protective and not a marker of tissue state or damage, makes a biopsychosocial approach sensible.[94]

In sports and exercise medicine, clinical assessment is generally aimed at establishing a structural diagnosis to guide a management plan in the hope that the patient will fully recover. The contemporary clinician should:

- understand the flaws in a narrow and linear model of care approach
- have a broader view considering appropriate value and validity data
- adhere to the "null hypothesis" science requirement, which is to continue asking questions as opposed to accepting established beliefs that don't stand up to analytic scrutiny
- appreciate pain as a protective output with a dynamic spectrum of manifestations
- assess the various recognisable contributors to the patient's pain while also appreciating that much is not recognisable, yet still influential
- refrain from "nocebic" contribution
- attempt to facilitate and empower an optimal re-adaptive outcome.

This approach, which incorporates advances in pain science, will mean fewer patients are given inappropriate and potentially harmful treatment that is missing an important element of their condition.

The concept that persistent pain management nirvana lies in the next pharmacy-based or interventional technique is perplexing because of (1) the central biology discussed, (2) the track record of this approach over many years and (3) the monetary ramifications.

Instead of repeating such processes hoping for a different overall "greater good" outcome, perhaps by converting to the model of care discussed here and in a way that aligns well with fundamental sports and exercise medicine principles, it will be possible to reverse the trajectory of persistent musculoskeletal pain.

## KEY POINTS

- Pain is a critical protective response.

- Tissue injuries and changes do not produce pain directly. They only produce signalling contribution to pain processing (nociception) along with many other contributing elements (e.g. contextual influences, psychosociocultural factors, beliefs, clinician advice), which influence protective responses in a powerful and commonly under-appreciated manner.

- Pain is a poor marker of physical injury/damage; it is robustly aligned with the conscious or subconscious perception of the need for protection. In other words, pain depends on how much danger your brain processes you to be in, not how much you are really in.

- Pain is one of an array of protective biological processes (inflammation, muscular spasm, immune and sympathetic nervous system changes, somatoform disorganisation etc.).

- Context, beliefs and expectations are powerfully influential in pain and outcomes. This is problematic when pain is conceptualised by prioritising a reductionist biomedical model of care.

- The safest and best outcomes are achieved when all involved stakeholder beliefs and expectations align broadly in an adaptive direction. The opposite occurs when these are maladaptive, divergent or influenced by fear and confusion.

- Be careful what you believe; your beliefs and what you inform can become your patient's reality.

- Exercise rehabilitation and normalisation of activity are safe, work and are encouraged by contemporary guidelines.

- The type of exercise rehabilitation seems to not be as important as the context in which it is delivered.

- Exercise rehabilitation benefits are likely to be augmented if the neurobiology is integrated and the patient is educated about its involvement.

- Contemporary, best-evidence guidelines indicate that there is a need to shift away from imaging, interventions and a reductionist model of care for better "greater good" outcomes to be achieved.

- The future in terms of a recommended model of care and funding of this model is very likely to lie in this direction as current, commonly used methods are associated with harms and monetary waste.

- Clinical sports and exercise medicine is ideally placed to implement an approach that manages physical injuries optimally but also manages the pain component by prioritising the neurobiology, a biopsychosocial model of care and re-adaptive exercise rehabilitation based on contemporary guidelines.

## REFERENCES

References for this chapter can be found at www.mhprofessional.com/CSM6e

## ADDITIONAL CONTENT

 Scan here to access additional resources for this topic and more provided by the authors

## CHAPTER 12

# Introduction to clinical biomechanics

with **ELANNA ARHOS** and **RICHARD WILLY**

*No matter what your sport, correct biomechanics is key.*

FAYE PATTISON (UK PHYSIOTHERAPIST)

## CHAPTER OUTLINE

Key concepts in biomechanics
Measurement of muscle performance
Tissue-specific tolerance to loads
Tissue homeostasis and mechanotherapy
How do we obtain biomechanical data?

## LEARNING OBJECTIVES

By the end of this chapter you should be able to:

- explain several basic biomechanical concepts in the context of sport and physical activity
- apply biomechanical principles to design and implement safe and effective training and rehabilitation programs
- discuss the broad mechanisms of sports injuries using biomechanical terminology
- list ways in which biomechanical data can be collected in the sports and exercise setting.

B

The field of biomechanics is broad, ranging from tissue mechanics to describing the movement of the human body. In this book, biomechanics refers to the interactions of the musculoskeletal system with (1) the laws of motion and (2) internal and external forces. Broadly, this chapter aims to provide you with a working knowledge of the principles of kinematics (visible movement of a body, joints and segments), kinetics (forces resulting from and driving movements) and neuromotor activity (muscle actions that generate and control forces and movements). Clinical examples demonstrate the applicability of these key biomechanical principles.

## KEY CONCEPTS IN BIOMECHANICS

Before you can understand joint kinematics and kinetics and how they relate to patient care, it is important to familiarise yourself with definitions related to data interpretation.

Often, motion is described with respect to either a joint within the body (e.g. glenohumeral joint, tibiofemoral joint) or segments within the body that make up that joint (e.g. scapula, thorax, thigh, shank). Movement can therefore be described as segments with respect to other segments, such as the position of the humerus with respect to the glenoid of the scapula, or segments with respect to the environment.

Osteokinematics describes relative motion between segments. For example, flexion, extension, abduction, adduction, internal rotation and external rotation all refer to osteokinematic motion and can be quantified clinically with a goniometer or inclinometer on a mobile app.

Arthrokinematics describes movement occurring between joint surfaces, such as rolls, spins and glides. It is assessed using joint mobilisation to test mobility within the joint itself.

In the biomechanics literature, there are references to both kinematics and kinetics.

## Kinematics

Kinematics typically has to do with joint angles and positions and is the study of movement without considering the contribution of the forces causing movement. When movement is considered in the context of the segments of the human body, it is typically either linear (i.e. translational) or rotational (i.e. angular):

- *Linear motion* (Fig. 12.1a) refers to a translational motion where each point of the segment moves at the same time and with the same speed. There is no axis of rotation. An example is scapular elevation and depression, where you have translation of the scapula in a superior or inferior direction over the thorax. Another great way to consider linear motion is when performing joint mobilisation with patients; for example, a posterior to anterior glide of the tibia on the femur to improve knee extension (Fig. 12.1a).
- *Rotational motion* (Fig. 12.1b) refers to when a segment rotates about a pivot point or an axis (e.g. longitudinal or vertical axis). In true isolated rotation, the points on the segment do not get closer to or further from the axis of rotation.
- *Curvilinear motion* is a combination of linear and rotational motion (Fig. 12.1c), where a segment moves along a curved path. Curvilinear motion is not as common as linear or rotational motion.[1]

We can think of movement as translational motion that occurs within a plane and rotational movement that occurs around an axis. We have the frontal (coronal) plane, vertical (sagittal) plane and horizontal (transverse) plane, about which movement occurs (Fig. 12.2).

- In the frontal (coronal) plane, movement occurs about the anterior-posterior axis (e.g. shoulder and hip abduction or adduction).

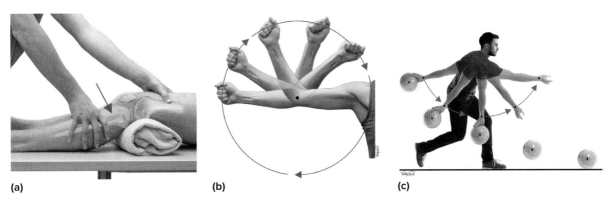

(a)     (b)     (c)

**Figure 12.1** Types of movement: (a) linear, (b) rotational and (c) curvilinear
ARTWORK BY VICKY EARLE. PHOTO CONTRIBUTOR (C): ISTOCK/4X6

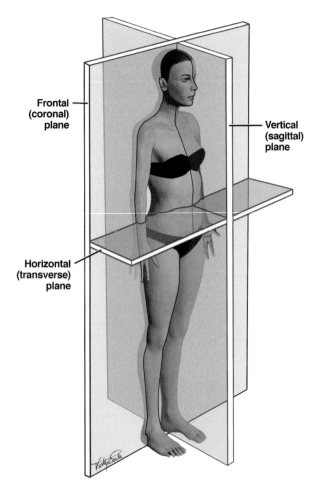

**Figure 12.2** Cardinal planes of movement with axis drawn through each plane

Frontal (coronal) plane

Vertical (sagittal) plane

Horizontal (transverse) plane

- In the vertical (sagittal) plane, rotation occurs about the medial to lateral axis (e.g. flexion and extension of the hip).
- In the horizontal (transverse) plane, rotation occurs about the longitudinal axis (e.g. hip internal and external rotation).[1]

Individual planes of movement contribute to multiplanar motion and enable clinicians to break motion down into individual components when assessing movement quality. For example, when assessing a single limb squat, a patient's movement can be broken down into the contribution of hip flexion, internal rotation and adduction.

## Kinetics

Kinetics describes the effect of forces on movement or tissues.[2] Kinetics is an integral part of describing motion of the human body. Forces (unit = Newtons [N]) are defined as external or internal push or pull that change the state of motion of the body. External forces are caused by the gravity of objects applying force against the body. Internal forces come from muscles, tendons, bones and joints. The application of force to a unit of area results in pressure, also known as stress (unit = megapascals [MPa]):

$$\text{Tissue stress (MPa)} = \frac{\text{Applied force (N)}}{\text{Surface area (cm}^2\text{)}}$$

Applied forces and stresses can be from an external source (e.g. gravity) or an internal source (e.g. muscle force). For example, when pushing off the ground during running, the ground reacts and pushes back against the foot (known as a ground reaction force) resulting in pressure (i.e. stress) on the plantar surface of the foot.

Figure 12.3 compares the vertical ground reaction forces between walking and running. During running (red dotted line) the stance phase is shorter and you will often see an initial impact peak followed by the maximal peak ground reaction force. During walking (black solid line) you will see two peaks with higher force, the first during weight acceptance and the second during push-off (plantar pressure).

If the foot's contact area is reduced but the ground reaction forces are maintained, plantar pressure increases, as can be measured with instrumented-pressure insole devices. High regional plantar pressures may play an important role in certain injuries, such as high lateral

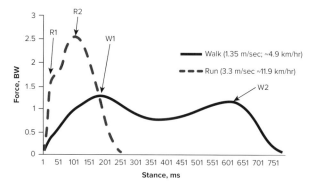

**Figure 12.3** Vertical ground reaction forces during walking (black) and running (red). Forces are normalised to body weight (BW) during the stance phase (in milliseconds). During walking, the first force peak (W1) corresponds with heel strike and the second force peak (W2) corresponds with the propulsive phase prior to toe-off. During running, there is an initial impact transient (R1) as the heel strikes, followed by a larger force peak (R2) associated with the propulsive phase.

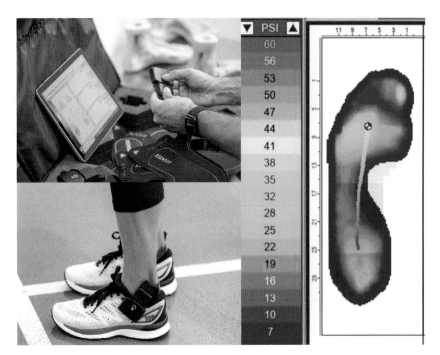

**Figure 12.4** Modern plantar pressure sensors enable remote data logging to assess pressures during field manoeuvres. Plantar pressure data from an instrumented pressure insole of a healthy subject during walking is shown here. Note the cursor, which shows the path of the centre of pressure from heel-strike to toe-off. Brighter colours overlayed on the insole are indicative of higher, localised plantar pressures. Centre of pressure data can be helpful in determining areas of high plantar stresses that might be seen clinically in individuals with a history of metatarsal bone stress injury, for example.
COURTESY OF RICHARD WILLY

plantar pressures in individuals who go on to develop 5th metatarsal bone stress injuries (Fig. 12.4).[3]

A clinical example of the importance of understanding internal forces and stresses can be seen when considering the Achilles tendon during a dynamic activity such as running. Consider two runners of the same height and mass, running the same speed, side by side. Runner A has a larger cross-sectional area of the Achilles tendon compared with runner B's tendon. During the stance phase of running, the plantarflexors contract and transmit force to the calcaneal tuberosity via the Achilles tendon. This plantarflexes the ankle to generate propulsive forces. Even though their Achilles tendon forces are the same during running, runner B will experience considerably greater Achilles tendon stress, because of their smaller Achilles tendon, compared with runner A who has a larger Achilles tendon to distribute the same force.[4]

## Tissue strain

You should also be familiar with the concept of tissue strain, which is the amount of deformation a tissue experiences when force is applied.[5] Tissue strain is calculated using the change in length of a material under load relative to its initial resting length. For example, if you wanted to measure patellar tendon strain during an isometric knee extension effort, you would first measure the resting tendon length and then the length of the tendon while loaded. From there you would use this equation to estimate the percentage of patellar tendon strain:

$$\text{Tissue strain} = \frac{\text{Loaded length (cm)} - \text{resting length (cm)}}{\text{resting length (cm)}}$$

## Force and torque

An important definition to clarify when interpreting clinical biomechanics is force compared with torque. You may hear the terms "force" and "torque" being used interchangeably but there is a fundamental difference between the two: muscles exert force internally at the point of muscle attachment; torque refers to the force applied to a segment rotating about an axis (usually the joint centre), or angular motion.

"Torque" and "moment" (units = Nm) are equivalent terms and are commonly used interchangeably. The moment arm (units = m) is an important part of the torque calculation and is defined as the perpendicular distance from the joint axis of rotation to the point of force application.[2] The formula for moment (or torque) is calculated with this equation:

$$\text{Moment (Nm)} = \text{force (N)} * \text{moment arm (m)}$$

Using a clinical example, when measuring quadriceps muscle performance on an isometric dynamometer, the quadriceps are producing a force attempting to rotate the tibia around the knee joint centre to extend the leg. The centre of the pad placement of the dynamometer lever is the point of force application. The distance between the centre of the pad placement and the knee joint centre of rotation is the moment arm of the external load (Fig. 12.5).

## Joint moments

Joint moments are often described in two ways: external moment, which is calculated using external forces (e.g. gravity, an externally applied force, objects, ground); and internal moment (e.g. muscles, ligaments, capsule, bone[2]).

We can use walking gait to illustrate the difference between external and internal moments. During the loading response phase of gait, there is an external knee flexion moment of gravity trying to bring the knee into flexion, which is countered by an equal, but opposite, internal knee extension moment produced by the quadriceps.

When we consider moment arms in a clinical setting, there are both internal (e.g. joint centre to internal line of action of the biceps muscle) and external (e.g. joint centre to external load of weight at the hand) moment arms. For instance, imagine holding your arm flexed in a stationary position of 90° elbow flexion (i.e. an isometric contraction) (Fig. 12.6). Gravity creates an external elbow extension moment and your bicep muscles create an *equal and opposite* internal elbow flexion moment to maintain a static position of 90° elbow flexion.

Isometric contraction
External moment (Nm) = Internal moment (Nm)
External moment arm (m) * External force (N) =
Internal moment arm (m) * Internal force (N)

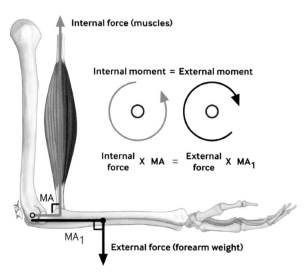

**Figure 12.6** Internal vs external moment arm

Concentric elbow flexion (flexing your elbow) is characterised by an internal elbow flexion moment generated by your biceps that is slightly greater than, but opposite of, the external elbow extension moment. Eccentric

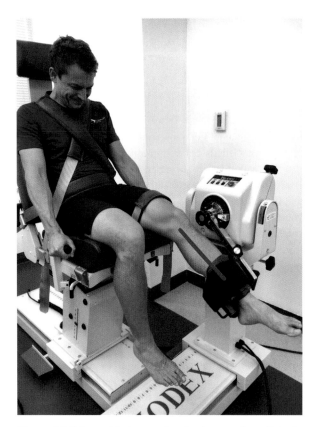

**Figure 12.5** Isometric knee extension torque strength test using an isokinetic dynamometer with moment arm shown (red)

elbow flexion (lowering your arm with active resistance by the biceps/brachialis) is characterised by an external elbow extension moment that is slightly greater than the internal elbow flexion moment generated by your biceps.

Moment arms are particularly important to consider when dosing exercises or using a handheld dynamometer to measure muscle performance. We will use two different types of open chain knee extension machines to illustrate the effect that moment arms can have on the external moment of an exercise:

- In the first example the external moment arm changes but the applied external force does not. Consider an athlete who is sitting on a bench wearing an ankle cuff weight (which remains firmly velcroed at the ankle). There is zero extensor moment at rest but as the athlete progressively extends their knee, the external moment arm lengthens to the maximal point where the knee is fully extended–parallel to the ground (Fig. 12.7a). The moment arm is the length from the knee joint to the

ankle weight. Note that the amount of applied external force (the weight) did not change but the athlete needed to increase their internal quadriceps force considerably as the knee extended.

- Next, consider equipment that uses a cable and weight stack system or a cable-resisted machine where the external moment arm remains constant throughout the range of motion (i.e. the position of the external load does not change; Fig. 12.7b). Since the magnitude of the external applied force does not change (the weight stack stays the same) and the external moment arm remains constant (the weight stack does not move), the athlete's internal quadriceps force remains fairly constant throughout the range of motion.

Knowing the biomechanical differences between these two knee extension machines can help explain how a patient may respond to treatment, particularly in the event of muscle and joint soreness.

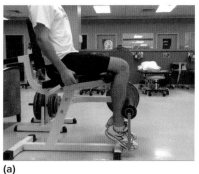 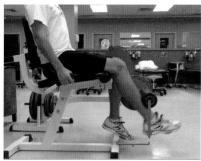 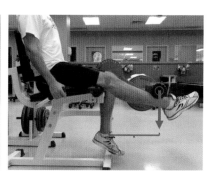

(a)

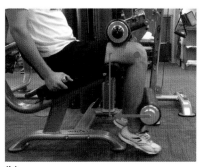 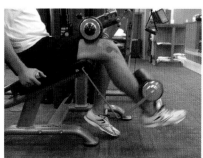 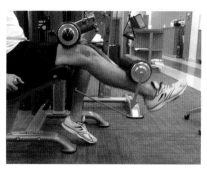

(b)

**Figure 12.7** (a) Variable moment arm knee extension machine. A weight is attached at the end of the swing arm of the knee extension machine, adjacent to the shin pad. Note how the external moment arm increases as the knee extends, resulting in an increasing external knee flexion moment. An opposite internal knee extension moment is created by the quadriceps to extend the knee. Because the external moment increases as the knee is extended, quadriceps force must also increase. (b) Constant moment arm knee extension machine. Resistance is provided by a cabled pulley and weight stack system. The resistance is applied perpendicular to the lower leg as the knee extends, resulting in a constant external knee flexion moment. Since the external knee flexion moment remains constant throughout the range of motion, the internal knee flexion moment also remains constant, resulting in constant quadriceps force demand throughout the range of motion.
COURTESY OF RICHARD WILLY

## Contact force

The last key concept we consider is internal loading, known as joint contact force (units = body weight or N). Joint contact forces are the forces acting on the articulating surfaces of a joint. This is the sum of the net joint reaction force plus the forces produced by muscles that are crossing the joint. This measure is typically derived using more advanced computational models that input patient-specific parameters such as joint angles, moments and muscle forces. Joint contact forces must be known to calculate joint stresses.

An example of the importance of considering internal muscle forces, joint contact forces and joint stress can be seen when performing a step-up manoeuvre. When the athlete steps up, their quadriceps musculature contracts, exerting force through the quadriceps tendon-patella-patellar tendon complex. During the step-up, or any other activity that requires a quadriceps contraction, the articular/articulating surfaces of the patella is contracted forcefully against the femoral trochlea. The force between the patella and the femoral trochlea is known as patellofemoral joint contact force.

Consider two athletes of the same height and mass, who are ascending a flight of steps together. Athlete A has a smaller contact area between the patella and the femoral trochlea compared with athlete B. Since they have the same dimensions and are ascending the stairs at the same rate, we can assume that their quadriceps forces and resulting patellofemoral contact forces are not different. However, athlete A will experience higher patellofemoral joint stress during the step ascent; athlete B will experience lower patellofemoral joint stress compared with athlete A,[6] because of their larger contact area. Individuals with patellofemoral pain often exhibit higher patellofemoral joint stress during routine activities compared with their nonpainful counterparts.[6]

Now consider two athletes with similar dimensions and patellofemoral contact areas as they ascend the same flight of steps. Athlete C is holding two 10-kg hand weights. Since athlete C is carrying added weight, they need greater quadriceps force compared with athlete D to extend their knee as they ascend a step. Athlete C will exhibit greater patellofemoral contact force because of the greater quadriceps contraction. Even though their contact area is the same as athlete D, athlete C will experience greater patellofemoral joint stress because their patellofemoral contact force is greater during the step up.

It is important to consider what factors may be playing into joint stresses when evaluating a patient with joint pain during routine functional activities.

## MEASUREMENT OF MUSCLE PERFORMANCE

A sound understanding of the measurement of force, external moment arms, the axis of rotation and the subsequent calculation of torque is essential to assess an athlete's muscle performance. Peak force production and the rate of force development are the most relevant clinical examples for measuring muscle force capacity. Modern, affordable dynamometers (also known as strain gauges) can be linked to proprietary mobile apps to quantify peak force production and rate of force development.

To measure an athlete's peak isometric torque (the maximal voluntary isometric contraction):

1. locate the joint centre
2. place the joint in a standardised and repeatable position
3. align the dynamometer so that it is positioned perpendicular to the distal segment
4. measure the external moment arm as the distance from the joint centre to the centre of the cuff attached to the dynamometer
5. collect force data (Fig. 12.8).

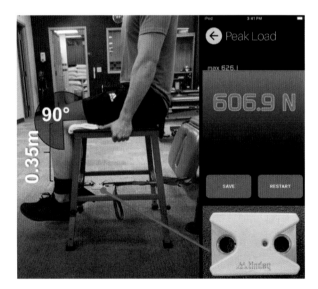

**Figure 12.8** Measurement of isometric knee extensor torque using a commercially available Bluetooth-equipped, dynamometer (Tindeq Progressor™; 300 kg force capacity) and associated device. Note that the knee joint centre has been identified (lateral femoral epicondyle), the knee is placed in a standard and repeatable position of 90° knee flexion and the dynamometer is attached with the line of force application perpendicular to the tibia. Peak isometric torque can be calculated as the product of force (606.9 N) and the external moment arm length (0.35 m), yielding 219.1 Nm of torque.

COURTESY OF RICHARD WILLY

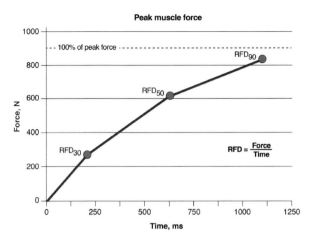

**Figure 12.9** Rate of force development is a measure of explosive strength or simply how fast an athlete can develop force

Peak isometric torque can be calculated using the formula: torque = isometric force × external moment arm length. Note that an alternative and more proximal placement of the dynamometer will yield *a greater force value,* with a smaller external moment arm, but the calculated torque will be the same between the two dynamometer placements.

Using the force (N)-time (s) curve, the rate that force is developed (units = N/s)–can be also calculated. Rate of force development is the average slope of the leading portion of the isometric force seen in Figure 12.9, calculated as follows:

$$\text{Rate of force development (N/s)} = \frac{\text{Force (N)}}{\text{Time to peak force (s)}}$$

Rate of force development is an important component of muscle performance in athletes, particularly when an athlete needs to generate an opposing force to recover from contact with an opposing player or when making a sudden manoeuvre such as a cut or pivot.[7]

## TISSUE-SPECIFIC TOLERANCE TO LOADS

Loading is an integral ingredient guiding a tissue's mechanical response. Tissues are routinely subjected to different types of forces (also known as loads), including tension, compression, bending, shear, torsion and combined loading (Fig. 12.10). Regular exposure to routine types, magnitudes and volumes of loads maintains tissue health, creates a state of tissue homeostasis and ensures the ability to resist loads, a concept known as capacity. Tissues have greater capacity for specific types of loads, with lower capacity for other loads. To illustrate this concept,

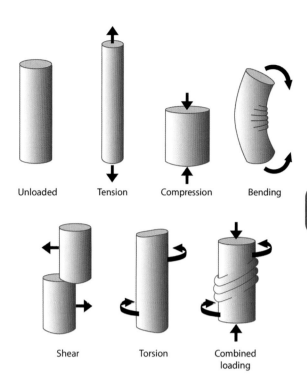

**Figure 12.10** Different types of forces (loads)

we will contrast the ability of bone and tendon to resist compression and tension loads.

Bone is optimally designed to resist compression, but has a much lower capacity to tolerate tensile loads. Bone's ability to resist compression is not surprising considering that bone is constantly under compression during weight-bearing. Tensile loads can occur at sites of tendon insertion on a bone, particularly when a tendon wraps around a bony prominence, but also on the convex side of a bone that experiences bending (Fig. 12.11).[8]

Sites of bone stress injuries that are subject to tension forces are highly prone to non-union or delayed union and require careful clinical management.

In contrast, bending results in compression on the concave side of a bone. As a result, bone stress injuries on the concave (compression) side are considered low risk and their management is typically uncomplicated, often taking 4–12 weeks to heal.[9] Compared with low-risk bone stress injuries, high-risk bone stress injuries take 2–4 times longer to achieve suitable healing to enable a return to sports participation.[10]

In contrast to bone, tendon is optimally structured to transmit tensile forces from muscle to the associated bony insertion. Tendon tolerates and responds well to tensile loads in training and therapeutic interventions. However,

171

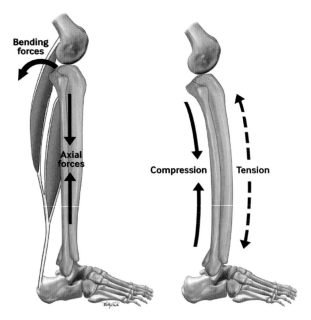

**Figure 12.11** Bone loading. Weight-bearing places a tensile load on the anterior tibia. Stress fractures heal poorly there. (See also bone stress injuries in Chapter 9.)

tendon has a low tolerance for compressive loads and can develop a pathological tissue response by replacing type I collagen typical of tendons with cartilage-like proteoglycans, type II collagen and fibrocartilage.[11]

Tendon compression is considered the primary mechanism of insertional tendinopathies such as proximal hamstring and insertional Achilles tendinopathies.

Notably, insertional tendinopathies require more nuanced rehabilitation to control compressive loads. The rehabilitation of mid-substance tendinopathies, which are not subject to compressive loads, is much less complicated.[12]

## TISSUE HOMEOSTASIS AND MECHANOTHERAPY

By manipulating the kinetics experienced by an athlete's tissues, we can control training loads to avoid tissue overload, while also prescribing therapeutic doses to improve training and rehabilitation outcomes. During sustained training, an athlete is exposed to a variety of applied biomechanical loads of a certain frequency, volume and magnitude. These sustained training loads promote a normal amount of tissue turnover, or renewal, known as tissue homeostasis (Fig. 12.12).[13, 14]

However, a reduction in training loads may create a state of "stress shielding" and tissues will negatively adapt by reducing their capacity to tolerate higher loads.[15] Stress shielding can be seen when there are large reductions in typical training volumes or when a certain training stimulus, such as high-speed running, is avoided. A more extreme example is when a limb is immobilised in a cast and tissues within the limb lose loading capacity.

Medical conditions and side effects of medications can also reduce a tissue's tolerance to loads. While healthy tissue can resist these forces within the bounds of physiological limitations, once tissue develops pathology or is subjected to stress shielding, daily forces may lead to tissue injury such as muscle strains, tendon ruptures and bone fractures.

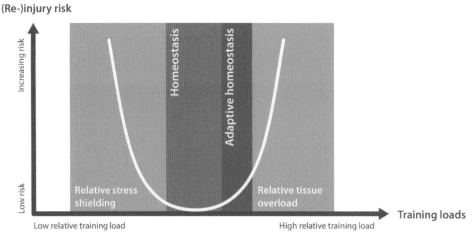

**Figure 12.12** Tissue homeostasis model. Relative stress shielding, tissue unloading, occurs when an athlete limits their use of certain muscles because of an injury. Adaptive homeostasis occurs during high-load phases of training. This type of training promotes tissue becoming more resilient. Note the y-axis—as the athlete adapts to the exercise, the risk of injury decreases.

To illustrate the concept of tissue homeostasis, consider a throwing athlete whose throwing activities consist of 4 hours of their normal 10 hours per week of training during the season. If the athlete's training load remains consistent, their shoulder structure will be in a state of tissue homeostasis. If the athlete ceases training during the off-season, their throwing musculature, tendons, shoulder capsule and associated ligaments will move to a state of stress shielding.

If the stress shielding continues, these structures will lose capacity. And if the athlete fails to resume training prior to rejoining their team at the start of the season, the throwing loads experienced during their training regimen will quickly overwhelm their shoulder structure, likely resulting in a relative tissue overload injury.

## Mechanotherapy

On the other hand, training loads can also result in adaptive tissue responses through a process known as mechanotherapy.[16, 17] When loads are applied to a limb, the muscles, tendons, bone, articular cartilage and ligaments experience tension, compression, bending, shear, torsion and combined loading forces. These applied forces harness the specific tissue's mechanosensitivities to trigger tissue adaptation (Fig. 12.13).

By prescribing applied loads that are slightly greater than those typically experienced by the tissue, adaptive homeostasis results. Over a period of time, adaptive homeostasis drives adaptations to muscles, tendons, bone, articular cartilage and ligaments that improve their ability to tolerate tension, compression, bending, shear, torsion and combined loading forces.[16, 17]

A working understanding of biomechanics allows you to prescribe appropriate loads during rehabilitation—that's mechanotherapy. In sum, forces applied to tissues can result in an adaptive response but can also result in injury if the applied force exceeds that tissue's capacity to tolerate load.[18]

Imagine that the throwing athlete now has an injured shoulder due to the relative tissue overload experienced at the start of the season. The physiotherapist prescribes progressively greater resistance exercises so that the athlete's shoulder structure will undergo adaptive homeostasis. By prescribing exercises such as a forward shoulder raise with resistance, the athlete's deltoid and rotator cuff musculature will increase in strength. If the athlete continues to perform these exercises, their bone, tendon, ligaments and cartilage will also adapt. However, if the physiotherapist instead prescribes protected rest without a progressive resistance program, the athlete will fall further into a stress-shielded state, unnecessarily prolonging their recovery.

Muscle performance (i.e. force production) is influenced by the velocity of the change in the muscle's length and the length of the muscle during contraction, known as the force-velocity relationship and the length-tension relationship, respectively (Fig. 12.14).

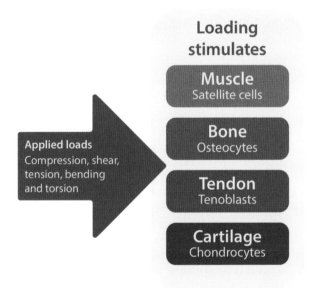
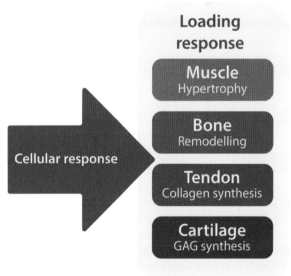

GAG, glycosaminoglycans

**Figure 12.13** The process of mechanotherapy

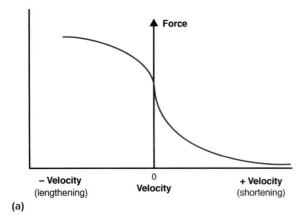

**(a)**

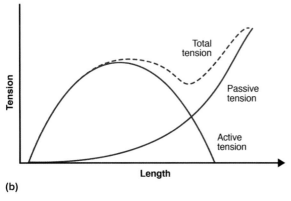

**(b)**

**Figure 12.14** (a) Force-velocity curve; (b) length-tension curve

## Force-velocity relationship

The force-velocity relationship describes how muscle force production changes as a muscle actively shortens (i.e. concentric contraction), maintains its length (i.e. isometric contraction) or lengthens (i.e. eccentric contraction). During these contractions, the velocity of the change in muscle length influences the muscle's maximal force production.

Consider the example of progressively adding load to an athlete while they are completing a maximal back squat. Initially, the athlete can quickly complete the lifting phase (i.e. concentric phase), since the force is moderate. As the weight increases, the velocity of the lifting phase decreases: the recruited muscle, such as the gluteus maximus, experiences a decrease in contraction velocity as the muscle force demands increase. If the coaching staff prescribe faster back squats, the weight on the barbell must be reduced for the gluteus maximus to complete the lifting phase. If the added weight continues to increase, the muscle will no longer be able to shorten, resulting in an isometric contraction.

In contrast, gluteus muscle contraction is forcefully lengthened during the lower phase of the lift (i.e. eccentric phase). The athlete is capable of eccentrically lowering the squat with greater weight than during the concentric phase of the lift. Furthermore, the athlete must eccentrically lower the barbell faster if the added weight is increased.

## Length-tension relationship

The length-tension relationship describes the relationship between a muscle's length and the force that the muscle can produce. The resting length of muscle is the length that provides the greatest number of actin-myosin cross-bridges, providing the greatest force-generating potential. The resting length is commonly known as the optimal length of a muscle. Optimal length differs greatly between muscles.

For instance, the optimal length of the quadriceps musculature corresponds with approximately 60–90° of knee flexion,[19] the optimal length of the soleus is near full dorsiflexion[20] and the optimal length of the biceps brachii is 110°.[21]

> **PRACTICE PEARL**
>
> Since assessing a muscle's performance is often done isometrically, it is critical to know the optimal length of the muscle as this will determine the testing position to obtain the muscle's peak performance.

## Muscle insufficiency

It is also important to understand when muscles are in a position of active or passive insufficiency:

- Active insufficiency occurs when a multi-joint muscle is placed in a shortened position across both joints at the same time, causing excessive overlap of myosin and actin cross-bridges. Muscles placed in a position of active insufficiency have a diminished ability to generate muscle force. An example of this is when you flex your shoulder and elbow joints simultaneously, losing the ability to generate maximal muscle tension in your biceps brachii.
- Passive insufficiency occurs when a multi-joint muscle lengthens to its full extent over both joints, preventing a full range of motion at each joint. For example, combined hip extension and knee flexion places the rectus femoris in passive insufficiency. Besides limiting hip extension and knee flexion range of motion, the resulting passive tension in the rectus femoris will limit hip extension and knee flexion torque capability in the compound position of knee flexion and hip extension.

## HOW DO WE OBTAIN BIOMECHANICAL DATA?

One of the most common ways that biomechanical data are measured in a laboratory or clinical environment is using 2-dimensional (2D) or 3-dimensional (3D) motion analysis:

- In 2D motion analysis, a video is captured with a phone or computer software, showing single plane movement (e.g. frontal plane only).
- 3D motion analysis typically includes a multiple camera motion capture system with retroreflective markers placed on bony landmarks of the body, showing multi-planar movement.

Many motion analysis labs also have embedded force plates used to derive joint moments that complement joint kinematics. These force plates measure ground reaction forces using load cells and can be used for movement such as walking, running, cutting, pivoting or jumping.

More recently, wearable devices have enabled the collection of biomechanical data outside of the laboratory or clinical environment. Wearable devices are surrogate measures for a gold standard, laboratory motion capture system. Because wearable devices are used most often to capture biomechanics during routine athletics activities on the field of play, they are designed to be lightweight, unobtrusive and able to perform onboard data logging.[22] One of the most common types of wearable devices are accelerometers, which measure segmental or body accelerations. Typically, accelerometers are embedded in an insole, ankle or chest strap (Fig. 12.15), helmet or mouthpiece.

Accelerometers are often worn by runners to assess tibial shock, which is postulated to be a risk factor for tibial bone stress injuries. Accelerometers can also be used to assess head impacts in contact sports with a high risk of concussion, and to assess player acceleration in sports that put a premium on sprinting and cutting, such as rugby and basketball. Other common wearable devices include global positioning systems (GPS), pressure-sensing insoles, smart garments and inertial measurement units.

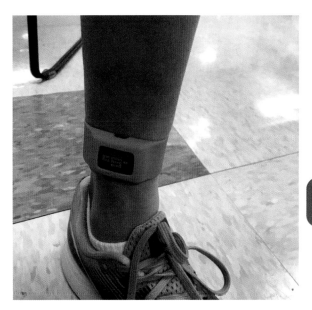

**Figure 12.15** This wearable device measures tibial shock (acceleration) during running and sporting activities outside the laboratory
COURTESY OF RICHARD WILLY

While wearable devices are intriguing, any device should be validated against a reference standard (i.e. the best available measure, usually 3-D motion capture) before use.[23] Table 12.1 outlines criteria to determine whether a wearable device should be used.

Finally, electromyography (EMG) can measure muscle activity through surface electrodes applied to muscle bellies. Muscle activity can be used to quantify muscle timing (e.g. muscle on and off) and to determine when peak muscle activity occurs. There is ample evidence in the research literature that can help delineate which muscles are active during different exercises to ensure that the appropriate muscles are being targeted for rehabilitation.

Assessing muscle activation through EMG is not the same as muscle force production. EMG measures the activity of muscle and is a helpful tool to determine muscle

**TABLE 12.1** Criteria to determine whether a wearable device should be used to quantify biomechanics on the field

| | |
|---|---|
| Has criterion validity been established? | The device compares favourably with the reference standard |
| Is the device reliable? | The device provides similar measurement between days |
| Do the wearable metrics matter? | The device quantifies biomechanics that are related to injury or sporting performance |
| Can it be easily worn and operated? | The wearable device should require minimal training to operate, and should be inconspicuous, without restricting the athlete's performance |

Source: Adapted from Willy RW. Innovations and pitfalls in the use of wearable devices in the prevention and rehabilitation of running related injuries. *Phys Ther Sport* 2018;29:26–33.

timing and activity, but this does not equate to the onset of force due to electromechanical delay. There are many ways that an EMG signal can increase, including the recruitment of more motor neurons, but this does not necessarily mean that more force is being generated. For example, at the same muscle activation level, a muscle with a larger cross-sectional area will produce more force than a smaller muscle.

## KEY POINTS

- The field of biomechanics helps clinicians understand how human tissues (e.g. bone, tendon, muscle) respond to the stress of physical activity, exercise and sport.

- Force and torque are sometimes used interchangeably, but this is incorrect of course. Torque and moment are synonymous terms.

- The concepts of external and internal moment arms are useful in understanding the distinctions between isometric, concentric and eccentric muscle contractions.

- Quantifying important sport-performance measures like maximal voluntary isometric contraction and rate of force development require a basic understanding of biomechanical principles.

- Different tissue types have individual strengths and weaknesses in absorbing various types of force. While bone may better withstand compressive forces, tendon tissue is better suited to sustaining tensile forces.

- The concept of mechanotherapy underpins our understanding of how progressive exercise facilitates strengthening of healthy tissue and rehabilitation of injured tissue.

- Finding the optimal body position to accomplish sport and exercise-related tasks relies on an understanding of passive and active insufficiency.

- Collecting biomechanical data is becoming more common. Strategies include motion capture systems, force plates and wearable devices.

## REFERENCES

References for this chapter can be found at www.mhprofessional.com/CSM6e

## ADDITIONAL CONTENT

Scan here to access additional resources for this topic and more provided by the authors

## CHAPTER 13

# Biomechanical aspects of injury in nine specific sports

*99% of my training is falling. Training for climbing means falling over and over again.*

JANJA GRANBRET (SLOVENIAN OLYMPIC GOLD MEDALLIST, 2020)

## CHAPTER OUTLINE

| | |
|---|---|
| Baseball | Rowing |
| Climbing | Swimming |
| Cricket (fast bowling) | Tennis |
| Cycling | Volleyball |
| Golf | Running shoes |

## LEARNING OBJECTIVES

By the end of this chapter you should be able to:

- identify common sport-related movement patterns in selected sports
- describe those movements using biomechanical terminology
- analyse sport-related movements and recognise features that may increase an athlete's risk of injury
- explain the connection between sport-related biomechanics and risk of injury
- list common intrinsic and extrinsic risk factors that may interact with biomechanics in determining an athlete's risk of injury
- develop an injury prevention and/or injury treatment program that addresses biomechanical risk factors
- discuss the key elements of the modern carbon-fibre running shoe.

This chapter outlines the key biomechanical factors that influence performance and predispose to injuries in nine popular sports: baseball, climbing, cricket (fast bowling), cycling, golf, rowing, swimming, tennis and volleyball. We also discuss the revolution in modern running shoes ("supershoes"). Management of specific injuries is covered in *Clinical Sports Medicine 6e: Managing Injuries*

## BASEBALL

There are whole textbooks on baseball medicine and we encourage you to pursue the quality free and paywalled learning opportunities in this field that has evolved decade by decade. Our aim here is to introduce you to the foundations of assessing the baseball player who presents to your clinical setting. We focus on pitching but don't limit ourselves to that position. In addition, some of the biomechanical principles described here are also relevant to other overhead sports activities, such as the javelin throw, volleyball spike and tennis serve.

### The foundation: biomechanics of throwing

Throwing is a whole-body activity that flows from the large muscles of the leg through rotation of the pelvis and trunk and continues on via the shoulder girdle. It continues with a whip-like transfer of momentum funnelled into elbow extension and onward to the small muscles of the forearm and hand. When done expertly, this remarkable process can propel a baseball at speeds of more than 160 km/hr.

We consider throwing as having six phases: wind up, stride, arm cocking, arm acceleration, arm deceleration, follow-through. These phases are outlined below and in Tables 13.1 and 13.2.

### 1. Wind-up

Wind-up (Fig. 13.1a) establishes the rhythm of the throw. During wind-up, the body rotates so that the hip and shoulders are at 90° to the target. The forces that launch a powerful pitch arise in the lower half of the body and develop a forward-moving "controlled fall".[1] In pitching, hip flexion of the lead leg raises the centre of gravity.

### 2. Stride

The stride (Fig. 13.1b) refers to the phase where the pitcher's front leg goes down and forward, the hands and arms separate, and the pitching arm swings down then up. Decrease in stride length is associated with decreased velocity of the pitch. Top (right-handed) pitchers turn their landing (left) foot in (somewhat towards 3rd base). Faster pitchers have a greater range of pelvic rotation between foot contact and ball release.

### 3. Arm cocking

The cocking movement (Fig. 13.1c) positions the body to enable all body segments to contribute to ball propulsion. In cocking, the humerus abducts through full horizontal extension ($27 \pm 10°$) and then into maximal external rotation ($45 \pm 19°$). When the scapula is maximally retracted, the acromion starts to elevate. With maximal external rotation, the shoulder is "loaded", with the anterior capsule coiled tightly in the apprehension position, storing elastic energy. The internal rotator muscles are stretched.[2]

**TABLE 13.1**   The six phases of throwing

| Phase | Defined by | Percentage of throw sequence |
|---|---|---|
| 1. Wind-up | Begins with the initial movement of the contralateral leg lower limb, and ends when the lead leg reaches its highest point and with separation of the throwing hand from the glove | 80% |
| 2. Stride | Begins at the end of wind-up and ends when the lead foot contacts the pitching mound | |
| 3. Arm cocking | Early cocking begins with the stride phase; late cocking occurs between lead foot contact and the point of maximal external rotation of the throwing shoulder | |
| 4. Arm acceleration | Occurs between maximum external rotation of the shoulder and ball release | 2% |
| 5. Arm deceleration | Occurs between ball release and maximum humeral internal rotation and elbow extension | 18% |
| 6. Follow-through | The body continues to move forward with the arm until motion has ceased; arm horizontal adduction increases to 60°; culminates with the pitcher in a fielding position | |

**TABLE 13.2**    The biomechanics of throwing

| Phase/event | Proper mechanics | Pathomechanics → consequences |
| --- | --- | --- |
| **1. Wind-up** | • Lift front leg | N/A |
| Maximum knee height | • Pitcher is balanced | N/A |
| <br>Figure 13.1(a) | | |
| **2. Stride** | • Front leg goes down and forward<br>• Arms separate, swing down and up | • ↓ Push off rubber → ↓ ball velocity |
| Foot contact 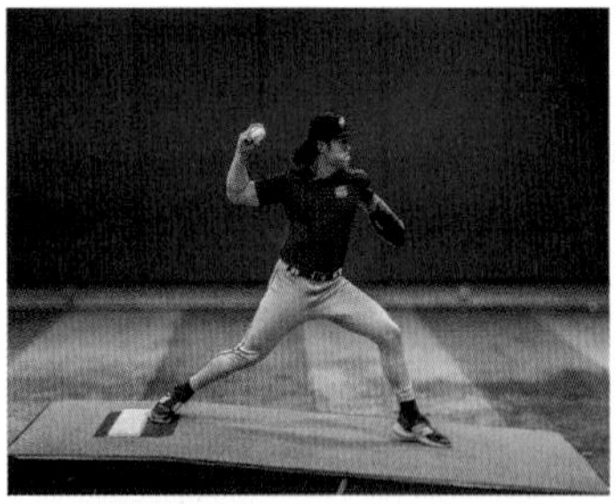<br><br>Figure 13.1(b) | • Front foot is planted slightly to third-base side (for a right-handed pitcher)<br>• Front foot is pointed slightly inward<br>• Shoulder is abducted approximately 90°, with approximately 60° of external rotation | • ↓ Stride length → ↓ ball velocity<br>• Front foot open (position or angle) → ↑ shoulder and elbow force<br>• Improper shoulder external rotation → ↑ shoulder and elbow kinetics<br>• Excessive shoulder external rotation → ↓ ball velocity<br>• ↓ Shoulder horizontal abduction → ↓ ball velocity |
| **3. Arm cocking** | • Pelvis rotation, followed by upper trunk rotation<br>• Shoulder externally rotates and trunk arches | • Early pelvis rotation → ↓ ball velocity<br>• Late pelvis rotation → ↑ shoulder and elbow kinetics<br>• ↓ Pelvis rotation velocity → ↓ ball velocity<br>• Poor timing between pelvis rotation and upper trunk rotation → ↓ ball velocity<br>• Poor timing between pelvis rotation and upper trunk rotation → ↑ Shoulder internal rotation torque |
| Maximum external rotation 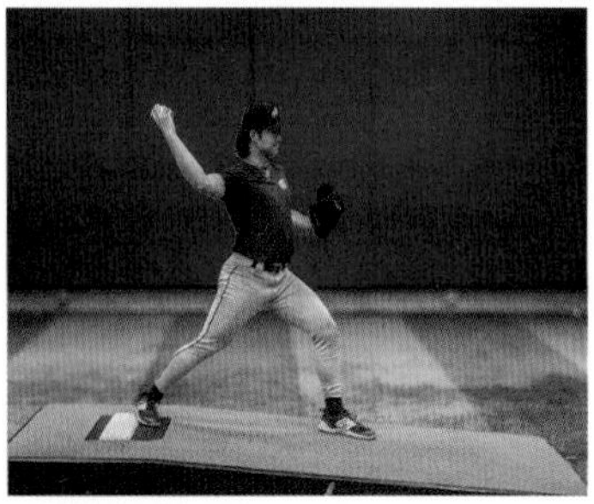<br><br>Figure 13.1(c) | • Shoulder external rotation is approximately 180°<br>• Elbow flexion is approximately 90° | • ↓ Shoulder external rotation → ↓ ball velocity<br>• Excessive shoulder horizontal adduction and elbow flexion → ↑ shoulder kinetics |

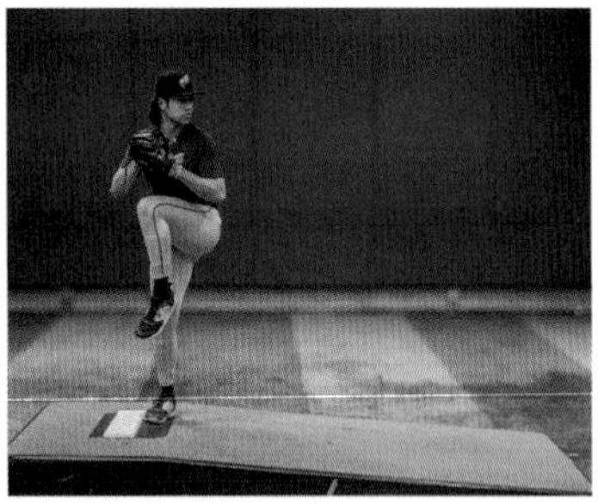

| Phase/event | Proper mechanics | Pathomechanics → consequences |
| --- | --- | --- |
| **4. Arm acceleration** | • Elbow extends, followed by shoulder internal rotation<br>• Front knee extends | N/A |
| Ball release 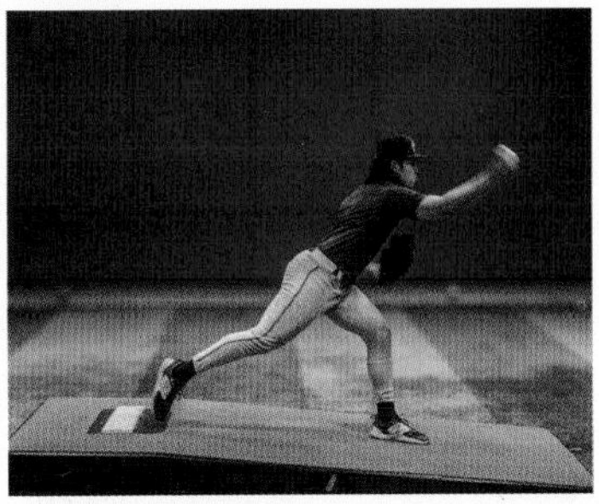<br>**Figure 13.1(d)** | • Throwing shoulder is abducted approximately 90° | • ↓ Knee extension velocity → ↓ ball velocity<br>• Improper shoulder abduction → ↓ ball velocity<br>• Improper shoulder abduction → ↑ elbow varus torque<br>• ↓ Forward trunk tilt → ↓ ball velocity |
| **5. Arm deceleration** | • Shoulder internal rotation and front knee extension continue<br>• Trunk tilts forward | N/A |
| Maximum internal rotation 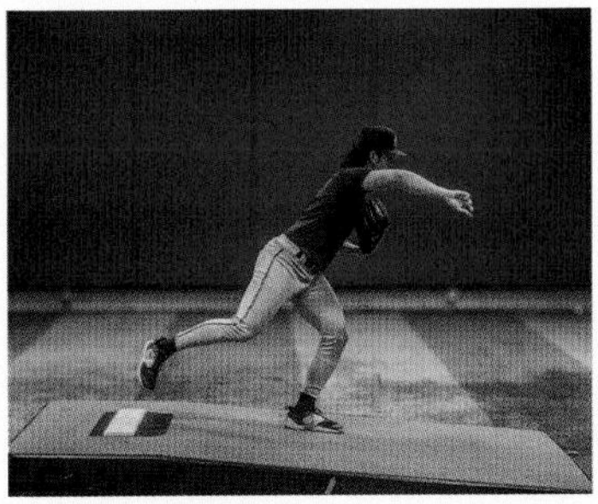<br>**Figure 13.1(e)** | • Shoulder external rotation is approximately 0° | N/A |
| **6. Follow-through** 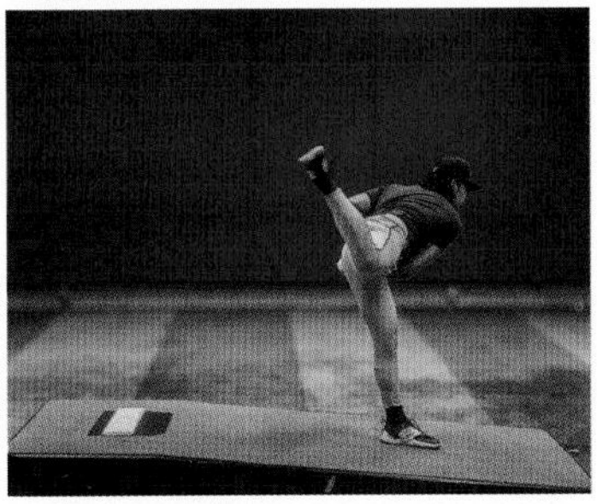<br>**Figure 13.1(f)** | • Arm crosses in front of body<br>• Trunk flexes forward | N/A |

PHOTOS COURTESY OF RYLAND HAGGIS AND VICARTE DOMINGO

The static anterior restraints (anterior inferior glenohumeral ligament and anterior inferior capsule) are under the greatest strain. At this stage, anterior joint forces are maximal and can exceed 350 Newtons (N)—equivalent to a weight of about 75 kg pulling the humerus backward (tending to dislocate the shoulder anteriorly). Because of the repetitive nature of throwing, the ligaments and muscles that restrain the humeral head in the glenoid (secondary and primary restraints, respectively) can stretch slightly and lead to subtle shoulder instability.[3]

The cocking phase ends with the planting of the lead leg–foot contact. This is an important landmark in throwing as it also marks the start of the critical acceleration phase. Now the body is positioned for energy transfer through the leg lower limbs, trunk and arms to the ball.

### 4. Arm acceleration

The acceleration phase (Fig. 13.1d) is extremely explosive. It consists of the rapid release of two forces: the stored elastic force of the tightly bound ligaments of the shoulder capsule, and forceful muscular internal rotation (subscapularis, pectoralis major, latissimus dorsi, teres major). This generates very high forces at the glenohumeral joint,[4] and places great demands on the rotator cuff musculature to keep the humeral head enlocated in the glenoid. Note that it is the large muscles *outside* the rotator cuff that are responsible for this massive acceleration of the arm—pectoralis major, latissimus dorsi, teres major.

At the shoulder, acceleration is the shortest phase of the throwing motion, lasting only 50 milliseconds (2% of the overall throwing time). In both the acceleration and the late cocking phases, muscle fatigue (which is accelerated if there is mild instability due to weakened static restraints) can lead to loss of coordinated rotator cuff motion.

The acceleration phase concludes with ball release. This occurs when the hand is at approximately ear level. The movements involved in acceleration also place enormous valgus forces on the (medial) elbow, which tends to lag behind the inwardly rotating shoulder.

### 5. Arm deceleration

Deceleration is the most violent phase of the throwing cycle, resulting in the greatest amount of joint loading. Very large forces pull forward on the glenohumeral joint following ball release, which stresses the posterior shoulder structures (Fig. 13.1e). Both intrinsic and extrinsic shoulder muscles fire at significant percentages of their maximum, to oppose the force tending to pull the humerus out of the shoulder socket. This force can exceed 500 N (roughly equivalent to 135 kg). The eccentric contraction of the rotator cuff external rotators decelerates the rapid internal rotation of the shoulder, as does eccentric contraction of the scapular stabilisers and posterior deltoid. In the properly thrown pitch, the spine and its musculature act as substantial force attenuators.

Towards the end of the pitching motion, the torso, having decelerated so that the arm could acquire kinetic energy in the arm acceleration phase, begins to rotate forward. The forward rotation of this larger link segment helps reacquire some of this energy. This theoretically reduces the burden on the serratus anterior and other stabilisers, which are attempting to eccentrically maintain the position of the scapula and maintain the humeral head within the glenoid.

In addition to the high stresses on the posterior shoulder structures, the deceleration phase stresses the elbow flexors that limit rapid elbow extension. This phase lasts approximately 350 milliseconds and constitutes approximately 18% of the total throwing time.

### 6. Follow-through

Follow-through (Fig. 13.1f) proceeds and trunk rotation helps to reacquire some of the energy generated. Eventually movement ceases and the pitcher is in a fielding position. This phase is rarely associated with injury.

## The kinetic chain

The kinetic chain is a term clinicians use to make the point that optimal function of a distal structure relies on well-functioning proximal elements. Consider the hand/fingers in throwing as a "distal" structure. The kinetic chain that underpins successful throwing includes the lower limb (the very beginning of the chain), the muscles that envelop the torso, the scapula and shoulder muscles, and finally the upper arm and forearm that connect to the hand (Fig. 13.2). It does not require much imagination to see these elements (links) working like a whip or a dynamic chain to allow very speedy release of a baseball, cricket ball or tennis ball (with the racquet extending the chain even further).

Let us illustrate the concept more specifically using the scapula as a model. It links the proximal-to-distal sequencing of velocity, energy and forces that optimise shoulder function. For most shoulder activities, this sequencing starts at the ground. Individual body segments, or links, move in a coordinated way to generate, summate and transfer force through various body segments to the terminal link. Large proximal body segments provide the bulk of the force.

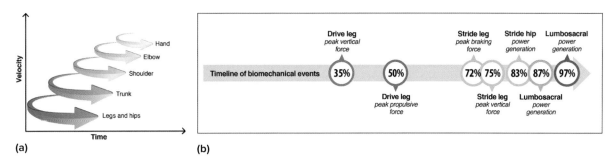

**Figure 13.2** The kinetic chain in throwing. (a) In a well-coordinated throw, each body segment generates additional force (velocity, y-axis) in a shorter and shorter time (x-axis). These forces sum. Ultimately all the forces are funnelled into a very fast hand release. (b) A timeline showing when biomechanical events occur during the pitch (in a developmental aged pitcher). Source: (b) Pryhoda MK, Sabick MB. Lower body energy generation, absorption, and transfer in youth baseball pitchers. *Front Sports Act Living* 2022;4.

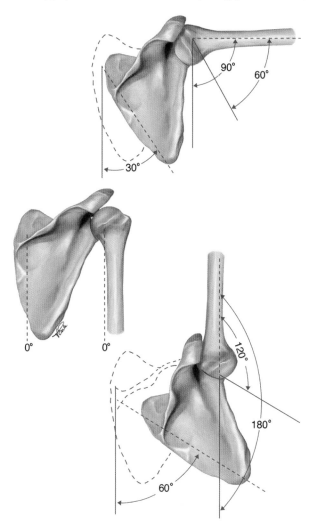

**Figure 13.3** Normal scapulothoracic rhythm allows the scapula to rotate upwardly during abduction, bringing the glenoid fossa directly under the humeral head to lend stability to the glenohumeral joint.

Why is the kinetic chain concept important? Because it highlights that treatment should not merely address local symptoms. Right shoulder tendon pain in a right arm bowling/throwing athlete may arise because of calf muscle weakness, hip joint tightness and incoordination of the scapular movements. You should look for causes of symptoms along the entire kinetic chain and treat all contributing links.

## Normal biomechanics of the scapula in throwing

The importance of the scapula in normal throwing biomechanics is well-recognised. For optimal shoulder function, and to decrease injury risk, the scapula must move in a coordinated way (Fig. 13.3). This section outlines Ben Kibler's[5] description of the role of the scapula in throwing (Box 13.1). If you understand normal scapular biomechanics, you will be able to detect abnormal scapular biomechanics in your patients with upper limb injuries.

> **BOX 13.1** Scapular function in normal shoulder mechanics
>
> 1. Provides a stable socket for the humerus
> 2. Retracts and protracts along the thoracic wall
> 3. Rotates to elevate the acromion
> 4. Provides a base for muscle attachment
> 5. Provides a key link in the kinetic chain

## Abnormal scapular biomechanics and physiology

The scapular roles can be altered by many anatomical factors to create abnormal biomechanics, both locally and in the kinetic chain (Table 13.3).

**TABLE 13.3**   Factors that can impair scapular function and potentially cause the athlete to have symptoms or limit their performance

| Scapular function alteration | How this can lead to symptoms/poor performance |
| --- | --- |
| **Anatomical factors** | |
| Cervical spine lordosis | Excessive scapular protraction—leads to impingement with elevation |
| Thoracic spine kyphosis | Excessive scapular protraction—leads to impingement with elevation |
| Shoulder asymmetry (i.e. drooping of the shoulder or "tennis shoulder") | Impingement/muscle function and fatigue |
| Injuries of scapula, clavicle | Alters orientation of scapula, length of clavicular strut; painful conditions that inhibit muscle function |
| **Factors that impair muscle function** | |
| Overuse, direct trauma, glenohumeral causes (instability, labral lesions, arthrosis) | Muscle weakness or force couple imbalances; serratus anterior and lower trapezius are particularly susceptible; can be a non-specific response to a variety of glenohumeral pathologies (this can be seen as analogous to the knee in that weakness of the vastus medialis obliquus can result in the patellofemoral syndrome) |
| Glenohumeral inflexibility, posterior (capsular or muscular) | Limits smooth glenohumeral joint motion and creates wind-up effect so that the glenoid and scapula get pulled in forward and inferiorly by the moving arm, leading to excessive protraction which, in turn, holds the scapula and importantly the acromion inferiorly and thus makes it prone to impingement |
| Nerve injury (causes less than 5% of abnormal muscle function in shoulder problems) | Long thoracic nerve-serratus anterior inhibited; accessory nerve—trapezius function inhibited |

## Clinical significance of scapular biomechanics in shoulder injuries

Abnormal shoulder biomechanics can compromise normal shoulder function. This observation has various descriptive titles, such as scapulothoracic dyskinesis, floating scapula or lateral scapular slide. These are merely titles for the same phenomenon: abnormal scapular function. We provide examples of how abnormal biomechanics can cause shoulder and elbow problems.

Lack of full retraction of the scapula on the thorax destabilises the cocking point and prevents acceleration out of a fully cocked position. Lack of full scapular protraction increases the deceleration forces on the shoulder and alters the normal safe zone between the glenoid and the humerus as the arm moves through the acceleration phase. Too much protraction because of tightness in the glenohumeral capsule causes impingement as the scapula rotates down and forward. These cumulatively lead to abnormalities in concavity/compression due to the changes in the safe zone of the glenohumeral angle.

Loss of coordinated retraction/protraction in throwing opens up the front of the glenohumeral joint and thus provides an insufficient anterior bony buttress to anterior translation of the humeral head. This increases shear stress on the rest of the anterior stabilising structures, the labrum and glenohumeral ligaments, which further decreases the stability of the glenoid for the rotating humerus.

Lack of acromial elevation leads to impingement in the cocking and follow-through phases. Impingement can also occur secondary to painful shoulder conditions that inhibit the function of the serratus and lower trapezius muscles. As these muscles normally act as a force couple to elevate the acromion, their inhibition commonly causes impingement. Thus, detecting and, if necessary, reversing serratus and trapezius inhibition is an important step in treating shoulder conditions.

If the scapula is unstable, the lack of an anchor affects the function of all scapular muscles. Muscles without a stable origin cannot develop appropriate or maximal torque and are predisposed to suffering muscular imbalance. If the scapula is truly unstable on the thoracic wall, as in spinal accessory nerve palsies or in extremely inhibited muscles, the muscle origins and insertions are effectively reversed and the distal end of the muscle becomes the origin. The scapula is then pulled laterally by the muscle, which contracts from the more stable distal humeral end rather than from the proximal scapular end.

A further problem of the unstable scapula is that it does not provide a stable base for glenohumeral rotation during link sequencing. Therefore, the arm works on an unstable platform and loses mechanical efficiency.

One of the most important scapular biomechanical abnormalities is the loss of the link function in the kinetic chain. The kinetic chain transfers energy and force to the hand. The scapula and shoulder funnel forces from the large segments, the legs and trunk, to the smaller, rapidly moving small segments of the arm.

Scapular dysfunction impairs force transmission from the lower to the upper extremity. This reduces the force delivered to the hand or creates a situation of "catch-up" in which the more distal links have to overwork to compensate for the loss of the proximally generated force. The distal links have neither the size, the muscle cross-sectional area, nor the time in which to develop these larger forces efficiently. For example, a 20% decrease in kinetic energy delivered from the hip and trunk to the arm necessitates an 80% increase in muscle mass or a 34% increase in rotational velocity at the shoulder to deliver the same amount of resultant force to the hand. Such an adaptation would predispose to overload problems.

This explains why injuries apparently unrelated to the upper limb—for example, decreased push-off due to Achilles tendinopathy, decreased quadriceps drive after a muscle strain or decreased segmental trunk rotation secondary to thoracic segmental hypomobility—can affect upper limb throwing mechanics and predispose to further, or more serious, upper limb injury.

## Changes in throwing arm with repeated throwing

Repeated throwing causes adaptive changes to gradually develop in the shoulder and elbow. Changes occur in flexibility, soft-tissue/muscle strength and bony contour.

At the shoulder, long-term throwing athletes have increased range of external rotation. This arises because of the repeated stress to the anterior capsule in the cocking phase and stretch or breakdown in the anterior static stabilisers of the shoulder joint (the inferior glenohumeral ligaments). This may compromise the dynamic balance that exists between shoulder function and stability. The combination of increased shoulder external rotation range of motion and breakdown of the static stabilisers may lead to anterior instability of the shoulder and secondary impingement.

The normal strength ratio of internal rotators to external rotators is approximately 3:2 but in throwers this imbalance is exaggerated and, over time, a relative lack of external rotation strength may increase vulnerability to injury. These dynamic changes in the shoulder joint highlight the need for a structured exercise program to prevent or correct muscle imbalances.

Throwing also produces structural changes at the elbow. Due to the valgus stress applied in the throwing action there is a breakdown of the medial stabilising structures (medial collateral ligament, joint capsule, flexor muscles). This leads to the development of an increased carrying angle at the elbow.

Less frequently, the eccentric overload on elbow structures causes anterior capsular strains, posterior impingement or forearm flexor strains and, subsequently, a fixed flexion deformity.

## Biomechanical patterns associated with injury

One of the most common biomechanical problems seen in throwing sports such as cricket, baseball and water polo is caused by the throwing athlete "opening up too soon". Normally the body rotates out of the cocking phase when the arm is fully cocked (externally rotated). If the body opens up too soon, the arm lags behind and is not fully externally rotated. This results in increased stress to the anterior shoulder structures and an increased eccentric load to the shoulder external rotators. It also results in increased valgus stress at the elbow.

The other common abnormality seen in throwing athletes is known as "hanging", which is a characteristic sign of fatigue. Fatigue results from excessive intensity, frequency or duration of throwing. Decreased shoulder abduction leads to dropping of the elbow and slower pitches. There is an associated increase in injury risk, particularly to the rotator cuff as well as to the shoulder joint and the elbow.

In baseball, the type of pitch is determined by the spin imparted onto the ball by the hands and fingers at ball release. The normal follow-through involves forearm pronation. In "breaking" pitches, the forearm is relatively supinated at release and then pronates. Breaking pitches are associated with an increased risk of injury. Some pitchers incorrectly forcefully supinate against the normal pronation of follow-through.

Baseball biomechanics authority Dr Fleisig debunked the fear that curveballs predisposed to injury with comprehensive biomechanical analysis and injury surveillance.[1] To prevent injury, fastball training is key (so that the tissue adapts). It is recognised that independent of biomechanics, throwing injuries in children are a result of super-specialisation. Among professional players, problems generally result from not varying the intensity of throwing.

To address biomechanical issues in baseball, it is essential that you work with the coach and expert biomechanical analysis. The latter is available in the elite baseball setting.

Remember that baseball team members have varying roles. This affects their workload (throwing volume and intensity) and their risk of injury (Table 13.4).

**TABLE 13.4**   How a baseball player's position is associated with workload and injury risk

| Position and typical anthropometry | Volume and intensity of throwing | Injury predisposition/clinical pearls |
| --- | --- | --- |
| Corners: 1st and 3rd base; bigger more powerful players | Can get away with easier throws if they have ulnar collateral ligament sprain | Position players more prone to hook of hamate injury/fracture because of the force of check swings |
| Up the middle (centre field, short stop, left fielder), smaller players | Fewer throws, but more intense | Short stop: flexor tendon injuries because they throw from different angles which loads the forearm, wrist and hand |
| Catchers (stockier) | Most low effort throws and most max effort throws | Ulnar collateral ligament injury; labral and rotator cuff injury; knee injuries as a result of repeated squatting |
| Pitchers | High volume and high intensity (see text) | UCL injury; labral and rotator cuff injury |

# CLIMBING

## with VOLKER SCHÖFFL and CHRISTOPH LUTTER

Olympic climbing debuted in 2021 at the Tokyo Olympic Games and consists of various disciplines:

- lead (climbing with rope protection)
- speed (maximum speed climbing on a standardised route in 1-on-1 mode)
- bouldering (climbing at lower heights with mattress floor protection).

For 2021 a triathlon of all three disciplines was chosen, and in Paris 2024 the competition was divided into a combination of lead and bouldering with a separate speed competition.

In lead climbing, the upper extremities are the most common site of injury; injuries usually occur while the climber is performing a strenuous move.[6] Bouldering shows an almost even injury distribution between fall injuries (sprains and strains) and overstrain.[6] There are few data specifically on speed climbing to date. It appears to have a lower burden of injury than bouldering.

Overall, climbing can be considered a low-injury sport when compared with other Olympic sports such as rugby and badminton. At the 2018 Youth Olympic Games, athletes' injury incidence was 43% of all players in rugby, 24% in badminton and <5% in swimming, equestrian, climbing and rowing.[7]

Table 13.5 shows the 10 most common diagnoses clinicians made in competitive climbers at one specialised clinic.

## Finger injuries

Climbing causes high biomechanical stress on the hands and fingers. Table 13.5 shows the four most frequent finger injuries. The two most important climbing-specific finger injuries are detailed below.

**TABLE 13.5**   Distribution of diagnoses among competition climbers treated in a specialised climbing clinic or during national and international climbing competitions such as the International Federation of World Climbing World Cup series

| Injuries 2017—2019 (n = 262) | n | % |
| --- | --- | --- |
| Tenosynovitis (finger) | 37 | 14 |
| Pulley injury (finger) | 33 | 13 |
| Acute ankle injury (sprain, fracture) | 30 | 12 |
| SLAP tear (shoulder) | 21 | 8 |
| Knee injury | 20 | 8 |
| Growth plate injury (finger) | 18 | 7 |
| Wrist sprain | 18 | 7 |
| Capsulitis (finger) | 17 | 7 |
| Impingement (shoulder) | 15 | 6 |
| Lumbrical muscle injury | 10 | 4 |

SLAP, superior labrum anterior to posterior
Source: Lutter C, Tischer T, Schöffl VR. Olympic competition climbing: the beginning of a new era-a narrative review. *Br J Sports Med* 2021; 55(15):857–64. © 2021 BMJ Publishing Group Ltd & British Association of Sport and Exercise Medicine. All rights reserved.

This QR code takes you to a great introduction to sport climbing, including the different types of climbing, why injuries occur and how to build a clinical relationship with climbers. Dr Carrie Cooper, a climber and physiotherapist, squeezes more than 20 years of experience into this 20-minute podcast:

## Pulley injuries

The pulley system of the 2nd to 5th fingers consists of five annular (A1–5) and three cross (C1–3) ligaments (pulleys) (Fig. 13.4). Mainly due to the crimping position, the A2, A3 or A4 pulleys, considered to be the most important ones, can either be strained or ruptured. The most frequently injured pulley is the A2.

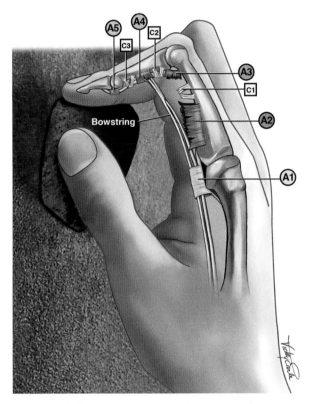

**Figure 13.4** Crimping posture with bowstringing in an A2 pulley rupture

Mostly, climbers report an acute onset of pain while crimping, and a loud "snapping" sound can be heard in many cases. After clinical suspicion and exclusion of a fracture, ultrasound examination is the diagnostic tool of choice. If multiple pulleys are ruptured, a clinical "bowstring" becomes visible. With the ultrasound an enhanced distance of the flexor tendons to the phalanx can be observed. If ultrasound fails to give an exact diagnosis, an MRI should be performed.

Based on a grading system and an algorithm,[8,9] single ruptures are treated conservatively and multiple ruptures surgically (Table 13.6). Biomechanical analyses and strength measurements after conservative management of single-pulley injuries show no strength deficit of the injured finger and typically climbers gain their original climbing level back after a year.[10]

The outcome after surgical repair of multiple pulley injuries is good, with most regaining full climbing ability. Nevertheless, a minor restricted range of motion often persists.[11] After pulley injury protective taping using "H-tape" is recommended; this taping technique has been evaluated biomechanically.[12]

### Epiphyseal fractures in adolescent climbers

Epiphyseal fracture of the base of the middle phalanx of the finger (Fig. 13.5) is specific to high-level adolescent climbers[8] and recent reports show an increase in incidence.[13,14] Patients are typically between 13 and 15 years old and in the pubertal growth spurt.[15]

The fractures are mostly "transient", meaning fractures during the phase of growth plate closure, where the palmar part of the growth plate is already fused and the dorsal part is still open.[16] The middle and ring fingers are most commonly affected (Fig. 13.5).[17] These fractures are caused by the high pressure onto the dorsal aspect of the growth plate in a crimping position,[17] in addition to the pulling forces of the extensor tendon central slip at the dorsal growth plate.[16,18,19]

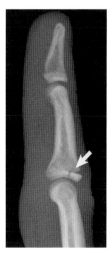

**Figure 13.5** Radiograph of epiphysial growth plate injury (epiphysial stress fracture) in a 15-year-old male athlete (arrowhead indicates fracture). This type of fracture is a common injury in competitive adolescent sport climbers.
IMAGE COURTESY OF VOLKER SCHÖFFL

If plain radiographs don't show any pathology where there is a high suspicion of fracture, CT scan and/or MRI should be performed to rule out an occult fracture. Therapy is mostly conservative, although displaced fractures or non-healing undisplaced fractures receive surgery.[20]

## Shoulder injuries

Shoulder injuries are the second most common pathology in climbing. Within our own patient cohort, shoulder injuries increased in prevalence from 5% in 1998–2001 to 20% in 2017–2018.[21]

SLAP lesions are the fifth most common diagnosis (5.8%) of all climbing-related pathologies.[21] Shoulder-demanding moves are particularly stressful for the insertion of the long

**TABLE 13.6**    Therapeutic guidelines for pulley injuries of the fingers in rock climbers

| | Grade I | Grade II | Grade III | Grade IVa | Grade IVb |
|---|---|---|---|---|---|
| **Injury** | Pulley strain | Complete tear of A3 or A4 Partial tear of A2 | Complete tear of A2 | Multiple ruptures: A2/A3 or A3/A4 rupture if:<br>• No major clinical bowstring<br>• Ultrasound proven possibility of reposition of the flexor tendon to the bone<br>• No contracture | Multiple ruptures: A2/A3 or A3/4 with obvious clinical bowstring A2/A3/A4 rupture Singular pulley rupture with flap irritation phenomenon Singular rupture with increasing contracture Singular rupture with secondary, therapy resistant, tenosynovitis |
| **Therapy** | Conservative | Conservative | Conservative | Conservative, if secondary onset of PIP contracture >20° then secondary surgical Therapy starting <10 days after injury | Surgical |
| **Immobilisation** | None | Optional, <5 days | Optional, <5 days | Optional, <5 days | Postsurgical 14 days |
| **Functional therapy with pulley protection (defined)** | 2–4 weeks H-tape (during day time) or thermoplastic ring | 6 weeks thermoplastic pulley ring | 6–8 weeks thermoplastic pulley ring | 8 weeks thermoplastic pulley ring | 4 weeks thermoplastic ring (after 2 weeks of immobilisation) |
| **Easy sport-specific activities** | After 4 weeks | After 6 weeks | After 8 weeks | After 10 weeks | After 4 months |
| **Full sport-specific activities** | After 6 weeks | After 8–10 weeks | After 3 months | After 4 months | After 6 months |
| **H-taping during climbing** | 3 months | 3 months | 3 months | >12 months | >12 months |

Source: Schöffl V, Hochholzer T, El-Sheikh Y, et al. Hand and fingers. In: Schöffl V, Schöffl I, Hochholzer T, et al., eds. *Climbing Medicine: A Practical Guide*. Heidelberg: Springer, 2022. © 2022 BMJ Publishing Group Ltd & British Association of Sport and Exercise Medicine. All rights reserved.

head of biceps tendon. During these moves, internal rotation and anterior tilt of the shoulder under load increase tensile strain on the pulley system and the labro-bicipital complex. Nevertheless, SLAP injuries in climbers are usually caused by repetitive microtrauma rather than one single incident.

The other prevalent shoulder pathology relates to overuse of the rotator cuff itself. There has been longstanding debate about the nomenclature of these conditions and we refer you to the shoulder chapters in *Managing Injuries* for a more detailed discussion. The important point from a climbing biomechanics perspective is to be aware of dynamic moves ("dynos"). These refer to the climber jumping from one set of holds to another. The rotator cuff is loaded more when the climber catches themselves on the wall—not when they are launching. As in other sports, force is high because of the eccentric load placed on the tissue over a very short

period of time. Dynos are used particularly in vertical and overhanging climbs. The rotator cuff will also be forced to contract rapidly if the climber's foot slips unexpectedly.

## CRICKET (FAST BOWLING)

### with KEVIN SIMS and ALEX KOUNTOURIS

Cricket fast bowling involves a combination of rapid near-end-range trunk movements (rotation, side flexion and extension) while absorbing high vertical and horizontal impact forces.[22–24] Elite fast bowlers bowl in excess of 300 deliveries in a single 4–5 day game and have the highest rate of injury among cricket players.[25]

### Injury epidemiology and risk factors

Soft-tissue and bone injuries are typically reported in injury surveillance studies of fast bowlers.[26] Lumbar spine injuries have received the most attention, mostly because bone stress injuries of the posterior vertebral elements (pedicle, pars interarticularis and lamina) require lengthy recovery periods and are particularly common.[25]

There are modifiable and non-modifiable risk factors for cricket injuries, particularly for lumbar spine injuries.[26,27] Traditionally, age, workload and bowling biomechanics are highlighted and it is likely that a combination of these factors determines the injury risk for fast bowlers. However, a recent study in a young cohort (average age 17.4 years) of variables reflecting bowling technique, bowling workload, physical competencies and anthropometric measurements was able to explain only 36% of lumbar bone stress injury risk.[28] Factors such as growth rate, genetics, anatomical variations, specific bone adaptations, skill level and nutrition may all be risk factors not easily accounted for in cricket research to date.

Adolescent fast bowlers have a higher incidence of lumbar bone stress injuries than adult bowlers[29] and a disproportionally high rate of lumbar spine radiological abnormalities for their age.[30] The pars interarticularis is particularly susceptible to repetitive loading into lumbar extension, rotation and lateral flexion.[31,32] Technique (biomechanical) faults that exaggerate these movements may therefore increase the load on the already susceptible musculoskeletal structures like the intervertebral disc and posterior vertebral arch.

Bowling workload is a modifiable risk factor associated with injuries in both adolescent and adult fast bowlers.[23,29,33–35] Workload spikes (rapid increases in workload) have been associated with fast-bowling injuries and particularly lumbar spine injuries.[29,36,37] It is also likely that bowlers with a technique that is biomechanically sound may be able to tolerate higher workloads than those with "less safe" techniques because they are better equipped to dissipate forces.

This relationship could be further complicated when considering age and that some structures may not have the resilience to absorb repetitive load (e.g. the posterior vertebral arch) until full maturity is reached. For example, in the lumbar spine peak bone mineral density is not attained until the early to mid-20s in females and males, respectively.[38]

Furthermore, specific asymmetrical increases in lumbar spine bone mineral density on the contralateral side to the bowling arm are observed in adolescence[39] and become even more evident in mature fast bowlers.[40] Other parameters such as vertebral height and width continue to develop until age 25,[41] at which point bowlers appear to become less likely to develop lumbar bone stress and other lumbar spine injuries.

The relative impact of workload and age as risk factors needs to be considered along with bowling technique, because technical faults that result in excessive end-range spinal motion and higher impact forces can magnify the impact of other risk factors. Fast-bowling technical faults

are modifiable risk factors although making meaningful technical change can be difficult.[42] Below we review the patterns of movement (kinematics) and forces (kinetics) that occur during the fast-bowling action.

## Fast-bowling biomechanics and injury

The fast-bowling action combines trunk rotation, lateral flexion and extension during the delivery stride.[22–24] The sequence of movements and associated ground reaction forces during the delivery stride can be broadly categorised into four bowling techniques: front-on, side-on, semi-open (semi-on) and mixed.[43] These techniques are defined by the position of the feet, pelvis, trunk and shoulders at specific times during the delivery stride and assessed using video (2D) or, ideally, 3D computer analysis.[43]

The fast-bowling action has three components that are interrelated and important for both performance and injury:[44]

- The run-up is important as it allows bowlers to generate linear momentum, which can be converted into angular momentum and transferred to the ball during the delivery stride.[45]
- The delivery stride is the last ground contact of the back foot, known as back-foot contact (BFC), then the transition to front-foot contact (FFC), and ends with ball release (Fig. 13.6). The highest ground reaction forces, between six to nine times bodyweight, occur during the period between FFC and ball release.[22,23,46]

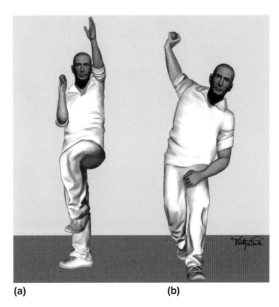

(a)                        (b)

**Figure 13.6** Cricket fast-bowling components: (a) BFC and (b) FFC
Source: Drawings adapted from Portus M, Mason BR, Elliott BC, et al. Technique factors related to ball release speed and trunk injuries in high performance cricket fast bowlers. *Sports Biomech* 2004;3(2):263–84.

- Follow-through begins at ball release and involves deceleration of the bowler until they come to a stop.

Bowlers are categorised into a bowling technique based on the positions and movements that occur during the delivery stride.[44] The four main bowling techniques are outlined in Figure 13.7.

Of the four bowling actions, the mixed technique has historically been identified as having the greatest association with lumbar spine injury and abnormal radiological features,[47,48] although more recent evidence has not substantiated this link.[49] The maximum amount of shoulder–pelvis separation angle occurs just after FFC,[43] and possibly represents the period that places the bowler at greatest risk of injury, especially as it is also the time when the greatest ground impact forces are being absorbed.[23,46] Initial work found bowlers using the mixed technique had higher rates of trunk contralateral side flexion and hyperextension compared with other bowling actions and this was proposed to place greater stress through the lumbar spine.[50] However, more recent work has not been able to replicate this finding,[43,51] probably due to differences in age, skill level and methods of data capture between the two cohorts.

Another biomechanical aspect that has been associated with lumbar spine injuries in fast bowlers is shoulder counter-rotation (SCR), which is the change in shoulder alignment between BFC and FFC, from a more front-on to a more side-on alignment (Fig. 13.8).[43,44] SCR has historically been associated with the mixed technique and several studies have linked higher ($>30°$) SCR during the delivery stride with a significantly higher incidence of lumbar bone stress injuries and abnormal radiological features.[22,23,44,48,52] However, subsequent studies using 3D motion capture cameras have demonstrated no association between lumbar bone stress injuries and SCR in male fast bowlers[49,53,54] or between SCR and low back pain in female fast bowlers.[51]

One of the limitations of SCR is that it represents whole trunk (and shoulder girdle) rotation rather than specific spinal kinematics.[55] A recent study using inertial measurement units demonstrated that junior bowlers with a history of low back pain had less rotation of the thoracic spine relative to the lumbar spine than those with no low back pain history,[56] suggesting that the movement of one spinal region relative to an adjacent region is relevant to a better understanding of fast-bowling pathomechanics.

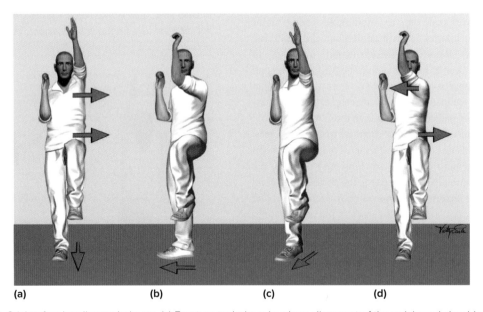

(a)    (b)    (c)    (d)

**Figure 13.7** Cricket fast-bowling techniques. (a) Front-on technique involves alignment of the pelvis and shoulders parallel to the batter at BFC. (b) Side-on technique involves alignment of the bowler's shoulders and pelvis perpendicular to the batter at BFC. (c) Semi-on or semi-open technique is defined as both shoulder and pelvis alignment somewhere between front-on and side-on positions at BFC. (d) Mixed technique involves dissociation between the shoulder and pelvis alignment at BFC, known as the shoulder—pelvis separation angle, e.g. a front-on pelvis alignment and side-on shoulder alignment at BFC, or side-on pelvis position and front-on shoulder position at BFC. A shoulder—pelvis separation angle of 30° has been used to classify bowlers as having a mixed technique.
Source: Drawings adapted from Portus M, Mason BR, Elliott BC, et al. Technique factors related to ball release speed and trunk injuries in high performance cricket fast bowlers. *Sports Biomech* 2004;3(2):263—84.

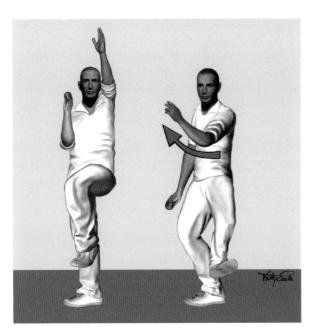

**Figure 13.8** Shoulder counter rotation during delivery stride
Source: Drawings adapted from Portus M, Mason BR, Elliott BC, et al. Technique factors related to ball release speed and trunk injuries in high performance cricket fast bowlers. *Sports Biomech* 2004;3(2):263—84.

B

The multifactorial nature of lumbar spine injuries has led to disagreement whether one particular bowling trunk position is associated with lumbar bone stress injuries or if a combination of movements is required to exceed load tolerance. Some of the earlier studies proposed that lumbar extension was most likely to be associated with lumbar bone stress injury in fast bowlers, based on cadaver studies highlighting an increased load on the posterior vertebral arch in a hyperextended position.[22, 57]

This is consistent with more recent modelling studies[31, 32] and biomechanical research (using 3D optoelectrical systems) identifying increased lumbo-pelvic extension at FFC as a risk factor for lumbar bone stress injuries in a group of early senior fast-bowlers (age 18.9 ± 1.9) prospectively followed over a 2-year period.[49] Increased lumbar extension at BFC was also identified in a small subset of senior fast bowlers (24.1 ± 4.3) who prospectively developed low back pain.[56]

The role of trunk side flexion and rotation has also received attention, with fast bowlers exhibiting greater ranges of thoraco-pelvic lateral flexion at FFC (proportional to their overall range in standing) than thoraco-pelvic extension (129% vs 26%, respectively).[53] The study authors concluded that the combination of high amounts of contralateral side flexion, ipsilateral rotation and the large impact forces would be most likely to be associated

with lumbar bone stress injuries in fast bowlers,[53] although there was no injury follow-up in the study and the measure of thorax motion relative to the pelvis may not be a true reflection of the kinematics of the lumbar spine.

A more recent biomechanical study (using 3D optoelectric systems) of young fast bowlers (aged 15—19) also identified higher amounts of thoracic lateral flexion in a group who prospectively sustained a low back injury over the next season.[54] It is most likely that a combination of trunk positions is responsible for the high force required to develop lumbar spine injuries, particularly bone stress injuries, and the individual contribution of each movement to injury risk could be associated with the bowling technique used.

Apart from the spine and trunk positions adopted during the delivery stride, lower limb joint kinematics have also been linked with fast-bowling injuries. In a prospective study, greater amounts of hip flexion at BFC were the best injury predictor, correctly identifying 76% of subsequent lumbar bone stress injuries.[49] The study authors proposed that this might reflect an inefficiency controlling the momentum of the run-up (too fast) or poor alignment of the run-up requiring a redirection of the centre of mass towards the target.[49] Additionally, it is consistent with a reduced ability to control the movement of the femur relative to the pelvis using functional movement screening tests identified in a previous study.[54]

The amount of knee extension at FFC influences the distribution of forces and the height at which the ball is released, so that a higher release height requires less knee flexion (straighter knee).[23, 58] The increase in front-foot knee extension leads to a stiffer knee segment and greater impact forces.[44, 58]

One study reported a relationship between a more extended front knee at FFC and ball release, and higher braking and vertical impact forces.[44] It also demonstrated that bowlers with greater knee extension also reached peak forces more quickly than those with a more flexed knee at ball release. The higher forces associated with a more extended front knee may increase injury risk but also allow bowlers to deliver the ball at faster bowling speeds.[44] This is an important performance benefit and needs to be considered if technique modification is contemplated. It is therefore possible that there may be a trade-off between faster bowling speeds and higher injury risk.

In summary, it is important to consider bowling biomechanics as one of the important risk factors for fast-bowling injuries. The relative impact of biomechanical errors on injury risk should be considered along with bowling workload and the age of the bowler, as there appears to be a delicate interplay between these key risk factors.

# CYCLING

## with BEN CLARSEN and F.C. DU TOIT

The demands and injury risks differ greatly across the various cycling disciplines:

- Traditional road cycling involves long-duration sub-maximal effort and places stresses on the body due to monotonous loading and the maintenance of static postures for extended periods.
- BMX and track sprint cycling require maximal effort over a short duration. Riders from these disciplines are more likely to suffer traumatic injuries or overuse injuries related to strength and power training.
- The various sub-disciplines of mountain biking encompass a wide range of demands, and both acute and overuse injuries are common.

The next section focuses on sub-maximal cycling, as this represents the mainstay of the sport's participants.

## Relationship between risk factors and loading

Overuse injuries in cycling are commonly blamed on extrinsic factors such as bike position or shoe and pedal setup, as well as intrinsic factors such as anatomical anomalies, poor cycling technique and reduced neuromuscular control. These factors may certainly be important due to the repetitive, uniplanar nature of the sport. However, it is important to recognise that even among top professionals, a wide variation of anatomy, techniques and bike setups is normally well-tolerated without injuries occurring. In almost all cases of cycling-related overuse injuries, symptom onset can be linked to a mismanagement of training and racing loads.

Cyclists are most likely to develop an injury following a rapid increase in load, such as when pre-season training is resumed after a winter break, or during intense periods of the season. When injuries are apparently "caused" by a change in equipment, it is normally because the change was made when the cyclist was already close to their limit of load tolerance.

A key to successful management of cycling injuries is load management (Chapter 15). You should establish with the cyclist and their coach the volume, intensity and frequency of cycling that they can tolerate, and create a systematic plan to increase these parameters over time. Wherever possible, loading should be quantified using a power meter, and training software should be used to monitor acute and chronic training loads during rehabilitation. Once an appropriate training plan has been established, intrinsic and extrinsic risk factors should be assessed.

The following sections cover biomechanical factors thought to be associated with the most common cycling injuries. There is little high-level evidence in the field of cycling injuries, with current practice largely based on indirect evidence and expert opinion. It is therefore necessary to take a trial-and-error approach; to be worthwhile, modification in technique or equipment should lead to an obvious improvement in symptoms (Box 13.2).

## Knee pain

The knee is the most common site of overuse injury among cyclists of all levels.[59–63] The majority of knee complaints are related to the patellofemoral joint.[64] However, there are a range of differential diagnoses including iliotibial band (ITB) syndrome, infrapatellar fat pad impingement, medial plica irritations and medial patellofemoral ligament sprains.[64–66] Although tendinopathy is generally rare in cyclists, pain can arise from the quadriceps tendon enthesis on the superolateral or superomedial patella.

Various biomechanical factors contribute to patellofemoral pain in cyclists, including patellofemoral joint compression forces, knee kinematics in the frontal plane and rotational torques in the lower limb.[67–70] Patellofemoral joint contact pressure is inversely related to saddle height,[67] leading to the common belief that cycling with a lower saddle height increases the risk of patellofemoral pain.[66,69–71] However, this remains to be confirmed in high-quality studies, and one study found that altering the saddle height within the normal ranges used in rehabilitation led to negligible changes in patellofemoral joint contact pressure.[72] Nevertheless, we advise that cyclists with patellofemoral pain ride in a relatively high saddle position, with maximal knee extension of approximately 30° (Fig. 13.10).

Excessive medial motion of the knee in the frontal plane (Fig. 13.11a) may also be a risk factor for patellofemoral pain, as this position encourages lateralisation of the patella in the femoral trochlea, increased lateral joint contact pressure and increased stress on medial soft tissues. This theory is supported by studies showing that cyclists with a history of knee pain adopt a more medial knee position compared with uninjured cyclists,[68] and that "normalising" frontal-plane motion (Fig. 13.11b) can lead to symptomatic improvement.[73]

Knee motion may be altered by motor control training or through manipulation of the cyclist's shoes and pedals. For example, foot position can be adjusted using small-angled wedges between the shoe and the pedal cleat or underneath the forefoot, or by using custom-made insoles. However, manipulation of cycling shoes and pedals has an unpredictable effect on knee motion.[74,75] It is therefore important to test each individual's response, making sure that adjustments lead to symptomatic improvement.

## BOX 13.2 Bike fitting

There are many approaches to bike fitting, ranging from simple anthropometry-based formulae to dynamic approaches using high-tech equipment (Table 13.7). As bike fitting involves optimisation of a wide range of competing variables (e.g. aerodynamics, comfort and control), it always requires compromise.

Despite the rapid pace of technological development in the cycling industry, there remains little research into bicycle equipment and injuries, and bike fitting remains just as much an art as it is a science.

You should aim to work closely with bike fitters who take a trial-and-error approach, considering the cyclist's previous and current injuries, cycling goals and physical limitations (Fig. 13.9).

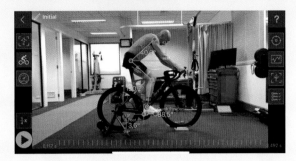

**Figure 13.9** Contemporary bike fitting includes motion analysis, pressure measurement in the saddle and analysis of power in each pedal
IMAGE COURTESY OF PAUL VISENTINI

**TABLE 13.7    Advantages and limitations of modern bike-fitting methods**

| Approach | Description | Advantages | Limitations |
|---|---|---|---|
| Formula-based approach | A number of formula-based approaches convert anthropometric measurements (e.g. inseam height) to bicycle setup parameters; the most well-known is named after two-time Tour de France winner Greg LeMond | Quick and easy: cyclists can perform measurements themselves | Highly unreliable, does not consider the cyclist's physical limitations[85] |
| Static angle-based approach (sometimes referred to as the Holmes method) | The cyclist's major joint angles are measured with a goniometer while they sit on the bike without cycling; the bike is adjusted to position each joint within a predetermined "optimal" range of motion | Good reliability[86] | Does not consider dynamic cycling technique |
| Dynamic angle-based approach | Combination of data streams such as power, pedal forces and saddle pressure with motion analysis | Good reliability;[86] accounts for the rider's technique and physical limitations | Does not consider kinetic variables such as power distribution between the legs |
| Combined-input approach | Combination of data streams such as power, pedal forces and saddle pressure with motion analysis | Multiple sources of data can lead to more informed clinical reasoned decisions | More data do not always lead to better clinical decisions; little research to assist data interpretation; validity and reliability unknown |

Rotational torque at the knee caused by fixation of the shoes to the pedals may also be a factor in patellofemoral pain in cycling. After the introduction of modern cleated pedals in the 1980s there were anecdotal reports of an increase in the prevalence of knee injuries among cyclists.[64, 70] It was thought that the natural rotation of the lower limb during pedalling was constrained by fixing the shoe, leading to increased stress at the knee joint.

Therefore, "float" pedals were designed to allow a small degree of axial rotation, which attenuated the rotational torque at the knee (Fig. 13.12).[70] Although there is no direct evidence that float pedals reduce injury, their design has been widely accepted and they remain the most popular type used by cyclists today.

ITB syndrome, often called "runner's knee", is also common among cyclists.[64, 76] Intrinsic factors thought to contribute to ITB syndrome include large leg-length discrepancies, external tibial torsion of greater than 20° and excessive subtalar pronation.[76] High saddle height, a "toe-in, heel-out" foot position and excessive medial knee

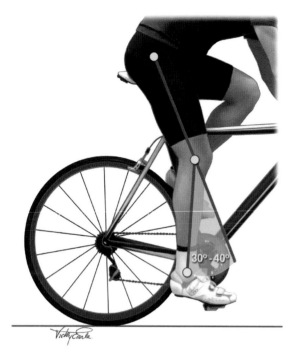

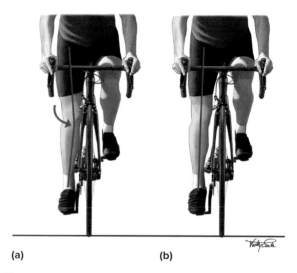

**Figure 13.11** Frontal-plane knee motion in cycling. (a) Excessive valgus motion of the knee is thought to contribute to a range of knee injuries. (b) Improving the alignment of the hip, knee and ankle may lead to symptomatic improvement.

**Figure 13.10** Maximum knee extension is a key bike-fitting parameter, which typically ranges from 35° to 40° among professional riders. Patellofemoral joint contact pressure may be minimised by selecting a higher saddle position, with maximum knee extension between 30° and 35°.

motion also increase the stress on the ITB.[77] Therefore, cyclists with lateral knee pain should be instructed to ride with a relatively low saddle (maximum knee extension

approximately 40°), keep their feet straight or pointed slightly outwards, and avoid a knee-in position.

## Low back pain

Although transient back discomfort can be considered normal in cycling, performance-limiting low back pain is common among amateur[78] and elite cyclists.[59,79] Cyclists with low back pain typically present with non-specific symptoms provoked by the maintenance of sustained

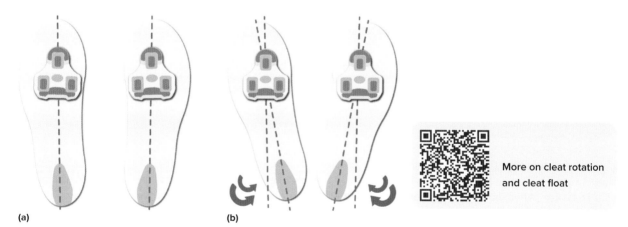

More on cleat rotation and cleat float

**Figure 13.12** Cleat rotation and float pedals. (a) Cleat rotation (a static angle) refers to the angle the cleats make—riders who walk with an out-toe gait often prefer their cleats to be rotated outwards. Riders who walk in-toed often have their cleats more inwardly rotated. (b) Float pedals refer to the type of cleat set-up that allows movement of the foot in the cleat: blue arrows show the long axis of the foot (blue dotted line) being able to rotate so that the toes face further out (red dotted line). This doesn't obviate the need to try to have accurate cleat rotation as the base.
ADAPTED FROM BIKEFIT (WWW.BIKEFIT.COM)

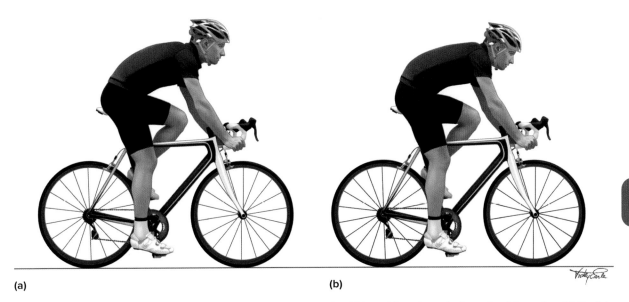

**(a)**    **(b)**

**Figure 13.13** Spinal position in cycling. (a) Ideally, forward bend should be achieved evenly throughout the spine. (b) Cyclists with low back pain often adopt a more flexed lumbar spine, with less anterior pelvic tilt and a more extended thoracic spine.

flexion positions, and they can often be classified as having a flexion-pattern motor control dysfunction.[80]

Careful biomechanical assessment of the cyclist is key to identifying the relevant dysfunction and then addressing it. Using a remote posture monitoring system, it has been shown that cyclists with low back pain adopt a more flexed position in their lumbar spine than do pain-free cyclists (Fig. 13.13).[81] This may be related to a number of pathomechanical mechanisms of low back pain,[80, 82] such as flexion/relaxation inhibition or fatigue of the erector spinae muscles and mechanical creep of the spine's viscoelastic tissues. However, these theories remain largely untested.

Encouraging a relaxed, anteriorly tilted pelvic position, with an even distribution of flexion throughout the spine is often important in the overall management of cyclists with low back pain. A number of equipment modifications may help facilitate this, including lowering the saddle, raising the handlebars and shortening or lengthening the overall reach. Adjusting the saddle to a slightly nose-down position (2°–4°) may be particularly helpful in achieving greater anterior pelvic tilt and reducing back pain.[83]

Excessive lateral flexion and/or rotation of the spine while cycling may also contribute to back pain, particularly if it is asymmetrical. This can be caused by a range of factors, such as large leg-length differences, hip range of motion limitations and asymmetrical muscle activation patterns. These should be considered as a part of the comprehensive management of the cyclist with low back pain.

## Ulnar neuropathy

The ulnar nerve may be compressed at the wrist as it passes through Guyon's canal, sometimes with ulnar artery thrombosis. This is known as "hypothenar hammer" syndrome and is most commonly seen in cyclists due to supporting body weight over a long duration ride,[84] because of poor bike fit or due to a failure to use several relaxed handlebar grip positions (Fig. 13.14). Within Guyon's canal, the nerve lies with the ulnar artery between the pisiform bone on the ulnar side and the hamate radially.

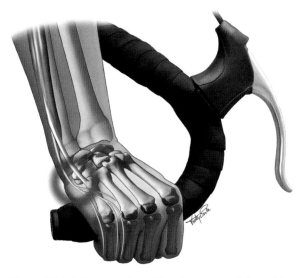

**Figure 13.14** Compression of the ulnar nerve at the wrist

Symptoms include pain and paraesthesia to the little finger and ulnar side of the fourth finger. Weakness usually develops later. Non-surgical treatment involves splinting, NSAIDs, postural strengthening and changes to bicycle setup. In particular, the grip position should be assessed, and moving the saddle backwards may reduce the amount of weight going through the cyclist's upper limbs. Surgical exploration of Guyon's canal may be required.

# GOLF

## with ANDREW MURRAY and ROGER HAWKES

Golf has social, mental wellbeing, physical health and longevity benefits and is a sport played globally by more than 66 million people of all ages.[87] Although injury incidence is low at 0.28–0.60 per thousand playing hours,[88] injuries are common because of the popularity of the sport and the long duration of play. More than half of all golfers will sustain a musculoskeletal injury during their playing career. Patterns of injury differ between professional and amateur golfers.

Table 13.8 shows career injury prevalence for amateur and professional golfers,[89] noting the hands and wrists, lower back and shoulders as the leading regions for symptoms in professionals, and elbow and forearm issues as common among amateur players.

Injuries are generally due to chronic biomechanical overload rather than acute injury. There are three main factors to consider:

1. volume of practice
2. internal biomechanical factors (e.g. golf swing biomechanics)
3. external biomechanical factors (e.g. type of golf equipment, firmness of ground and length of grass—fairways and rough).

Golf relies on a coordinated and repeated swing in which energy is generated in the lower body and trunk. In long hitters, the force is transferred efficiently into the upper limbs and ultimately the club head, which can travel at speeds of >200 km/hr.

Professional tournaments usually consist of a daily round of 18 holes over a 3- or 4-day period during which the player also includes considerable golf practice, physical and mental preparation, and recovery. Around 75% of professionals hit more than 200 shots per day,[90] with professionals hitting 10 times as many balls as amateurs. Average drives by amateur and professional golfers range from 180 m to 275 m, respectively.[91]

This section focuses on the most common golf injuries to the wrist, low back, shoulder and hip, as well as briefly mentioning elbow pain, which is also common.

## Wrist pain

Good amateurs and professional players require considerable practice and intentionally take ground divots to impart backspin on the ball. In the winter professional players often practise on mats. As a result, the leading wrist of professional players is subject to greater forces than in amateur players.[92]

### The leading wrist

The leading wrist is the more vulnerable of the two wrists during the golf swing because it moves from radial deviation

**TABLE 13.8**   Career injury prevalence with relative risk analyses by individual anatomical region for amateur and professional golfers

| Injury site | Career injury prevalence, % (95% CI) | | Relative risk (95% CI) | p-value |
|---|---|---|---|---|
| | **Amateurs** | **Professionals** | | |
| Neck | 4.4 (1.0–9.9) | 10.5 (1.2–26.5) | 1.84 (0.11–30.78) | 0.670 |
| Lower back | 16.2 (11.2–22.0) | 40.9 (35.2–46.7) | 3.05 (2.14–4.34) | <0.001* |
| Shoulder | 11.1 (6.7–16.4) | 18.4 (12.3–25.3) | 1.79 (0.71–4.52) | 0.216 |
| Elbow and forearm | 20.5 (18.7–22.4) | 13.6 (7.7–20.8) | 0.88 (0.53–1.47) | 0.628 |
| Hand and wrist | 13.2 (9.5–17.4) | 51.5 (24.6–78.0) | 3.33 (2.28–4.86) | <0.001* |
| Hip | 2.1 (1.4–2.8) | 4.0 (1.9–6.7) | 1.68 (0.07–39.14) | 0.746 |
| Knee | 3.0 (0.9–7.7) | 11.1 (7.6–15.0) | 4.02 (0.55–29.4) | 0.170 |
| Foot and ankle | 3.6 (2.3–5.2) | 5.4 (0.4–14.6) | 1.91 (0.20–18.21) | 0.574 |
| Other | 5.4 (4.2–6.8) | 13.8 (1.0–36.8) | 1.85 (0.16–21.65) | 0.943 |

*Statistically significant (p <0.05)

Source: Williamson KR, Robinson P, Murray A, et al. The epidemiology of musculoskeletal injury in professional and amateur golfers: a systematic review and meta-analysis. *Br J Sports Med* 2024;58. © 2024 BMJ Publishing Group Ltd & British Association of Sport and Exercise Medicine. All rights reserved.

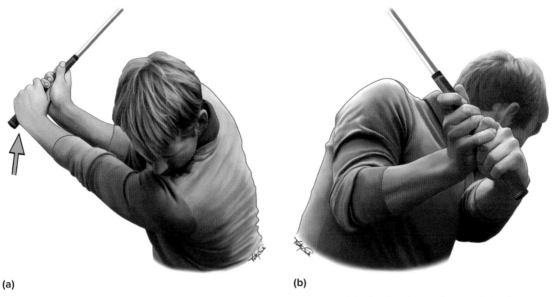

(a)                                                                                      (b)

**Figure 13.15** (a) The leading wrist is in maximal radial deviation at the top of the back swing and moves into ulnar deviation during the follow-through. (b) The trailing wrist is in maximal extension at the top of the back swing and moves into flexion during the follow-through.

at the top of the backswing (Fig. 13.15a) to ulnar deviation during follow-through. The trailing wrist follows a less stressful extension/flexion movement pattern (Fig. 13.15b).

At ball impact, force is transmitted through the ulnar side of the leading wrist and the extensor carpi ulnaris (ECU) tendon, which is thus susceptible to tenosynovitis and tendinopathy from tissue overload. More rarely when a player hits an obstruction (tree root or stone), it can rupture the ECU sub-sheath which holds its position at the lower end of the ulna. This structure is particularly vulnerable in supination, which occurs during the golf swing and results in a large angle between the muscle axis and the tendon as it inserts onto the 5th metacarpal.[93]

As a result of repetitive movement, the leading wrist is also susceptible to bone stress reactions, particularly of the hamate. Due to chronic biomechanical load, older players may develop osteoarthritic changes in the carpus, and players with long ulnas (either constitutionally or acquired after radial fracture) may be susceptible to ulnocarpal synovitis or other ulnar-sided wrist pain as a result of impaction.

Fractures of the hook of hamate are rare, but they can occur.[94] The hook of hamate is particularly vulnerable when a tall player uses standard-length clubs: the end of the club may press onto the hook of hamate (Fig. 13.16) or pisohamate ligament. Acute fractures can occur if the club hits the ground or an object and with repetitive impacts the hook is also susceptible to bone stress injuries. Players who have had hook of hamate stress reactions or fractures may need to use longer clubs.

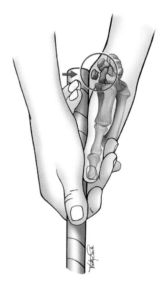

**Figure 13.16** Fracture of the hook of hamate. Possible mechanism—when the golf club is suddenly decelerated (e.g. hitting the ground), the grip is forced against the hook of hamate.

### The trailing wrist

The trailing wrist extends during the back swing and flexes during the follow-through (Fig. 13.15b). Players with dorsal rim impaction syndrome[95] pinpoint pain at the radial carpal joint in loaded extension, but often have no pain in passive extension. This condition results from nipping of the synovium, which can become inflamed and hypertrophied.

It often occurs in players who still have an extended wrist at impact and those with a steep downswing.

Ultrasound is a good starting investigation as it may identify the hypertrophied synovium with colour-flow Doppler but can also be normal. MRI is the examination of choice as it can definitively show hypertrophy of the synovium (Fig. 13.17) and loose bodies, which can be confirmed by CT if necessary.

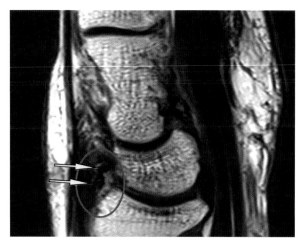

**Figure 13.17** Dorsal rim impaction syndrome. Sagittal MRI showing capsular hypertrophy (arrows) of the dorsal aspect of the radiocarpal synovium. On MRI, a normal capsule appears as a thin low signal line.

Players with dorsal or ulnar-sided pain due to tenosynovitis reduce practice (load manage) to reduce pain. Amateur players may also choose a more forgiving shaft, such as those made of graphite. They may improve the sweet spot by using hollow back clubs rather than blades.

Players who acutely sublux their ECU tendons generally prefer to have the subsheath repaired; on the other hand, we have treated tennis players conservatively with good results, with no apparent increased time away from their sport. Some players have asymptomatic subluxing ECU tendons and do not require treatment.[92]

## Low back pain

As back pain is common in the general population, recreational golfers often attribute back pain to activities of daily living or sports other than golf.[96] In recreational golfers, a contributor to back pain is carrying a heavy golf bag on one shoulder, rather than using a double shoulder strap or push-cart.

Good recreational and professional players develop low back pain more frequently than those who practise less.[89] This is not surprising given practice volume and the forces generated to increase swing/clubhead speed. A potent golf swing generates an 8-times bodyweight force on the player's lumbar spine. In the modern backswing (Fig. 13.18) the player aims to rotate the shoulders maximally on the hips to increase potential energy. Club speed is generated on the

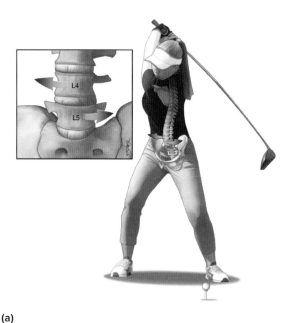

(a)

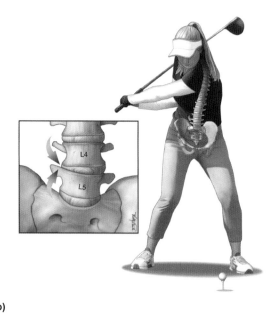

(b)

**Figure 13.18** Forces at the spine during the phases of the golf swing. (a) At the point of full backswing, the shoulders are maximally rotated on a stable pelvis. This creates rotary forces at various levels including L4—L5 (illustrated). (b) As the player generates club speed on the downswing, they generate large lateral flexion forces, as shown.

downswing with aggressive lateral flexion and axial rotation ("a crunch" of the joints on the trailing side).

Lack of internal rotation in the leading hip increases stress on the thoracolumbar spine, as the follow-through rotation is transferred higher up the kinetic chain. Tight hip flexors promote more anterior pelvic tilt and therefore "jam" the facets in the lumbar spine.[97]

Golf swing biomechanics and its possible relation to injury in golf legend Tiger Woods is discussed here:[98]

Biomechanics of the modern golf swing

## Shoulder pain

The forces acting on the leading shoulder in golf are almost opposite to those involved in throwing. The shoulder hyperadducts during the backswing, which can overstretch the posterior structures. During the follow-through, the anterior structures work eccentrically to slow the shoulder down. The resultant combination of anterior capsular tightness and posterior laxity pushes the humeral head posteriorly and stresses the labrum, which can lead to posterior instability.[99]

Acromioclavicular joint pathology may occur in golfers. It is aggravated by joint compression, which occurs during the backswing for the leading shoulder and during the follow-through for the trailing shoulder. Due to repeated overhead and rotatory activity, golfers of all abilities frequently develop rotator cuff tendinopathy, or subacromial or other bursitis.

Players who are recovering from shoulder injuries often need to limit golf participation in the early phases of rehabilitation. Their progression towards return to sport begins with putting and small chips with high irons, before gradually increasing the swing and playing with progressively longer clubs. Following this, the volume and speed of shot increase gradually before a return to competition.

## Hip pain

Hip pain is prevalent in recreational golfers[96] but much of this is due to hip pain of daily life that affects their ability to play golf freely. Loss of range of movement at the hips can predispose to low back pain. A systematic review and meta-analysis of injuries in golfers reported that hip pain due to playing golf is less frequent.[100] Common hip diagnoses in golfers include labrum pathology, FAI syndrome and osteoarthritis.

In the golf swing, the leading hip[100] rotates rapidly and moves through a much greater range of motion than the trailing hip.[101, 102] However, both hips need to move freely to facilitate an effective swing, particularly into internal rotation. The trailing hip goes into internal rotation at the top of the backswing and the leading hip is at maximum internal rotation at the end of the follow-through. Players with osteoarthritis and femoroacetabular impingement may present with hip pain at either end of the swing.

## Overall assessment and treatment considerations

When assessing or treating a golfer, it is vital to look with them (and where relevant, their coach) at any change in the volume of balls hit, and at their internal and external biomechanical factors. Injuries can be predicted and prevented by close attention to volume, and limiting any increase in practice when there is a change in equipment or ground conditions. Similarly, any change in swing biomechanics should be integrated gradually to avoid increased injury risk.

When an injury does occur, managing load and considering biomechanical factors can help find the root cause of the symptoms. Often, slightly changing these mechanics, or for example strapping to limit ulnar deviation in a painful lead wrist, can assist the golfer in being able to compete and train.

## ROWING

### with FIONA WILSON and JANE THORNTON

The biomechanics of rowing are complex, with many variables contributing to the speed of the boat. The legs, trunk and arms each contribute approximately one-third of the stroke length. Contrary to common belief, the legs are the greatest source of power, increasing their contribution as the stroke rate increases.[103] Different technical styles (e.g. simultaneous or sequential use of the legs and trunk) can influence this distribution.[104]

High forces are generated at several anatomical sites. Due to the cyclical movement pattern and high volume of training, these forces are repeated hundreds of times during a typical training session. There are three scenarios in which the rower is particularly at risk:

1. during abrupt changes in training volume, intensity or type
2. when there are changes in the rower's load through equipment/crew changes
3. at the transition between dry land and on-water training.[105]

This section focuses on three of the most common regions of rowing-related overuse injury: the lower back, chest wall and wrist/forearm.

## Low back pain

On average, 61% of adult rowers experience an episode of low back pain in a 12-month period. Risk factors for rowing-related low back pain are a previous history of low back pain, ergometer training (particularly training sessions that last longer than 30 minutes) and rapid increase in training load.[106] These risk factors are important to note at pre-season screening/periodic health assessment (Chapter 18).

A number of biomechanical factors are thought to contribute to the development of low back pain. The spine is maximally loaded at the front of the stroke (known as the "catch" position) where the blade of the oar is placed in the water and force is applied through the trunk, arms and legs. Ideally, forward reach at the catch is achieved through maximal hip (at least 130°), knee and ankle flexion, with the lumbar spine in slight flexion and the pelvis in anterior rotation (Fig. 13.19a).

However, inadequate lumbopelvic control or limitations in hip, knee or ankle range of motion may lead to a position of extreme lumbar flexion at the catch, with the pelvis in posterior rotation (Fig. 13.19b). In this position the intervertebral discs and posterior elements of the spine may be more vulnerable to injury. A focus on achieving greater hip range of motion and neutral or anterior pelvic rotation at the catch may be an important strategy to reduce the risk of low back pain.

Rowing technique deteriorates during continuous rowing, leading to increased lumbar flexion and frontal plane motion, which is attributed to fatigue. Fatigue is associated with increased spinal flexion at the catch, and training the trunk muscles to withhold forces over long durations and with increased load may be protective. The extensor muscles of the trunk dominate the rowing stroke and this should be considered in training.[107]

Good lumbopelvic control is also important in the finish position. Here, a neutral lumbar spine is ideal (Fig. 13.20a), whereas collapsing into lumbar flexion increases stress on the spine (Fig. 13.20b). Novice rowers use high levels of lumbar flexion with limited pelvic rotation, deteriorating further with

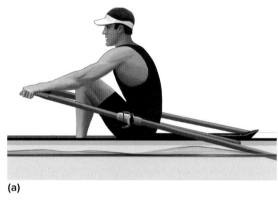

(a)

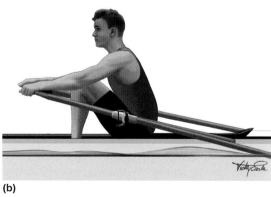

(b)

**Figure 13.19** The catch position: (a) pelvis in relative anterior rotation with an even distribution of flexion throughout the spine; (b) pelvis in relative posterior rotation increases the stress on the lumbar spine.

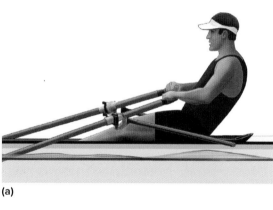

(a)

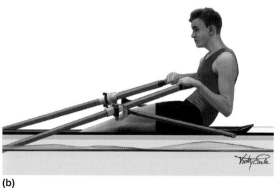

(b)

**Figure 13.20** The finish position: (a) lumbar spine in a neutral position; (b) lumbar spine collapsed into flexion.

higher work intensities.[108] While similar changes are seen in elite rowers, these are of a much lower magnitude.[109]

Another factor is time spent ergometer training. Lumbar kinematics are different in ergometer rowing compared with rowing in the boat: increased lumbar flexion associated with prolonged rowing and fatigue is a greater problem in ergometer rowing.[110] Therefore, rowers with low back pain should reduce their time on the ergometer and pay close attention to their lumbopelvic control while rowing, ideally using some form of biofeedback (mirror, video or electrogoniometer).

A majority of rowers with low back pain present with flexion-pattern motor control dysfunction.[111] As for other patient groups, a multidimensional cognitive functional approach has been shown to have the best efficacy in rowers.[112, 113] However, a number of specific considerations should be applied to the rowing population. An exercise approach that focuses on optimal position of the trunk and pelvis throughout the stroke should underpin rehabilitation. Excellent range of motion, particularly at the hips, knees and ankles, should be emphasised.

A mistake made by many clinicians who guide rehabilitation in low back pain in rowing is poor specificity in exercise prescription, particularly overemphasis of isometric exercise in the trunk such as the "plank" exercise. Rowing is a dynamic sport and rehabilitation exercises aimed at improving trunk endurance should allow fluid movement. Being able to hold static positions for long periods does not result in rowing medals.

### Management principles

First-line non-operative treatment includes early unloading, maintaining physical activity and physiotherapy,[114] and early and effective pain relief.[106] Dynamic, endurance-based training is preferable to static core stability during regular training.[106]

Other strategies include using a lower load setting on the ergometer and correcting any underlying hip range of motion and/or strength and flexibility deficiencies.[114, 115] Behavioural therapies to address biopsychosocial elements of low back pain are key.[116] Surgery may be considered in rare cases of significant nerve damage, progressive pain and disability, or non-response to treatment.

As a clinician, encourage rowers to report episodes of pain early to allow you to modify load as a first-line strategy. There is stigma and secrecy surrounding the disclosure of low back pain so try to encourage a clinical alliance between the medical staff, coaches, managers and rowers.[117]

Figure 13.21 summarises the 2021 consensus statement for preventing and managing rowing-related low back pain.[117]

## Chest wall pain

Chest wall pain is particularly common in elite rowers,[118] but may occur in rowers of all levels. While the risk is low, chest pain that is due to cardiac or respiratory origins must first be ruled out. Most often chest pain is rib-related, such as intercostal muscle strain, costochondritis or rib stress injury,[119] in particular in the anterolateral portion of the 4th to 8th ribs.

### Risk factors for rib stress injury

The mechanism of rib stress injury is likely to include mechanical loading of the chest wall as well as individual intrinsic factors such as bone mineral density.[119–121] A combination of force vectors acting on the ribs from the scapula retractors, external obliques and rectus abdominis may lead to the stress fracture. Training volume (particularly a sharp load increase) and equipment issues such as blade size and type have also been implicated.[119, 121] Thoracic hypomobility, primarily limited extension, is common among rowers who sustain bone stress injuries.

As with any stress injury, low energy (relative energy deficiency in sport [REDs]; Chapter 9) is implicated as a causal factor. Bone mineral density, weight category and menstrual function are factors that should be considered in management.[122]

Emerging research has noted an increased risk of stress fracture in Para rowing athletes.[123] This may reflect low thoracic bone mineral density in athletes with spinal cord injuries because of reduced skeletal loading.

### Clinical features

Rowers with bone stress injuries typically present with pain in the anterolateral chest wall that is initially aggravated by rowing. As the condition worsens, other activities become painful, point tenderness develops and pain becomes aggravated by deep breathing, coughing, rolling over in bed and rising from supine.

Examination may reveal a positive rib spring and reproduction of pain during movements mimicking the rowing stroke,[119, 121] particularly on isometric resistance. Diagnosis is primarily from symptoms and examination, and may be confirmed with MRI.[124, 125]

### Management

The primary approach to management is 2–6 weeks of relative unloading while staying active. Exercise such as cycling can be maintained during this phase. Monitor symptoms and allow the athlete to return to training gradually, depending on pain.

Many rowers report ongoing symptoms for months (sometimes intermittently for longer) despite achieving

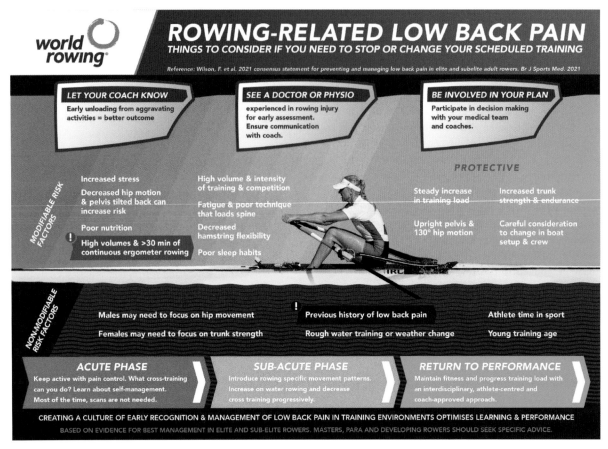

**Figure 13.21** 2021 consensus statement for preventing and managing rowing-related low back pain
Source: Wilson F, et al. 2021 consensus statement for preventing and managing low back pain in elite and subelite adult rowers. *Br J Sports Med* 2021.
© 2021 BMJ Publishing Group Ltd & British Association of Sport and Exercise Medicine. All rights reserved.

good function. Replacing use of traditional stationary rowing ergometers with dynamic ergometers may provide a protective element due to lower peak forces at the handle, without compromising performance.[126]

Biomechanical factors such as poor thoracic extension or altered movement control should be corrected. Manual therapy of the thoracic spine can be very useful, although compression of the rib cage should be avoided. Taping for proprioceptive feedback may aid comfort. Liaising with the coach and video analysis can be very useful in identifying correctable faults, such as overreaching or poor scapula control at the catch position.

The medical staff of the Great Britain Rowing Team have published clinical guidelines for the diagnosis and management of rib stress injuries in rowers (Fig. 13.22).[127, 128]

### Wrist and forearm injuries

Common wrist and forearm injuries in rowers include intersection syndrome, de Quervain tenosynovitis, and exertional compartment syndrome. All of these conditions are associated with incorrect or excessive loading of the forearm musculature, which is influenced by a variety of factors.

Rowing requires the athlete to rotate the oar handle after taking it out of the water (feathering the blade) and again prior to the blade re-entering the water (squaring the blade). Ideally, the blade should be feathered and squared using a combination of wrist and metacarpophalangeal joint movement. However, a common technical mistake, particularly among novice rowers, is to use wrist motion only during this action.

High grip pressure is also linked with the development of forearm injury. This is a particular problem when rowing in poor weather conditions and among beginners, who tend to grip the oar more firmly. Oar handle size and grip should be considered. Modern oar handles have synthetic grips and may be custom-fitted in different sizes; however, non-elite rowers are more likely to use oars that may be worn down or are not customisable.

# Rib Stress Injury: Guidelines for Diagnosis and Management

Definition: Rib stress injury is the development of pain due to bone oedema caused by overload along the bone shaft

## Chest wall pain

## Diagnostic features for rib stress injury (and clinical markers*)

### History

- Insidious  sudden onset or crescendo pain over a few days or weeks
- Pain on deep breathing*
- Pain on pushing/pulling doors*
- Difficulty rolling over in bed or sitting up from a lying position*
- Unable to sleep on affected side*
- Possible cough/sneeze pain*

### Examination

- Tenderness commonly mid axillary line of chest wall
- Ribs 5-8 in particular
- Tender spot over oedema and sometimes palpable callous
- +ve spring/compression of ribcage (AP & lateral)*
- Pain with press up or resisted serratus anterior testing*
- Pain on initiating trunk flexion (sit up position including oblique bias)*

## Severity of injury

### Mild

- VAS score 2-3/10**
- Rib pain towards end of activity
- 'Can row through it'
- 'Tightness or soreness'
- Mild tenderness
- Compression test may be negative
- May only be stiff splinted rib cage without pain
- Often not all clinical markers* present

** Interpret VAS score cautiously as can be highly subjective to individual

### Moderate

- VAS score 4-6/10**
- Rib pain on movements
- Unable to complete training/racing
- Tender on palpation and compression test positive
- Most clinical markers* will be present

### Severe

- VAS score 7-10/10**
- Rib pain at rest
- Painful on deep inspiration/coughing
- Pain on simple movements/lying/reaching
- Unable to train or race
- Compression test positive
- All clinical markers* likely to be present

Early investigations may be normal and therefore not helpful

## Investigations:
### Usually CLINICAL DIAGNOSIS

Consider MRI or bone scan if unclear diagnosis. Bone oedema may be present beyond resolution of symptoms so imaging may be misleading

## Management

### Stage 1

- Offload rib – stop all rowing mechanics both in a boat and on the ergo
- Initiate pain free cross training
- Analgesia for comfort but not NSAIDs as impede recovery
- Consider taping for comfort
- Soft tissue work helpful to alleviate symptoms of protective mechanism
- Ultrasound/Laser treatment may shorten recovery period if available but not essential
- Gradual return to activity ensuring load kept low and under supervision
- Ensure resolution of all clinical markers*
- Time frame 3-6 weeks

### Stage 2

- Biomechanical assessment by physiotherapist and coach
- Improvement of thoracic mobility and maintenance of mobility as load increases
- Assess rowing technique and correct to reduce areas of overload if possible
- Consider all intrinsic and extrinsic risk factors (see overleaf)
- Consider implementing prevention program

N.B. Stage 2 may be started early in rehabilitation process and does not necessarily require completion of stage 1

*See overleaf for intrinsic and extrinsic risk factors for rib stress injury*

**The GB RowingTeam is the High PerformanceArm of British Rowing**

**Figure 13.22** Clinical guidelines for the diagnosis and management of rib stress injuries in rowers
Source: Evans G, Redgrave A. Great Britain Rowing Team Guideline for Diagnosis and Management of Rib Stress Injury: Part 2 – The Guideline itself. *Br J Sports Med* 2015;50(5).

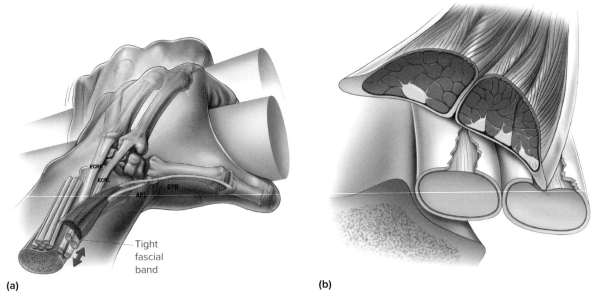

APL, abductor policies longs; EPB, extensor pollicis brevis; ECRB, extensor carpi radialis brevis; ECRL, extensor carpi radialis longus

**Figure 13.23** Injury at the crossing point of the 1st dorsal compartment (APL and EPB) and the 2nd dorsal compartment (ECRL, ECRB): (a) tight fascial band rubbing on tendons; (b) close up of pathology.
COURTESY OF DR GREG HOY

Sweep-oar rowers, who row with only one oar, are more likely to suffer from intersection syndrome (Fig. 13.23) and de Quervain tenosynovitis on their inside arm, as that wrist is in a greater degree of ulnar deviation. Changing sides may help alleviate pain.

In this setting, experienced clinicians recommend the rower switch to the ergometer (at the lowest drag factor setting with grip modification). This allows earlier return to rowing with a moderate load. The rower should avoid feathering and ulnar deviation. Non-operative management is first-line treatment but in one study Australian rowing clinicians reported encouraging results from early surgery among 6 rowers with intersection syndrome.[129]

## SWIMMING

### with ELSBETH VAN DORSSEN

Clinical management of swimmers is a challenge. Swimmers begin their career earlier than many athletes (typically between 8 and 12 years) and often train twice a day for 3–6 hours. Elite swimmers perform 1.5 million strokes per arm every year.

### Swimming biomechanics

In freestyle, backstroke and butterfly the swimmer's arms generate approximately 80% of the propulsion. The swimmer tries to generate propulsive force, while reducing resistance to forward motion. Drag forces (friction drag, form drag and wave drag) are extremely important at all swimming speeds; when you double the speed in water, you quadruple the form drag force.

Achieving a hydrodynamically efficient swimming position (long and lean body position, aligned with the direction of travel), while still being able to generate the propulsive forces requires specific strengths, flexibilities and skills. Swimmers will try to increase the length of the propulsive phase (when the arm is in the water), combined with a fast but "relaxed" recovery phase (above the water).

Swimmers compete in 4 strokes: freestyle, butterfly, backstroke and breaststroke. However, irrespective of a swimmer's preferred stroke, more than 50% of their training will be spent doing freestyle.[130]

When assessing the freestyle stroke, it is helpful to consider it in four phases (Fig. 13.24):

- hand entry
- reach/glide
- pull-through
- recovery phase.

The following sections consider the most common swimming injuries: shoulder pain, low back pain and medial knee pain.

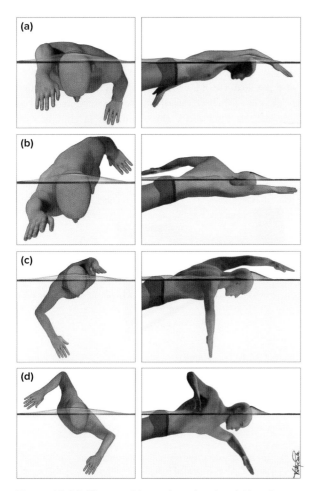

**Figure 13.24** Phases of freestyle swimming: (a) hand entry (b) reach/glide (c) pull-through (d) recovery

## Shoulder pain

The shoulder is by far the most common site of injury in swimmers, accounting for 31–39% of all injuries.[131, 132] The prevalence of shoulder pain in elite swimmers can be as high as 91%,[130] with 10–31% needing to stop training for some time during the year due to shoulder pain.[131–135]

There is a higher risk for shoulder injuries:

- after an abrupt increase in training volume or intensity[136]
- with a training volume over 35 km (or 15 hours) per week[130]
- when a unilateral breathing pattern is used[137]
- after a recent change of stroke technique—ask about any technical flaws that have been pointed out by the coach[138]
- when crossing the midline during pull-through
- with a history of shoulder injuries[134]
- with a recent change in coach (and therefore changed training load)
- after increased use of hand paddles[133, 139]

- with the use of drag-increasing training devices (bags, elastic cords, drag suits, propellers, power racks, etc.).

The term "swimmer's shoulder" is no longer appropriate (see Box 13.3). Rotator cuff tendinopathy is the most common shoulder pathology seen in swimmers.[140] Tendinopathy of the long head of the biceps and impingement against the anterior third of the coracoacromial arch are also frequent diagnoses. However, a clear pathoanatomical diagnosis is often difficult to achieve; it is more important to diagnose and understand the underlying functional or pathomechanical reasons for the "structural failure" and address these in the management plan.

> **BOX 13.3** Shoulder pain in swimmers: diagnostic terminology
>
> The term "swimmer's shoulder" was introduced by Kennedy and Hawkins 50 years ago.[140] It is a nondescript catch-all term that doesn't really advance our understanding. We believe this term should be replaced by an individualised and more specific diagnosis that accounts for the individual contributing factors (extrinsic and intrinsic) and suspected pathology of each injured swimmer. For example, supraspinatus tendinopathy with:
>
> - hypomobility of the cervicothoracic junction
> - insufficient scapular upward rotation, loss of internal rotation of the glenohumeral joint
> - greater internal rotation strength, due to sudden increase of intensity of training and possible overload in the use of hand paddles and drag suits.
>
> Note that this more precise diagnosis relies on skilled assessment but it allows for a clearer approach and tailored treatment.

### Assessing the swimmer with shoulder pain

You should aim to assess the entire kinetic chain thoroughly looking for those intrinsic factors that predispose to injury and persistent pain. Swimmers must be capable of extreme ranges of motion, especially in the shoulder girdle,[137] and they must be able to reach these positions easily. Swimmers who do not have such range of motion have a mechanical cost of:

- unnecessary extra movements and drag
- suboptimal use and possible overload of musculoskeletal structures.

Modelling studies suggest that, on average, the supraspinatus tendon is already in a position of potential mechanical impingement for nearly 25% of the freestyle arm stroke cycle.[137]

If swimmers are not flexible enough in the glenohumeral joint, they tend to pass this motion requirement to the scapulothoracic joint or the spine. On the other hand, hypermobility can also increase the potential for injury due to excessive translation of the humeral head. There might be a range of "optimal motion" in swimmers.

One study found that those with more than 100° or less than 93° of external rotation had a greater risk of shoulder impingement symptoms.[134] Internal rotation is the most important, as it allows the swimmer to have an early catch and high elbow. A measure between 40° and 50° seems to be necessary for freestyle, backstroke and butterfly. Breaststroke swimmers can have a little less.

Testing abduction with internal rotation gives important information about the swimmer's ability to achieve and maintain a high elbow. For this the swimmer sits on a bench, while you abduct both arms passively, with the elbows maintained in 90° flexion (Fig. 13.25). Their forearm must be perpendicular to the plane of abduction (causing internal rotation). The angle measured is the line of the humerus to the straight spine: an appropriate range is between 150° and 170°.[141]

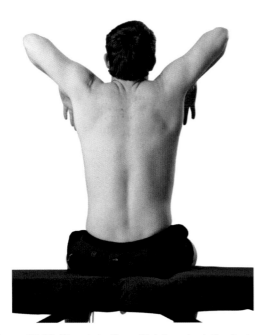

**Figure 13.25** The abduction with internal rotation test. The tester abducts both arms at the same time, while the swimmer sits on a bench, keeping the elbows in 90° flexion and the forearms perpendicular to the plane of abduction. Do not allow the arms to move forward of the plane of the body, or to be in less internal rotation than perpendicular. The tester then measures the angle of the line of the humerus to the straight spine.

The combined elevation test can give more information about the swimmer's ability to achieve a high elbow position at the start of the stroke, recovery and streamline. The swimmer lies in a prone position with both arms elevated above the head (with locked thumbs together and extended elbows). They then elevate their arms as high as they can while keeping their head, chest and legs in contact with the bench (Fig. 13.26). An angle between the line of the humerus and the horizontal axis of 5° to 15° is appropriate.[141]

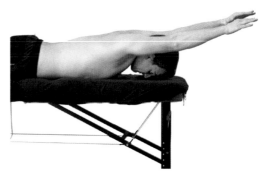

**Figure 13.26** The combined elevation test. The swimmer lies in a prone position and is asked to lock their thumbs together, extend their elbows and elevate the arms as high as they can while keeping their head, chest and legs in contact with the bench. The humerus angle is measured relative to horizontal.

To maintain a streamlined position, core stability is important and should be assessed. Swimmers need to transfer load efficiently between the arms and the legs under internally generated flexion torques.

### Managing shoulder pain in swimmers

Individualised rehabilitation programs emphasising range of motion, flexibility, muscle balance and motor control of the glenohumeral and scapulothoracic joints are the key features in the management of shoulder pain in swimmers.[142] Modification of training load is often necessary.

Most commonly, the entire kinetic chain is involved, with multiple intrinsic and extrinsic contributing factors such as:

- reduced rotation and/or extension of the thoracic spine—important in relation to body roll
- tightness or improper motor control around the scapula
- muscular imbalance around the shoulder; in particular, internal and external rotators
- incorrect swimming technique (Table 13.9)
- too much training with hand paddles or drag-increasing devices
- improper land training, weight training or stretching (individual training plans for dry land and weight

**TABLE 13.9** Technique factors related to shoulder pain in freestyle swimming

| Presentation | Possible cause | Solution |
|---|---|---|
| Shoulder pain at hand entry | • Thumb-first hand entry—excessive internal rotation in full elevation<br>• Crossing the midline with the hand at hand entry<br>• Lateral deviation of the trunk | • Palm-down hand entry<br>• Ensure adequate abduction/internal rotation range of motion<br>• Avoid crossing the midline<br>• Improve mobility in the kinetic chain, improve core stability |
| | • Insufficient upward rotation of the scapula | • Address scapulohumeral muscle flexibility<br>• Train scapular upward rotation in overhead exercises |
| Shoulder pain during pull-through | • Dropped elbow—elbow-first water entry or elbow below the level of the shoulder and wrist during early pull-through | • Improve internal rotation ROM—sleepers stretch and cross-body stretch—check kinetic chain |
| | • Crossing the midline with the hand during pull-through | • Avoid crossing the midline |
| | • Insufficient or excessive body roll | • Body roll should be approximately 45°; this can be limited by thoracic rotation and core stability |
| Shoulder pain during recovery | • Excessive horizontal abduction due to insufficient body roll—posterior cuff impingement | • Increase body roll<br>• Optimise mobility of cervicothoracic spine |
| | • Unilateral breathing pattern (pain on same side) | • Strive for a bilateral breathing pattern |

training are important to optimise the "weakest links" in the kinetic chain)

• sub-optimal core strength and/or control.

Take a team approach: look at technical stroke analysis and adjustment with the coach and physiotherapist, keeping the findings during the consultation in mind.

Swimmers with shoulder complaints should avoid the following drills:

• long leg drills with a kick board, as arms are maintained in maximum shoulder flexion—this can aggravate impingement symptoms
• hand paddles, as these increase the load on the shoulder during the pull-through
• pull buoy—the legs are held together without kicking, so 100% of the propulsion is generated by the arms.

## Low back pain

Low back pain is common in swimmers. Back muscle strains are the most common diagnosis. Because of development in the sport with start devices and limited underwater phase, coaches and swimmers are keen to generate lower extremity power. Whereas strength training was once mainly focused on core and upper extremity, nowadays gym sessions focus on jump strength and powerful kicking. Where swimmers need to have extreme range of motion to generate propulsion in the water, on dry land with closed chain and jumps, they need to develop "functional" stiffness. When

swimmers perform weight training, lifting technique and appropriate periodisation are very important. Butterfly and breaststroke swimmers are especially at risk of developing a low back injury, due to the repetitive flexion and extension of the back.

Low back pain usually doesn't start during swimming sessions, but during dry-land training, weight training or recreational activities.[143, 144] Although swimming is not usually the primary mechanism of developing lower back complaints, swimmers often describe lower back pain being aggravated while swimming. In particular, rotation in freestyle, turns, diving and underwater phases can create pain and/or motion restriction if the lower back is injured.

Don't only ask questions about low back pain for your diagnosis but also ask about swimming-specific factors (intrinsic and extrinsic). Assess the use of drag-increasing training devices and training devices such as kick boards, fins or zoomers, pull-buoys and hand paddles as these may contribute to excessive hyperextension of the lower back. For example, the pull-buoy, which is placed between the legs to swim with the arms only, places the legs in a higher position in relation to the surface of the water, resulting in an increase in forced hyperextension of the lower back.

Focus on the whole kinetic chain, not just the back. Look for a rounded shoulder posture, standing with a hyperlordosis or hyperkyphosis (swayback posture). Assess for lumbar spine hypermobility, and cervical spine and thoracic spine mobility. Core stability is highly important, so assess whether the swimmer is able to actively stabilise the core and how is the muscular control around the core. Forces for strong kicks are anchored by the core muscles.

Chronic degenerative disc lesions, especially in the L5–S1 discs, as well as spondylolysis/listhesis, are seen in swimmers (perhaps due to repetitive extension loading of the spine). The repetitive extension with rotation movements can result in pars stress fractures. Don't forget to rule out Scheuermann's kyphosis, intra-articular hip pathology and nerve root compression as causes of back pain.

Principles of management of acute lumbar spine strains are detailed in Chapter 15 in *Managing Injuries*. Education is an important part of treatment. Emphasise muscle strengthening, and core- and pelvic-stability exercises. Consider advising the swimmer to modify the use of training devices and advise about body position when using these devices. Modify butterfly and/or breaststroke training, underwater kicking, weight and dry-land training. Also have the swimmer work kinetic chain function (especially thoracic extension), shoulder flexion and hip extension.

## Medial knee pain

Medial knee pain is common in breaststroke swimmers.[145] Although the term "breaststroker's knee" is non-specific, it usually refers to overuse injury of the medial collateral ligament. However, the medial patellofemoral joint, pes anserine tendon or bursa and adductor muscles may also be involved.

The medial knee is highly loaded at the beginning of the breaststroke thrust phase, where the knee is flexed and externally rotated and the hips are flexed and internally rotated. The knee undergoes valgus loading throughout the leg thrust. A number of intrinsic factors and technique flaws can increase the valgus load and contribute to medial knee pain, including:

* valgus alignment of the lower limb
* inadequate or asymmetrical hip internal rotation or tibial external rotation
* large abduction angle of the hips during the kick (>30°)
* ineffective arm–leg coordination, which may increase loads on the lower limbs
* sudden increase in the amount or intensity of training
* hip extension and ability to achieve core and pelvic stability.

Clinical assessment of the lower back, hips, knees and ankles is important, particularly the range of hip internal rotation and tibial external rotation. These two measures should add up to approximately 90°, so that at the beginning of the thrust phase the feet are square to the line of progression.

This results in the biggest area to use to propel in the kick with the knees closer together, thus reducing form drag.[141]

As in shoulder injuries, you should focus on both intrinsic and extrinsic factors during the rehabilitation process. Breaststroke training should be reduced, and exercises that place a valgus load on the knee should be avoided during dry-land and weight training. Hip rotation range of motion should be optimised and the load capacity of the knee should be increased through progressive lower limb strengthening.

## TENNIS

### with BABETTE PLUIM

In a typical tennis match, players hit the ball 300–500 times and run 2.5–3.5 km in high-intensity 3-m bursts. Due to the game's explosive, intermittent and repetitive nature, both acute and overuse injuries are common. Groups particularly at risk include elite players, who often train up to 5–6 hours per day, deconditioned players who suddenly increase their training load, and young players who play more than 4 matches per week.[146]

The main biomechanics-related tennis injuries are those of the lateral elbow, shoulder and back: these represent approximately 30–40% of all tennis injuries[147]

### Lateral elbow pain

Lateral epicondylalgia is colloquially referred to as "tennis elbow" and has been estimated to affect up to 50% of active tennis players at some point in their career.[148, 149] Its prevalence among tennis players seems to be declining, and this may be related to increasing use of the two-handed backhand.

The condition is caused by a tendinopathy of the common extensor tendon, in particular the extensor carpi radialis brevis, at the insertion on the lateral humeral epicondyle. Here, forces are greatest during one-handed backhand shots, as the wrist extensors contract eccentrically at impact with the ball.

Lateral elbow pain is much more common in beginners and players over 40 years of age;[150] it is usually attributed to a combination of overuse and poor stroke biomechanics. Skilled players hit the ball with an extended wrist and extend the hand through impact (Fig. 13.27a), whereas novice players often hit the backhand with a flexed wrist, resulting in an eccentric contraction and less strength at impact (Fig. 13.27b).[151, 152]

However, the relationship between this technique flaw and elbow injury remains unclear,[153] and other potential factors include hitting the ball off-centre and squeezing the grip too tightly during follow-through.[154] The topspin

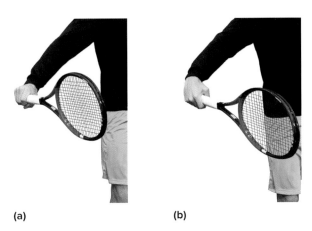

**(a)**                 **(b)**

**Figure 13.27** One-handed backhand technique. (a) An extended wrist at impact reduces stress at the lateral epicondyle. (b) A flexed wrist at impact increases stress at the lateral epicondyle.

backhand usually provokes more complaints than the slice backhand.[155] Tennis elbow is very rare in players with a two-handed backhand.

Tennis racquet grip size is traditionally considered to be a risk factor for lateral elbow pain, as grip sizes that are too small or too large may lead to extra strain on the forearm muscles. It is therefore important to optimise the racquet grip size to the player.[156] Other common recommendations to reduce load on the forearm muscles include using a larger racquet head, a flexible racquet, lower string tension (with high-quality strings) and pressurised tennis balls. Playing with heavy, wet tennis balls, long hours of play or a sudden increase in volume or intensity of play may lead to sudden overuse and the development of lateral elbow problems.

The general management principles for lateral epicondylalgia are covered in detail in Chapter 10 in *Managing Injuries*. However, tennis-specific management should include developing muscular strength to better cope with the racquet–ball impact and an analysis of backhand technique, with effort focused on using the correct grip and achieving concentric wrist extension at the point of impact.

Video analysis may be a useful biofeedback tool to help players change technique. This can be done with various apps that help analyse the stroke during slow-motion video (e.g. Swing Vision, Dartfish, Kinovea, SevenSix Tennis, Tennis Commander). Low-compression balls should also be considered during the early phase of treatment.

## Shoulder injuries

The shoulder is subjected to high loads in tennis, particularly during the serve where the shoulder is abducted to 140°–160° and rotates 160°–180° at a rate of up to 2400° per second.[157] As a player serves approximately 100-120 times in an average match,[158] it is not surprising that overuse shoulder injuries are common. The causes and pathology of shoulder injuries in tennis players are similar to those in other overhead and throwing sports; common diagnoses include internal impingement, rotator cuff and biceps tendinopathy, and glenoid labrum injuries.[159, 160]

During the cocking phase of the serve, the supraspinatus, infraspinatus and serratus anterior all contract concentrically to stabilise the scapula and glenohumeral joint. This is followed by a rapid eccentric contraction of the rotator cuff and serratus anterior to decelerate the arm during the follow-through. These repetitive concentric and eccentric demands, which occur during both serving and groundstrokes, may lead to muscular fatigue and so-called eccentric failure of the tendons.

Adding further stress, the supraspinatus and infraspinatus tendons can become compressed between the humeral head and the posterosuperior rim of the glenoid during the cocking phase of the serve, when the glenohumeral joint is in maximal external rotation and horizontal abduction. This is often referred to as internal impingement.

Local factors that contribute to internal impingement include muscular imbalances (external rotator weakness or dysfunction compared with the internal rotators), weakness or dysfunction of the scapular stabilisers (scapular dyskinesis) and tightness of the posterior capsule, resulting in reduced internal rotation range of motion (glenohumeral internal rotation deficit). These factors should all be considered when treating shoulder injuries in tennis players.

Remote factors also play an important role in the development of shoulder injuries in tennis players. In order to create optimal power during the serve, there should be coordinated activation of a number of body segments (legs, hips, trunk, shoulder, arm and hand—the kinetic chain) in order to achieve a high racket speed at impact.[161] Suboptimal kinetic chain mechanics may lead to overload of the upper limb as it tries to make up for lost energy production.[162] This is referred to as the catch-up phenomenon.[160]

Common clues that a player has suboptimal use of the kinetic chain during serving include:[163]

- insufficient knee bend: the front knee should flex >15° during the loading phase
- inadequate rotation: the player should be coiled enough such that they show their back to their opponent (Fig. 13.28)
- inadequate shoulder and pelvis tilt during the loading phase.

B

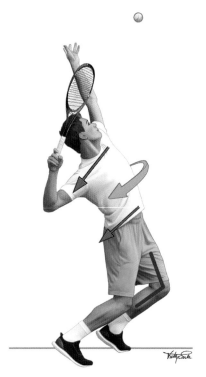

**Figure 13.28** Optimal tennis serve technique, loading phase; note the deep knee bend, rotated trunk and tilted shoulders and pelvis

## Back injuries

### with BEHNAM LIAGAT

Back injuries such as spondylolysis, lumbar strains and disc degenerative pathologies are common in tennis—a sport that demands repetitive flexion, extension, rotation and lateral flexion.[164] Serving imposes lateral flexion loads on the spine that are eight times greater than those experienced while running.[165, 166] The topspin "kick" serve transmits the highest forces to the lumbar spine.[167] Groundstrokes impose a relatively lower load on the spine, but their repetitive nature affects total load.[168]

A 5-year summary of injuries among male professional tennis players, based on data from the Association of Tennis Professionals, confirms that the spine is the most frequently injured area. Furthermore, back injuries are reported as the primary reason for match departures (i.e. retirement, withdrawals and "lucky losers") due to injuries, accounting for 18.6% of all injuries among professional male players.[169]

Interestingly, back injuries occur more often on grass courts like Wimbledon than on clay and hard courts. This is potentially due to the shorter rallies and higher frequency of serves and successful serve aces, resulting in short and intensive loads.[170, 171]

The presence of underlying spinal pathology is observed in tennis players, even without clinical symptoms, which is similar to the general population.[172] Structural changes in the spine of non-symptomatic young tennis players are quite common and include facet joint arthropathy and disc degeneration, with a much higher prevalence (62.2%) compared with similar non-elite athlete groups (37%). Disc herniation occurs more frequently (6.1%) in young tennis players due to repetitive axial loading and rotation during serves and groundstrokes. Abnormalities in the pars interarticularis are also prevalent, with a higher prevalence (29.6%) than in elite athletes of similar ages (20.3%).

Possible contributing factors include sudden spine hyperextension during serving and groundstroke motions, increased repetitive motion associated with double-handed ground strokes, and greater use of topspin on hard courts. Female players exhibit a lower prevalence of these structural changes than males, possibly owing to the slower pace of the female game resulting in less stress on the spine. Additionally, younger players under the age of 16 demonstrate a lower prevalence of these issues than those over 20 years, suggesting a gradual progression of spondylotic changes with age.

While these issues may not directly affect daily player activities, they underscore the significant musculoskeletal impact of tennis training on young players. Detecting these structural changes is crucial for appropriate prehabilitation to prevent potential career-ending injuries and loss of playing time.

To assess back injuries in tennis players, the focus should be on evaluating trunk endurance, spinal mobility, motor control, and muscle activation patterns.[173] For example, adolescents who are more susceptible to back injuries could undergo tests such as the prone plank and side plank; they should be able to maintain these positions for at least 30 seconds.[174]

Players with a history of recurrent back injuries or pain often move beyond their lower lumbar range during groundstroke execution. Symptomatic players experiencing back pain tend to display lower activation of the extensor muscles, reduced co-contraction patterns and decreased abdominal endurance.[173]

Key components in the treatment of back injuries include structuring the training schedule to prevent rapid increases in weekly training load, as well as implementing coaching and rehabilitation strategies aimed at maximising spine mobility and optimising load and movement distribution throughout the entire kinetic chain, including the hips, thorax and shoulder girdle.[168, 175] Additionally, you should prioritise enhancing abdominal endurance and ensuring proper muscle activation during lumbar stability exercises.

The goal is to minimise end-range strain on the lumbar spine, particularly during complex movements such as the serve.

Spondylolysis can be treated using different types of braces.[176] These braces may be rigid or elastic and can provide support or limit lumbar extension. Activities that exacerbate lumbar pain should be avoided, and lumbar rehabilitation exercises should be incorporated into the treatment plan to facilitate recovery. Surgical intervention may become necessary when conservative treatments fail, especially in cases of progressive slippage, untreatable pain and back pain associated with neurological deficits or vertebral instability. The choice of treatment depends on the nature and severity of the injury, with the ultimate goal of relieving pain and enabling the player to continue their sport successfully.

## VOLLEYBALL

### with CHRISTOPHER SKAZALSKI and KERRY MACDONALD

The repetitive nature of volleyball requires players to perform a large number of jumps and overhead attacks. Professional men's players may perform 100 jumps per training session or match, and accumulate well over 10,000 jumps per year.[177] The knee (20–33%), shoulder (20–32%) and low back (18–32%)[178, 179] are the primary locations for overuse injuries.[180, 181]

While not all physical complaints result in time lost from sport, the majority of elite men's university and professional players report some level of knee (79%), shoulder (67%) or low back (71%) pain during the season, with an average weekly prevalence of knee complaints of 31%, shoulder complaints of 19% and low back complaints of 21%.[182]

The emphasis on jumping to hit in volleyball leads to biomechanical adaptations within the body's lower and upper halves to provide enough explosiveness to jump high and contact the ball with force. The lumbar spine links the two halves; it must be flexible enough to allow the player to react to the ball's location while allowing forces to transfer from the lower half to the upper half.

### Knee injuries

Patellar tendinopathy, or jumper's knee, is the most common knee injury in volleyball (prevalence: 45–51%); it is more commonly observed in volleyball than in basketball and athletics.[183, 184] It is characterised by activity-related pain from the patellar or quadriceps tendon, usually accompanied by localised tenderness and structural changes in the tendon on ultrasound or MRI.[185]

This injury is related to jumping load.[186, 187] One study of patellar tendinopathy reported a dose–response relationship in which the more days of training and matches per week, the greater the prevalence of patellar tendinopathy complaints

(2×/week: 3%; 3×/week: 15%; 4×/week: 29%; >4×/week: 42%).[188] There is also a relationship between patellar tendinopathy and training load at the elite junior level: match exposure increases injury odds ratio 4 times for every extra set per week and training exposure increases injury odds 1.7 times for every extra hour of training per week.[189]

If you are working with junior level players you have an important role—this is the level at which patellar tendinopathy symptoms often begin. Note the patellar tendinopathy paradox in which the best and most-talented jumpers are at the greatest risk—jumping ability is a risk factor for tendinopathy.[190]

The jumping load in volleyball comprises several jump types with distinct biomechanical elements and is dependent on the game context and skill being performed. The spike approach (Fig. 13.29) is the jump type with the greatest jump height, whereas jump sets frequently exhibit the lowest. While substantial loads are placed on the knee extensors during the propulsion phase of jumping, the clinical focus should be on the landing phase, as this is when the tendon is exposed to forces that are often several magnitudes greater.[191] Little is known regarding the prospective relationship between landing technique and complaints.

One study examining landing strategy during drop jumps found players with current patellar tendon symptoms used an altered landing technique that avoided tendon loading, while players with a history of previous patellar tendinopathy complaints, but no recent symptoms, used a stiffer strategy.[192] Although it is unclear what effect traditional approaches emphasising good landing biomechanics may have in preventing symptoms, you should examine landing strategy in players with a history of complaints.

A biomechanical consideration specific to volleyball is that spike jumps that occur close to the net tend to have less forward displacement but greater vertical heights; jumps further from the net (i.e. back-row attacks and spike serving) have greater forward displacement and lower vertical heights. Blocking and setting jumps rarely exhibit large forward displacement but they may exhibit other rotational forces while jumping. Spike jumps with forward displacement subject the patellar tendon to greater forces during the landing phase compared with vertical spike jumps of similar height that lack forward displacement.[193]

While patellar tendinopathy has often been thought of as a jump landing problem, it is still important to consider the take-off, specifically during the spike approach. During a traditional 2- to 3-step approach, the player's last step will include planting both feet on the ground and a lowering of their centre of mass. This results in the front foot being partially internally rotated, as the player applies a partial

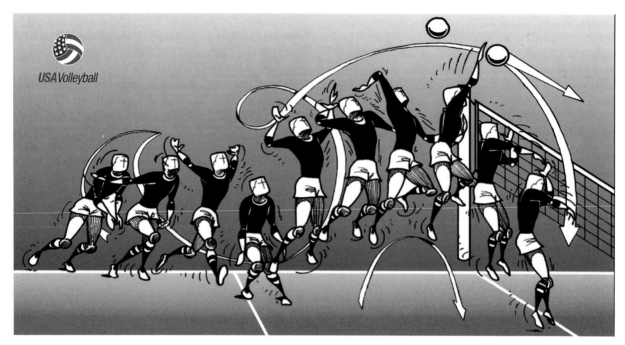

**Figure 13.29** Biomechanical considerations for players with knee or shoulder complaints during a typical 2- to 3-step spike approach. Players with knee complaints may want to consider the positioning of their front foot and leg during the last step of the approach in addition to evaluating their most commonly used landing techniques. Those with shoulder complaints might assess the position and amount of elbow elevation during arm cocking to avoid problematic shoulder positions.
COURTESY OF USA VOLLEYBALL

breaking force to absorb their forward momentum in transition for maximum vertical displacement.

You should carefully examine a player's biomechanics when they present with early tendinopathy. Small biomechanical adjustments, combined with the monitoring of jump load and the response to loading, may improve performance and/or decrease knee complaints. When you assess or prescribe jump loads for players with and without knee complaints, take into account both the size of jumps and the specific types of jumps.

During the landing phase of a jump, the ankle dorsiflexes and absorbs impact force[192] so hypomobility may limit the ability of the ankle joint to absorb force.[194] Limited ankle dorsiflexion has been associated with overuse knee injuries in volleyball players[194–196] and it likely increases force on the knee joint.[197]

## Shoulder injuries

An efficient volleyball attack is a key component to a team's success.[198] Two important elements are a high jump and high arm velocities as these allow the player to contact the ball at a height that provides the greatest strategic

advantage with a powerful hit over the net and past the opposing blockers.[199]

The volleyball attack can be divided into four phases: (1) the approach, (2) arm cocking, (3) arm acceleration and (4) ball contact and follow-through.[200] While the general movement pattern is similar between a volleyball spike and serve compared with other overhead actions such as a baseball fastball pitch or a first serve in tennis, the volleyball spike and serve are performed with greater shoulder abduction (~130°) and horizontal adduction (~30°) at the moment of ball contact.[201]

This is important to keep in mind during the rehabilitation and return to sport of volleyball players, as players require this additional overhead range of motion and need to be able to generate and withstand substantial overhead forces within this available range. It has been speculated that this may be related to the higher prevalence of infraspinatus muscle atrophy observed within the sport.[201]

Volleyball players use different types of arm swings, specifically during the cocking phase, to get their arms into an overhead position in preparation for ball contact. Historically, young players were instructed in the use of a traditional arm swing that elevates the elbow above shoulder level through use of a straight or bow-and-arrow technique.[202,203] The elbow is brought back, and a brief pause occurs before the hand is brought overhead and accelerated into ball contact.

However, a large proportion (65%) of elite indoor players now use an alternative technique (snap or circular), which does not elevate the elbow as high; this may be more forgiving for the shoulder. The circular technique allows for continuous arm movement during the entire attack.[202]

You can learn more about swing techniques from this excellent YouTube video:

Volleyball swing techniques

There is no known relationship between arm swing technique and injury, but training players in a range of swing techniques may help those with a history of shoulder complaints to avoid glenohumeral end-ranges and generate greater ball speed.[203]

Similar to other overhead athletes, volleyball players often present with more shoulder external rotation and less internal rotation range of motion in the dominant arm compared with the non-dominant arm.[204] This appears to be a natural adaptation of increased humeral torsion in the dominant arm.[205]

Of interest to clinicians, players with current or previous shoulder complaints often have ongoing strength imbalances—particularly decreased external rotation strength relative to internal rotation strength.[205–208] There is, however, no clear relation between shoulder strength and injury. A one-time strength or screening assessment is probably not sensitive enough to detect problems that may develop in weeks and months. Therefore, you may prefer to monitor physiological changes in response to sports participation (e.g. strength, range of motion) on a daily or weekly basis.

It is normal for asymptomatic elite-level players to have shoulder joint "pathology" when their dominant arm is imaged for another reason or in a research study. Morphological changes in the rotator cuff and labrum are prevalent; this does not limit these players in any way and is not a risk factor for imminent injury.[209]

## Indoor vs beach volleyball

Indoor and beach volleyball share similar techniques and gameplay but players have made biomechanical adaptations in the sports. Beach volleyball (teams of 2 people on the court compared with 6 in indoor volleyball) requires a much larger number of ball contacts per player. As a result, beach players tend to lower their centre of mass and slow their movements compared with indoor players.[210] This allows for maximum jump height while minimising their sinking into the sand.

Another difference is in the arm swing. Most beach volleyball players (73%) use a traditional technique (i.e. bow-and-arrow or straight) rather than an alternative technique.[211] Of those players who choose an alternative technique, men most commonly use a circular technique (24%) whereas women use a snap technique (30%).[212]

The use of more traditional, bow-and-arrow techniques is not surprising as beach volleyball players tend to use more soft roll- or cut-shots (men: 41%, women: 50%).[212] As indoor players have more defenders on the court to contend with, and as sets are more predictable, the players adopt alternative swing techniques to generate high-velocity attacks.

## RUNNING SHOES

Running shoes with carbon-fibre plates first appeared at events such as world marathons and the Olympics in 2016. Since their introduction, the shoes have created much controversy, particularly from 2016 to 2020 when World Athletics had not yet regulated elements of the shoes such as stack height and number of carbon plates in a single shoe (one). Box 13.4 looks at whether carbon-plated "supershoes" increase the risk of injury in athletes.

## BOX 13.4 Supershoes: how they work and what to advise runners
### with PAUL BLAZEY

Recent advances in shoe technology enable distance runners to run faster. The use of new resilient foams (e.g. polyether block amide) combined with different varieties of carbon fibre plate encased in the shoe sole have earned many shoes the nickname "supershoes". This name was coined after multiple new world records were set by athletes using the new shoe technology.[213,214] That athletes run faster is not in question—but should supershoes come with an injury warning?

Figure 13.30 depicts the structure of these new shoes.[215] To encase the curved carbon plates and as much "bouncy" energy-returning foam as possible, the shoes have greater stack heights (the amount of shoe material between your foot and the ground) than previous generations of running shoes, which were generally known as "racing flats". Stack heights on the new shoes are up to 40 mm (or 30 mm for track spikes).[216]

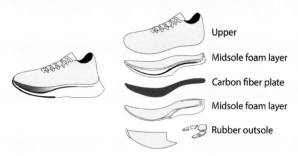

Upper

Midsole foam layer

Carbon fiber plate

Midsole foam layer

Rubber outsole

**Figure 13.30** How supershoes are constructed. Image also demonstrates a 31 mm stack height.
Source: Burns GT, Tam N. Is it the shoes? A simple proposal for regulating footwear in road running. *Br J Sports Med* 2020;54(8):439—40.

This has affected runners' biomechanics.[217] The increased stack height artificially elongates the athlete's lower limbs. This, coupled with the plate and bouncy (more resilient) foam, has resulted in increased stride length, reduced cadence, longer flight times, higher peak vertical ground reaction forces, and other kinetic and kinematic changes.[218,219]

### Potential benefits
The new foam has left many runners from elite to novice reporting a reduction in muscle soreness from efforts that previously resulted in delayed-onset muscle soreness. Runners can also spend greater time at higher speeds due to the reduced energy costs associated with running

at the same speeds, and there is anecdotal evidence of improved recovery between running sessions.

The stiff carbon-fibre plate shifts forces away from the 1st metatarsophalangeal joint. This has potential advantages for those suffering from conditions such as hallux rigidus or limitus and flexor hallucis longus tendinopathy, as the joint and muscle acting around the 1st ray is relatively protected by the new shoe design.

### Potential drawbacks
To best take advantage of the curved plate, biomechanists suggest that runners land with a rear- or mid-foot strike to roll through the gait cycle (coined the "teeter-totter effect").[220] The shift in internal joint forces to more proximal areas such as the ankle—knee and hip (and potentially lumbar spine when running downhill), combined with the increased time at faster speeds, may make runners more susceptible to aggravating existing conditions (e.g. low back pain or labral tears of the hip) or developing new concerns such Achilles or patellar tendinopathy.

Increased speed (or time spent at the higher end of an athlete's maximum speed) can also increase bone-related loads. Coupled with the altered running mechanics caused by the carbon-fibre plate, there are concerns for athletes recovering from, or who have a history of, lower limb stress fractures. Navicular stress fractures have been reported in elite runners using the new shoes due to the changes in foot mechanics.[221]

The increased stack height has also anecdotally resulted in an increase in runners sustaining ankle sprain injuries due to a decrease in shoe stability, especially when runners are performing on uneven terrain (e.g. running over cobblestones or trail running). The reduced stability may be a consideration for athletes recovering from conditions impacted by ankle instability such as peroneal or tibialis posterior tendinopathy.

### Clinical tips
New shoe technologies are here to stay. Consider how you can support athletes to transition to these new technologies. Explain the need to manage load and suggest a gradual transition into the new shoes.[222] Runners may wish to avoid using shoes with high stack height on uneven courses.

There may be risks using supershoes during a runner's rehabilitation period if shoe-related mechanical changes increase stress on the healing area (e.g. peroneal tendons post ankle sprain or navicular following a bone stress injury).

## KEY POINTS

- Knowing the demands specific to a sport/position gives you much-needed context when assessing and planning treatment for an injured athlete.

- Common sport-related movements (e.g. overhead throwing, swimming strokes) can be broken down into stages or phases. This helps to identify specific points in a movement when the athlete may be most vulnerable to tissue stress or the possibility of injury.

- Older, non-clinical terms such as "tennis elbow" and "jumper's knee" lack specificity and may be confusing. We recommend contemporary consensus-based terminology to describe common sport-related injuries.

- Sports such as cycling and climbing are not a single activity. There are important differences in the biomechanics of mountain biking and road cycling; and in bouldering and speed climbing. Within team sports, there are important differences in the demands across positions. Knowing these differences is important for clinicians.

- Very few sport-related movements are isolated to a single joint or body region. When assessing the injured athlete, keep in mind the entire kinetic chain. Be sure to assess both proximal and distal structures.

- Structural anatomical changes can occur in the competitive athlete. For example, overhead throwing athletes often demonstrate an increase in external rotation range of motion at the shoulder (coupled with a decrease in strength) and a decrease in internal rotation.

- Atypical sport-related biomechanics do not necessarily directly provoke an injury. Players may demonstrate deviations from normal form and remain asymptomatic.

- Deviations from typical biomechanics may contribute to the development of overload injuries. In addition to correcting biomechanical issues, load management is an important part of injury prevention and treatment.

- When athletes develop an overuse injury without a clear inciting event, consider lifestyle and environmental factors that may need to be addressed. For example, the way a golfer carries their bag may influence the development of chronic back pain.

- Due to the many variables that contribute to developing on overload injury, a direct line between biomechanics and injury is difficult to draw. Consider a comprehensive list of intrinsic, extrinsic and environmental risk factors during your assessment.

- There are vulnerable periods during which an athlete is more susceptible to injury. Across sports, these often include times when load is significantly increased, after periods of detraining and after changes in technique.

- Age interacts with biomechanics in the development of sport-related injuries. In many cases, the adolescent athlete and the ageing athlete are at an increased risk.

- Biomechanical analysis can be aided by video capture and biofeedback technologies. Equipment specialists can also be helpful.

## REFERENCES

References for this chapter can be found at www.mhprofessional.com/CSM6e

## ADDITIONAL CONTENT

Scan here to access additional resources for this topic and more provided by the authors

**B**

## CHAPTER 14

# Training principles, programming and prescription

with DARREN BURGESS

*Success is no accident. It is hard work, perseverance, learning, studying, sacrifice, and most of all, love of what you are doing or learning to do.*

BRAZILIAN FOOTBALLER PELE (1940–2022)

## CHAPTER OUTLINE

Principles of training
Conditioning training
Endurance training
Speed training
Agility training
Resistance training
Flexibility training
Putting it all together: designing the training program

## LEARNING OBJECTIVES

By the end of this chapter you should be able to:

- explain ways in which the principles of training coincide with sports injury prevention and rehabilitation
- define basic concepts related to exercise training
- provide examples of various types of training, as well as how to safely employ them with athletes
- give examples of how our understanding of training in sport has evolved over time
- discuss the areas of sport-related training where there are scientific debates or controversy.

The sport and exercise clinician should understand the different elements of training and their possible relationship to injury. This facilitates you obtaining a full training history from an injured athlete and learning about training strategy from a coach or fitness practitioner and enhances your understanding of the phases of rehabilitation outlined in Chapter 27. This chapter reviews the principles of training and outlines some more common training programming and assessment practices. You are directed to other sources for more detailed outlines of the various types of training.

## PRINCIPLES OF TRAINING

Training is the pursuit of activity that will ultimately lead to improved performance in a given sport. A number of general principles of training apply to all sports:

- periodisation
- overload
- specificity
- individualisation.

### Periodisation

Periodisation is an important component of all training programs in both the long and short term. Training can be divided into three distinct phases (Table 14.1):

- During the conditioning (preparation) phase the emphasis is on the athlete developing the fundamental components of fitness relative to the sport they play. In field-based sports this is generally centred around development of aerobic and anaerobic fitness, strength and power. Often during this period, the athlete is training under fatigue and if required to compete would probably perform poorly. Careful monitoring of athlete response to training during this period is advised to prevent overtraining and/or injury.[1]
- During the pre-competition (transitional) phase, the emphasis switches from pure conditioning and prevention to more technical work.
- During the competition phase, the emphasis is on competitive performance while maintaining basic conditioning.

In many sports (e.g. football, basketball, hockey), a 4–6-month competition season is usual. Sometimes, an athlete may be required to undertake two periods of competition in the one year. A suggested program for athletes in these two situations is outlined in Figure 14.1. In other instances, the competition period may last as long as 8–10 months and conditioning work can extend into the competitive season. However, in all of these scenarios the same principles of training periodisation apply.

To ensure complete recovery from the physical and mental stress of competition, adequate time should be allowed between the end of one season or competition phase and the start of the next season or phase. This period may last 4–6 weeks but is dependent on when the next competition begins.

In the intermediate time frame, it is important to introduce easy weeks into the training program; these give the athlete time to recover, allow the body to absorb the training stimulus and diminish risk of injury. During these easy weeks, the volume of training is typically reduced; however, intensity should be maintained to prevent detraining.[2]

In the short term, the training program must allow for adequate recovery between training sessions. This ensures that the athlete is able to train at appropriate intensities throughout the week and reduces the risk of injury.[2]

### Overload

Overload is a variable that coaches manipulate to allow the athlete to perform work at a greater intensity or to perform a greater volume of work at a given intensity. Practically speaking, overloading an athlete involves applying stress to the body over and above that which is normally, or has been recently, encountered. If increased stress is not excessive and adequate adaptation time is allowed, the athlete's work capacity will be increased (supercompensation). Athletes should be carefully monitored during periods of overload to prevent injury, overtraining or even poor performance.

### Specificity

Specificity refers to the principle of directing training to performance in the athlete's given sport. It is important to identify the most important components of fitness for each

**TABLE 14.1** Different types of training performed during the three phases of the yearly cycle

| Training phase | Aerobic training | Anaerobic training | Plyometrics training | Weight training | Technique training |
|---|---|---|---|---|---|
| Conditioning | +++ | ++ | ++ | +++ | + |
| Pre-competition | ++ | +++ | ++ | ++ | +++ |
| Competition | + | + | − | + | ++ |

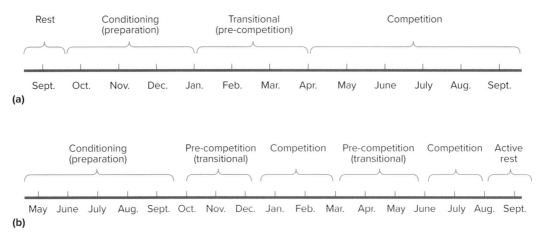

**Figure 14.1** Periodisation of training showing (a) a single cycle annual program and (b) a dual cycle annual program

particular sport and to tailor the athlete's training towards improving these particular components. For example, there is no advantage for a strictly power athlete in doing large amounts of endurance training.

Specificity can refer to both training the specific fitness demands of a sport and the athlete's role/position and training the direct movement patterns of the sport to improve the athlete's fitness. Those choosing the latter method argue that specific training in this way has the advantage of training skills and decision making while improving fitness.[3] Most field sports require a complex combination of strength and endurance training and therefore specificity should include a combination of fitness training and training for the particular movements of the sport.

### Individualisation

As individual differences between athletes are great, training must be tailored to the individual's needs. Individuals differ in their tolerance of particular training loads, response to specific training stimuli, speed of recovery, psychological make-up, nutritional intake and lifestyle habits. Individual responses to training are influenced by previous training history, age, current state of fitness, genetic make-up and so on. Even in a team setting, it is vital that players are treated as individuals and trained accordingly.

## CONDITIONING TRAINING

Maintenance of fitness is not only crucial to sporting success and injury prevention, it is also an essential component of the rehabilitation process. Regardless of the injury an athlete has sustained, exercises to maintain fitness should be incorporated as soon as possible. For example,

with injuries to a lower limb, cardiovascular fitness may be maintained by performing activities such as swimming with a pool buoy or arm "grinder" work. Depending on the athlete's particular sport, this may include a combination of endurance, interval, anaerobic and power work. It is important to maintain alternative training methods for cardiovascular fitness, to encourage motivation and compliance with general fitness goals.

We have divided conditioning into five separate types of training—endurance, speed, agility, resistance and flexibility. In practice these methods are often combined for a more global conditioning effect.

## ENDURANCE TRAINING

Technically, endurance training aims to increase oxygen delivery to the working muscles and thereby increase aerobic capacity. Adaptations to endurance training include an increase in maximal oxygen uptake ($VO_2max$) and an increased ability of skeletal muscle to generate energy via oxidative metabolism.[4,5]

The long-term consequences of prolonged endurance training have been debated, with proposed cardiovascular risks associated with cardiac fatigue.[6,7] However, a study of young Olympic athletes subjected to extreme uninterrupted endurance training over prolonged periods (up to 17 years) found that endurance training was not associated with significant changes in left ventricular morphology, deterioration in left ventricular function or occurrence of cardiovascular symptoms or events.[7] Endurance sports include long-distance running (greater than 5 km), cross-country skiing, cycling, rowing and triathlon.

It is important to be aware of the many benefits that increased aerobic capacity can have for a range of different sports. Enhanced aerobic capacity will improve not only the efficiency of oxygen delivery but also the regeneration of anaerobic energy pathways. This means that performance in intermittent sports such as ice hockey, soccer, American football and netball—all traditionally thought of as strictly anaerobic sports—will be improved with enhanced aerobic capacity. This is important to remember when prescribing or reviewing rehabilitation programs for athletes in these sports.

There are numerous methods to train endurance capacity. This section focuses on the more popular techniques.

## Interval training

Interval training involves numerous sessions of high-intensity effort for set times or distances. Both effort duration and recovery time in between sets dictate the intensity of each session. An endurance interval session might be 6 sets of 1-minute running. For a high-intensity session, 2 minutes recovery could be prescribed in between sets. To challenge the aerobic capacity to recover more quickly, 1-minute recovery between sets could be prescribed. These repeat-effort intervals have been shown to dramatically increase $VO_2max$.[8]

## Fartlek training

Fartlek, which means "speed play" in Swedish, is a popular form of endurance training that involves high-intensity effort interspersed between constant-paced exercise. A typical fartlek session on a bike might involve 30 seconds of high-intensity cycling every 2.5 minutes for 30 minutes. This would provide the cyclist with 10 high-intensity sets during the 30-minute ride. In some sports, athletes may be unaware of the duration and intensity of sets and have to respond to the coach's feedback during the session.

## Maximal aerobic speed training

Maximal aerobic speed training involves calculating an athlete's maximal aerobic speed and then prescribing a certain percentage of this within an interval training session.[9] Typically, the speed an athlete can complete a 2 km (or similar distance) time trial is used as that athlete's maximal aerobic speed. Precise distances and expected times can then be calculated for each athlete. The most common time periods for maximal aerobic speed are 15 seconds of work followed by 15 seconds of recovery (15:15).

## Cross-training

To prevent injury, it may be beneficial to reduce the amount of weight-bearing exercise. Cross-training, involving activities other than the athlete's usual sport, enables the athlete to maintain aerobic fitness while reducing stress on

weight-bearing joints, muscles and tendons. For athletes with a chronic condition such as articular cartilage damage to a weight-bearing joint, cross-training may be used to reduce the impact load while maintaining adequate training volume.

Similarly, for someone returning to sport from an overuse injury (such as a stress fracture), cross-training can reduce the risk of recurrence. Runners may wish to introduce one to two sessions per week of activities such as cycling, swimming or water running. These alternative workouts can mirror the athlete's usual training session (e.g. interval, fartlek).

## Skill training for endurance

It is important to realise that a skill drill or indeed an entire skill session can enhance endurance capacity. There are numerous ways to alter skill drills to emphasise endurance while maintaining the important aspects of the skill (e.g. decision making, team combinations, specific skill execution).[10] For example, a simple soccer game could be altered to increase the aerobic requirements of the exercise by:

- increasing the size of the field
- decreasing the number of players
- requiring that, for a goal to be scored, all players must be over the half-way line
- having the coach blow the whistle every 1 minute to signal that one player from each team must run to a specified marker outside of the field.

## SPEED TRAINING

Running speed, an important component of many sports, is influenced by genetic factors. However, athletes can improve their speed by enhancing their muscular power and strength, as well as by improving their technique, which increases the efficiency of ground coverage. Therefore, running speed can be increased by undertaking resistance and power training and by performing technical running drills.

There is debate regarding how much speed can be developed or improved in a mature athlete. Speed can arguably be enhanced, or at the very least maintained, with an appropriate strength and power program (see later in the chapter). However, debate remains about the extent to which speed can be improved through technical modification or repeated exposure to a speed stimulus.

## Technique training

Improving the technical aspect of speed requires spending significant time analysing athlete running mechanics and performing extensive corrective exercises as required. Within most sports, time dedicated specifically to work on technical speed is often at the expense of other conditioning, strength training or even skill training. As a result, most work on speed technique is confined to small amounts of time with large groups of players during warm-up activities or in the pre-season.

This requires a broad approach where emphasis is placed on high knee drive, exaggerated heel lift and horizontal foot position throughout the sprint motion. An ideal opportunity exists to improve speed technique during the rehabilitation process, where a more individualised approach can be taken.

Of course, in sports such as running and long jump, a large percentage of training time should be devoted to technical speed drills.

## Speed intervals

Appropriate exposure to speed not only will maintain speed qualities but also may prevent soft-tissue injury,[11] particularly in the hamstrings.[12] These "unpractised" movements that occur in games often cause muscle injury.

### PRACTICE PEARL

Regular speed interval work, particularly during weekly competition cycles, will ensure that the muscles and tendons are not "shocked" into unfamiliar explosive movements during competitions or games.

Remember, absolute speed intervals should be performed while the athlete is fresh; however, speed exposure in training should also occur under fatigue to prepare the body for what it may encounter during competition.

## Skill training at speed

In most sports, speed training can and should be integrated into skill training. This can easily be achieved by executing simple skills at the end of sprinting activities. Care should be taken in programming these drills, however, as they can be quite physically and structurally demanding.

## AGILITY TRAINING

Agility in sport can be defined as a player's ability to alter direction to achieve a specific goal (e.g. evade/react to an opponent, create space). Agility and rapid reflexes are often inherited characteristics. However, like speed they can be improved somewhat by training and thus are included in many training programs. Agility training has also been implemented for seniors to prevent falls.[13]

Agility training often involves stationary objects (e.g. cones, poles, ladders), which may allow the coach to teach the athlete correct foot placement or stride mechanics. However, more complete agility training requires a reaction and therefore a decision-making component.[14]

## Technique training

Training agility technique may be appropriate in the initial stages of rehabilitation or perhaps within adolescent programs. The coach can spend some time on effective techniques to approach a known object. However, this type of training should be limited as it often leads to inappropriate habits such as a player keeping their head down to review foot placement.

## Agility drills

A reaction component should always be included in agility drills, such as reacting to a particular movement, command, opponent or teammate. Advanced agility drills should also include a decision-making element.

## Skill training with agility

Most sports skill training could be counted as agility training, as most field sports training involves reacting to opponents, the ball or teammates. Any additional agility-specific training should be programmed carefully, as repeated changes of direction could cause overload issues to the pelvic region.

## RESISTANCE TRAINING

Resistance training can be used to enhance athletic performance, improve musculoskeletal health and correct muscle imbalances.[15, 16] Resistance training is often used in rehabilitation when weakness compromises function and sports performance. This is particularly true following periods of immobilisation, injury or pain.

The primary goal of resistance training is normally to increase muscle size (hypertrophy), strength or power. Increases in muscle hypertrophy and strength depend on five biochemical and physiological factors that are all stimulated and enhanced by appropriate resistance training:

- increased glycogen and protein storage in muscle
- increased vascularisation
- biochemical changes affecting the enzymes of energy metabolism
- increased number of myofibrils
- recruitment of neighbouring motor units.

It is important that athletes are provided with the correct resistance training environment (e.g. an appropriate progression of weights, benches that can be configured at various angles). To maximise gains from resistance training, the athlete should:

- warm-up adequately to increase body temperature and metabolic efficiency
- perform exercises with control and using correct form
- perform exercises without feeling pain
- use slow, controlled exercise initially, with little or no resistance, to develop a good base for neural patterning
- stretch purposefully to restore/maintain full range of motion
- pre-activate muscles that will be used for ballistic movements (part of the warm-up)
- strengthen muscles throughout the entire available range of motion
- place gym sessions appropriately in relation to running and skills training (e.g. if the main priority is strength in younger players, consider strength before running training).

Additionally, there is a training crossover effect—that is, when one limb is trained, strength gains will also be recorded in the contralateral limb.[15, 16] This is known as central adaptation and reflects the important role the central nervous system plays in motor unit firing, as well as the bracing role the contralateral limb plays in most single-limb exercises.

## Types of exercise used in resistance training

The three main types of exercise used in resistance training are isometric, isotonic and isokinetic.

### Isometric exercise

In an isometric exercise, a muscle contracts without associated movement of the joint on which the muscle acts. Isometric exercises are often the first form of strengthening exercise used after injury, especially if the region is excessively painful or immobilised. These exercises are commenced as soon as the athlete can perform them without pain.

Isometric exercises are used when a muscle is too weak to perform range of motion exercises, in conditions where other forms of exercise are not possible (such as patellar dislocation or shoulder dislocation) or when isometric contraction is required in activities (e.g. stabilising). Isometric exercises can minimise muscle atrophy associated with immobilisation and injury by maintaining or improving static strength, minimising swelling via the muscle pump action, and enhancing neural and proprioceptive inputs to the muscle.

Ideally, isometric exercises are held initially for 5–45 seconds, with contraction time increasing as the athlete becomes more tolerant. They can be performed frequently during the day as pain permits. The number of sets will vary at different stages of the rehabilitation program. If an athlete has difficulty, exercises may be performed against resistance or against an immovable object. It is important to remember that the quality of the exercise is more important than the quantity.

Isometric exercises should be carried out at multiple angles, if possible, as strength gain can be specific to the angle of exercise. The athlete should progress from submaximal to maximal isometric exercises slowly within the limitations of pain and function.

Isometric exercises have proven useful in the rehabilitation of tendon injuries (see Chapter 9) and should form a large component of any musculotendinous rehabilitation program.[17]

When significant isometric effort is tolerated at multiple joint angles, dynamic exercises may begin. An example of an isometric exercise for the lower limb is shown in Figure 14.2.

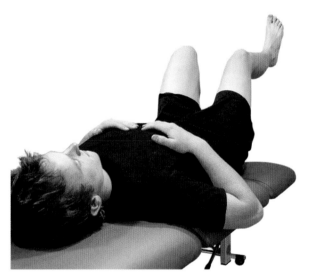

**Figure 14.2** Isometric co-contraction of the hamstrings, gluteal and quadriceps muscles with the patient pushing their foot into a wall

### Isotonic exercise

In isotonic exercises, the joint moves through a range of motion against a constant resistance or weight. Isotonic exercises may be performed with free weights such as dumbbells, pulleys or sandbags (Fig. 14.3). Free weights encourage natural movement patterns and require muscle coordination and joint stability in all planes of movement and therefore may transfer strength gains more readily to the playing field.[18]

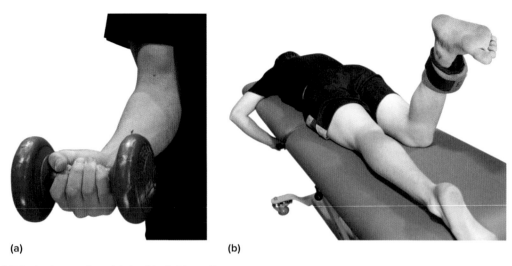

(a)                                   (b)

**Figure 14.3** Isotonic exercises: (a) dumbbell, (b) sandbag

With free weights it is possible to simulate athletic activities as the body position can be varied. Isotonic exercises may be:

- *concentric*—a shortening isotonic contraction in which the origin and insertion of the muscles approximate; the individual muscle fibres shorten during concentric contraction
- *eccentric*—a lengthening isotonic contraction where the origin and insertion of the muscles separate; the individual muscle fibres lengthen during eccentric contraction.

Concentric and eccentric exercises for the quadriceps are shown in Figure 14.4.

The intramuscular force produced per motor unit during an eccentric contraction is larger than that during a concentric contraction.[16] Eccentric contractions may generate high tension within the series elastic component, which consists of connective tissue and the actin–myosin cross-bridges in muscles. It has been observed that eccentric exercise results in higher rates of delayed-onset muscle soreness and even muscle damage if used inappropriately.[19, 20] Consequently, eccentric programs should commence at very low levels and progress gradually to higher intensity and volume.

The use of eccentric exercise programs may help prevent recurrence of musculotendinous injuries. Eccentric training has been advocated in the rehabilitation of tendon injuries, due to the proposed facilitation of tendon remodelling through promotion of collagen fibres within the injured tendon.[20-22] There is evidence that Achilles, patellar and lateral elbow tendinopathies respond well to an eccentric rehabilitation program.[22, 23]

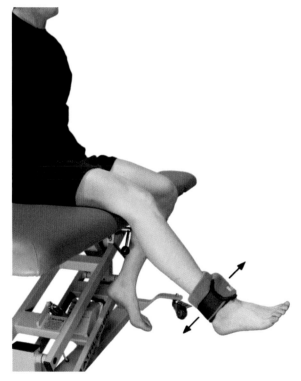

**Figure 14.4** Concentric (white arrow) and eccentric (black arrow) quadriceps exercises

However, not all tendon injuries benefit from eccentric exercises. Specifically, eccentric exercises have shown poor success rates for rotator cuff tendinopathy and for insertional Achilles tendinopathy, compared with mid-tendon Achilles lesions.[20, 24] Therefore, the site of tendon pathology should be considered when prescribing eccentric exercises.

Practically, there are some potential dangers with isotonic resistance training. Athletes require adequate supervision in the gym and should never attempt to lift a maximal weight without a spotter (an assistant who is able to help the athlete if problems arise). Isotonic machines such as Keiser® equipment may provide a safe alternative to free weights, but they limit range of motion and are generally unable to provide truly constant resistance through the lift.

Isotonic exercises in which the body weight of the individual is used as resistance are also safer than free weights and are often more convenient to perform. Exercises such as squats, lunges, push-ups and chin-ups can be done almost anywhere and require no supervision. However, it is difficult to increase the resistance of the exercise and the only way to increase effort is to increase the number of repetitions performed.

### Isokinetic exercises

Isokinetic exercises are performed on devices at a fixed speed with a variable resistance that is totally accommodative to the individual throughout the range of motion. The velocity is therefore constant at a preselected dynamic rate, while the resistance varies to match the force applied at every point in the range of motion. This enables the individual to perform more work than is possible with either constant or variable resistance isotonic exercise.

Isokinetic testing can highlight imbalances, such as scapular muscle imbalances in overhead athletes with chronic impingement signs.[25] A number of isokinetic devices are available and include the Ariel®, Biodex®, Cybex®, KinCom®, Lido and Merac® machines. However, these machines do come at a cost, which may explain why they are more commonplace in research than in clinical settings.

### Open and closed chain exercises

An open chain exercise often involves a single joint movement performed in a non-weight-bearing position where the distal extremity freely moves through space.[26] Closed chain exercises involve multiple joints and are performed in weight-bearing positions with a fixed distal extremity. Closed chain exercises are thought to be more functional, provide more proprioceptive feedback and cause less shear joint force than open chain exercises.[26]

Although some studies promote closed chain over open chain exercises,[26, 27] others advocate that both types of exercise play a beneficial role in rehabilitation, especially in regards to anterior cruciate rehabilitation and patellofemoral pain.[28-30] Proposed advantages and disadvantages of open and closed chain exercises are shown in Table 14.2.

Examples of these exercises are illustrated in Figure 14.5. Figure 14.5(c) shows an example of open (right arm) and closed (left arm) chain exercises for the shoulder girdle. Closed chain upper limb exercises are particularly useful during the early recovery period after shoulder surgery (Chapter 24). Excessive mobility and compromised static stability within the glenohumeral joint have been linked to capsular, labral and musculotendinous injuries in throwing athletes.[31] The positive benefits of closed chain exercises, performed under load-bearing positions, are thought to stimulate joint receptors and facilitate muscle co-contractions around the shoulder and therefore enhance joint stability.[25, 31]

## Types of resistance training

There are four main types of resistance training:

- strength
- power
- endurance
- hypertrophy.

### Strength training

Muscle strength is the muscle's ability to exert force. Strength gains can be seen quickly, even before physiological hypertrophy occurs. The initial strength gain in response to exercise is thought to be related to increased neuromuscular facilitation (i.e. the nervous system enhances the motor

**TABLE 14.2** Advantages and disadvantages of open and closed chain exercises

| | Advantages | Disadvantages |
|---|---|---|
| Open chain exercises | • Decreased joint compression<br>• Can exercise in non-weight-bearing positions<br>• Able to exercise through increased range of motion<br>• Able to isolate individual muscles | • Increased joint translation<br>• Decreased functionality |
| Closed chain exercises | • Decreased joint forces in secondary joints (e.g. less patellofemoral force with squat)<br>• Decreased joint translation<br>• Increased functionality | • Increased joint compression<br>• Not able to exercise through increased range of motion<br>• Not able to isolate individual muscles |

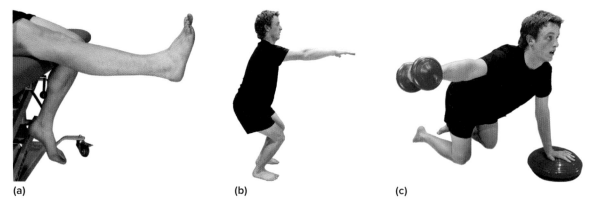

(a)                                    (b)                                    (c)

**Figure 14.5** Open and closed chain exercises. (a) Open chain knee extension with the foot moving freely. (b) Closed chain knee extension with the feet immobile. (c) Open chain (right arm) and closed chain (left arm) exercises on an unstable surface.

pathways so that the muscle group becomes more neurologically efficient).[15, 16, 32] Neural adaptations facilitate changes in coordination and learning that enhance the recruitment and activation of muscles during a strength task.[15]

Typical loading patterns for strength training can be seen in Table 14.3. Most importantly, the resistance needs to be at or near maximal levels with large rest periods in between sets. This enables the muscles to recuperate adequately in between sets.

Strength training is generally the base from which all other resistance training emanates so it generally occurs at the beginning of pre-season training.

### Power training

Muscle power is the muscle's rate of doing work. Similar to strength training, the initial power gains observed with power training result from improvements in neuromuscular efficiency.[33] Specifically, initial improvements in power can be attributed to improved muscle coordination between agonist and antagonist muscles. Power exercises may include:

- fast-speed isotonic or isokinetic exercises (concentric and/or eccentric)
- increased speed of functional exercises (e.g. faster reverse calf raise, drop squat)
- plyometric exercises (e.g. hopping, bounding).

Most sports involve a combination of strength and power, so profiling where athletes are on the strength–power continuum is important to designing a program.

Power exercises often involve functional and sport-specific exercises. Exercises should be appropriate to the athlete's sport to gain optimal benefits (e.g. bounding for a sprinter, jump and land for a basketballer).

Another technique for increasing power is plyometric training. Plyometric exercises (plyometrics) use the natural elastic recoil elements of human muscle and the neurological stretch reflex to produce a stronger, faster muscle response. Plyometrics combine a rapid eccentric muscle contraction with a rapid concentric contraction to produce a fast, forceful movement. Plyometric exercises must be performed in conjunction with a resistance training program, as athletes need to have minimum basic strength levels before commencing plyometrics.

### PRACTICE PEARL

Because of their explosive nature, plyometrics have a great potential for injury, so an athlete's plyometrics program should be carefully supervised.

**TABLE 14.3**   Resistance training loading patterns

|  | Sets | Reps | Rest (s) | % RM | Speed |
|---|---|---|---|---|---|
| Strength | 3–5 | 3–6 | 90–120 | 90–100 | Controlled |
| Power | 3–4 | 8–12 | 45–60 | 40–60 | Explosive |
| Endurance | 1–2 | 15–30 | 45–60 | 50–70 | Sport-specific |
| Hypertrophy | 2–3 | 8–12 | 60–75 | 70–90 | Slow on eccentric |

RM refers to the maximum amount of weight you can lift for one repetition of a given exercise.

Plyometric exercises include hopping and bounding drills, jumps over hurdles and depth jumps. These activities emphasise spending as little time as possible in contact with the ground. This form of exercise can cause delayed-onset muscle soreness (Chapter 8). Plyometric training should be performed only when the athlete is fresh and the volume of work should be built up gradually. The training surface must be firm but forgiving, such as a sprung basketball floor. When technique begins to deteriorate, the exercise should be stopped.

Olympic-type weightlifting is often used as part of a power training program. Olympic lifting involves explosively lifting a weight from the floor to a position above the ground using the entire body. Typical Olympic lifts include the power clean, snatch, and clean and jerk. These lifts exercise a greater number of muscle groups than conventional weightlifting, exercising them both concentrically and eccentrically. The potential for injury is high and athletes must learn correct lifting technique before attempting these lifts.

When injury has decreased muscle power or the athlete's sport includes periods of explosive power, the rehabilitation program should incorporate power exercises. Commonly, power-focused exercises are incorporated into the later stages of rehabilitation due to the potential for re-injury and the explosive nature of this training.

Typical loading patterns for a power program are shown in Table 14.3. The most important factor in a power development program is the speed of movement, which must be as explosive as possible.

Similar gains have been observed when comparing power exercises in the form of plyometrics with Olympic weight-lifting. This can be useful when equipment is limited.[34]

### Muscular endurance training

Muscle endurance is the muscle's ability to sustain contraction or perform repeated contractions. The aim of muscular endurance training is to increase the capacity to sustain repetitive, high-intensity, low-resistance exercise such as running, cycling and swimming.[4] Excessive bouts of muscular endurance training can result in fatigue and reduced sporting performance. Therefore, you should take care when incorporating this type of training into a resistance training program, especially during prolonged pre-season training.

Typical loading patterns for muscular endurance training are shown in Table 14.3. This type of training involves high repetitions with very little rest.

### Hypertrophy training

Hypertrophy training aims to increase muscle size. This is important particularly for combative sports where increased muscle mass can be advantageous. Generally, hypertrophy occurs through an increase in the size or cross-sectional area of the muscle cells rather than an increase in the number of muscle cells.

Typical loading patterns for hypertrophy are shown in Table 14.3. As the table demonstrates, the eccentric or lowering component should be slower than the concentric component. This will create additional muscle damage and take greater time for the muscle to repair and regenerate. As a result, care must be taken when prescribing additional speed or resistance training around hypertrophy sessions.

## FLEXIBILITY TRAINING

Athletes are susceptible to injury if they lack sufficient flexibility to meet the specific demands of their sport. Stretching and range of motion exercises increase joint range of motion. The acute effects of stretching include:[35, 36]

- decreased muscle stiffness through viscoelastic deformation of the muscle tissue (this is likely to be extremely transient)
- increased muscle length through serial addition of sarcomeres
- altering sensation, thereby increasing stretch tolerance.

Traditionally, stretching has been widely promoted for injury prevention and to enhance performance for sporting activity. However, some researchers have suggested that stretching does not prevent injury in otherwise healthy individuals.[37] Others have noted that it is important to differentiate between pre-exercise stretching (where stretching does not appear to prevent injury)[38] and regular stretching outside periods of exercise (where there is some clinical and basic science evidence suggesting that stretching may prevent injury).[39, 40] Additionally, stretching does not seem to reduce the effects of delayed-onset muscle soreness.[41]

Furthermore, the acute effects of stretching can cause temporary strength deficits and reduce sporting performance.[42] These deficits seem to be associated with stretches performed for more than 60 seconds, while stretches of shorter duration may have less significant deficits.[42] As traditional stretching routines are performed during warm-up sessions prior to playing sport, the amount of time athletes stretch should be taken into consideration.

Stretching is often promoted as having a number of beneficial effects,[43, 44] although not all of the following have been appropriately studied:

- increases muscle and joint flexibility
- increases muscle relaxation
- decreases muscle soreness
- improves circulation
- helps prevent excessive adhesion
- promotes a flexible, strong scar.

> **BOX 14.1** Recommendations for effective stretching
>
> - A gentle warm-up before stretching increases tissue temperature and facilitates stretching. This may include activities such as jogging or cycling.
> - Superficial or deep heat modalities may be applied to the area prior to stretching to increase tissue temperature.
> - Cryotherapy may reduce pain and muscle spasm and thereby enhance the overall stretch of a muscle in the initial stages after an injury, even though the temperature is decreased (i.e. opposite to heat).
> - Incorrect positioning may cause injury, so athletes should be carefully instructed regarding the correct stretching position.
> - Different muscles seem to require different durations of stretch. In general, a slow sustained stretch should be held for a minimum of 10–15 seconds and progressed for 1 minute or longer. The athlete should feel the stretch in the appropriate area.
> - As the athlete's flexibility improves, increases in the intensity, duration, frequency and type of stretch can be considered.
> - Stretching should always be pain-free—that is, "tightness" without pain.

Recommendations for effective stretching are shown in Box 14.1.

## Types of stretching

There are four main types of stretching: static, dynamic, ballistic and proprioceptive neuromuscular facilitation.

### Static stretching

Static stretching involves moving a muscle or joint into an elongated position and holding that position for an extended period. Historically, this type of stretching has been used to prepare muscles for exercise; however, research has consistently demonstrated a reduction in power immediately after static stretching.[45] As a result, the more contemporary practice for athletic populations is to use static stretching post-training for recovery and away from training to improve flexibility.

### Dynamic stretching

In dynamic stretching, the muscles and joints are taken through their range of motion during movement. Unlike static stretching where you hold a position for an extended period, dynamic stretching is characterised by continuous, rhythmic motions. They mimic movements that will be performed during exercise, such as leg swings, arm circles or walking lunges. Dynamic stretching is often used as a warm-up before a workout or physical activity. It helps increase blood flow to the muscles and prepares them for more intense movements. Dynamic stretches have been shown to significantly increase tendon flexibility and elasticity and have been promoted for end-stage rehabilitation of tendon injuries.

### Ballistic stretching

Ballistic stretching involves rapid, bouncing movements to force a muscle into an extended range of motion. It involves eccentric contractions during the stretch phase, which may result in soreness or injury. Because of its forceful nature, ballistic stretching carries a higher risk of injury, including muscle strains, tears and joint sprains, and is considered more suitable for advanced athletes who require extreme flexibility for their specific sport or activity.

### Proprioceptive neuromuscular facilitation stretching

Proprioceptive neuromuscular facilitation stretching involves a combination of contracting the antagonist (opposite) muscle and excessively stretching the agonist muscle. This type of stretching is quite aggressive but can result in rapid increases in flexibility. Proprioceptive neuromuscular facilitation flexibility sessions should not be performed more than 1–2 times per week and should be cycled into and out of training as they can cause some muscle damage.

## Flexibility in the rehabilitation process

Regaining or maintaining full flexibility of joints and soft tissues is an essential component of the rehabilitation process. Following injury, musculotendinous flexibility often decreases as a result of spasm of surrounding muscles. Inflammation, pain and/or stiffness can limit joint range of motion and the normal extensibility of the musculotendinous unit can be compromised. This may result in dysfunction of adjacent joints and soft tissues. For example, the lumbar spine may be restricted in range of motion and the paraspinal muscles may spasm following knee or hip surgery, especially after periods of restricted mobilisation. Adequate soft-tissue extensibility after injury is essential to encourage pain-free range of movement. Stretching muscles and joints is one way of improving tissue and joint extensibility.

## PUTTING IT ALL TOGETHER: DESIGNING THE TRAINING PROGRAM

Integrating all aspects of training into a weekly, monthly or annual program is complex. In isolation, the various training principles we have outlined are relatively simple to program. However, when combined together, as well as the numerous other influences on a training schedule, designing the complete program can be more complex.

Numerous factors influence the design of a team or individual program. These include:

• individual versus team goals—some players might require strength as a focus whereas others require endurance as a focus; prioritising these in the schedule may not suit all team members

• external schedule influences—coach/athlete preferences, competition fixtures, player association guidelines and stage of season can all influence the schedule and therefore the programming priorities

• weather—hot/cold weather may affect training time and intensity in various parts of the season

• training age/injury history—an athlete's injury history and years spent training will influence which factors should be prioritised.

While this is not an exhaustive list, these factors can greatly affect the training program in the team setting as well as for individual athletes. In both the team and the individual setting, be sure to engage all parties (e.g. team coach(es), other relevant practitioners) in your plans so there is shared buy-in. Communication is a key skill.

## KEY POINTS

• The principles of sport-related training (overload, specificity, etc.) are often discussed in the context of improving athletes' performance. The same principles can be applied to structure injury prevention and treatment programs.

• After a sport-related injury, maintaining the athlete's fitness should be a priority. While protecting the injured tissues, various forms of cross-training can be used to limit deconditioning.

• Speed and agility are largely inherited qualities, but can be improved by addressing subcomponents such as strength, technique and power.

• Resistance training is important not only for sport performance, but also in preventing and managing overuse injuries. This is site and tissue specific.

• Loading patterns during resistance training vary based on the desired outcome (e.g. strength, power, endurance).

• Isometric, isokinetic and isotonic exercises have a role in distinct phases of injury prevention and rehabilitation. Isometric exercises are effective after periods of immobilisation or early after injury, while isokinetic exercises are a subsequent progression.

• Building and maintaining flexibility are an important part of overall training. However, acute pre-exercise stretching does not prevent injury or delayed-onset muscle soreness.

## REFERENCES

References for this chapter can be found at www.mhprofessional.com/CSM6e

## ADDITIONAL CONTENT

Scan here to access additional resources for this topic and more provided by the authors

## CHAPTER 15

# Load management

with **TORSTEIN DALEN-LORENTSEN**

*I don't know who created the term 'load management' for guys sitting out games or this narrative that continues to play on about star players or guys not being available. I don't know who started the narrative, but it's completely run amok. I think it has dehumanized some of us in terms of just the way we prepare ourselves day to day.*

**DALLAS MAVERICKS GUARD KYRIE IRVING (*BLEACHER REPORT*, 18 FEBRUARY 2023)**

## CHAPTER OUTLINE

Collecting training load data
Analysing training load data
Decision making with training load data
Why load management remains more art than science

## LEARNING OBJECTIVES

By the end of this chapter you should be able to:

- explain the overarching goals of training load management
- discuss the limitations of training load management in terms of injury prevention
- categorise types of training loads and provide examples
- contrast the approach to training load management in team versus individual sports
- define/operationalise several commonly used terms in training load management
- construct an individualised training load management plan that incorporates appropriate contextual factors.

Managing an athlete's training load is common practice to enhance performance and help prevent injuries. The process is performed in three steps:

1. data collection (monitoring, e.g. from smartwatches or questionnaires)
2. data analysis (transforming the findings from raw data into tangible insights)
3. decision making (changes in training informed by the data, including load management).

Load management refers to the use of data to inform decisions that may improve the athlete's performance and/ or reduce health issues. The meticulous and time-consuming nature of the steps varies based on factors such as the specific sport, the athlete involved, available resources and the ambitions of the team or organisation. One size does not fit all: the approach to load management must be customised.

Planning an athlete's training based on various forms of feedback is well established. However, load management based on new forms of data remains relatively new in the sporting world. Athletes who are advised to sit out a game or practice may disagree with the decision when it is based on the data alone (as highlighted by the opening quote). Therefore, in the final section of this chapter we touch on the "science" of using data-driven insights to support the "art" of helping athletes to remain at the peak of their performance. Load management is not about restraining athletes, but rather helping them to train more and with higher quality.

## COLLECTING TRAINING LOAD DATA

Athletes participating in training or competitions experience a psychophysiological stimulus that can be termed "load".[1, 2] Load can be divided into two main categories: non-sport-related load and training load. The sum of these is often referred to as the total load. It is essential that athletes have control over the total load.

### Non-sport-related load

Non-sport-related load is important but often more challenging to quantify and therefore more difficult to monitor. It includes everything that affects athletes outside of training and competition (such as non-exercise-related physical activity).

It can also arise from stressful family events—both good and bad—and other everyday life circumstances. Examples are school exam periods for young athletes, and the arrival of a new family member for older athletes. Such situations can increase the total load on the athlete but may not be detected by traditional load monitoring tools (such as wearables or self-reported athlete questionnaires).

### Training load

Training load is any stimulus placed on an athlete from training or competition, as all activities performed in training or competition will elicit a physiological response.[3, 4] Although training load has recently been investigated in relation to injury, its use stems from the prescription and evaluation of training.[5] Using a practical approach, training load can be seen as the input variable to elicit a training response.[6]

Training load has been categorised according to various dimensions, and below we look at three of them.

#### External and internal loads

The most common categorisation is the division into external and internal loads.[7, 8] External load is considered the physical work an athlete performs during a training session or match. It can be measured using various methods but is often expressed as numerical data.

When we have information about the physical work the athlete has done, we want to examine their response to this work—this is the internal load. The most common way of measuring internal load is through heart rate monitors and the rate of perceived exertion (RPE).[9]

Training monitoring should ideally capture external and internal loads. Examples of the differences between internal and external loads, and their measurement, are shown in Figure 15.1.

Failure to match the external load placed on an athlete to their internal load responses can result in an injury or drop in performance (often known as a training error). Errors in matching external load placed versus internal load experienced can be used to modify the training plan as part of a feedback loop (e.g. if an athlete does not have enough minutes in the target heart rate zone, the following day's training could be changed to compensate). Historically, training monitoring provides important feedback to complement the athlete and coach's assessment of whether the athlete is responding to the training program.

The importance of athlete availability for team success has led to interest in training monitoring rising exponentially over recent years. Monitoring is now frequently used to plan training and decide how much competitive exposure a team and the individuals on the team are exposed to. For instance, chronic exposure to repeated sprints of short (15–20 m) and long duration (>30 m) can be tracked to enhance performance outcomes in team-based sports.[10, 11] The impact of these decisions on a team's success has made load monitoring and management a key component of both short- and long-term decision making on athlete management.

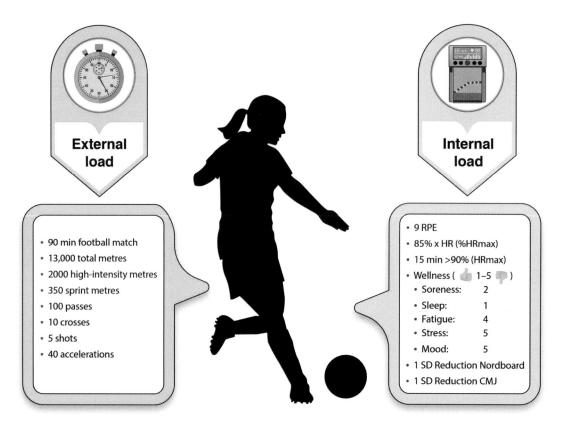

RPE, rate of perceived exertion; HR, heart rate; HRmax, heart rate maximum; SD, standard deviation; CMJ, counter movement jump

**Figure 15.1** Examples of external and internal loads in a footballer

### Mechanical and physiological loads

The training load imposed on athletes through training and competition can be divided into two main load-adaptation pathways: mechanical (or biomechanical) load and physiological load.[12] Mechanical load predominantly leads to stresses in the musculoskeletal system (e.g. cartilage, bone, tendons and muscle tissue). Physiological load mainly affects metabolic systems (e.g. oxygen uptake, heart rate and kinetic energy).

Vanrenterghem and colleagues propose the following analogy: consider the impact of training load on an athlete as you would the load you place on a car.[12] The physiological parameters focus on how the car consumes energy. The mechanical parameters are intended to capture aspects like how the shock absorbers and suspension work (in other words, the mechanical properties of the car).

The relationship between mechanical, physiological, external and internal loads is depicted in Figure 15.2.

Traditionally, it is common to monitor physiological parameters (such as total distance run or heart rate achieved during exercise) since these can easily be measured with a watch or monitor. Evolution in technologies such as global positioning systems (GPS) and inertial measurement units means we can also track external mechanical load parameters such as acceleration and deceleration. The use of wearable technology and the development of sophisticated algorithms have made measuring changes in internal mechanical loads such as the percentage change in performance measures (e.g. counter movement jump) more accessible to those without expensive equipment such as force plates.

### Specific and general loads

It is possible to distinguish between the specific load on an individual structure (e.g. the hamstring muscles) and the general load placed on the entire body. In sports that primarily involve single movements (such as high jump, javelin throw, ski jumping), general load measures are of little value.

For instance, imagine collecting load data for a baseball pitcher using the session rating of perceived exertion (sRPE) method (this uses a subjective questionnaire and asks the athlete to score their effort between 1 and 10). This would poorly represent the actual load on the key structures

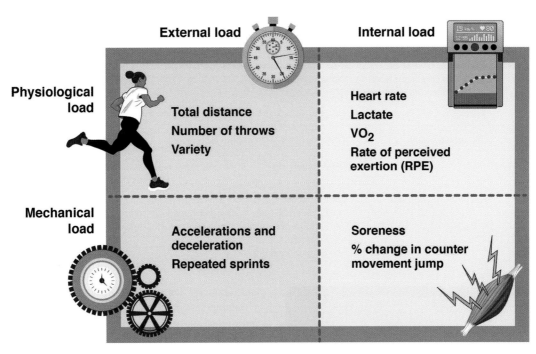

**Figure 15.2** Differences between physiological, mechanical, internal and external loads

such as the rotator cuff muscles during a training session or in competition. It would be more appropriate to measure the cumulative force generated by the shoulder joint.

## Team sports

Team sports involve a variety of complex movements, making it a challenge to find parameters that cover everything. When monitoring 15–30 athletes simultaneously, careful parameter selection is necessary to make the most practical use of the data you have available.

The parameters commonly used in team sports are often indirect measures of general load. They are seldom sufficient to cover both general and specific loads. For instance, the use of microsensors (GPS, local positioning system [LPS] and inertial measurement units[13]) in sports like handball and football provides good oversight of the general load from running and other movements but does not provide insights into the specific load on a group of tissues from kicking or throwing.

Despite the large numbers of individuals in teams or squads, individual monitoring is essential to enable informed decision making. Internal load can vary significantly between athletes, even if a training session involves a similar amount of total work for each athlete. Internal load depends on factors such as age, physiological condition, mental state, sleep, stress level and skills. External load can also vary significantly within a team, even in training sessions where all athletes have similar tasks and in theory should do the same amount of work. Variation may occur due to an athlete's motivation to perform, patterns of play and so on.

The resources available to the team will dictate the type of monitoring that is used and/or suitable to support load management decisions. Table 15.1 suggests a tiered approach to training load monitoring at different competition levels from community to elite.

For amateur teams, sRPE offers a useful option. It is a combination of external load (duration, most often measured in minutes) and internal load (RPE). Originally proposed by Foster and colleagues, sRPE consists of quantifying the athlete's perceived exertion in a session using a category scale (Borg CR10 scale) and multiplying it by the session duration. The product of this calculation gives a "load figure" or an arbitrary unit of measurement that can be used in context to decide whether a session or group of sessions is placing greater load on the athlete.[9] sRPE is a straightforward, reliable and validated way to monitor load.[9, 14, 15] By monitoring sRPE, you can get an overview of the general load an athlete is experiencing. See Box 15.1 for an example of using sRPE.

In professional teams with dedicated staff to manage load and access to expensive equipment, many parameters can be monitored.[16] External parameters are often measured using sensors attached to the athletes. The most common are GPS/LPS and accelerometers. These devices consist of

**TABLE 15.1**  A tiered approach to training load monitoring at different competition levels

| Competition level | Person responsible for data collection | Systems commonly available | Recommended approach |
|---|---|---|---|
| Community | Head coach or physio/ medical staff or athlete themselves | Smartphone app | Observation and awareness, communication with athletes, sRPE registration and evaluation |
| Medium resource | Performance coach or medical staff | Smartphone app, GPS, basic physiological and strength testing (e.g. heart rate and 1 repetition maximum) | All the above + use of athlete management system to compile data from tracking technology, testing and subjective questionnaires. Use data as decision support to plan training. |
| Elite | Performance staff | Smartphone app, GPS/LPS system, VO$_2$max and lactate testing, advanced strength/power testing equipment (e.g. force platforms), indirect calorimetry and more | All the above + data streams from more advanced measurements and testing |

---

**BOX 15.1**  Example of using sRPE to measure load

Athlete A plays a 90-minute football match and rates the match using sRPE as an 8 out of 10. Athlete B also plays 90 minutes but rates the match as 10 out of 10. Athlete C is returning from an injury so plays only one half (45 minutes) and rates it as 10 out of 10.

The calculations are as follows:

- Athlete A: 90 × 8  = 720
- Athlete B: 90 × 10 = 900
- Athlete C: 45 × 10 = 450

The data show the different loads (calculated in arbitrary units) placed on each player despite the similarities and differences in the total time played. These calculations may also be affected by each athlete's physiological and psychological state.

---

a chip that connects to a global or local satellite system, an accelerometer (which measures force), a gyroscope (which measures angle) and magnetometers (which measure direction). The devices collect vast amounts of data (between 10 and 1000 recordings per second) and the manufacturers' systems convert the raw data into parameters such as total distance and number of accelerations.

The choice of parameters depends on the sport, but typically around 5–10 variables are monitored closely, covering the most important physiological and mechanical external loads. For professional settings, several internal parameters will also be collected.

In addition to RPE, a wellness questionnaire can be valuable. In this questionnaire, athletes rate themselves from 1 to 5 in categories such as mood, sleep, stress, soreness and tiredness. The questionnaire may be completed before a training session to assess an athlete's overall response to training and non-sport-related load, or post-training or competition to provide information on how the athlete responded to the training session or competition. Wellness is one of the few parameters that can provide information about non-sport-related loads. Wellness may be used as an early warning system to discuss non-sport-related factors with an athlete to help address and/or mitigate their impact on performance or injury risk, or simply to provide more holistic care to the athlete.

**PRACTICE PEARL**

In addition to being a measure of sport-related load, wellness scores taken on a daily basis provide a measure of non-sport-related load. A drop in scores may prompt discussion about the athlete's wider health or lifestyle choices and how to support the athlete in aspects of their life outside of the competitive environment.

Internal load can also be estimated by testing performance capabilities pre- and post-training or competition. This can be achieved by comparing the maximum vertical jump (on a force platform) with the athlete's normal (average) vertical jump following training or a competitive event. This enables you to evaluate the athlete's response to the work they have done: for instance, a drop in jump height compared with the athlete's normal jump height may indicate that the athlete has significant fatigue and may require additional recovery in the future training plan.

Heart rate monitoring is another internal parameter that can easily be tracked, and in team sports particularly, time spent in the higher intensity zones may be relevant in deciding whether additional recovery is required.

## Individual sports

For some individual sports, movements are more uniform, making it easier to define a precise measure of load. For instance, for a recreational runner, the information from a simple GPS watch gives relatively precise measures of distances run at different paces. With this information, you would have a very good estimate of the total distance run and the duration, providing two ways to estimate the total external load placed on the runner.

Distance running athletes place a high demand on the lower leg muscles in particular.[17] However, as running movement patterns tend to be relatively uniform (e.g. there is less load placed on the athlete related to the acceleration and deceleration forces associated with changing direction), it is often unnecessary to track as many parameters as in a team-based sport. This gives recreational and amateur runners greater control over the most important loads placed on their body (distance run, speed and running duration). Similar to team sports monitoring, sRPE is useful for tracking load over time in distance running athletes.[18, 19]

In more complex individual sports such as alpine skiing, decathlon or triathlon, you will often need to increase the number of parameters that you monitor and attempt to control because of the diverse demands these sports put on the athlete.

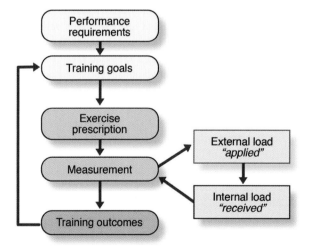

**Figure 15.3** Framework of the training process showing the relationship between goals, exercise prescription, measurement and outcomes. This is an important iterative feedback loop.
Source: Adapted with permission from Impellizzeri FM, Marcora SM, Coutts AJ. Internal and external training load: 15 years on. *Int J Sports Physiol Perform* 2019;14(2):270–3.

Although there are different groups of training load, we recommend tracking a mix between (1) subjective and objective, (2) internal and external, and (3) biomechanical and physiological.[20-22] Figure 15.3 illustrates the cycle between training goals, exercise (external load, internal load) and training outcomes.[8] Monitoring these components helps the coach/practitioner understand whether the prescribed training (external load) has induced the planned response (internal load) and whether that response has induced the planned training adaptations (training outcomes).[23, 24]

## ANALYSING TRAINING LOAD DATA

After collecting the data, the next step is to transform the information into tangible insights. The method you use to do this depends on the sport, expertise, resources and ambitions of the team or individual athlete and their support staff. One useful way of analysing training data is into absolute and relative loads.

### Absolute load

The absolute load is simply the amount of load performed over a period of time—for a distance runner it might be 100 km during that week. The best measure of absolute load should be sport-specific. Contrast baseball (162 games in Major League Baseball before playoffs) and some combat sports (1–2 bouts per year).

Shorter periods (i.e. 1–9 days) are typically known as acute periods and extended periods (i.e. >9 days) are known as chronic periods. Absolute load can also be analysed as the number of matches played during a time period, referred to as "match/fixture density". (We prefer the objective term "density", although "fixture congestion" has become synonymous with "density" in some sports.)

### Relative load

The relative load relates to a reference value (a denominator in maths). The most commonly used references are competition demand (i.e. loads athletes received in previous competitive events) and training load history. When using competition demand as a reference, the absolute load is divided by the competition demand to give the relative load (e.g. the athlete this week performed 500 m of sprinting or 120% of the demand that will usually be asked of them in competition). The competition demand reference is most often used as a whole competition (or match) average; it can also be a "worst-case" period (e.g. calculated based upon the most demanding 60-second period), but the usefulness of this is debated.[25]

You can also use an athlete's individual training load history to establish relative load; this is referred to as "change-in-load" analysis. There are three common options for performing this analysis:

- Option A is to analyse monotony and strain. Monotony is the daily training load average divided by the standard deviation, and strain is the average weekly training load multiplied by monotony.
- Option B is to calculate basic differences between periods, such as week-to-week change. This can be done as the absolute change in load (e.g. the increase from week 4 to week 5 was 200 m) or the percentage change in load (i.e. 100% increase).
- Option C is to use the acute:chronic workload ratio. This was introduced by Hulin and colleagues as a modification of Banister's fitness-fatigue model.[5, 26] It is calculated by dividing the total amount of training an athlete has recently completed (e.g. the past 3–9 days) by the amount they have completed over a longer period (e.g. 14–28 days). The acute:chronic workload ratio intends to reflect preparedness for training by accounting for both positive and negative training effects (i.e. fitness and fatigue). There has been a lot of debate regarding this approach.

Experienced practitioners appreciate the pros and cons of these approaches and will select the calculations that make most sense for them or their athletes. The choice of a "change-in-load" calculation will vary depending on factors such as the intensity of the training session being developed and the potential injury risk for a particular athlete.

## DECISION MAKING WITH TRAINING LOAD DATA

Once you have monitored and analysed the athlete's load, the final step is decision making (load management). The monitoring and analysis steps can provide information about training and competition but if this is not used to make decisions about the athlete's training, it has very limited value.

---

### PRACTICE PEARL

The burden to collect data should always be weighed against its usefulness; i.e. the capacity of the data to inform coaches or clinicians to make athlete-centred decisions about future load prescription.

---

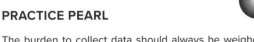

### Relationship between training load, injury and performance

Creating an accurate framework of the relationship between training load, injury and performance is difficult, mainly because of the multifactorial nature of both injuries and performance. Injuries and performance are complex and dynamic outcomes influenced by a multitude of factors, often without a predictable pattern.

Bittencourt and colleagues exemplified this by their complex model for sports injuries, which outlines a web of determinants that display a dynamic and open structure with inherent nonlinearity due to recursive loops and interactions between risk factors.[27] While the complex nature of injury makes prediction extremely difficult, recognising and measuring known risk factors may help determine specific periods when athletes may be at an increased risk of injuries.[28]

Meeuwisse and colleagues have demonstrated how intrinsic and extrinsic risk factors influence risk and are dynamic.[29] For non-modifiable risk factors (e.g. age, sex), single baseline values can be enough. For modifiable risk factors that change over time, we must use repeated measures that coincide with the change. Some modifiable risk factors are slow to change, such as athlete strength, muscle balance and fitness level. This means that they can be measured over a longer period (e.g. every 3 months). Fast-changing risk factors such as training load must be updated daily (or even every minute in certain elite sports).[28]

Many studies have attempted to find a relationship between training load and injuries. One of the most studied concepts is the acute:chronic workload ratio. After initial praise and endorsement,[4] there has been increased scrutiny of this concept. This scrutiny can broadly be divided into two categories: studies highlighting methodological weaknesses, and studies questioning the validity of the entire concept.

The methodological criticism has focused on the calculation,[30-33] the statistical and analytical approaches[23, 33] and other questionable research practises.[23, 32] The acute:chronic workload ratio also lacks conceptual and theoretical models.[23, 34] Most acute:chronic workload ratio studies looking to assess its relationship to health or injury are descriptive, meaning they cannot make conclusions on causality.[35]

The acute:chronic workload ratio is not a one-size-fits-all metric to measure the risk of training load increases (or decreases) and cannot be relied on to prevent injuries. This problem is not isolated to the acute:chronic workload ratio, which to its credit has been well studied. Almost all of the literature evaluating relationships between training load and injury suffer from similar problems.

---

### PRACTICE PEARL

We caution against using the acute:chronic workload ratio as a standalone measure to assess the risk of increases or decreases in training volume.

---

## WHY LOAD MANAGEMENT REMAINS MORE ART THAN SCIENCE

Although no causal link has been established between training load and injury, the consensus among practitioners is that training load data should still be used to support informed decisions when prescribing future training sessions. Training load data can help:

- inform decisions on the amount of load an athlete needs to be prepared to withstand in competition, or how much absolute load they need to perform to compete with their peers
- balance the load an athlete is prescribed with their response to that load.[28]

The rationale behind load management is to carefully progress the training stimuli to allow the player's body and mind time to adapt. This can reduce fatigue, which may improve performance and reduce the risk of injuries and/or illness. The physiological systems will then either go through a recovery period and adapt to the increased demand (i.e. increase their capacity) or undergo maladaptation if the stimulus was excessive (i.e. tissue damage).[36]

If the training load takes key contextual factors into account, the athlete is more likely to perform better and have fewer injuries. These contextual factors can be thought of as relating to the athlete, the coach and the training/match environment.[28] Some examples (not exhaustive):

- athlete factors include age, injury history, subjective (mental) wellness and non-sporting load, attitudes and beliefs to screening and/or strength test data
- coach factors include experience, preferences relating to training methods, team standing in the competition, job security
- training/match factors include the physical sporting environment, the importance of the upcoming match/competition, as well as the context of that match/competition in relation to the season calendar.[28]

A selection of these factors is depicted alongside training load in Figure 15.4.

Currently we do not know which contextual factors are most important, or how they interact. We therefore cannot measure their influence on training load, or their influence on performance and injury. However, great practitioners are still able to manage training load and balance the contextual factors so that training will increase performance and reduce the potential for injury. This has historically been achieved on an intuitive basis (i.e. based on coach/athlete experience), but more recently has been described using frameworks.

We and others[8] propose that both external load and internal load be used to link the training data with how the

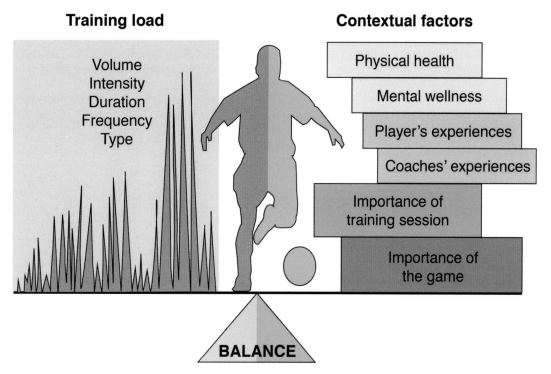

**Figure 15.4** The balance between training load and a selection of contextual factors

athlete performs (Fig. 15.3). The first step is to identify the key determinants of performance, before setting training goals and prescribing training. External load is used to ensure that the training went as planned, and internal load is used to ensure that the athlete's psychophysiological response to the training was as planned.

There are five overarching levels for training load management decisions,[28] ranging from long term to short term:

- long-term use (e.g. managing the athlete across several seasons)
- season planning (e.g. preparing for game demands)
- day-to-day planning (e.g. planning and performing the training session to fit the weekly periodisation)
- in-session adjustment (e.g. live evaluation of and intervention on the athlete's physical outputs)
- feedback (e.g. how we can learn from this training session for the next session).[28]

Long-term management includes the use of data that are not required in day-to-day practice, but provide insights into trends and tendencies in the training adaptation and performance of an athlete. An example might be an analysis of the external load versus the internal load across different periods of the season, which may help to identify times when the athlete is not coping.

Short-term management is the most resource-intensive and consists of everything from macrocycle (i.e. months) planning to within-session adjustments. Macrocycle planning and evaluation are key to keeping athletes fit and injury-free. Unlike microcycles (i.e. weeks) that must taper into the games or competitions, macrocycles need to ensure that athletes either build or maintain their fitness over time. This is done by administering appropriate amounts of load to each athlete.

Box 15.2 highlights the recent increase in the use of microdosing load exposures with the aim of maintaining performance and reducing injury risk.

---

**BOX 15.2** Microdosing: applying load management in practice to maintain performance and reduce the risk of injury
**with PAUL BLAZEY**

Chapter 14 covers the traditional approach to athlete strength and conditioning, including how athletes periodise their training around the competitive season. A gold-standard example might include Olympic track and field athletes who periodise their training to focus on specific training adaptations over a 4-year cycle (the macrocycle). In team-based sports, athletes often maximise strength, power, and aerobic and anaerobic performance during the pre-season, so that they can better tolerate the stresses of in-season competition. This is illustrated by Figure 14.1.

Athletes need regular exposure to physiological stimuli (such as training at or around their $VO_2max$ or performing heavy resistance training) to maintain the physical capabilities that they build up in their conditioning or pre-competitive phases. This supports them to maintain performance and potentially reduces their risk of injury.[37] However, during the competitive phase exposure to high amounts of heavy resistance, plyometric or anaerobic speed work can also present a risk to athletes who need to balance the loads incurred in training with the demands of competitive sport.

It is a challenge to maintain performance while avoiding injury or illness. An overcautious athlete can underload (e.g. not perform enough high-intensity outputs), resulting in decreased performance.[37]

### Building a case for microdosing using the principles of load management

Recent studies recommend more frequent exposure to training stimuli, such as heavy resistance training throughout the competitive season.[38, 39] This is where collecting, analysing and applying load management can support decision making.

Microdosing (sometimes called microloading) involves partitioning training load into smaller, more frequent bouts. This can be achieved around competitive events, which dictate how and when microdosing will occur.

For example, a team sport athlete who works to build their anaerobic capacity (sprint speed and volume) may require short but regular bouts of sprint speed training in-season to maintain or increase their capacity.[40] If the athlete does not reach their usual sprint speed during competition (due to variations in play or tactical decisions by the team coach), they will already have had small exposures the day before their game, so will maintain their performance capacity.

An example of when microdosing might occur in relation to competition and training is given in Figure 15.5.

Load management (based on quality data monitoring) enables us to understand what the athlete's regular competitive output would be, and to prescribe microdoses that match the athlete's "standard" physical output for a given variable (e.g. sprint intensity).

Microdosing is useful at the team level, especially during intense blocks of competitive play, where a group of athletes need to maintain maximal aerobic, anaerobic and strength capacity without impeding their performance in an upcoming event. Microdosing allows a whole squad of athletes to be subject to "high enough" levels of load, supporting all athletes to maintain their physical capability and to be ready when called on.

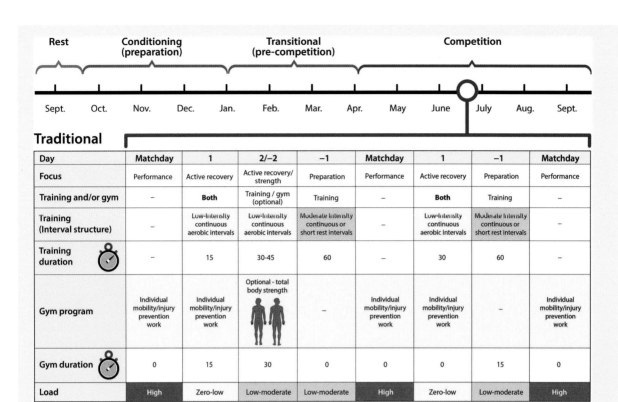

**Figure 15.5** An example of microdosing implemented into a training week schedule based around two different competitive patterns

## Traditional

| Day | Matchday | 1 | 2/–2 | –1 | Matchday | 1 | –1 | Matchday |
|---|---|---|---|---|---|---|---|---|
| Focus | Performance | Active recovery | Active recovery/strength | Preparation | Performance | Active recovery | Preparation | Performance |
| Training and/or gym | – | **Both** | Training / gym (optional) | Training | – | **Both** | Training | – |
| Training (Interval structure) | – | Low-intensity continuous aerobic intervals | Low-intensity continuous aerobic intervals | Moderate intensity continuous or short rest intervals | – | Low-intensity continuous aerobic intervals | Moderate intensity continuous or short rest intervals | – |
| Training duration | – | 15 | 30-45 | 60 | – | 30 | 60 | – |
| Gym program | Individual mobility/injury prevention work | Individual mobility/injury prevention work | Optional - total body strength | – | Individual mobility/injury prevention work | Individual mobility/injury prevention work | – | Individual mobility/injury prevention work |
| Gym duration | 0 | 15 | 30 | 0 | 0 | 0 | 15 | 0 |
| Load | High | Zero-low | Low-moderate | Low-moderate | High | Zero-low | Low-moderate | High |

## Microdosed

| Day | Matchday | 1 | 2/–2 | –1 | Matchday | 1 | –1 | Matchday |
|---|---|---|---|---|---|---|---|---|
| Focus | Performance | Active recovery | Active recovery/strength | Preparation | Performance | Active recovery | Preparation | Performance |
| Training and/or gym | **Both** | **Both** | **Both** | **Both** | **Both** | **Both** | **Both** | **Both** |
| Training (Interval structure) | – | Low-intensity continuous aerobic intervals | Low-intensity continuous aerobic intervals | Moderate intensity continuous or short rest intervals | – | Low-intensity continuous aerobic intervals | Moderate intensity continuous or short rest intervals | – |
| Training duration | – | 15 | 30-45 | 60 | – | 30 | 60 | – |
| Gym program | Lower body strength (post game) | Individual mobility/injury prevention work | Upper body strength | Upper body power | Lower body strength (post game) | Individual mobility/injury prevention work | Upper body strength | Lower body strength (post game) |
| Gym duration | 15 | 10 | 15 | 15 | 15 | 10 | 15 | 15 |
| Load | High | Low | Moderate | Moderate | High | Low | Moderate | High |

Dr Mathew Cuthbert has discussed the application of microdosing in a team-based environment (the English Football Association):

Implementing microdosing in practice

## Balancing load management with competitive excellence

While recent framing may have overemphasised a medicalised rationale for load management, leading to practitioners focusing too much on reducing loads, it is equally important that athletes are exposed to sufficient loads. Not allowing an athlete to push beyond their boundaries may impair their ability to prepare for the demands of competition, or worse still may prevent them from reaching their athletic potential. Athletes must train *enough,* often equating to several times their competition requirements per week.

For example, team sports athletes often train 2–3 times their match requirements in a training week when there is one match per week. In individual sports, elite marathon runners will often train upwards of 5 times the marathon distance in a single training week, with many kilometres run at speeds higher than their target marathon speed. The principle is the same: the body and mind must have sufficient progression with time for adaptation, and this progression must be significantly above competition requirements.

In a rehabilitation context, load management is a crucial tool to ensure that an athlete returns to their sport

**PRACTICE PEARL**

Training or competitive load data alone should never be used to make decisions about when an athlete does or does not compete; instead, data should be used to inform decisions that are made collaboratively between clinicians, coaches, high-performance staff and the athlete.

quickly and safely. One of the challenges of rehabilitation is to ensure that both the injured structure and the non-injured structures have a suitable load progression. Again, a method with relative load as a basis can be used to find a suitable progression.

The relationship between training load, performance and injury is complex. However, until precise models can explain the relationship and experimental studies can document effectiveness, practitioners must embrace uncertainty and move back to basics. Trust your expertise and use the skill and art of coaching to make shared decisions on training load management.

## KEY POINTS

- Managing an athlete's training load involves three steps: (1) collecting data, (2) analysing the data and (3) decision making.

- The overarching goal of managing an athlete's training load is to allow them to train more and at a higher quality, not to restrain them. Load management can take place over the short- and long-term training cycle.

- The total load for an athlete includes their training load and their non-sport-related load. Both must be addressed.

- There are multiple approaches to categorising load, including internal versus external load, mechanical versus physiological load, and specific versus general load.

- Individual monitoring is still required in the team setting. Even if all athletes are engaged in the same training program, there will be variations in internal and external loads across the athletes.

- A range of load monitoring tools are available, depending on the resources available to a team. Relatively simple, low-resource tools can be effective.

- The frequency with which you monitor any given variable for an athlete should correspond with how quickly your variable of interest can change.

- There are several ways to use an athlete's training load history as a reference when determining a change in their training load. One method is the acute:chronic workload ratio. However, while widely adopted, there are important limitations to its usefulness.

- To date, training load has not been directly (causally) linked to athletic performance or risk of injury. This is due to the multifactorial nature of performance and injury. Managing training load can, however, help inform decisions about the load necessary for an athlete to reach their performance goals and how to match the athlete's load with their training response.

- When making load management decisions, use shared decision making and consider contextual factors like the athlete's injury history, age, attitudes, beliefs and self-reported wellness, as well as the importance of the competition ahead.

## REFERENCES

References for this chapter can be found at www.mhprofessional.com/CSM6e

## ADDITIONAL CONTENT

Scan here to access additional resources for this topic and more provided by the authors

**B**

## CHAPTER 16

# Recovery

with SHONA HALSON, CAS FUCHS, JAMES BROATCH, SUZANNA RUSSELL, MATTHEW DRILLER and GRAEME CLOSE

*I've been very consistent with training my body, rehabbing my body, eating, having my body be very clean throughout this journey because I've always wanted to have a long career, or as long as I could be in this space.*

LEBRON JAMES (AMERICAN PROFESSIONAL BASKETBALL PLAYER ON *THE TIM FERRISS SHOW*)

## CHAPTER OUTLINE

Cooling
Heating
Contrast therapy
Hydrostatic pressure
Compression
Nutrition
Mental recovery
Sleep
Practical strategies: putting it all together
Conclusion

## LEARNING OBJECTIVES

By the end of this chapter you should be able to:

- list the most common recovery techniques used in sport and the basic protocols for their use
- explain the physiological basis behind these recovery techniques
- discuss the discrepancies behind the effects of a given recovery technique and the scientific evidence
- discuss how nutrition recovery strategies can help athletes' performance
- describe the emerging focus on sleep and mental restoration as recovery strategies
- offer recommendations for practical application of recovery strategies in the athletic population.

The rate and quality of recovery are extremely important for the high-performance athlete in terms of enhancing performance and reducing risk of injury. Effective recovery should seek to address the physiological, nutritional, structural, neural and psychological effects of training and competition. A range of modalities have been purported to facilitate various aspects of recovery; however, at times the evidence is conflicting.

As there are also a myriad of new and unproven recovery strategies and devices, in this chapter we focus on established recovery strategies. What is the mechanism of action? What evidence is there in the field? Our aim is to assist you, the clinician, to make quality decisions regarding the type and timing of recovery strategies for individual athletes.

> **PRACTICE PEARL**
>
> The most appropriate blend of recovery strategies depends on a detailed understanding of the sport, the individual athlete and the relative benefits of the recovery modality.

## COOLING

Cooling, also referred to as cold therapy or cryotherapy, is a popular and widely applied recovery strategy. Cooling strategies include cold water immersion, ice application and whole-body or partial-body cryotherapy.

- With cold water immersion, the individual typically submerges their limbs or body (excluding the head) in water 5–15°C for a duration of 5–20 min.[1]
- Applying ice (e.g. ice pack or crushed ice) allows for a more targeted cooling of specific localised areas, typically for 10–20 min.
- Whole-body or partial-body cryotherapy is a method by which the individual is exposed to cold air in a closed chamber system (i.e. whole-body cryotherapy in a cryochamber) or vaporised liquid nitrogen in a head-free cabin system (i.e. partial-body cryotherapy in a cryosauna). During the session the athlete may be exposed to very low temperatures (below –110°C) for a relatively short duration (2–5 min).[2-4]

Despite some differences among these strategies, their primary aim is to decrease tissue temperature,[5] thereby reducing blood flow, tissue perfusion and tissue metabolic rate.[6-8] Cold-induced decrements in tissue temperature may lower acetylcholine production and nerve conduction velocity,[9, 10] exerting an analgesic effect, especially when skin temperature is below 13°C.[11, 12]

These mechanisms explain, at least partly, the reported benefits of cooling on reducing the sense of fatigue, delayed-onset muscle soreness, swelling and (secondary) exercise-induced muscle damage.[13-19] Probably due to cooling alleviating feelings of discomfort, several studies have shown that cooling can improve recovery of muscle function/performance after exercise.[1, 15, 16, 20, 21] Post-exercise cooling may support muscle conditioning by stimulating mitochondrial biogenesis and angiogenesis.[22-24]

However, several other studies have failed to observe benefits of cooling on various aspects of post-exercise recovery.[25-30] These conflicting results may reflect differences in study design and of course a placebo effect must be considered as it is very difficult to control for, or blind from, a cooling intervention.[29-31]

The traditional belief that cooling reduces inflammation after regular exercise has recently been challenged,[32] with evidence indicating no impact of post-exercise cooling on inflammatory markers.[33] Moreover, a decline in muscle temperature and its associated reduction in metabolic activity and/or blood flow may compromise other key aspects of post-exercise recovery, such as attenuating the post-exercise increase in muscle glycogen repletion[34, 35] and muscle protein synthesis rates for tissue repair.[36]

Overall, whether cooling is recommended depends on the goal (e.g. reducing pain vs increasing muscle protein synthesis rates) (Fig. 16.1). Therefore, it is important to consider both the primary recovery objective as well as the cooling strategy.

## HEATING

Heating, also referred to as heat therapy or thermotherapy, has been used since ancient times for medicinal purposes such as the treatment of muscle disorders.[37, 38] Like cooling, heating can be applied using various strategies, including hot water immersion, heat pack/pad application and sauna.

- With hot water immersion, the individual typically submerges their limbs or entire body (excluding the head) in water ≥36°C for a duration of 10–24 min.[1]
- Heat pack or heat pad application allows for a more targeted heating of specific localised areas, and the duration varies based on the intensity of the heat.
- Depending on the type of sauna (e.g. infrared vs Finnish sauna), the individual is exposed for a brief duration (e.g. 10–30 min) to high temperatures typically ranging from 40 to 110°C.

Despite its longstanding use and popularity, the benefits of heating on muscle tissue have remained largely unknown until recently. Heating elevates skeletal muscle temperature and may increase muscle blood flow/perfusion and intramuscular metabolism.[39-42] Heating also promotes capillary growth, attenuates disuse muscle atrophy, enhances mitochondrial content and function, and improves glucose metabolism and insulin signalling.[43-47]

Given these beneficial physiological effects, heating has been tested as a means to accelerate muscle recovery and tissue conditioning following exercise.[48-50] However, recovery markers such as reducing delayed-onset muscle soreness, lowering limb swelling and aiding performance recovery do not point to substantial benefits—heating appears to be less effective than cooling for these elements of recovery.[1, 15, 51-53]

Because heating may augment the delivery and uptake of nutrients like glucose and amino acids as well as increasing

anabolic signalling in muscle tissue,[43, 48, 54] it has been tested for its ability to enhance glycogen and muscle protein synthesis. The results of post-exercise heat application on muscle glycogen replenishment are mixed: studies have indicated a positive,[55] neutral[56] and negative[57] effect. Post-exercise hot water immersion did not modulate postprandial muscle protein synthesis rates or help incorporate dietary protein-derived amino acids in muscle tissue during post-exercise recovery.[42]

Overall, despite its physiological effects and reported benefits on specific aspects of muscle conditioning (e.g. increased capillarisation), heating has so far not proven to be an effective recovery strategy following exercise (Fig. 16.1).

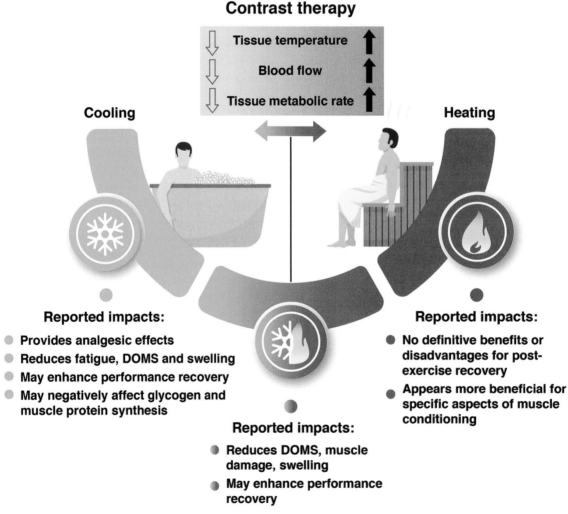

DOMS, delayed-onset muscle soreness

**Figure 16.1** The proposed physiological effects and effectiveness for post-exercise recovery of cooling, heating and contrast therapy

## CONTRAST THERAPY

Contrast therapy is a treatment modality in which parts of the body are exposed to contrasting temperatures, alternating between cold and hot. It can be performed in a variety of ways, including cold and hot packs, cold and hot showers, and cold and hot baths. The individual typically alternates continuously (e.g. every min) between cold and hot water for up to 15 min.[1]

Given that cooling restricts and heating opens the vascular bed within muscle tissue, it has been suggested that alternating between cold and hot water may induce a "pump" effect, which could then stimulate blood flow in the applied area. Theoretically, this could improve post-exercise recovery by accelerating the removal of metabolic by-products as well as increasing the supply of nutrients.

However, previous studies have shown, at best, only small increases in arterial blood flow following contrast water therapy,[58, 59] and no substantial changes in muscle temperature.[60-62] This questions the proposed physiological mechanism of contrast therapy.

Yet there is evidence that contrast therapy reduces delayed-onset muscle soreness, muscle damage markers (i.e. creatine kinase) and swelling, and enhances performance recovery.[1, 15, 63, 64] Therefore, despite the absence of a clear physiological mechanism, contrast therapy could be considered as an effective strategy for some aspects of recovery (Fig. 16.1).

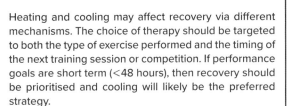

**PRACTICE PEARL**

Heating and cooling may affect recovery via different mechanisms. The choice of therapy should be targeted to both the type of exercise performed and the timing of the next training session or competition. If performance goals are short term (<48 hours), then recovery should be prioritised and cooling will likely be the preferred strategy.

## HYDROSTATIC PRESSURE

When an athlete is immersed in water, a compressive force is exerted on their body—this is referred to as hydrostatic pressure.[65] The degree of pressure exerted depends on immersion depth and, to a lesser extent, factors like atmospheric pressure and water density.[1, 65]

Hydrostatic pressure causes an upward and inward displacement of body fluid, aiding the return of fluid from the muscles to the blood.[65, 66] Central blood volume increases as a result,[67, 68] which in turn may improve diffusion gradients.[69]

When used in recovery from exercise, hydrostatic pressure may improve the transport of substrates and metabolites, as evidenced by faster blood lactate clearance following post-exercise water immersion.[70, 71] These benefits may be particularly favourable following exercise that severely depletes muscle energy stores and increases metabolic by-products, such as repeated high-intensity bouts.[65]

The shift of fluid from muscles to blood also reduces exercise-induced muscle oedema (which slows substrate transportation).[72] Reduced muscle oedema can assist nutrient delivery and aid muscle function and repair.[65] The benefits associated with hydrostatic pressure from water immersion also occur without a compensatory increase in heart rate or energy expenditure, as would be expected with low-intensity active recovery.[71, 73]

Another potential benefit of increased hydrostatic pressure during recovery is the feeling of buoyancy. When immersed in water, the body receives an upward thrust proportional to the immersion depth.[65] This net upward force makes the body buoyant, which may reduce the athlete's perception of fatigue.

Immersion in water may conserve energy required by gravitational and postural muscles,[65] reduce neuromuscular signal magnitudes[74] and modify peripheral processes associated with muscle contraction[75]—all factors that may aid recovery.

## COMPRESSION

Compression is traditionally used in medicine to treat circulatory pathologies, including lymphoedema, pulmonary embolism and deep vein thrombosis.[76] More recently, athletes have used compression to try to accelerate recovery after exercise. The rationale is that compression improves venous return and reduces exercise-induced swelling and inflammation.

The primary mechanism by which compression improves post-exercise recovery is an improvement in venous return. The external pressure applied to the limb causes a mechanical reduction in vein diameter and subsequent improvement in valve competence,[77, 78] mimicking the muscle pump action. This diverts blood from superficial veins to deep veins, which increases deep venous velocity, reduces venous pooling and improves venous return.[77, 79, 80]

From a recovery perspective, increased venous blood flow may accelerate the removal of myofibrillar proteins and metabolic by-products from the exercised muscle. This is evidenced by lower concentrations of plasma creatine kinase and lactate dehydrogenase when compression garments are worn after exercise.[81-84] Compression garments worn

**TABLE 16.1**   Practical issues to consider when using hydrostatic pressure and compression techniques

| Strategy | Practical considerations |
|---|---|
| Water immersion | • Athletes should opt for whole-body, "head out" water immersion where possible, maximising the hydrostatic pressure effects.<br>• Hydrostatic pressure decreases as temperature increases, meaning there will be a larger (but minimal) hydrostatic pressure as water temperature decreases. |
| Sports compression garments | • Encourage athletes to choose garments that cover and apply pressure to most of the exercised limb (e.g. full-length tights).<br>• There is no consensus regarding the best level of pressure for sports compression garments in recovery. The limited evidence suggests 15–20 mmHg at the thigh and calf, respectively. There are likely diminished returns as these values increase or decrease.<br>• The level of pressure applied varies considerably between garment brands, and given anthropometric differences between individuals, athletes are advised to ensure that the garments they use provide a positive pressure gradient (i.e. a decrease in pressure from distal to proximal) to reduce distal pooling of blood and fluids.<br>• Applying compression for up to 4 h after exercise appears to enhance recovery indices. This may help athletes who train multiple times in the same day (e.g. morning and evening sessions), or those in competition settings with minimal rest periods. |
| Pneumatic compression | • Evidence to support the use of intermittent pneumatic compression pumps for recovery purposes is limited.<br>• Preliminary evidence suggests that these devices can improve post-exercise blood flow and reduce swelling and soreness to about the same extent as compression garments.<br>• Because pneumatic compression pumps apply high pressure (70–110 mmHg), their effect can occur in a comparatively short period of time (30 min). |

during recovery may also reduce the risk of post-exercise hypotension, which can persist for several hours.[85]

In addition to venous return, compression increases arterial perfusion and subsequent muscle blood flow. Applying compression to an exercised limb will reduce arteriolar transmural pressure, subsequently resulting in reflex vasodilation of underlying arteries, reduced arterial flow resistance and increased arterial blood flow.[86]

Considering limb blood flow is a critical moderator of muscle regeneration,[87] compression-induced increases in muscle blood flow may aid in muscle recovery after exercise.[88] However, a recent meta-analysis suggests that the effect of compression is most evident during exercise itself—there were no benefits for the post-exercise recovery period.[77] Note that any improvements in arterial perfusion may be offset by a lower microvascular blood flow,[89] the site at which oxygen and nutrients, critical for muscle regeneration, are delivered.

Apart from alterations in blood flow itself, compression of an exercised limb during recovery also limits the space available for exercise-induced muscle oedema to form, in a similar fashion to mechanisms discussed above for hydrostatic pressure. For athletes recovering from exercise, compression-induced reductions in limb swelling will improve joint range of motion and alleviate muscle soreness, allowing them to recover faster and train sooner. Additionally, compression results in a shift of fluid from the exercised muscle back to the blood, thereby removing mediators of muscle inflammation and secondary muscle damage.[90, 91]

Lastly, compression may also aid recovery via psychological means, as compression garments have been reported to reduce feelings of fatigue and muscle soreness following exercise. A number of factors may explain the improvements in psychological variables in recovery, including a reduction in muscle swelling, inflammation and associated soreness.[92] Psychological wellbeing may also be a result of positive perceptions and belief in their efficacy; these are still benefits, nonetheless.

Table 16.1 outlines practical considerations regarding hydrostatic pressure and compression based on recovery strategy.

## NUTRITION

Nutrition is essential for complete recovery. Recovery eating and drinking should help meet the athlete's nutritional goals in terms of energy needs, desire to manipulate physique and overall requirements for nutrients. It should also be practical; for example, it should be affordable, fit in with the daily timetable and social commitments, and contain food and drinks that are acceptable and readily available.

### Replacing fluids

Substantial fluid loss should be replaced. The simplest way to determine the amount of fluid lost is by weighing the athlete pre- and post-event. Every 1 kg of weight loss equates to 1 L of fluid loss. The athlete should consume (via drinks and meals) water and sodium at a modest rate that minimises diuresis/urinary losses.[93]

> **PRACTICE PEARL**
>
> Because sweat and urine losses continue during the post-exercise phase, effective rehydration requires an intake of 125–150% of the final fluid deficit (e.g. 1.25–1.5 L fluid for every 1 kg of body weight lost).[94, 95]

Dietary sodium/sodium chloride (from food or fluids) helps to retain ingested fluids, especially extracellular fluids including plasma volume, so athletes should include sodium in their post-exercise nutrition. The optimal sodium level in a rehydration drink appears to be close to the sodium content of sweat[96] and may be as high as 50–80 mmol/L. This is higher than the sodium concentration of typical sports drinks and is close to the level found in oral rehydration solutions manufactured for the treatment of diarrhoea, but a growing number of sports electrolyte products, often in effervescent tablet form, are now commercially available with sodium concentrations in the 50 mmol/L range.

Fluids can be consumed with meals or snacks that include salt-rich foods (e.g. bread, breakfast cereals, crackers, cheese, preserved meats) or that have been seasoned with added salt. Milk is a better sports drink for rehydration than many commercial products because of its sodium content; it also contains protein and fat, which may aid fluid retention.[97, 98]

The beverage rehydration index (BHI)[99] classifies drinks based on the volume of urine produced 2 hours after drinking a product, expressed relative to regular still water. Most drinks including cola, tea, beer, orange juice and commercially available sports drinks are no different to regular still water; only oral rehydration solutions and milk (including skimmed milk) provide a greater BHI than water.

Alcohol is a diuretic, so consumption is discouraged in the recovery period. However, previous warnings about caffeine as a diuretic appear to be overstated when it is habitually consumed in moderate amounts (e.g. <180 mg = 1–2 standard brewed cups).[94] There is emerging evidence that low-/zero-alcohol beers, especially those with a higher sodium content, could provide a more socially acceptable rehydration option in some situations, with significantly enhanced net fluid balance compared with regular beer.[100]

The athlete should start to consume fluids on finishing activity and aim to consume the target volume over the next 2–4 hours. Spreading fluid intake over time promotes gastrointestinal comfort and maximises retention via smaller urine losses.[101] When the athlete's total energy needs are low, low-energy fluids such as water, low-energy soft drinks and mineral water are recommended. When energy needs are higher, fluids can be combined with other energy sources.

## Replacing fuel

Most athletes use carbohydrates as their major fuel supply, so glycogen restoration is often a goal of post-exercise recovery, particularly between two rounds of exercise when there is a priority for performance in the second session. Refuelling requires adequate carbohydrate intake and time. Provided that total energy intake is adequate,[102, 103] increasing carbohydrate intake increases muscle glycogen storage until an upper limit for glycogen synthesis is reached.[104] Current guidelines for post-exercise glycogen storage recognise a scaling of requirements according to the fuel cost of training or competition and the athlete's body size (Fig. 16.2).[105, 106]

The mean hourly rate of glycogen restoration is about 2% of the total glycogen capacity per hour and the maximum rate is around 5%. Thus, it can take approximately 24 hours to normalise stores after substantial levels of depletion.[101] During the 2–4-hour period after exercise, there is the potential for high rates of muscle glycogen storage as a result of depletion-activated stimulation of the glycogen synthase enzyme and exercise-induced increases in muscle membrane permeability and insulin sensitivity.[107]

This potential can be realised only if carbohydrates are consumed during this period; otherwise, refuelling rates are very low.[108] Indeed, following a simulated rugby game, simply delaying the first carbohydrate-based meal for 2 hours post-game significantly reduced muscle glycogen resynthesis 48 hours later,[109] which could affect future training and performance.

Meals and snacks can be chosen according to personal preference and timing of intake.[104, 105] The athlete should aim to consume recovery drinks, snacks or meals providing carbohydrate equal to approximately 1 g/kg/hour body mass for the first 4 hours post-exercise.

Over the last decade there has been growing interest in the source of carbohydrate consumed post-exercise to facilitate glycogen resynthesis. Consuming glucose with fructose may help the athlete to replace liver glycogen at a rate greater than 1.2 g/kg/hour in the post-exercise recovery window while minimising the risk of gastrointestinal distress.[110]

There is some evidence to suggest that carbohydrate consumed in the first few hours post-exercise should be from high glycaemic index (GI) sources due to greater muscle glycogen resynthesis over the following 24 hours compared with low GI foods.[111] High GI foods may be more

**B**

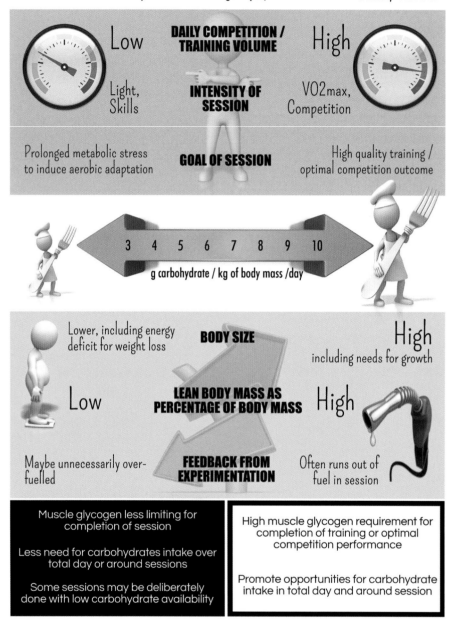

**Figure 16.2** An athlete's daily carbohydrate target will vary from day to day. The top (blue) panel highlights the major factors that determine carbohydrate targets in swimmers. The lower panel (orange) lists factors that will modify the target (think of a dimmer switch that provides fine control).

REPRODUCED WITH PERMISSION FROM DR YANN LE MEUR

**TABLE 16.2** Typical carbohydrate-based foods consumed post-exercise

The foods below are rarely eaten in isolation, and often athletes will achieve their carbohydrate goal through both eating and drinking

| Food | Volume required to provide 50 g carbohydrate | Approximate GI |
|---|---|---|
| Wholegrain bread | 3 × medium slices | 68 |
| White bread | 3 × medium slices | 100 |
| Banana | 2 × large | 57 |
| Spaghetti | 180 g | 68 |
| White rice | 160 g | 72 |
| Muesli | 70 g | 69 |
| Corn flakes | 60 g | 75 |
| Orange juice | 568 mL | 48 |
| Energy gel | 20–30 g per gel | Varies, typically high up to 100 |
| Chocolate muffin | 105 g (1 muffin) | 60 |

palatable post-exercise and include foods that the athlete restricted in the days prior to competition.

There does not appear to be any advantage in consuming the carbohydrate in either solid or liquid form[112] and so this should be left to the athlete's preference. In practice, a selection of high GI snacks and drinks should be available post-exercise (Table 16.2). A GI >70 is high; values of 56–69 are moderate.

## Repair

Exercise-induced muscle damage is a common consequence of exercise, especially if it involves a high number of eccentric contractions or a substantial increase in training load and/or intensity.[113, 114] Exercise-induced muscle damage often results in muscle soreness and impairments in muscle contractile activity that can last for several days. As a consequence, a key component is to introduce strategies that may attenuate muscle damage and increase recovery.[115]

Dietary protein is essential in the regulation of muscle protein synthesis and has therefore been the focus of attention regarding nutrition to facilitate muscle repair post-exercise. Although post-exercise protein is crucial to muscle adaptation, whether protein also reduces muscle damage and soreness is less clear.[114] Some studies have suggested that post-exercise protein can reduce muscle soreness,[116] while others have shown no benefit.[117]

The most relevant meta-analysis suggests that protein supplementation post-exercise, while increasing protein synthesis and intracellular signalling, does not result in measurable reductions in muscle soreness.[118] This is logical given the differing time course of muscle protein turnover (days) and muscle protein soreness (hours). Practically speaking though, even if protein does not help reduce muscle soreness, appropriate consumption of protein post-exercise is still essential for muscle adaptions and remodelling so it is crucial that protein is provided in the correct amount and at the correct time post-exercise.

There has been considerable debate on the theoretical maximal protein synthetic response to a resistance exercise bout. Early work suggested that an intake of 20–25 g of high-quality protein[119] or 0.3 g/kg body mass was needed to maximise muscle protein synthesis. This work was predominantly performed using isolated single-leg exercise. More recent studies suggest that this may be doubled to 40 g when whole-body exercise is performed.[120]

Excess protein stimulates increased rates of irreversible protein oxidation and may be considered wasteful,[119] although it is unlikely to be harmful[121] unless the excess protein is consumed to the detriment of other nutrients. The pattern of protein intake should probably involve a series of meals or snacks every 3–5 hours providing 20–40 g of protein rather than frequent consumption of smaller protein doses or infrequent meals with larger protein doses.[122] Consuming protein just before bedtime may be valuable because it can increase muscle protein synthesis at a time when it would otherwise be low.[123-25]

The important characteristics of protein-rich foods are its digestibility and its content of essential amino acids, especially leucine. High-quality protein-rich foods such as milk (or whey), eggs and meat are all associated with significant increases in muscle protein synthesis after exercise.[126, 127] Immediately after exercise at least, there is superior muscle protein synthesis with an intake of rapidly digested, or "fast", protein to provide a rapid rise in plasma leucine concentrations; this includes whey and liquid protein.[128]

There is growing interest in plant-based protein sources. Many plant-based proteins, especially when combined or eaten in slightly greater absolute amounts, provide comparable muscle protein synthesis to animal protein.[129] Researchers have tested this for protein from peas,[130] potatoes[131] and mycoprotein[132] (protein from fungus, technically not "plant").

Unlike carbohydrates, which appear to have an optimal post-exercise consumption window, protein has a longer lasting anabolic response period.[133] Nevertheless, it makes sense to start the recovery process immediately post-exercise if possible. Table 16.3 provides a list of protein-rich foods giving approximately 30 g of protein, an amount that would appear to be sufficient for most athletes post-exercise.

**TABLE 16.3** Protein-based foods that might be consumed post-exercise

| Food | Volume required to provide 30 g protein |
| --- | --- |
| Chicken satay skewers | 120 g |
| Chocolate milk | 650 mL |
| Typical protein shake | 1 serving |
| Salmon steak | 130 g |
| Greek yoghurt | 375 g |
| Eggs | 4–5 eggs |
| Beef fillet steak | 140 g |

### PRACTICE PEARL

Protein alone is insufficient for optimum recovery post-exercise—there is a strong scientific rationale to include carbohydrate as well as protein.[134]

A number of sports recovery drinks provide carbohydrates, protein and hydration in one convenient format. While most sports dietitians and nutritionists correctly adopt a food first philosophy, there are times when supplements may be convenient.[135] Many athletes find it difficult to eat post-exercise, especially on hot days; in such situations, sports supplements may be warranted rather

than not consuming anything. Any supplements should be from manufacturers that use third-party testing to check for supplement contamination. A food first option is chocolate milk: this excellent recovery drink combines carbohydrates and protein, while also helping with rehydration given its high ranking on the BHI.[136]

Aside from the key macronutrients, a growing number of functional foods have received attention due to their potential to assist in post-exercise muscle soreness and recovery. The most studied of these are Montmorency cherries, alongside other reported high-polyphenol foods.[137]

In many of these studies, polyphenols were removed from participants' diets prior to the trial. It may be that the addition of polyphenols could be most effective for athletes with diets lacking such foods, whereas athletes who consume them regularly do not gain the same benefit. For example, a rugby player fed a high polyphenol diet did not demonstrate any improved markers of recovery or inflammation following cherry juice supplements.[138]

### PRACTICE PEARL

Athletes should try to achieve a high polyphenol diet to aid recovery by consuming a diet rich in fruit and vegetables; where this is not possible, the use of specific polyphenol supplements could be explored.

Finally, it is important to mention vitamin D. Many athletes present with vitamin D deficiencies due to a lack of adequate sunlight exposure.[139] Vitamin D deficiencies can delay muscle repair.[140] It is crucial that athletes are checked for vitamin D deficiencies,[141] with target 25(OH)D concentrations of >75 nmol/L.

## MENTAL RECOVERY

Mental recovery is a facet of recovery that has gained recent scientific and practitioner attention. It is defined as the process of regaining allostatic balance and replenishing cognitive resources and capabilities through restorative processes.[142] It is important for practitioners to appreciate the enormous mental demands placed upon athletes during their daily training, competition and lifestyle practices. This generates the need for psychological recovery.[143]

Mental fatigue results in impairments in physical, psychological, tactical and technical aspects of performance.[144-146] Beyond the known performance impairments, elevated mental demands can also compromise subsequent physical recovery,[147] further supporting the need for athletes to prioritise mental recovery.

Athlete- and practitioner-identified sport-specific factors that contribute to mental fatigue include:[148]

- Changes in the immediate sporting environment, including exposure to scenarios where athletes may experience something for the first time or encounter a lack of stability in their immediate environment, resulting in a lack of comfort and consistency. This points to athletes prioritising mental recovery when travel is required for competition or training is undertaken away from a regular venue, such as away matches, major competitions or tours.[149]
- The professional aspects of sport, such as requirements from individual sponsors, commercial partnerships and interview commitments, as well as contract negotiations.
- Activities beyond direct athlete training and competition demands, such as external study or emotionally challenging work, driving or transportation between commitments under time pressure, and managing relationship dynamics.

Further contributors include over-analysis, information overload, a need for regular problem solving without clear outcomes, and lengthy team meetings.[149] Athletes also suffer mental fatigue if they constantly think about their sport and are unable to switch off.[148, 149] Combined, these perceptions identify numerous factors that contribute to the occurrence of mental fatigue and emphasise the importance of prioritising athlete mental recovery together with physical recovery.

Information regarding the specific time course of athlete mental fatigue is largely elusive. Laboratory evidence has traditionally investigated mental fatigue over an acute time course, but mental fatigue may remain elevated over an extended time course.[150] Athletes and support staff perceive mental fatigue in both an acute and cumulative manner.[148]

Evidence from athletes during pre-season, in-season and camp periods supports this, with reports of mental fatigue tending to fluctuate and accumulate when assessed over extended periods.[151-153] Accordingly, in addition to the rapid onset of mental fatigue, repetitive bouts of exposure without adequate prioritisation of mental recovery may lead to cumulative or sustained mental fatigue.

Following periods where cognitive and emotional demands are high, athletes may benefit from several mental recovery strategies that minimise the impact of mental fatigue on performance.[154] Since mental recovery is emerging as an area of importance, the evidence base for athlete-specific interventions is still developing.

However, research has explored mental recovery using exercise and sports-centric research designs to develop guidelines that may support the application of protocols to athletes. The enhancement of mental recovery for cognitive and emotional restoration includes interventions with a physiological, behavioural or psychological basis. Common strategies include:

- a power nap
- systematic breathing intervention
- listening to binaural beats
- exposure to naturally restorative environments (either physically or virtually)
- mental imagery and detachment and exposure to odours.

Such interventions should be applied considering the source of mental demand and any situational factors including the timing of subsequent training or competition. For example, it may be appropriate to place increased emphasis on mental recovery during congested fixture periods.

As with all recovery, athlete preference and beliefs may play a role in the efficacy of the chosen strategies.[155] Individual athletes vary greatly in both susceptibility to feeling mental fatigue and subsequent impact on performance.[156, 157] Mental recovery strategies may be most effective when individualised to the specific sources of cognitive demand and chosen in accordance with athlete self-preference and beliefs. Facilitating athlete input and agency to select from the range of available evidence-based mental recovery strategies may provide additional benefit.

**PRACTICE PEARL**

Implementing effective mental recovery strategies provides a potential competitive advantage for athletes. Practitioners should be aware of the range of evidence-based strategies and apply these in an individualised manner (considering athlete preferences and beliefs).

Athletes and support staff perceive mental fatigue to negatively impact aspects of performance; conversely, practitioners perceive mental recovery as an opportunity to facilitate athlete performance in training and competition. Such perceptions include the athlete being better able to perform and having improved energy and mood; greater self-awareness and self-regulation; enhanced adaptation, learning and growth; and improved information-processing decision making, response time and skill execution.

Furthermore, perceptions of improved motivation and willingness to exert effort, and increased energy and athlete freshness have been reported. Despite this, empirical evidence indicates that a large percentage of practitioners do not deliberately manage mental fatigue in their athletes. Approaches that are currently used by practitioners to manage mental recovery are indicated in Table 16.4.[158]

**TABLE 16.4**   Approaches used by practitioners to manage mental recovery in athletes

| Enhancement of mental recovery | Practitioner use: % (raw number) |
| --- | --- |
| Mindfulness | 13.4 (58) |
| Directing time away from daily training or competition environment | 12.4 (54) |
| Breathing techniques | 11.8 (51) |
| Debriefing | 11.8 (51) |
| Avoidance of social media | 9.4 (41) |
| Exposure to restorative environments | 8.3 (36) |
| Power naps | 8.1 (35) |
| Mental imagery | 6.5 (28) |
| Avoidance of media engagement | 5.8 (25) |
| Music—other | 4.1 (18) |
| Mental detachment | 3.9 (17) |
| Other | 2.3 (10) |
| Psychological techniques—other | 2.1 (9) |
| Music—binaural beats | 0.2 (1) |
| Transcranial direct current stimulation | 0.0 (0) |

Source: Adapted from Russell S, Johnston R, Stanimirovic R, Halson S. Global practitioner assessment and management of mental fatigue and mental recovery in high-performance sport: a need for evidence-based best-practice guidelines. *Scand J Med Sci Sports* 2023; 34(1) e14491.

## SLEEP

Sleep is increasingly recognised as the foundation of athlete recovery. This is based on the role that sleep plays in muscle repair, cognitive function, immune function, metabolism and mood.[159] Research in both Australian[160] and British[161] athletes suggests that athletes have less sleep than the general population—and athletes' sleep is of a lower quality.

There are differences in sleep duration between team and individual sport athletes: team sport athletes appear to sleep 30 minutes longer than individual sport athletes.[160] This may be due to the earlier training start times for individual sport athletes. Early morning start times compromise sleep, and inconsistent bed and wake times impair sleep quality.[162] Poor sleep in athletes may be sport-related (travel, late competition and training times), but many causes are behavioural and therefore give the practitioner an opportunity to see whether the athlete is open to trialling changes in sleep hygiene.

Other reasons for disturbed sleep include nervousness and stress around competition,[163] stress and anxiety from other sources such as team selection, sponsorship arrangements, work or school stress, and relationship issues. In addition, caffeine intake, muscle soreness, current injury, travel, jetlag, sleeping in foreign environments, social media and gaming are anecdotally reported to negatively affect an athlete's sleep if not managed appropriately.

### Managing sleep in athletes

Athletes aiming to improve their sleep quality and/or quantity may benefit from sleep monitoring, feedback and education. Figure 16.3 outlines a series of steps to identify poor sleepers and a process for feedback and education:

1. Using a questionnaire-based tool such as the Athlete Sleep Screening Questionnaire (ASSQ),[164] the Athlete Sleep Behaviour Questionnaire (ASBQ)[165] or the Pittsburgh Sleep Quality Index (PSQI)[166] can help quickly identify an athlete with sleep issues and potentially determine some of the reasons for poor sleep (i.e. behaviours that are not conducive to optimal sleep).

   The ASSQ and ASBQ were specifically developed for use in athletes. The ASSQ is typically used as a screening tool to determine which athletes require further intervention, while the ASBQ assesses behaviours that may disturb sleep. The PSQI is the most commonly used sleep questionnaire and provides a global sleep quality score as well as component scores that contribute to the global score (sleep duration, sleep disturbance, sleep latency, daytime dysfunction, sleep efficiency, overall sleep quality and sleep medication use).

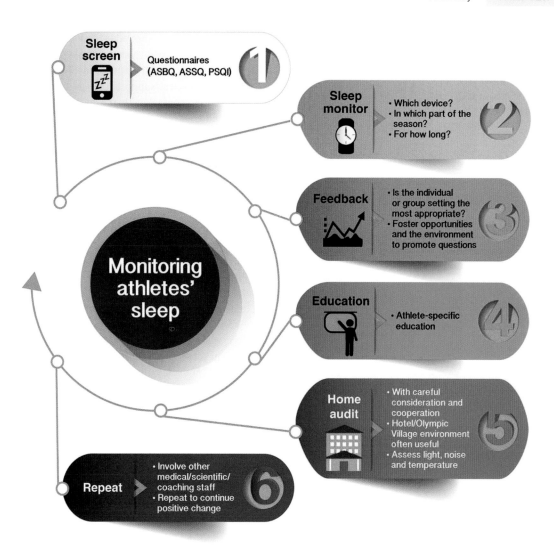

**Figure 16.3** Steps to identify poor sleepers and a process for feedback and education
ARTWORK BY VICKY EARLE. PHOTO CONTRIBUTOR: GREEN.SHUT/SHUTTERSTOCK

2. Monitoring sleep can provide objective data on a range of sleep characteristics including sleep onset latency (time taken to fall asleep), sleep efficiency (sleep quality), sleep onset time (bedtime), sleep offset time (wake time) and sleep duration as well as consistency of bed and wake times. Combined with a simple sleep diary that captures relevant information such as caffeine intake, smartphone/computer use prior to sleep and alertness upon waking, monitoring can provide invaluable information to an athlete to identify and target sleep concerns.

Identify a suitable monitoring device (e.g. Oura Ring), the duration of monitoring (a minimum of 2 weeks is ideal) and the relevant time period for monitoring during the training/competition season. Remember that with the proliferation of wearable devices and the substantial amount of data they collect, some athletes may not respond positively to, or may feel overwhelmed by, the amount of data provided by the device, especially in the absence of individual feedback and recommendations.

3. As with all forms of monitoring, relevant feedback should be timely and thoughtful. Focus on sleep concerns that can be practically addressed. Fostering an environment that is conducive to questioning and communication allows the athlete to answer relevant yet potentially personal questions regarding sleep habits and behaviours.

4. Sleep education sessions improve sleep and typically provide information regarding strategies to optimise sleep quantity, quality and timing as well as behaviours that may interfere with sleep (caffeine intake, smartphone/computer use, etc.). Providing education regarding the relationship between sleep and performance may also be useful to create long-term behaviour change.

**BOX 16.1** Practical tips for sleep

To assist with both the consistency and duration of sleep, athletes should:

- supplement with a daytime nap when there is insufficient opportunity for sleep at night (due to early-morning training or late-night competition); ideal nap times are between 1 and 4 pm and of 20–90 min in duration
- observe caffeine intake and its effects on night-time sleep, as individual responses to caffeine intake are highly variable; caffeine intake should ideally cease prior to 2 pm, but observing effects on the time taken to fall asleep and sleep quality are a priority
- ensure consistency of bed and wake times, and minimise very early-morning training start times
- avoid consuming alcohol prior to sleep and avoid using computer or smartphone screens in the hour before bed
- create an optimal sleep environment: a cool (approx. 19–21°C), dark and quiet bedroom is ideal; eye masks and ear plugs are useful for travel or when exposed to excess light/noise
- try not to force sleep; going to bed when sleepy is important and if periods of time are spent awake during the night, getting up and out of bed until sleepy is recommended.

5. Assessing the athlete's sleep environment in a "sleep audit" can aid in the identification of potential sleep disruptors such as light, noise and temperature. This can be particularly useful in an Olympic Village or longer-term accommodation facility. An audit of the athlete's home environment may also be useful, but of course must be conducted with the athlete's cooperation and support.

6. While monitoring and education can improve sleep, the athlete may need repeated messaging to ensure that positive changes are continued. Involving and educating other practitioners/support staff (particularly those with very regular contact with the athlete) can also aid in reinforcing messaging.

Box 16.1 offers some practical tips to help athletes with sleep.

## PRACTICAL STRATEGIES: PUTTING IT ALL TOGETHER

Recovery modalities are implemented to act across various physiological, biomechanical, neurological and psychological domains (Table 16.5), although athletes primarily report reducing muscle soreness as the main purpose of implementing recovery strategies.[167] While muscle soreness is unlikely to significantly impact athletic performance, excessive levels of muscle soreness may discourage athletes from engaging in further exercise or lead them to reduce the intensity in subsequent training sessions.[168]

Without implementing any recovery interventions, individuals will naturally recover at their own rate following exercise. However, the underlying theory behind using recovery interventions is that they have the potential to expedite this process.[169]

Incorporating different recovery strategies might permit an athlete to minimise muscle soreness and perceived fatigue and allow them to train and perform better. If a particular strategy alleviates muscle soreness, for example, this may allow the athlete to train sooner, with greater quality and/or with higher volume/intensity.

Unfortunately, athletes' perceptions of recovery methods often do not align with current scientific evidence[170] and, as such, they may overlook some of the well-established methods of recovery in favour of new or novel recovery

**TABLE 16.5** Overview of how recovery modalities may act on various domains

| Physiological | Biomechanical | Neurological | Psychological |
|---|---|---|---|
| • Improved blood flow<br>• Reduced heart rate<br>• Increased heart rate variability<br>• Decreased blood pressure<br>• Reduced skin and core body temperature<br>• Hormonal changes (e.g. reduced cortisol, increased growth hormone)<br>• Reduced oedema<br>• Improved removal of metabolic by-products | • Improved muscle-tendon compliance<br>• Improved limb/joint range of motion<br>• Restoration of isometric strength and peak torque<br>• Decreased active and passive stiffness<br>• Decreased tissue adhesion | • Reduced muscle tension and spasm<br>• Reduced neuromuscular excitability<br>• Reduced pain response | • Improved mood state<br>• Reduced anxiety<br>• Reduced feelings of fatigue<br>• Increased feelings of relaxation<br>• Decreased perceived muscle soreness |

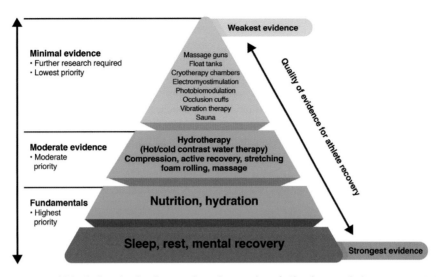

**Figure 16.4** Recovery pyramid, including the fundamentals and examples of other lower priority recovery strategies for athletes
ARTWORK BY VICKY EARLE. PHOTO CONTRIBUTOR: GREEN.SHUT/SHUTTERSTOCK

technologies. While research evidence is weak or sparse on many of the newer technologies like massage guns, occlusion cuffs, float tanks and pneumatic compression, there is a greater level of empirical support for some of the fundamental recovery strategies discussed in this chapter and their role in athletic recovery.

These fundamentals (Fig. 16.4) make a much greater overall contribution to athletic recovery and performance than any potential marginal improvements from devices/tools and must therefore be prioritised before considering further strategies or devices (referred to as moderate or minimal evidence strategies in Fig. 16.4).

The selection and application of recovery strategies throughout the training cycle are influenced by the preferences of both the coach and the athlete, as well as the desired physiological and psychological outcomes. Yet aside from cold water immersion, our understanding of prolonged use of recovery methods during extended periods of athletic training remains limited.

One recent comprehensive analysis of eight studies highlighted that consistent use of cold water immersion following resistance training could dampen the development of maximum strength, without affecting endurance exercise performance.[171] This finding underscores the need for a discerning approach to the use of cold water immersion, based on the training phase and objectives, which has been termed "recovery periodisation".[171]

Our knowledge of the chronic application of other recovery modalities, such as compression garments, saunas and cryotherapy chambers, and their potential to either help or hinder long-term physiological adaptations is currently limited. Despite the gaps in our knowledge, athletes should not be dissuaded from using recovery strategies that facilitate their continued training participation and, consequently, the stimulation of physiological adaptations. Table 16.6 outlines considerations for the timing of incorporating recovery strategies during different training phases.[172]

**TABLE 16.6** Suggestions for recovery strategies across training phases

| General preparation/pre-season | Specific preparation | Taper/pre-competition | Competition/major event |
|---|---|---|---|
| • Appropriate use of recovery strategies to maximise training adaptation and goals of general preparation/pre-season phase.<br>• May involve withholding recovery strategies (e.g. cold water immersion) to maximise adaptation (especially following resistance training). | • Recovery strategies after key sessions, particularly when subsequent sessions require high levels of skill and/or high-quality training.<br>• Recovery strategies may also be used to reduce fatigue and soreness in preparation for key sessions. | • Recovery strategies can be used to minimise fatigue. This may be useful to decrease the period of time required to taper effectively.<br>• Recovery strategies may be incorporated to maintain high-intensity training during this period. | • Recovery strategies can be used to minimise fatigue and maximise competition performance during a season or at a tournament/major event.<br>• Recovery strategies may help to manage fatigue around travel and jetlag. |

## CONCLUSION

We live in an age of significant growth in the array of recovery devices, technologies and strategies available to athletes. This growth is driven by athletes' pursuit of effective, time-saving and often portable methods to enhance their physical and psychological recovery post-training and competition. Social media has accelerated the popularity of new devices and strategies, and specialised "recovery centres" now cater to both athletes and the general public.

This rapid proliferation of options has made it challenging to assess the efficacy and potential risks of various strategies; there is limited published research on many of these techniques. Conversely, while research evidence is ideal, athletes and practitioners sometimes make informed decisions to adopt untested methods to stay ahead of the curve and gain a competitive edge.

Coaches and athletes frequently rely on their own intuition and past observations when employing recovery strategies.[173] In addition, preconceived notions, beliefs and expectations regarding recovery techniques can outweigh marginal recovery benefits[31] and should be factored into the decision-making process when selecting recovery strategies.

## KEY POINTS

- Cooling techniques offer analgesic benefits and have demonstrated effectiveness in reducing muscle fatigue and soreness, but may have no effect and may even compromise other important recovery aspects (e.g. glycogen and muscle protein synthesis).

- Heating techniques have potential for muscle conditioning but show less consistent effects on post-exercise (performance) recovery.

- Contrast therapy appears effective for reducing muscle soreness. The choice of recovery modality should align with specific recovery goals and individual variability.

- Compression and hydrostatic pressure may augment recovery due to changes in blood flow, as well as by reducing exercise-related swelling and inflammation.

- Nutrition is an essential part of recovery and tissue repair. There is a substantial body of evidence relating to fluid replacement and macronutrient intake. Nutrition plans need to be practical and affordable.

- Mental recovery should be prioritised to mitigate the potential negative effect of acute or cumulative mental fatigue on athletic performance. Mental fatigue may be induced by a range of factors, and it is recommended that management strategies be implemented in an individualised manner.

- Prioritising sleep is essential for athlete recovery. Practitioners should aim to identify behaviours that may interfere with sleep (e.g. caffeine) and strategies to protect sleep (i.e. delay early-morning training times).

- Fundamental recovery strategies (adequate sleep, rest, nutrition) should be prioritised before implementing any other recovery tools or techniques.

## REFERENCES

References for this chapter can be found at www.mhprofessional.com/CSM6e

## ADDITIONAL CONTENT

Scan here to access additional resources for this topic and more provided by the authors

# The clinical approach

# CHAPTER 17

# Preventing injury

with **CAROLYN EMERY, STEPHEN WEST, BEN CLARSEN** and **ROALD BAHR**

*Yes, I do play a contact sport, but I also feel I take more preventative measures than probably anybody in the world ... so I really don't have concerns.*

TOM BRADY (FORMER NFL PLAYER)

## CHAPTER OUTLINE

What has sport learned from injury-prevention science?
Reducing injury risk in your team
Sport policy and rules
Personal protective equipment
Embedding injury prevention in coach-led programs
The role of playing surfaces in injury prevention
Stretching

## LEARNING OBJECTIVES

By the end of this chapter you should be able to:

- differentiate between primary, secondary and tertiary prevention of sports injuries
- distinguish intrinsic from extrinsic and modifiable from non-modifiable risk factors
- list the five-step approach to reducing sports injury risk and explain each step
- cite examples of policies or rules that have reduced sport-related injuries or illness
- summarise the available evidence for personal protective equipment in sport and its ability to mitigate injury risk
- discuss the elements of an effective neuromuscular training program
- construct a comprehensive, sport-specific, evidence-informed injury prevention strategy.

Prevention is the best medicine. Sports injury prevention keeps athletes healthy and enables them to perform better, because they don't miss training and competitions. It also promotes lifelong participation in sport and physical activity.

The remarkable growth in sports injury-prevention research since the turn of the century means that we can prevent many sports injuries, such as concussion, knee, ankle and hamstring injuries. These advances apply across the continuum from grassroots/participatory sport to elite level.

## WHAT HAS SPORT LEARNED FROM INJURY-PREVENTION SCIENCE?

Sports injury prevention crosses the continuum of primary, secondary and tertiary prevention. We use the term "prevention" synonymously with what is technically known as "primary prevention" (Fig. 17.1).[1] *Primary prevention* reduces the risk of injury in a healthy athlete population. The word "healthy"–treating all involved–is the key element of primary prevention. Examples include sport rule changes, personal protective equipment and training strategies. Do these approaches work? Yes, they can! We and others have shown the effectiveness of:

- disallowing body checking in adolescent ice hockey[2]
- wearing ankle braces to reduce the risk of ankle sprains[1]
- neuromuscular training warm-up strategies to reduce the risk of injuries in youth team sports.[3]

> **PRACTICE PEARL**
>
> The greatest impact in reducing the burden and consequences of sports injuries can be made through primary prevention strategies.

*Secondary prevention* focuses on preventing injuries in those at greater risk than the healthy athlete population. For example, secondary prevention of ankle sprains in a team setting focuses on athletes who have already had an ankle sprain (an intrinsic risk factor, see below) or who have other risk factors (e.g. early detection). We refer to this as part of treatment in *Clinical Sports Medicine* (e.g. early treatment of an ankle sprain, see Chapter 24). In this example, ankle treatment is both management and a form of secondary prevention.

*Tertiary prevention* focuses on rehabilitation to reduce the consequences of a sports-related injury. For example, anterior cruciate ligament (ACL) rupture is associated with post-traumatic osteoarthritis; tertiary prevention after ACL rupture focuses on high-value rehabilitation to minimise/delay the onset of osteoarthritis. We refer to this as rehabilitation (Chapter 27). In this case, rehabilitation is both management and a form of tertiary prevention.

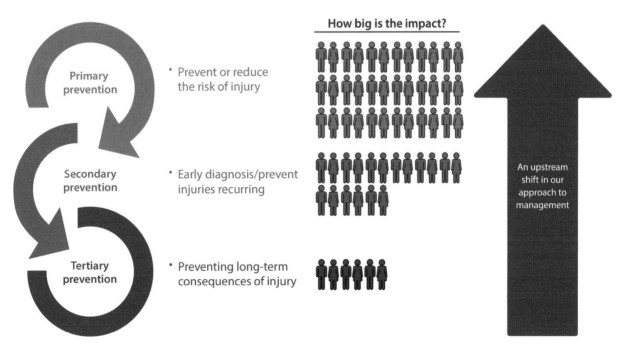

**Figure 17.1** Sports-related injury-prevention continuum: how the impact of primary, secondary and tertiary prevention compares. Outside of sports and exercise medicine, primary prevention includes public health measures such as clean water and vaccination programs.

## Risk factors: sport-related injuries are predictable and preventable

If you read widely, attend conferences or listen to podcasts, you might be familiar with the terms "intrinsic and extrinsic risk factors" and "modifiable and non-modifiable risk factors" and may prefer to skip this section. However, if you are new to this field these terms can seem confusing.

Think back to when injuries were thought of as essentially random "accidents". Persons A, C and L all had sporting accidents—an ankle sprain, a concussion and a ruptured knee ligament, respectively. They were just "unlucky". Fast forward, and we know now that certain factors may predispose individuals to ankle sprain, concussion and ligament sprain; for example, poor ankle proprioception, having had a previous concussion and having a family history of knee ligament rupture, respectively. Let's call them "risk factors".

### Intrinsic risk factors

Examples of intrinsic risk factors include:

- Poor ankle proprioception, having had a previous concussion and having a family history of knee ligament rupture are all examples of *intrinsic risk factors,* linked to the individual athlete. If an individual has several intrinsic risk factors, they are at more risk than if they only have one. Other examples of intrinsic risk factors include age, maturation, biological sex, body composition and fitness level. Here you can see the move away from an "unlucky" person to the concept of an "at-risk" person.
- Note that *previous injury* is an important risk factor regardless of the injury type. For example, previous dislocation is a risk factor for shoulder dislocation.
- Intrinsic risk factors can be modifiable and non-modifiable, and both are relevant to sports injuries:
  - *Modifiable risk factors* (e.g. muscle weakness) can be targeted (e.g. specific muscle training).
  - *Non-modifiable risk factors* (e.g. sex in the case of ACL injury) can be addressed indirectly. Female athletes can be offered a preventive exercise program that mitigates their increased risk of ACL injury without changing their sex.

### Extrinsic risk factors

Now consider three different "accidental" injuries: an ankle sprain when sliding to make a base in baseball, a concussion from an elbow to the head in a football heading duel, and a knee ligament injury when a player's boot got stuck on the playing surface. Were they just "unlucky" players? Victims of random events? No—external or *extrinsic risk factors* contributed to those injuries. Other examples of extrinsic risk factors include interactions with the environment such as floor friction in indoor team sports, snow conditions in alpine skiing, a slippery surface on a running track or very cold weather.

We now know that controlling extrinsic risk factors—making bases slide, awarding automatic red cards for elbow contact with the head and considering how a player's boots interact with variable surfaces—reduces injuries. We can't prevent all injuries, but we can reduce their incidence and severity.

Note that risk factors—both intrinsic (e.g. muscle strength, balance) and extrinsic (e.g. rules of the sport, helmet fit)—are not usually static and may change with time, even during one training session (e.g. due to fatigue).

## Connecting the dots: a basic injury-prevention model

Experts love models as they can depict a lot of information (and wisdom) visually.[4] A good model can make concepts gel. In Figure 17.2 we share Professor Winne Meeuwisse's models[5] of how intrinsic risk factors increase an athlete's risk—those factors *predispose* the person to injury. If there are also extrinsic risk factors this adds risk, which Dr Meeuwisse called "susceptible", but it's really just more risk. In this model we highlight previous injury within our examples of intrinsic risk factors because it's such a fundamental risk factor.

## The inciting event

The final catalyst for an injury, the injury mechanism in lay language, is known as the inciting event (Fig. 17.3). "Incite" has Latin roots of rousing and prompting, which seems apt. Just as forensic engineers seek clues when a plane crashes, injury researchers scrutinise events immediately before an injury (e.g. playing situation, player and opponent behaviour) and the forces that resulted at the time of injury (Chapter 12).[4]

If you think of shoulder dislocation, the typical inciting event is a fall on an outstretched and externally rotated arm. More complex mechanisms precede ACL injuries in soccer—at least four different mechanisms have been reported.[6–8] There are patterns of inciting events but they vary by injury type, sport (ACL injuries occur differently in skiing and soccer), age group and gender.

Researchers try to identify the key inciting event with the aim of changing the injury pathway. Clinicians are very aware of inciting event patterns as it helps them with diagnosis (e.g. a fall on an outstretched hand can lead to wrist extension

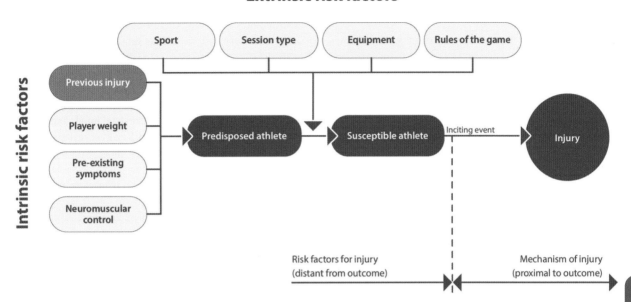

**Figure 17.2** Intrinsic risk factors (left) predispose an athlete to injury. Extrinsic risk factors (top) make an athlete even more predisposed ("susceptible") to injury. The inciting event is the event that triggers the injury.
Source: Adapted from Bahr R, Krosshaug T. Understanding injury mechanisms: a key component of preventing injuries in sport. *Br J Sports Med* 2005;39(6):324–9; and Meeuwisse WH, Tyreman H, Hagel B, et al. A dynamic model of etiology in sport injury: the recursive nature of risk and causation. *Clin J Sport Med* 2007;17(3):215–19. © 2007 BMJ Publishing Group Ltd & British Association of Sport and Exercise Medicine. All rights reserved.

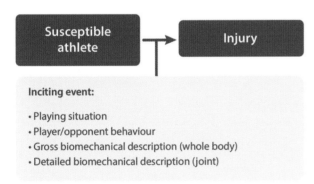

**Figure 17.3** Factors that contribute to the inciting event. In acute injuries the inciting event happens very close to the time of injury, whereas in overuse injuries the inciting event can precede the onset of pain by weeks or months.
Source: Adapted from Bahr R, Krosshaug T. Understanding injury mechanisms: a key component of preventing injuries in sport. *Br J Sports Med* 2005;39(6):324–9. © 2005 BMJ Publishing Group Ltd & British Association of Sport and Exercise Medicine. All rights reserved.

injuries, including a scaphoid fracture). Note the emphasis to date on acute/traumatic injuries (Chapter 8).

For overuse or gradual-onset injuries (e.g. bone stress injury, tendinopathy), the inciting event may occur well beforehand. For example, for a long-distance runner who sustains a stress fracture, the inciting event won't be the training session when they first felt pain, but their training and competition load over the previous weeks or months (Chapter 15).

## REDUCING INJURY RISK IN YOUR TEAM

As a clinician, you can benefit from the substantial knowledge of how to prevent injuries. You are way ahead of those who were trying to prevent injuries 20 or even 10 years ago.

We suggest the four key questions you need to ask yourself are:

1. What are the most common injuries?
2. Who is at increased risk?
3. Why are they at increased risk?
4. How do injuries typically occur?

When caring for a group of athletes such as a rugby team or an alpine skiing team, you can answer these questions (and then intervene) using a five-step approach to mitigate injury risk:[9]

1. Review the literature: what are the typical injury patterns for the sport, gender and age group specifically?
2. Develop an injury surveillance program where you work: record injury and participation data.

3. Perform a season analysis: look at the players'/team risk profile across the training and competition program (season plus).
4. Complete a periodic health assessment (Chapter 18): map current problems and intrinsic and extrinsic risk factors to inform individual and team-based training strategies (e.g. neuromuscular training, load management, personal protective equipment, shoe type, environmental factors).
5. Develop, implement and evaluate a targeted and/ or multifaceted injury-prevention program: based on the intrinsic and extrinsic modifiable risk factors identified and using injury surveillance, video analysis and wearable technologies to ideally evaluate targeted prevention strategies.

## 1. Review the literature

Each sport has a specific injury pattern. For example, "tennis elbow", "runner's knee" and "jumper's knee" got their names from the sports in which they were prevalent. For most sports, there are ample data in the literature to identify and assess the risks. When considering risk, you should also take factors such as gender, age and level (i.e. recreational vs professional) into account. Injury risk is not only related to injury frequency—you must also consider injury severity.

Injury data can be illustrated by a risk matrix that highlights risk in terms of injury likelihood and injury consequences.[10] We illustrate a risk matrix in Figure 17.4. Men's rugby injury data have been plotted on a y-axis of injury severity and an x-axis of injury incidence. Note that elbow and upper limb (shoulder) injuries cause mean absences of more than 40 days.

The injury with the greatest incidence, not surprisingly, was hamstring strain (x-axis). The green, amber and red regions of the matrix reflect the product (multiplication) of injury incidence and severity (burden; units are days absent per 1000 player-hours). The injuries with the highest burden

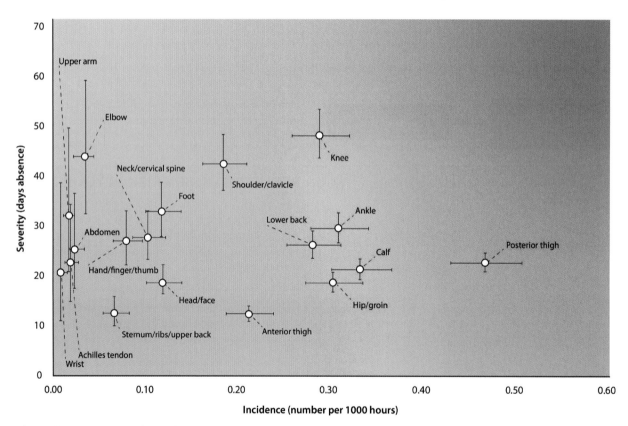

**Figure 17.4** A risk matrix for professional men's rugby illustrating the relationship between injury severity (consequence) and injury incidence (likelihood). The vertical and horizontal error bars represent 95% CIs. The red zone reflects the greatest severity and incidence (injury burden).

Source: Data from West SW, Williams S, Kemp SPT, et al. Patterns of training volume and injury risk in elite rugby union: an analysis of 1.5 million hours of training exposure over eleven seasons. *J Sports Sci* 2020;38(3):238–47.

are in the top-right quadrant (i.e. red)—in this case, knee and posterior thigh injuries have a similarly high burden of injury, even though one is associated with greater severity and the other with greater incidence.

## 2. Develop an injury surveillance program

One of our goals is to encourage you to monitor both *injuries* and *exposure* to assess risk in your own setting.

### Recording injuries

For medical staff, recording injuries is a relatively easy task as they are required to keep accurate records of all assessments and treatments provided to patients. Thus, establishing a surveillance system often involves analysing information that has already been captured. However, the commercial tools to do this are not ideal. The best examples are taking place in research settings.

Injury and illness surveillance definitions and data elements already exist. These are based on the International Olympic Committee Consensus Statement: Methods for Recording and Reporting of Epidemiological Data on Injury and Illness in Sport 2020.[11] Using this as a guide, you can compare data across sports and sports contexts internationally.

This foundational document is deliberately sport-agnostic—it is designed to work for all sports. It has been extended on by papers that provide more detailed advice in other sports (e.g. tennis, soccer).[12] There is a specific publication addressing special considerations for injury and illness surveillance for women and girls.[13]

### Recording individual player's training and competition hours (exposure)

This is a challenge for the medical team since they are not always present during practice or on road trips and the recording is done by other team personnel (e.g. strength and conditioning coach). Many injury-recording software programs record exposure data, which can then be entered based on the coaching records. Exposure data are essential as you need to calculate injury rates (e.g. number of injuries/1000 athlete competition-hours, number of injuries/1000 athlete practice-hours).

The standard method for reporting injury incidence rates typically used in team sports is the number of time-loss injuries per 1000 hours of exposure (e.g. games, practices). For some sports and specific player positions such as a baseball pitcher, injuries per 1000 pitches may be a more appropriate measure.

It may also be relevant to record exposure in relation to extrinsic risk factors, such as turf type (e.g. training on grass, gravel, artificial turf), use of personal protective equipment and whether the exposure happens during competition or training. Injury data are very difficult to interpret unless exposure data are collected. Consider as an example an increase of 30% in the number of match injuries from one season to the next. If the number of matches also increased by 30%, there is no increase in the injury incidence rate.

### What about overuse injuries?

A limitation with standard methods of injury registration (counting) is that they historically underestimate the gradual onset of overuse injuries. Symptoms such as pain and functional limitation often appear gradually and may be transient in nature. Therefore, athletes will continue to train and compete despite the presence of a gradual-onset injury, at least in the early phase. It's the same for minor illnesses such as the common cold. Many health problems, especially gradual-onset problems, do not lead to time loss from sport and are therefore not recorded in standard injury surveillance systems.[14]

Sports physiotherapist Dr Ben Clarsen and colleagues addressed this problem by developing the Oslo Sports Trauma Research Center (OSTRC) questionnaire/app on health problems (Table 17.1).[15-17] Rather than waiting for players to present to the medical team with injuries, the questionnaire/app enables engagement with athletes. The clinical team can therefore monitor all illnesses and injuries, not just those leading to time lost from sport (Box 17.1). This is useful across sports settings but particularly so for sports where overuse injuries and illnesses dominate.

## 3. Perform a season analysis

One helpful method to manage risk in sports is a pre-season review of the planned training and competition program to identify risks. The method of season analysis is therefore fundamentally different from injury surveillance, where data on injuries are collected as they happen. Season analysis represents an attempt to identify risks before they occur. Risks in the program can be related to the competition schedule, the training program, the possibilities for athlete recovery, travel or other issues.

The analysis is based on the idea that the risk of injuries is greater during transitional periods and that each stage has certain characteristics that may increase risk. Examples are when athletes switch from one training surface to another (e.g. from grass to artificial turf) or to new types of training (e.g. at the start of a strength training period).

## BOX 17.1 A questionnaire/app to capture health problems in real time

The OSTRC questionnaire on health problems is sent to athletes once a week to record the consequences of illnesses and injuries, including those that do not lead to time lost from sport.[17] It is generally delivered to athletes as an electronic questionnaire on their phone. The app directs athletes only to relevant questions, based on their responses.

The questionnaire begins with four key questions that all athletes should answer (Table 17.1). A health problem is defined as "any condition that you consider to be a reduction in your normal state of full health, irrespective of its consequences on your sports participation or performance, or whether you have sought medical attention". If athletes indicate a health problem in any

**TABLE 17.1    Updated Oslo Sports Trauma Research Center questionnaire on health problems (OSTRC-H2)**

Please answer all questions, regardless of whether you have experienced health problems in the past 7 days. Select the option that is most appropriate for you; if you are unsure, try to answer as best you can.

A health problem is any condition that you consider to be a reduction in your normal state of full health, irrespective of its consequences on your sports participation or performance, or whether you have sought medical attention. It may include injury, illness, pain or mental health conditions.

If you have several health problems, please begin by recording your worst problem in the past 7 days. You will have an opportunity to register other problems at the end of the questionnaire.

**Question 1—Participation**

Have you had any difficulties participating in normal training and competition due to injury, illness or other health problems during the past 7 days?

a. Full participation without health problems (0) ☐

b. Full participation, but with a health problem (8) ☐

c. Reduced participation due to a health problem (17) ☐

d. Could not participate due to a health problem (25) ☐

**Question 2—Modified training/competition**

To what extent have you modified your training or competition due to injury, illness or other health problems during the past 7 days?

a. No modification (0) ☐

b. To a minor extent (8) ☐

c. To a moderate extent (17) ☐

d. To a major extent (25) ☐

**Question 3—Performance**

To what extent has injury, illness or other health problems affected your performance during the past 7 days?

a. No effect (0) ☐

b. To a minor extent (8) ☐

c. To a moderate extent (17) ☐

d. To a major extent (25) ☐

**Question 4—Symptoms**

To what extent have you experienced symptoms/health complaints during the past 7 days?

a. No symptoms/health complaints (0) ☐

b. To a mild extent (8) ☐

c. To a moderate extent (17) ☐

d. To a severe extent (25) ☐

Source: Clarsen B, Bahr R, Myklebust G, et al. Improved reporting of overuse injuries and health problems in sport: an update of the Oslo Sport Trauma Research Center questionnaire. *Br J Sports Med* 2020;54(7):390–6. © 2020 BMJ Publishing Group Ltd & British Association of Sport and Exercise Medicine. All rights reserved.

question (i.e. any response except the minimum value), they are then asked:

- whether they are referring to an illness or an injury
- to provide the location (for injuries) or the symptoms (for illnesses)
- to indicate the number of days of time loss the problem has caused in the past week
- whether they have received medical attention for the problem
- whether they have any other health problems (in which case the questionnaire starts again).

In some teams and organisations, this weekly questionnaire is an important connection between athletes and clinicians, particularly when athletes are geographically dispersed and/or have inconsistent contact with their team's medical staff. In these cases, it may be useful to add extra questions such as "Who knows about this problem?" and "Do you have any comments for your team medical staff?"

The severity of each reported problem is rated using the scoring system shown in Table 17.1. The scores for questions 1–4 provide a severity score out of 100. This score is tracked over time to reflect the effect of the problem and how it is fluctuating. Figure 17.5(a) shows the severity score (y-axis) over time (x-axis) for one athlete's injuries. Summary data for the entire team can be collected. Figure 17.5(b) depicts the prevalence of injuries, not the individual severity score. Figure 17.5(c) is a screenshot of how one of the questions appears for the athlete.

You can listen to a masterclass on everything in this box. Dr Ben Clarsen from the Oslo Sports Trauma Research Centre speaks to *Clinical Sports Medicine* author Dr Liam West:

Dr Ben Clarsen and Dr Liam West walk you through Box 17.1 in a 20-min podcast

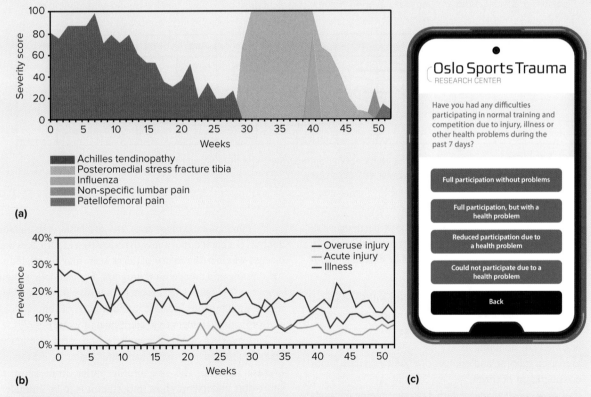

**Figure 17.5** Example data from injury surveillance using the OSTRC questionnaire on health problems. (a) Individual severity data (y-axis) from an athlete who reported five separate health problems during the past year (see legend); remember the y-axis depicts the severity of each problem on a scale from 0 to 100 based on the sum of the responses to each problem. (b) Data from a team of athletes showing the proportion of athletes reporting any health problem each week during the past year (prevalence of overuse injury, acute injury, illness). (c) How one of the questions appears for the athlete.
COURTESY OF THE OSLO SPORTS TRAUMA RESEARCH CENTER

**BOX 17.2** An example risk profile for a college basketball team

Risk profiling (Fig. 17.6) works best when the clinical team truly engages with coaches and players. Including them allows you to draw on their past experiences with the team; this is especially important if there are no injury surveillance data available from the past. Coaches and players are key for interventions—implementing preventive measures.

### Risks 1–8

1. Change in time zone, off-court training surface, climate and altitude during training camp in Colorado. Emphasis on defensive stance training and quick lateral movements could lead to several groin injuries. Players should not increase the amount or intensity of training too much.
2. Transition to greater amount of on-court training and intensity, combined with several practice games. Floor surface quite hard. Risk of lower limb injuries such as Achilles tendinopathy, medial tibial stress syndrome.
3. New training camp before beginning the competitive season; practice games on unusually slippery courts.

Training and practice matches are intense as players try to avoid being cut from the squad.

4. Beginning of the competitive season. A higher tempo and packed competitive schedule to which the player is unaccustomed. Risk of gradual-onset injury (e.g. patellar tendinopathy, tibial stress fracture) compounded by heavy academic periods (e.g. exams) leads to additional fatigue.
5. High risk of acute injuries during the competitive season, and a tough competition schedule at full intensity.
6. Interposed period of hard basic training with strength exercises to which the player is not accustomed and plyometric training increases risk of tendinopathy and muscle strain.
7. The end of the competitive season. Worn out and tired players? This is an important time to aggressively treat low-level "grumbling" injuries. Waiting for the injury to heal with rest alone is not recommended.
8. Transition to basic training period with running on trails.

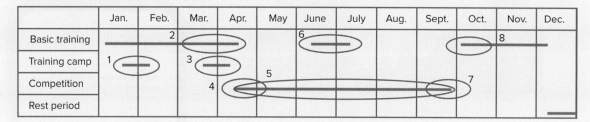

**Figure 17.6** One way of depicting the elements of training (rows) and the rhythm of the season (months/columns). The circles represent the injury risks outlined in this box.

Box 17.2 outlines how a team may be at particular risk of different types of injury at various stages of the season. Other examples of key events that could be correlated with increased injury risk include:

- poor sleep due to a tight schedule or time differences
- changeover from heavy pre-season training to competition
- return to sport after mid-season pause
- beginning of final rounds
- increased training and competition load associated with consideration of travel
- change of coach/manager with different training methods
- change in training volume
- change of climate (e.g. moving from a training camp in a warm climate to a colder climate)
- selection time for important matches (e.g. representative schedule—an athlete may hide early symptoms of an injury, thinking this may prevent selection).

If injury surveillance data are available, the season analysis is a great opportunity to review past experiences and discuss whether the injury patterns seen may be related to the training and competition program. For example, a surge in hamstring injuries in a soccer team may have coincided with a simultaneous increase in the volume of running load and/or tactical changes (e.g. additional pressing).

This type of analysis can help you plan preventive measures and it may have particular value in preventing overuse injuries. The risk profile varies from sport to sport—this underscores how important it is to be intimately familiar with the sport you cover.

## 4. Complete a periodic health assessment

Periodic health assessments (PHAs) are routinely performed on hundreds of thousands of athletes around the world every year; in some cases, this is required by sports regulations or even by law. The value of doing routine physical examinations on athletes is questionable.

**PRACTICE PEARL**

If periodic health assessments are done properly, they can represent a key ingredient in the risk management program. If done simply to clear athletes for participation, their value in injury prevention is limited.

In Chapter 18, we discuss the many potential objectives of performing a PHA. In this chapter we focus on two goals:

1. identifying current injuries, illnesses and chronic medical conditions
2. identifying factors that increase risk of future injury or illness.

The PHA has long been considered as a pre-participation or pre-season examination but this is not ideal. It is better performed at the end of the season, when there is still sufficient time to treat and rehabilitate ongoing problems and to work on correcting risk factors.

*Current injuries:* The high-value PHA should be tailored to your sport. Focus on conditions that are particularly prevalent (e.g. low back problems in rowers, eating disorders among female gymnasts, reduced pulmonary function among cross-country skiers), or where the physical requirements of the sport imply a higher risk of certain conditions (e.g. Marfan syndrome among basketball or volleyball players).

*Risk factors:* To identify risk factors to predict future injury requires two steps:

1. identify athletes with risk factors relevant to the sport in question
2. have a plan to follow up with athletes and mitigate risk if risk factors are identified.

### Identify athlete risk factors

Sadly, few PHAs are designed with real focus on the sport in question. In most team settings, the same screening examination is used across sports. This is inappropriate as injury patterns and risk factors differ among sports. To design a screening program for a particular sport, you need to define the main injury types and their risk factors.

Once you have defined the key risk factors, you need to select appropriate methods to screen for these factors. Screening methods should be valid, accurate, sensitive and specific.

A valid testing method measures the factor you wish to measure (e.g. if low hamstring strength is a risk factor for muscle strain, what method should be used to measure this

best?) An accurate (reliable) test yields the same result each time. Finding valid and accurate tests to measure relevant risk factors is difficult.

Predicting who may be at increased risk of injury is nearly impossible.[18] A testing method with high sensitivity will identify all players with increased risk. A test with high specificity will identify only players with increased risk (Chapter 21). Few, if any, tests can clearly distinguish between athletes with high and low risk of a sports injury. Therefore, you should interpret screening tests with caution.

**PRACTICE PEARL**

No test has high enough sensitivity *and* specificity to predict future injury.

### Plan to follow up risk factors

If a player's strength is inadequate, you need to follow up with a strength training program. If a player's balance is poor, a training program should rectify this. This might be done on an individual level, but in the absence of predictive screening tests, a team approach is more appropriate. As an example, in a team of female soccer players, preventive training programs to protect the knees should be offered to all players, not limited to players identified as being at risk on a screening test or those who have had previous ACL injuries.

## 5. Develop, implement and evaluate a targeted and/or multifaceted injury-prevention program

The final step in the risk management process is to take a broad view of the risks to the team and individual athletes and to plan. The injuries (and illnesses) to be targeted can be identified from the risk matrix, scientific literature and team injury surveillance data from past seasons. The season analysis may have identified specific risks associated with the training and competition program. Finally, the specific injury and risk profile for each athlete is mapped through the PHA.

Based on this assessment, you can construct a prevention program. A multifaceted program should target the risks that you have identified as being important for the team and individual athletes. You cannot implement a prevention program alone; however, you need to consider all stakeholders responsible for athlete sport safety. Figure 17.7 illustrates an ecological model based on an example of youth team handball.[19, 20] Note that there are barriers and facilitators to injury prevention among stakeholders at multiple levels.[19, 20]

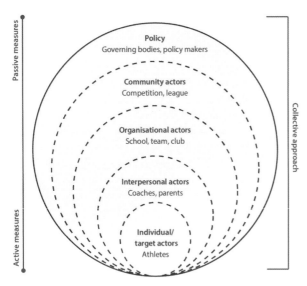

**Figure 17.7** An ecological model defining a responsibility hierarchy in preventing injuries in youth sport. The lowest level of responsibility is assigned to the child (player) and highest level to organisations with the potential to affect the most.
Source: Ageberg E, Bunke S, Lucander K, et al. Facilitators to support the implementation of injury prevention training in youth handball: a concept mapping approach. *Scand J Med Sci Sports* 2019;29(2):275–85.

## SPORT POLICY AND RULES

One impactful strategy to reduce injury rates in sport is through policy, rule or law changes. In this section, we illustrate how rule changes in several sports have led to fewer injuries. We also share how policy changes could be used to introduce full contact (e.g. body checking, tackling), argue that early sport specialisation is harmful and introduce the concept of bio-banding to reduce injury.

### Body checking policy in ice hockey

In ice hockey, body checking is an attempt by a player to gain an advantage over their opponent with deliberate use of the body. The burden of body checking-related injuries and concussions was found to be high at the grassroots (adolescent) level. Injury rates were three times higher and concussion rates four times higher in the leagues for 11–12-year-olds that allowed body checking compared with those that didn't.[21]

Informed by this evidence, policy makers in Canada (2013) and the US (2011) prohibited body checking in games in the leagues for 11–12-year-olds nationally. Injury and concussion rates fell by more than 50% in the leagues for 11–12-year-olds and also in the leagues for non-elite 13–17-year-olds where the rule had been introduced. This prevents more than 10,000 injuries annually in Canada alone.[22-25] When data across all studies of leagues

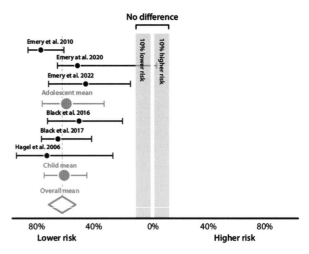

**Figure 17.8** The concussion rate is much lower in youth ice hockey when body checking is disallowed. The original studies are in black and the subgroup means are in light green. The combined point estimate for all studies is the open diamond.
Source: Data from Eliason PH, Galarneau JM, Kolstad AT, et al. Prevention strategies and modifiable risk factors for sport-related concussions and head impacts: a systematic review and meta-analysis. *Br J Sports Med* 2023;57(12):749–61.

that disallow body checking in youth ice hockey were combined, the concussion rate was 58% lower in leagues that disallowed body checking compared with leagues that permitted it (Fig. 17.8).[26]

Does eradicating body checking mean that players are more vulnerable to injuries when they progress to older age-group leagues (where body checking is part of the game)? No! The number of years of body checking experience in games in younger age groups was not associated with higher concussion rates in the leagues for elite 13–17-year-olds.[25, 26]

These impressive results are being considered by other contact sports (e.g. tackle football, rugby union, lacrosse). Rules that sports are considering include:

- setting a standardised age to introduce the tackle (e.g. football, rugby union) or body checking (e.g. lacrosse)
- limiting game-related tackling at younger ages
- introducing mandatory tackle training programs
- changing policies on the height of the tackle
- reducing full-contact practices.

### Preventing tackle injuries in rugby
#### with STEPHEN WEST and ISLA SHILL

World Rugby is working hard to minimise injuries and concussions through a number of measures, including (1) policy changes to lower the legal maximum height of the tackle and (2) education to support improved tackle technique and proficiency within the sport.

World Rugby recommends that irrespective of the level of player or previous player experience, tackling and contact should be introduced gradually with a focus on both the player making the tackle (tackler) and the player in possession of the ball (ball carrier). During its Tackle Ready program, over a number of weeks players (1) learn the correct technique, (2) refine their technical proficiency, (3) train so that they can follow this technique even while fatigued, (4) improve the quality of their skill and (5) learn to reproduce this skill numerous times in a game.

World Rugby Tackle Ready program

## Preventing concussion in youth American football

In youth American football, strategies to reduce head contacts and concussion in practices include:

- reduced number of contact practices
- reduced intensity of contact in practices
- restricted collision time in practices
- partial equipment practices (no helmets, no shoulder pads).

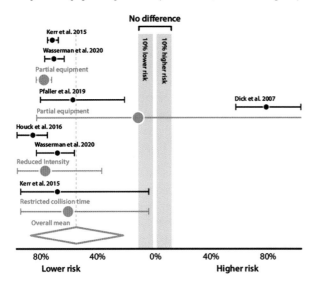

**Figure 17.9** Concussion rates are lower when teams implement strategies to reduce head contacts in practices in youth American football (compared with rates in teams that use no such strategies). The original studies are in black and the subgroup means are in light green.
Source: Data from Eliason PH, Galarneau JM, Kolstad AT, et al. (2023). Prevention strategies and modifiable risk factors for sport-related concussions and head impacts: a systematic review and meta-analysis. *Br J Sports Med* 2023;57(12):749–61. © 2023 BMJ Publishing Group Ltd & British Association of Sport and Exercise Medicine. All rights reserved.

The effectiveness of these programs has been measured through video analysis and/or wearable technologies (e.g. instrumented mouthguards):[2,27,28] combined, these interventions have lowered concussions by 62% (Fig. 17.9).[2]

> **PRACTICE PEARL**
>
> Clinicians can ensure that coaches know about strategies to reduce head contact and concussion in sport.

## Preventing knee ligament injuries in Australian Rules Football

The Australian Football League (AFL) had a high rate of posterior cruciate ligament injuries among ruckmen due to high-velocity collisions between players at starts in play (called centre bounces).[29,30] A simple rule change at the start of the 2005 season, limiting the run-up of the ruckmen, reduced the incidence of these injuries from 13 per 10,000 player-hours and 5.6 ruck injuries per 10,000 centre bounces in the six seasons prior to the rule change to 6 PCL injuries per 10,000 player-hours and 0.9 ruck injuries per 10,000 centre bounces in four seasons following the rule change.[31]

## Early specialisation in youth sport
### with CHRIS WHATMAN

Sport specialisation is intentional and focused participation in a single sport for the majority of a year that restricts opportunities for engagement in other sports and activities.[32] Sport specialisation and its repetitive, high-volume homogenous loads appear to increase injury risk.[33] Sport specialisation also reduces range of motor skill development.[34] The most common age-based threshold for defining early sport specialisation is before the age of 12;[35] many authorities advise delaying specialisation until the age of 16 or after the adolescent growth spurt.[34,36] This reflects a healthy focus on long-term development rather than short-term success.[33]

You can gauge the level of sport specialisation by asking three simple questions of a young person:

1. Can you choose one main sport that is more important than others?
2. Do you train/compete in one sport for more than 8 months of the year?
3. Have you quit all other sports to focus on your main sport?[37]

A young person who answers "yes" to all three questions is considered highly specialised and this should raise concern, especially if they have a pre-existing injury.

The athlete can reduce their injury risk by:

- taking breaks from the sport to avoid training or playing more hours per week than their age in years, more than 5 days in a week and more than 8 months in a year[38]
- modifying training to incorporate a wide range of movement challenges.

Parents can also be involved in explaining the benefits of the athlete participating in more than one sport and enjoying non-sport-related activities (including free play).[39] Importantly, early specialisation is not a requirement to attain high-level performance as an adult in most sports and may in fact be detrimental.[40,41] Although in certain cases injury risk may not be increased in highly specialised youth athletes, this is likely to be in settings (such as a sports academy) where highly trained practitioners provide an environment that mitigates negative consequences.[42] There are usually no highly trained practitioners in community sports settings led by volunteers. You thus have an important role to play in educating adolescent athletes and their families about the value of physical activity and sport.

## Bio-banding to reduce injuries
### with SEAN CUMMING

Bio-banding is the process of grouping athletes using biological rather than chronological age to mitigate the risk of growth-related injuries in young athletes.[43] The strategy is based on two premises about children: (1) they demonstrate marked differences in the age and rate at which they grow and mature, and (2) they are more susceptible to specific types of injury at different stages of maturity (i.e. pre-, circa-, post-puberty).

The incidence of growth-related and overuse injuries (e.g. Sever's, Osgood-Schlatter, Sinding-Larsen) peaks during the adolescent growth spurt and the burden of growth-related injuries is greatest in those athletes who grow the most rapidly during adolescence.[44] Also, the higher incidence of ACL injuries in female athletes emerges at the onset of puberty—a time when females gain strength and improve functional capacity. The incidence of muscle- and joint/tendon-related injuries in young athletes tends to increase after the growth spurt.[44]

By regularly assessing and monitoring growth, maturation and injuries, it is possible to group athletes by their developmental status. This process can be applied in training and competition and used to identify athletes at particular risk of specific types of injury and it can also be used to modify training load. The modified training focuses on movement competency, core and lower body strength, mobility, balance, coordination and lower load/intensity.[45,46] Using this approach, Bath University's Dr David Johnson and colleagues[47] reduced injury incidence and burden among English professional academy soccer players identified as experiencing the adolescent growth spurt.

Bio-banding may also reduce injury risk in competition, especially in collision and combat sports. Grouping athletes based on age and weight is accepted in combat sports and practised in some collision sports (e.g. American football, rugby), although this tends to be the exception rather than the rule.

Although there is limited evidence to suggest that smaller players are at greater risk of injury, the absence of an effect is potentially a result of differences in exposure (i.e. smaller players being less likely to play important roles). Children of the same chronological age can vary by as much as 5–6 years in skeletal age; weight differences of more than 70 kg have been reported between players competing within the same age grade in French academy rugby. If you are aware of the potential benefits of bio-banding, you can advocate for sport-specific recommendations.

## PERSONAL PROTECTIVE EQUIPMENT
### with ASH KOLSTAD

Personal protective equipment can prevent injuries in sport. This prevention strategy is relatively cheap by high-income country standards and doesn't require system-level support, unlike policy and training strategies. However, it is limited by the individual's attitude to wearing the equipment. In this section, we review the current evidence for the use of personal protective equipment in preventing injuries.

### Mouthguards

The use of mouthguards began in boxing in the 1890s.[48] Evidence across various sports (e.g. ice hockey, tackle football) indicates that wearing a mouthguard lowers the risk of both dental and orofacial injuries by 57%.[49]

Does wearing a mouthguard reduce concussion rates?[50] Three mechanisms have been proposed. It is plausible that wearing a mouthguard:

1. activates the player's neck and orofacial musculature when clenching to hold the mouthguard and this steadies the player's head
2. increases the space between the temporomandibular joint. which may dissipate force transmitted from the jaw up to the brain
3. provides shock absorption to protect against blows to the lower jaw.

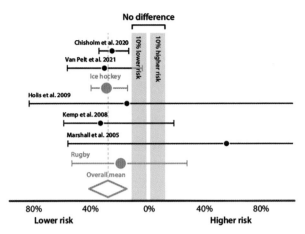

**Figure 17.10** Concussion rates are lower in ice hockey and rugby players who wear a mouthguard compared with those players who don't. The original studies are in black and the subgroup means are in light green.

Source: Data from Eliason PH, Galarneau JM, Kolstad AT, et al. (2023). Prevention strategies and modifiable risk factors for sport-related concussions and head impacts: a systematic review and meta-analysis. *Br J Sports Med* 2023;57(12):749–61. © 2023 BMJ Publishing Group Ltd & British Association of Sport and Exercise Medicine. All rights reserved.

In ice hockey, players who wear a mouthguard have a 28% lower concussion risk than those who don't (Fig. 17.10); however, results are inconclusive in other sports (e.g. rugby, basketball).[51] There is no evidence that wearing a mouthguard at the time of concussion affects the severity[52,53] of the concussion.

How does an athlete choose a mouthguard (Fig. 17.11)? What advice can you give? Mouthguards are either store-bought (e.g. no dental form-fitting, boil-and-bite/partial dental form-fitting) or custom-fitted by a dentist (perfect dental form-fitting). Evidence of the effectiveness of store-bought versus customised fit is largely mixed, so the decision which to choose should be based on the individual's price range, appeal and overall comfort.[2]

## Rigid helmets and soft-shell padded headgear

Rigid helmets are mandatory in sports such as motor racing, motor cycling, cycling, ice hockey, horse riding and American football. Wearing a helmet is effective in reducing head injuries in many settings. For example, wearing a helmet while recreationally cycling and skiing/snowboarding has reduced head injuries by 51% and 35%, respectively.[54,55]

Cricket batters face bowlers whose short-pitched deliveries rear at their heads at speeds greater than 140 km/hr. Helmets were only introduced to cricket in the 1970s and since then helmet design has advanced significantly

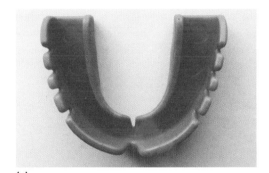

(a)

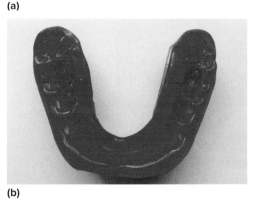

(b)

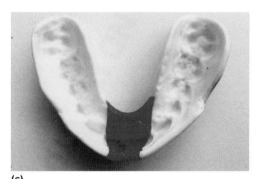

(c)

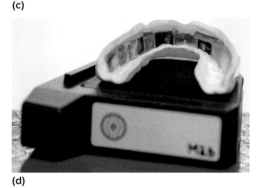

(d)

**Figure 17.11** Mouthguards: (a) stock mouth guard, (b) mouth-formed guard, (c) custom-made mouthguard, (d) instrumented mouthguard—note the embedded sensors that measure linear and angular kinematics of the head. They provide head impact data in possible concussive events.

**The evolution of protective headgear**

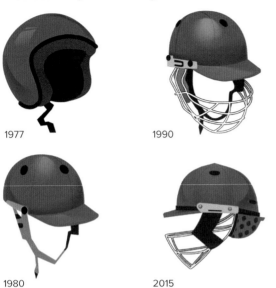

1977                1990

1980                2015

**Figure 17.12** Evolution of cricket helmets with protective face grille (1990 onwards) and more recently the addition of a wedge-shaped neck protector at the rear

(Fig. 17.12). In many countries it is compulsory to wear a helmet while batting, wicketkeeping up at the stumps and fielding close to the bat. Since the introduction of helmets, serious head injuries have virtually disappeared from cricket.

Interestingly, the frequency of batters being hit on the helmet nowadays is much higher than the relatively rare cases of batters being hit in the head in pre-helmet-wearing days. As a result, the incidence of concussion in cricket has increased in recent years.

Following the tragic death in 2014 of Australian batter Phil Hughes, who was struck in the neck and sustained a vertebral artery dissection, neck protection has been added to helmet design either as a separate guard or by extending the grill to cover the neck.

Poor helmet fit undercuts its protective value. In both youth ice hockey and high-school level American football, a properly fitted helmet has been shown to mitigate concussion risk and severity.[56] Note, though, that 80% of elite youth ice hockey players and 60% of youth football players have a poor-fitting helmet, commonly with a loose chin strap or chin piece (Fig. 17.13).

In sports where rigid helmets are not allowed, such as rugby and Australian Rules Football, some players use soft-shell padded headgear in the hope of preventing injury. The current evidence is mixed: wearing such headgear does not lower the risk of concussion in rugby but it may protect against scalp and ear lacerations;[57] on the other hand, in soccer and female lacrosse the concussion rate is lower using such headgear (Fig. 17.14).[2]

Much of the concern regarding the wearing of soft-shell padded headgear relates to the theory that the player may be "risk compensate" (feel invincible) while wearing it.[58] According to this theory, the "compensating" athlete responds to the false sense of security by engaging in more aggressive play and tackling harder.[58] This theory is entirely based on subjective self-reports.[59, 60]

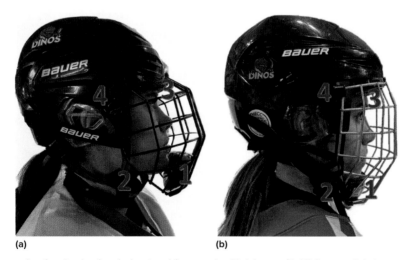

(a)                                    (b)

**Figure 17.13** An example of an ice hockey helmet and facemask with (a) poor fit: (1) facemask is loose on chin/cage hang, (2) chin strap >2.5 cm between strap and chin, (3) <2.5 cm between front of helmet shell and eyebrows (4) cage is loose against "J-clips"; and (b) good fit: (1) facemask is snug on chin, (2) 2.5 cm between chin strap and chin, (3) 5 cm between front of helmet shell and eyebrows, (4) cage is snug against "J-clips".
COURTESY OF ASHLEY KOLSTAD

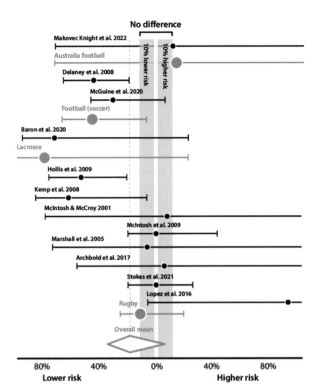

**Figure 17.14** The current evidence for soft-shell padded headgear use and concussion. Original studies are followed by subgroup point estimates.
Source: Data from Eliason PH, Galarneau JM, Kolstad AT, et al. (2023). Prevention strategies and modifiable risk factors for sport-related concussions and head impacts: a systematic review and meta-analysis. *Br J Sports Med* 2023;57(12):749–61. © 2023 BMJ Publishing Group Ltd & British Association of Sport and Exercise Medicine. All rights reserved.

## Prophylactic knee bracing

In recent decades, prophylactic use of knee braces in contact sport has increased, particularly in American football (linemen) (Fig. 17.15). Preventing medial collateral ligament and ACL sprains is the primary focus of implementing team- or position-wide rules that mandate the use of a knee brace, typically a double-hinged upright brace. These braces are costly and may cause skin irritation and other physical discomfort. The proposed mechanism of their action is to restrict range of motion at the knee, which has the potential to also limit sport performance.

The evidence for their effectiveness is largely mixed, inconclusive and subject to the limitations of many other injury-prevention strategies.[61,62] Observational data from the field lack controls and controlled laboratory studies lack real-world sporting conditions. In laboratory studies, knee braces reduce strain on the knee ligaments[63] and reduce frontal plane loading. Whether these findings translate to a decrease in serious knee injuries is unknown.

A recent low-quality retrospective cohort study[64] comparing professional footballers who did and did not

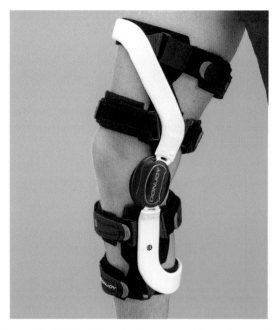

**Figure 17.15** Does knee bracing prevent knee ligament injury in American football? The jury is still out: it's a challenging question to study.
IMAGE COURTESY OF PARIS EVERYBODY. PHOTOGRAPHER RYLAND HAGGIS

wear prophylactic knee braces demonstrated a significant protective effect of these braces in terms of medial collateral ligament injury, but the quality of evidence is low. A player considering whether or not to adopt prophylactic knee braces as an injury-prevention strategy should consider cost, maintenance and possible impacts on performance alongside their personal preference.

## Ankle braces and taping

Ankle braces have been proven in randomised trials to reduce ankle sprains by 50–60%, particularly in athletes with a previous history of ankle sprain.[65,66] Taping has not been studied in such trials, but experts assume that tape has similar effectiveness. Ankle braces do not lose their ability to restrict inversion with time, whereas newly applied taping restricts inversion but the tape "loosens up" after several activity cycles. Braces and tape enhance proprioception[67] in addition to limiting ankle movement directly.

Other factors such as cost and skin care also affect a player's choice between tape and orthoses. Two myths can busted here:

- Does wearing an ankle orthosis increase the incidence of knee injuries? No.
- Do semi-rigid orthoses significantly impair athletic performance? This is difficult to study as performance has many domains, but no researchers have been able to show such impairment, so the answer is no.[68,69]

After an ankle sprain, the risk of injury is increased several-fold[70] and there is strong evidence that taping or bracing should be recommended for a period of up to 12 months (Fig. 17.16). Note that the preventive effect of taping or bracing is limited to players with previous injury, where proprioceptive function is reduced.[71-74] There are many different commercially available ankle supports. The equally important role of neuromuscular training for ankle sprains is discussed in Chapter 30 of *Managing Injuries*.

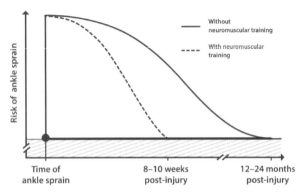

**Figure 17.16** The immediate effect of tape to prevent further ankle sprains. More risk is shown on the y-axis. Using a brace/tape keeps the risk line (red) at the baseline level.

## EMBEDDING INJURY PREVENTION IN COACH-LED PROGRAMS
### with BROOKE PATERSON and ISLA SHILL

For more than 20 years, warm-up programs that include aerobic, balance, strength and agility components have reduced lower extremity and specifically ACL injuries by more than 30%.[75] More recent programs have reduced upper limb injuries[76, 77] and there are ongoing studies aimed at reducing concussion rates in certain settings.

Thus, coach-led training strategies have the potential to reduce the rate of all injuries. Marshall and colleagues have demonstrated healthcare cost savings[78] in a range of team sports, community and school settings, and across different levels of play.

A non-exhaustive list of injury-prevention programs is shown in Table 17.2. They have common training elements including aerobic, agility (e.g. change of direction and deceleration, jumping and landing, high-speed run throughs), balance (e.g. single leg balance, dynamic balance) and eccentric strength (e.g. Nordic hamstring, lunges) exercises. Most of the programs aim to incorporate these elements within sport-specific skills[79-81] (i.e. partner ball exercises in ball sports). In sports such as rugby (see Activate program in Table 17.2), exercises that stabilise the head on the neck have been included to prevent concussion.[82] The listed programs are evidence-informed and were co-designed with community sport partners and/or coaches and/or athletes.

> **PRACTICE PEARL**
>
> Take-home message for coach-led prevention programs:
>
> - do something that's evidence-informed
> - incorporate into the warm-up and other training sessions
> - combine with education (practical coach training, athlete education)
> - try to provide players with technical feedback (peer-to-peer learning).

**TABLE 17.2** Sports and their evidence-informed injury-prevention programs

| Sport with QR code for the program | |
| --- | --- |
| **American football**<br><br>SHRed Injuries Football | **Australian Rules Football**<br><br>Footy First (men)* |
| **Basketball**<br><br>SHRed Injuries Basketball** | Prep to Play (women)**<br>(Box 17.3) |

## Sport with QR code for the program

### Gaelic football

GAA15

### General jumping, cutting and pivoting sports, and school sports

GET SET App

Prevent Injury Enhance Performance*

Harmonknee*

Sportsmetrics*

ISprint*

### Netball

The KNEE program

Netball Smart

### Handball and floorball

Knakontroll (and soccer, see below)*

### Hockey

Warm up Hockey (WUP)

SHRed Injuries Field Hockey**

SHRed Injuries Ice Hockey/ Ringette**

### Rugby

Activate*

SHRed Injuries Rugby**

Rugby Smart NZ

### Touch football

TouchFit

*continues*

| Sport with QR code for the program | | | |
|---|---|---|---|
| **Soccer** | | | |
| 11+* | | SHRed Injuries Soccer** (Box 17.4) | |
| 11+ Kids | | Knakontroll (soccer and handball)* | |
| Perform+ | | **Volleyball** | |
| | | VolleyVeilig** | |

*Injury prevention effect has been evaluated but not necessarily via randomised trials
**Injury prevention effect under investigation

---

**BOX 17.3** The Prep to Play warm-up program

Prep to Play was developed as a collaborative project between the Australian Football League and La Trobe University (Fig. 17.17).[83, 84] It includes the best available evidence at the time, as well as expert opinions from coaches, players and clinicians. The aim was to provide structure, guidance, education and resources for clubs as they were empowered to develop their existing programs. The Prep to Play program is informed by previous research designed to reduce the risk of injuries and enhance performance.

 Prep to Play manual

 Prep to Play instructional videos

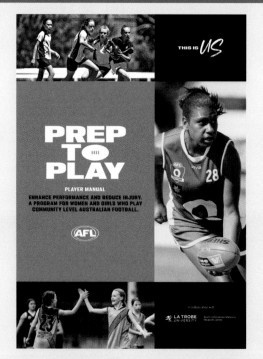

**Figure 17.17** Prep to Play is a coach-led program for women and girls who play Australian football at the community level

**BOX 17.4** The SHRed Injuries Soccer warm-up program

The SHRed Injuries Soccer warm-up program was developed based on several evidence-informed programs. One of them was a cluster randomised controlled trial undertaken in youth soccer in Canada.[85] The updated SHRed program provides different strength exercises, multiple progressions for each exercise, and drills incorporating a ball target concussion-specific prevention opportunities.

The program was developed with input from physiotherapists, technical coaches, strength and conditioning coaches, researchers and soccer players. It is designed to be completed in 10–12 minutes at the beginning of every practice and game (Fig. 17.18).

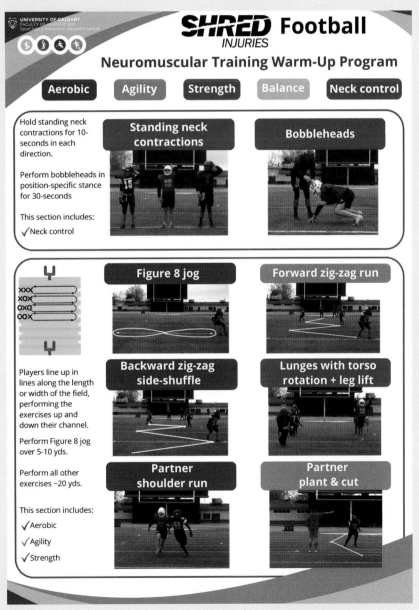

**Figure 17.18** The SHRed warm-up program for soccer includes a neck strengthening program (to prevent concussion) as well as aerobic training, strength training and neuromuscular training

IMAGE COURTESY OF DR CAROLYN EMERY

# THE ROLE OF PLAYING SURFACES IN INJURY PREVENTION

## with ATHOL THOMSON

In recent years, there has been increased interest in the role of playing surfaces in sports injuries. Researchers emphasise that when players obtain high (rotational) friction at the foot–surface interface, they feel that their performance increases–they can run faster and better change direction. Surface hardness also improves player speed, but harder surfaces are associated with a greater risk of lower limb injury.

Grass has entered the lexicon of professional football players as they try to match their footwear with the nature of the grass they play on. Grass isn't a uniform surface–different types of grass have different properties regarding traction and hardness. Although there are devices to measure rotational traction and hardness, many players use their experience and "feel" to test out which boots to wear on a field. This speaks to the importance of awareness that grass is a variable surface both at one venue and across venues. Many "grass" pitches are now hybrid–the natural grass is augmented by artificial polypropylene fibres (Fig. 17.19).

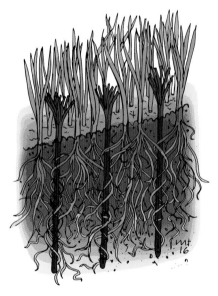

**Figure 17.19** Hybrid playing surfaces are those where natural grass has been reinforced with artificial fibres. It is created by a large, portable sewing machine stitching polypropylene fibres deep into the rootzone of the natural grass surface to provide an anchor for the natural grass roots to grow around.

ARTWORK BY THE LATE MICHAEL TODD AND IVAN STANKOVIC; REPRODUCED WITH THE PERMISSION OF THE ARTIST'S FAMILY AND THE *ASPETAR SPORTS MEDICINE JOURNAL*

## Does artificial turf carry a greater injury risk than natural grass?

The conclusion from a series of recent publications comparing injuries that various players sustained on third-generation turf and on natural grass is that:

- the rate of foot and ankle injuries is higher on artificial turf compared with natural grass[86, 87]
- the rates of (all) knee and hip injuries are essentially similar between playing surfaces.[86, 87]

However, in three studies of elite American football players, knee injury rates were higher on new-generation turf.[86] Similarly, Xiao[88] in subgroup analysis showed that the incidence of ACL injuries for female players in soccer matches on artificial turf was 1.2 times higher than that on natural grass.

With respect to sports-related concussion, Dr Paul Eliason and colleagues' meta-analysis combined estimates from nine studies. They found 40% lower concussion rates (CI:0.47–0.76) when matches were played on artificial turf compared with natural grass.[2]

## STRETCHING

Stretching is widely used before exercise to improve performance and/or prevent injury. Of the two types of stretching (dynamic and static; Box 17.5), static stretching has historically been the preferred method. Static stretching improves flexibility, but evidence for its impact on both performance and injury prevention is not strong.[89] As a result, static stretching is no longer widely used.

---

**BOX 17.5** Types of stretching

- Static stretching involves holding muscles in an elongated position. It is generally advised to hold the stretch for 30 seconds and repeat 2–3 times.
- Dynamic stretching involves active, repetitive controlled movement through a joint's range of motion.

---

The paradigm shift to dynamic stretching may be attributed to its improving athletes' range of movement, with a lack of negative or perhaps even positive effects on performance. Although very little research has investigated the effects of dynamic stretching, there is extensive evidence showing the positive injury attenuation effects of activity programs incorporating dynamic stretching and dynamic activity (e.g. FIFA 11+).[90] In sport, dynamic stretching is widely used as part of the warm-up, but further research is needed to determine whether it reduces injury and/or improves performance.

## KEY POINTS

- Primary prevention aims to reduce injury risk in healthy athletes; secondary prevention aims to reduce the risk of injury in high-risk athletes; tertiary prevention focuses on efforts to minimise or prevent the consequences of an injury after it has occurred.

- Intrinsic risk factors (e.g. biological sex) are related to the characteristics innate to an athlete, while extrinsic risk factors (e.g. environment) are external to the athlete. Modifiable risk factors (e.g. fitness level) are more easily targeted than non-modifiable risk factors (e.g. age).

- The first step in approaching injury risk reduction is conducting a review of the literature to identify risks inherent to the sport, gender or age group with which you are working.

- An injury surveillance program, which records exposure and injury/illness data, can help monitor trends in illness and injury. Consider outcome measures aside from just time loss from sport. The Oslo Sports Trauma Research Center questionnaire on health problems can be a helpful surveillance tool.

- Conducting a season analysis may help identify periods of heightened risk throughout the season (e.g. high schedule density, periods of transition), informing injury prevention efforts.

- The value of a periodic health assessment depends on how and when it is conducted, its specificity to the target population, and the extent to which the medical staff can and will follow up on flagged risks.

- There are currently no tests with both high sensitivity and high specificity in predicting a future sports injury.

- Sport-related policies/rules are one of our most effective tools in preventing sports injuries.

- Rules addressing body checking (ice hockey) and collisions resulting in head impact (American football) have effectively reduced sport-related concussions.

- In youth sport, rules that introduce bio-banding or address early sport specialisation have the ability to reduce sport-related injuries.

- Education and training in proper tackling have the potential to decrease injuries in collision sports.

- Personal protective equipment plays a role in reducing sports injuries. Helmets are effective in reducing skull injuries and associated lacerations. Mouthguards can prevent dental and facial injuries. The effects of helmets and mouthguards on concussion are less conclusive.

- Ankle taping and bracing seem to provide a protective effect on the recurrence of lateral ankle sprains. This seems to occur via improved proprioception, rather than purely mechanical support.

- Neuromuscular training programs, typically targeting the lower body, are effective in preventing lower body injuries. The goal is to ingrain safe movement patterns and avoid positions of vulnerability.

## REFERENCES

References for this chapter can be found at www.mhprofessional.com/CSM6e

## ADDITIONAL CONTENT

Scan here to access additional resources for this topic and more provided by the authors

## CHAPTER 18

# Periodic health assessment of athletes

with STEPHEN TARGETT, BEN CLARSEN and DUSTIN NABHAN

*Cardiac arrest can happen at any time.*

AMERICAN RED CROSS

## CHAPTER OUTLINE

Why perform the health assessment?
Who to assess
When to perform a PHA
What to include in the template
Other things to consider

## LEARNING OBJECTIVES

By the end of this chapter you should be able to:

- list the components and goals of the periodic health assessment (PHA)
- discuss the pros and cons of screening as part of the PHA
- identify available resources and templates for creating or implementing the PHA in sport practice
- detail how the principles of early disease detection apply in the sport setting
- explain why there is considerable variation in the PHA across sport, and why no single template will serve all athletes
- summarise the medico-legal considerations in the PHA.

Sport and exercise clinicians commonly perform standardised health evaluations of athletes and many different organisations around the world require that athletes undergo a pre-participation evaluation to be allowed to participate in sport. However, organisations rarely provide guidance regarding the content of the required evaluation, and the effectiveness of the approach in reducing the risk of injury, illness or sudden death in athletes remains controversial.

There are many different templates available for this evaluation, such as the FIFA pre-competition medical assessment (PCMA),[1] the IOC periodic health examination (PHE)[2] and the American Academy of Pediatrics (AAP) pre-participation physical evaluation (PPE).[3] It should be emphasised, however, that each of these is designed for different target groups and there is no one universal template that suits all situations.

In this chapter, we use the term "periodic health assessment (PHA)" to refer to the standardised health assessment of athletes, without being specific to any group's recommended template. The development of a template for the PHA of an athlete, whether elite or recreational, requires careful planning and gives an opportunity for all members of the sports medicine team and coaching staff to work in collaboration. Establishing the optimum template for each situation can be achieved by considering the following questions in turn:

- Why perform the health assessment?
- Who is being assessed?
- When and where should the assessment be performed, and by whom?
- What should be included in the assessment?
- Are there any other issues to consider?

## WHY PERFORM THE HEALTH ASSESSMENT?

The first step in planning a PHA template is to determine why you are performing the health assessment. The primary goal of the PHA is to make participation in sport safer, but there are a number of other valid reasons for wanting to perform a PHA such as assessing the status of known injuries and illnesses, screening for risk factors, reviewing medications and supplements, baseline testing, athlete education and establishing rapport with athletes (Table 18.1).

**TABLE 18.1    Objectives of the PHA**

| | |
|---|---|
| Current symptomatic health problems | • Determine general physical and psychological health |
| | • Determine eligibility for sport participation |
| | • Ensure current health problems are managed appropriately |
| Occult health problems | • Screen for silent medical conditions, with an emphasis on identifying conditions associated with sudden cardiac death |
| Risk factor identification | • Identify risk factors for future injury |
| | • Introduce prevention strategies for athletes at risk |
| | • Document and review the past medical history |
| Performance | • Identify barriers to performance |
| | • Undertake performance analysis in sport science disciplines (nutrition, biomechanics, physiology, psychology) |
| Baseline data collection | • Collect baseline data to use as a diagnostic tool in the event of future injury |
| | • Collect baseline data to use as a benchmark for return-to-sport decision making in the event of future injury |
| Education and relationships | • Develop relationships between athletes and medical staff |
| | • Serve as a portal of entry into the healthcare system |
| | • Provide education on health topics and available resources |
| Medico-legal and anti-doping | • Satisfy requirements of sport federations, local government and regional standards of care for periodic screening of athletes/employees |
| | • Review medications and vaccination history for medical and anti-doping risk management |

## Identifying medical conditions that contraindicate participation in sport

Some medical conditions may contraindicate participation in certain sports or recreational activities—for example, uncontrolled epilepsy in motor racing, cycling or swimming; or HIV infection in an amateur boxer. In many cases, such as asthma in a SCUBA diver, the medical condition is not an absolute contraindication and participation should be decided on a case-by-case basis.

Table 18.2 shows examples of medical conditions that contraindicate participation in certain sports; links to more comprehensive lists can be found in the recommended resources at the end of the chapter. It is important that the clinician performing the PHA understands the physical and mental demands of the sport in question, as well as its regulations.

It is important to identify medical conditions that may be made worse by intense exercise—for example, uncontrolled type 1 diabetes, poorly controlled asthma or uncontrolled hypertension. Although such conditions are usually not absolute contraindications to participation in sport, optimal control should be established prior to commencing intense training and competition.

### Assessing known injuries and illnesses

Athletes often have persisting or recurrent injury problems, and the PHA is a good opportunity to check that they are receiving optimal treatment. Recent studies of American college athletes and professional footballers in Qatar found that 11% and 17% had a current injury at the time of the PHA, respectively.[4,5]

All medical personnel involved in the care of each existing injury should be listed. The current level of symptoms should be ascertained, as well as the athlete's compliance to ongoing rehabilitation or prevention exercises. It is also important to check that exercises are being performed correctly.

The athlete's health history alone identifies 90% of health problems discovered during the PHA[6] and a history of prior injury is the strongest predictor of future injury.[7] After reviewing current complaints, review any known prior health problems the athlete has experienced. This is best performed by interviewing the athlete, as research shows that athletes report four times more previous health problems in interviews than on computerised health history forms.[8]

It is equally important to address chronic or recurrent illnesses. This involves checking for optimum treatment (e.g. measuring blood pressure for those with hypertension, asking about breakthrough symptoms in asthma or epilepsy, checking blood glucose control for diabetics), monitoring compliance with treatment (taking of medication, correct inhaler technique and attending follow-up appointments) and checking whether the athlete has any questions and/or adequately understands their condition.

### Reviewing current medications and supplements

This involves checking prescribed medications as well as over-the-counter medications or supplements that an athlete is currently taking, takes occasionally or is considering taking. Athletes sometimes neglect to inform their team medical staff about any changes to their medications and supplements, and these should be checked to ensure compliance with the current World Anti-Doping Agency (WADA) regulations and updated in their medical records.

While discussing medications it may be a good opportunity to remind athletes of their responsibilities under the WADA code (see *Recommended resources*). In particular, emphasise that they are ultimately responsible for all substances they ingest and may also be required to report their whereabouts to anti-doping authorities. Remind them about the potential hazards associated with taking supplements, minerals and non-prescription medications without first checking with medical staff.

**TABLE 18.2**    Medical conditions that contraindicate participation in certain sports

| Medical condition | Contraindicated sport/activity |
| --- | --- |
| Myocarditis | Any exercise |
| Herpes simplex or other infective skin conditions during contagious period | Wrestling and other contact sports |
| Infectious diarrhoea | Contact sports or sports with a risk of dehydration |
| Fever | Any exercise |
| Infectious mononucleosis—acute or with splenic enlargement | Any moderate exercise or contact sport |
| Bleeding disorders | Contact sport |

## Educating

In addition to providing education about anti-doping, medication use and supplements, other issues may be worth discussing with athletes depending on the local circumstances. Although sudden cardiac death is often discussed, the leading cause of death in teenagers and young adults is accidents, and in particular road traffic accidents,[9] meaning that education on drink driving, wearing seatbelts and safe driving practices should be considered.

Other lifestyle behaviours that may have a negative effect on health and/or performance include abuse of alcohol, use of recreational drugs or "legal highs", smoking or vaping (tobacco or shisha) and unsafe sexual practices. Carefully consider the best mode of delivery for these messages, such as on a one-to-one basis during the PHA or at a later date as a group lecture or interactive workshop. This will vary from situation to situation.

Other general health topics that may affect performance include basic nutrition and the importance of sleep and recovery.

## Baseline testing

The PHA can be used to perform baseline tests for a range of purposes, if appropriate. Examples include:

- neuropsychological testing for athletes involved in contact sports, to be used as a baseline post head injury (see *Clinical Sports Medicine 6e: Managing Injuries,* Chapter 2)
- tests used in the monitoring of fatigue and recovery in athletes throughout a season, such as blood and/or saliva biochemical, hormonal or haematological tests, aerobic or anaerobic fitness tests, psychological tests such as profile of mood states or tools to assess sleep and recovery (see Chapter 16)
- physical measures to be used as post-injury reference values (these can be important when making return-to-sport decisions—see Chapter 28), such as:

  - muscle strength (Fig. 18.1)
  - single-leg hop
  - vertical jump (counter movement jump)
  - agility T-test (Fig. 18.2)[10]
  - 30 m sprint time
  - glenohumeral joint range of motion (see *Managing Injuries,* Chapter 8).

## Developing athlete rapport

The PHA is often the only time for team medical personnel to have a one-on-one consultation with athletes and to be proactive rather than reactive. It is also an opportunity

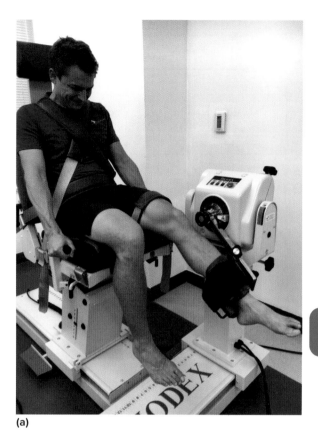

(a)

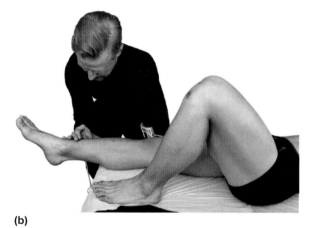

(b)

**Figure 18.1** Strength testing. (a) Quadriceps strength testing using an isokinetic dynamometer. (b) Testing hip abductor strength with a hand-held dynamometer.

for athletes to ask questions or discuss any matters that they have been hitherto unwilling to discuss and helps in improving rapport and building the clinician–patient relationship.

In some parts of the world, where a PHA is required for recreational athletes, it is the only contact that some athletes

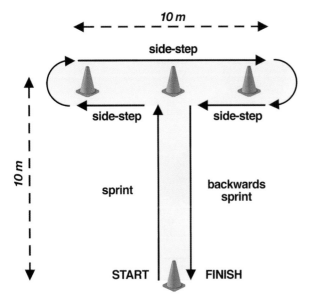

**Figure 18.2** The agility T-test

will have with the healthcare system and is an opportunity to establish a "medical home" and discuss general health issues, especially if performed by a family physician.

## Screening

Screening is traditionally defined as the identification of disease among apparently well people. In 1968 Wilson and Jungner described 10 principles of early disease detection that are still relevant today when considering a screening program for athletes (Box 18.1).[11] Although these principles are universal, two are worth considering more closely in the

context of sport, as they may be interpreted differently in athletes than in the general population.

First, the condition being screened for should be deemed "important". For athletes, particularly elite competitors, anything that negatively affects performance or leads to lost training time may be seen as very important, particularly during crucial periods of the season. In the general population, however, a 2% reduction in 5 km time or a 10% loss of strength may be insignificant.

Second, the screening program must be cost-effective. In professional sport, where athletes are often paid many thousands of dollars per week, even short periods of time loss or small performance reductions can be very costly. Prevention of minor injuries and illnesses among professional athletes may thus be highly cost-effective.

Screening is therefore commonly considered to be a valuable process for athletes and is standard practice in many elite sports. However, the actual preventive value of mass screening programs for athletes has been questioned.[12-15] We will examine this in greater detail in the following section where we review the most common types of athlete screening: cardiac screening, screening for unknown injuries and illnesses, and screening for risk factors for future injury.

### Cardiac screening

Several high-profile cases of sudden cardiac death in sportspeople over recent years, such as Norwegian swimmer Alexander Dale Oen, as well as the cases of Danish professional footballer Christian Eriksen and Buffalo Bills NFL player Damar Hamlin, who both survived sudden cardiac arrest after on-pitch resuscitation, have stimulated a healthy debate in both the medical community and the

---

### BOX 18.1 10 principles of early disease detection

1. The condition should be an important health problem.
2. There should be an accepted treatment for patients with recognised disease.
3. Facilities for diagnosis and treatment should be available.
4. There should be a recognisable latent or early symptomatic stage.
5. There should be a suitable test or examination.
6. The test should be acceptable to the population.
7. The natural history of the condition, including development from latent to declared disease, should be adequately understood.
8. There should be an agreed policy on whom to treat as patients.

9. The cost of case-finding (including diagnosis and treatment of patients diagnosed) should be economically balanced in relation to possible expenditure on medical care as a whole.
10. Case-finding should be a continuing process and not a "once and for all" project.

Wilson and Jungner state that the ability to be able to treat the condition adequately when discovered is perhaps the most important. For those conditions where there is no treatment or intervention that will offer a better prognosis, alerting a person to such a condition may cause actual harm. In order to know whether a treatment offers benefit, the natural history of a condition needs to be known.

Source: Wilson JM, Jungner YG. Principles and practice of mass screening for disease. *Bol Oficina Sanit Panam* 1968;65(4):281–393.

popular press about the pros and cons of cardiac screening. Despite all this debate there is no universal consensus on whether or how cardiac screening should be performed. The lack of agreement is because the context in which the PHA is being performed will affect the decision on whether or not to offer cardiac screening and thus this decision will likely remain an individual one for each organisation or country.[16]

Some of the many factors that have to be considered when deciding whether or not to offer cardiac screening and/or how to screen include:

- the population being studied (numbers, age group, gender, prevalence of conditions predisposing to sudden cardiac death)
- the screening tests being used (sensitivity and specificity)
- the resources available (money, equipment and access to cardiologists with expertise in conditions that predispose to sudden cardiac death).

When considering mass screening funded by the public purse, the cost-benefit of screening for conditions predisposing to sudden cardiac death versus other demands for the health dollar also needs to be considered. Many countries simply do not have the resources to be able to offer a large-scale screening program, particularly if it might place barriers to people partaking in exercise, which will actually reduce public health costs.

Cardiac screening usually consists of the following elements:

- targeted history for symptoms suggestive of cardiac disease, and for personal or family history of cardiac disease
- physical examination of the cardiovascular system
- special tests—for example, electrocardiograph (ECG), echocardiograph or stress test.

As mentioned above, there is no international consensus on which tests should routinely be used. Most of the debate, however, centres on the routine use of an ECG as part of cardiac screening. Those against the routine use of the ECG in cardiac screening point out that there is a high false-positive rate, there may be undue stress associated with further investigations of "abnormal" results, expertise is required to interpret the ECG and the costs are high.

Those in favour of the routine use of the ECG argue that the ECG is more sensitive and specific than a history and examination alone—a study of college athletes showed that 30% responded positive to at least one of the American Heart Association (AHA) cardiac questions, which reflects the high rate of false positives.[5] Furthermore, they argue that the use of standardised ECG criteria to interpret ECGs can improve the accuracy of ECG interpretation[17] and athletes feel reassured by ECG screening, not unduly stressed.[18, 19]

Echocardiography and stress tests are usually only routinely used as part of cardiac screening by professional sporting teams with sufficiently large budgets and access to expertise or when further investigation is indicated by an initial screening assessment.

Two of the most common causes of sudden cardiac death—hypertrophic cardiomyopathy and arrhythmogenic right ventricular cardiomyopathy—develop with age and may not be detectable on the initial screening. Therefore, cardiac screening is not a one-off process and must be repeated to detect cases that manifest at a later date.[20, 21] A negative screening may give false reassurance, so even after a normal cardiac screening, cardiovascular symptoms should be assessed according to standard practice.[20]

> **PRACTICE PEARL**
>
> An important part of the topic that often gets overlooked when considering cardiac screening, and arguably should be addressed even before considering cardiac screening, is being adequately prepared for a sudden cardiac arrest should one occur, since even a comprehensive cardiac screening program will not identify all those with conditions predisposing to sudden cardiac death.

High school studies in the US clearly show the benefit of having an automated external defibrillator (AED—Fig. 18.3) on site and that sudden cardiac arrest is survivable with an AED program. A study published in 2013 looking prospectively at 2149 high schools, 87% of which had an AED program, reported that 89% of athletes (including students and older athletes) survived to hospital discharge because of prompt CPR and early defibrillation.[22] Being prepared for a sudden cardiac arrest involves more than just having an AED on site. Staff also need adequate training in its use (see Chapter 2).

### Screening for unknown illnesses

In some situations, screening for the presence of unknown or "subclinical" medical conditions may be worthwhile. These include medical conditions that:

- have a negative effect on performance (e.g. iron deficiency anaemia or exercise-induced asthma)
- predispose athletes to injury (e.g. there is an association between vitamin D deficiency and stress fractures in military populations[23])
- might be hazardous to other athletes or medical staff (e.g. hepatitis B).

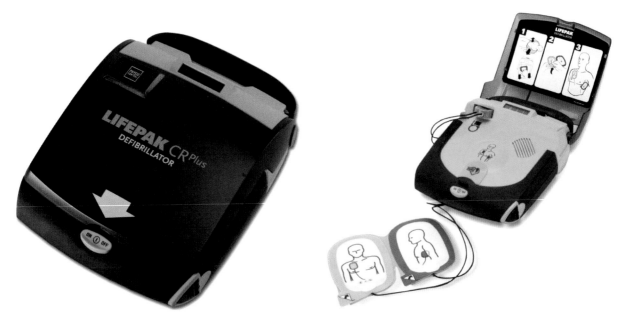

**Figure 18.3** AEDs are effective and increase the survival rate following sudden cardiac arrest
COURTESY OF PROFESSOR JONATHAN DREZNER, UNIVERSITY OF WASHINGTON CENTER FOR SPORTS CARDIOLOGY, WITH PERMISSION FROM PHYSIO-CONTROL, INC.

### Screening for risk factors for future injury

A comprehensive musculoskeletal examination is among the most common elements of a PHA. Typically, the athlete's strength and flexibility are measured and compared to normative values or pre-determined cut-off values to determine whether the athlete is at risk of future injury. Specific orthopaedic tests may also be performed to identify unknown existing injuries.

In recent years, however, there has been a trend away from static clinical measurements towards dynamic screening of the athlete's ability to perform a range of functional tasks. A number of similar systems are popular, all of which aim to identify "weak links" in strength, flexibility or motor control that can then be targeted by individualised injury prevention programs. These include the Functional Movement Screen (FMS),[24-26] the US Tennis Association High-Performance Profile[27] and the 9-test battery developed by physiotherapists at the Swedish Sports Confederation.[28]

Whether traditional clinical measurements or a qualitative approach is used, the goals of musculoskeletal screening remain the same: to identify athletes at risk of specific injuries and guide the development of individualised injury prevention training programs. Although this is a theoretically appealing approach, there are several reasons why it may not deliver the desired results in practice.

First, for most injuries very few intrinsic modifiable risk factors have been identified, and screening cut-off values are often based on expert opinion or assumed associations with injury risk. For example, athletes with poor hamstring flexibility are commonly advised to stretch to avoid hamstring strains. However, research into the link between hamstring flexibility and injury is inconclusive[29, 30] and there is no cut-off value for hamstring flexibility that can identify players at risk of future injury. This is the case for a majority of physical measures currently used to screen athletes.

Second, even in cases where significant associations have been established between risk factors and injury, such as eccentric knee flexor weakness for hamstring strains,[31] or glenohumeral joint stiffness for shoulder injuries in throwing athletes,[32-35] intrinsic risk factors are poor predictors of future injury. This is because they typically only explain a small part of an athlete's overall injury risk, and because cut-off values are likely to have low sensitivity (many false negatives) and/or low specificity (many false positives), depending on which value is used.[15]

Clearly, more high-quality research into injury risk factors is required, in particular into the combination of test findings in order to maximise their predictive value. It is likely that dynamic predictive models are necessary before athletes at risk of future injury can be successfully identified.[36]

Nevertheless, musculoskeletal screening remains a popular and potentially valuable tool, particularly in helping sport and exercise clinicians familiarise themselves with each athlete's physical attributes and limitations. The information obtained through these screenings can be helpful for baseline testing in the event an athlete suffers an injury, to profile an athlete's or group of athletes' function, and for research purposes for development of future prevention models. Care should be taken, however, in telling athletes that they are not at risk of injury or that they don't need to perform injury prevention training because they passed a particular screening test.

### Mental health screening

In 2019 the International Olympic Committee released a Consensus Statement on mental health in elite athletes.[37] Although exercise is considered to be somewhat protective against some mental health disorders such as depression and anxiety, the prevalence of mental health symptoms and disorders in elite athletes has been shown to be similar to that in the general population and may be higher in some situations.[38] One of the main recommendations of the Consensus Statement was the need to screen elite athletes for mental health symptoms or disorders. [37]

A two-step screening process known as the Sport Mental Health Assessment Tool 1 (SMHAT-1) has subsequently been developed (Fig. 18.4).[38] This starts with a triage using the Athlete Psychological Strain Questionnaire (APSQ), which is a brief questionnaire of 10 questions. If positive, further assessment using six existing validated disorder-specific questionnaires is recommended. Due to the serious nature of mental health conditions, it is important to build up a network of resources necessary to handle mental health emergencies.

**C**

# SMHAT-1

The International Olympic Committee Sport Mental Health Assessment Tool 1

DEVELOPED BY THE IOC MENTAL HEALTH WORKING GROUP

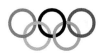

Athlete's name: _____     Athlete's ID number: _____

**What is the SMHAT-1**

The International Olympic Committee (IOC) Sport Mental Health Assessment Tool 1 (SMHAT-1) is a standardized assessment tool aiming to identify at an early stage elite athletes (defined as professional, Olympic, Paralympic and collegiate level; 16 and older) potentially at risk for or already experiencing mental health symptoms and disorders, in order to facilitate timely referral of those in need to adequate support and/or treatment.

**Who should use the SMHAT-1**

The SMHAT-1 can be used by sports medicine physicians and other licensed/registered health professionals, but the clinical assessment (and related management) within the SMHAT-1 (see step 3b) should be conducted by sports medicine physicians and/or licensed/registered mental health professionals. If you are not a sports medicine physician or other licensed/registered health professional, please use the IOC Sport Mental Health Recognition Tool 1 (SMHRT-1). Physical therapists or athletic trainers working with a sports medicine physician can use the SMHAT-1 but any guidance or intervention should remain the responsibility of their sports medicine physician.

*To use this paper version of the SMHAT-1, please print it single-sided. The SMHAT-1 in its current form can be freely copied for distribution to individuals, teams, groups and organizations. Any revision requires the specific approval by the IOC MHWG while any translation should be reported to the IOC MHWG. The SMHAT-1 should not be re-branded or sold for commercial gain. Further information about the development of the SMHAT-1 and related screening tools (including psychometric properties) is presented in the corresponding publication of the British Journal of Sports Medicine.*

**Why use the SMHAT-1**

Mental health symptoms and disorders are prevalent among active and former elite athletes. Mental health disorders are typically defined as conditions causing clinically significant distress or impairment that meet certain diagnostic criteria, such as in the Diagnostic and Statistical Manual of Mental Disorders 5th edition (DSM-5) or the International Classification of Diseases 10th revision (ICD-10), whereas mental health symptoms are self-reported, may be significant but do not occur in a pattern meeting specific diagnostic criteria and do not necessarily cause significant distress or functional impairment.

**When to use the SMHAT-1**

The SMHAT-1 should be ideally embedded within the pre-competition period (i.e., a few weeks after the start of sport training), as well as within the mid- and end-season period. The SMHAT-1 should also ideally be used when any significant event for athletes occurs such as injury, illness, surgery, unexplained performance concern, after a major competition, end of competitive cycle, suspected harassment/abuse, adverse life event and transitioning out of sport.

**Step 1: Triage Tool — Athlete's form 1**
Assessment with APSQ

**Score APSQ < 17** | **Score APSQ ≥ 17**

No further action needed

**Step 2: Screening Tools — Athlete's form 2**
Assessment with 6 screening instruments

Score ≥ 1
PHQ-9 item 9
= ACTION

**6 screening instruments under threshold** | **1 or more screening instruments at or above threshold**

**Step 3a: Brief intervention and monitoring**
- Single or combination of brief interventions
- Monitoring with APSQ (**Athlete's form 1**)

**Step 3b: Clinical assessment**
- Assessment (e.g., severity, complexity, diagnostic)
- Additional information (**Athlete's form 3**)
- Definition and application of treatment and support plan
- Referral to a mental health professional

**Figure 18.4** First page of the IOC's Sport Mental Health Assessment Tool 1
Source: Reproduced with permission from Prof Dr Vincent Gouttebarge

This screening process is expected to evolve over time with newer versions of the SMHAT-1 (like the Concussion in Sport SCAT tool—now on its sixth version, SCAT 6). In some situations, it may be appropriate to add the APSQ triage tool to a PHA.

## WHO TO ASSESS

There are numerous factors to consider about the population being assessed that can affect the content of the PHA.

### Sport and position

The incidence and types of injuries or medical issues vary widely between sports. For example, in soccer the major injuries are knee injuries (ligament and meniscal tears), ankle ligament sprains, thigh muscle strains (hamstrings and quadriceps) and groin injuries.[39] In some sports, such as rugby, the incidence of injuries differs between positions played. A study of professional rugby union players in the UK showed that anterior cruciate ligament (ACL) injuries cause the most time loss for forwards and hamstring injuries cause the most time loss for backs.[40]

It is important to know about the injury and illness epidemiology for the athlete's sport and position as the PHA should specifically look for any risk factors associated with the important injuries or medical issues connected with each athlete's sport and seek to address any that are modifiable. Some sporting bodies require athletes taking part in international competitions to undergo a health assessment prior to competing, such as the FIFA World Cup, the Rugby World Cup and the Olympics. A set template will usually be provided and should be followed.

### Geography

In some countries legislation dictates that athletes require a health assessment prior to playing sport. Since 1971 the Italian government has required the screening and medical clearance of all athletes with an annual physical examination, personal and family history and 12-lead ECG for all athletes aged 12–35 participating in competitive sport.

Local patterns of disease, both infective and genetic, vary from place to place around the world and should be taken into account when designing a PHA. For example, in certain parts of the world there is a high prevalence of hepatitis B.

The most recent guidelines from the US Preventive Services Task Force recommend screening adolescents and adults at increased risk of hepatitis B infection who are either living in areas or from important risk groups (e.g. men having sex with men or persons with injection drug use) with a prevalence of over 2% in the general population.[41] However, screening for hepatitis B immunity may be appropriate in order to be able to offer immunisation to those who are non-immune, even in countries with a lower prevalence rate for athletes involved in contact sports.

Athletes may experience extreme environmental conditions such as heat, cold and altitude when they play or compete in some geographical locations. When athletes are likely to encounter such environmental stresses, any previous history of complications associated with such conditions should be explored in the history.

### Age

There is no consensus on what age to start performing PHAs. The AAP recommends annual routine health screening for all healthy children and adolescents from age 6 but there is no evidence to support starting PHAs in sporting groups at any particular age.

In Italy an annual cardiac screening is mandatory for all competitive sport from age 12. The American Heart Association/American College of Cardiology statement on ECG screening[42] recommends starting at age 12, whereas the European Society of Cardiology makes no recommendation about which age to start screening.

Some sports have an increased risk of overuse injuries to certain growth plates (epiphysitis or apophysitis)—for example, the proximal humeral epiphysis or medial humeral epicondyle epiphysis in pitchers, and the distal radial epiphysis or calcaneal apophysis in gymnasts (see *Managing Injuries*, Chapter 33). During the PHA for a young athlete between the ages at which these different conditions occur, ask about symptoms of growth plate injuries associated with their sport, as a change in technique or training load may be required. Although the majority of these injuries heal with adequate rest, there have been reports of growth arrest of epiphyses when not treated properly.

If at all practicable a parent or legal guardian should accompany a child to the PHA. Studies of high school students undergoing a PPE have shown that only 19–33% of athletes' responses were the same as those given by their parents or legal guardians when completing the same form.[43,44] If a parent is unable to attend, they should complete the previous medical history and family history sections of the questionnaire prior to the consultation.

### Sex

Female athletes generally have the same basic PHA template as males playing the same sport, but the range of conditions associated with relative energy deficiency in sport (REDs, see Chapter 9) needs to be considered for female athletes,[45] particularly for those involved in high-risk sports (those with weight categories to meet or where the aesthetic can be judged, such as gymnastics or ballet). Several screening tools have been proposed to identify athletes with relative energy deficiency. However, none has been validated and a high index of suspicion is required. It should be noted that relative energy deficiency may also occur in male athletes.

Female athletes have a two- to threefold higher incidence of ACL injury than their male counterparts, and male athletes have a higher incidence of hamstring injuries. Such differences in injury rates, when present, should be reflected in the health assessment.

Compared with non-athletic women, female athletes have a higher risk of developing urinary incontinence,[46] with a prevalence of up to 80% in trampolinists. The prevalence of other pelvic floor dysfunctions is unknown. A screening tool for pelvic floor dysfunctions has been developed by Giagio and colleagues following an international Delphi consensus but is yet to be validated.[46]

## Available resources

At the end of the day, the available budget usually dictates the content of the PHA, irrespective of the desired components. A major hurdle for organisations considering developing a publicly funded PHA cardiac screening program for large numbers of athletes is the availability of cardiologists with expertise in sports cardiology who will be needed to follow up those with cardiovascular symptoms, abnormal physical examination findings or abnormal ECGs.

In elite or professional sport, where money may be less of an issue and there are often full-time medical staff available to perform health assessments, access to equipment (e.g. isokinetic testing equipment, $VO_2$ max testing equipment) or expertise (cardiologists with expertise in sports cardiology) may instead limit the content of the PHA.

## WHEN TO PERFORM A PHA

The timing of the PHA is often dictated by the sports organisation the athlete is competing for but the PHA is typically performed in the pre-season period. This is often the first time that the medical staff get to meet any new members of the squad who have joined in the off-season and is a good opportunity to develop a working relationship with new players.

It is a good idea for medical staff to engage coaching staff and management in the development and planning of the PHA. They will therefore understand the goals (and limitations), be encouraged to think about injury prevention

and be more likely to allow adequate time for medical staff to perform the medicals as well as being supportive with the delivery of any recommendations that might come out of the PHA, such as individual or team-wide injury prevention programs.

The value of engaging coaching staff has been clearly shown with the ACL injury prevention program in elite female handball players in Norway.[47] Despite the fact that an intervention study showed that a series of rehabilitation exercises done routinely as a part of team training significantly reduced the incidence of ACL injury, most teams stopped performing the exercises once the study was completed and the study personnel were removed from the clubs. ACL rates consequently rose in subsequent seasons. A reduction in injury rate was only seen again after the introduction of education sessions for coaches and a sport-specific website on injury prevention.[48]

Ideally, a shorter modified PHA is also performed at the end of the season to review any injuries that might have occurred during the season (including any that may not have been reported to medical staff), to possibly repeat some of the baseline musculoskeletal and/or laboratory measurements that were performed earlier in the season and to formulate a treatment or rehabilitation program for the off-season.

No research has conclusively shown that more frequent PHAs reduce the incidence of death or injury, and recommendations on frequency vary. The most common recommendation is that a comprehensive assessment be performed for adult athletes every 2–3 years with a shorter, annual questionnaire and targeted examination in between. However, practice varies depending on the context and available resources.

## WHAT TO INCLUDE IN THE TEMPLATE

The basic structure of the medical template consists of the history, examination and investigations. A detailed injury history is an important part of the assessment because the most consistent risk factor for injury across injury types is a previous history of injury.

Defining the goals of the PHA and considering the unique factors associated with the population in question, including the available resources, will allow you to select the appropriate tools for the task. The AAP PPE monograph is an excellent resource for anyone designing a PHA and contains sections on the history and a systems-based examination, as well as an example of a PHA form (see *Recommended resources*).

The temptation when designing a PHA template is to include too much, particularly in the musculoskeletal examination. For example, taking reliable measurements of strength or joint range of movement is time-consuming. It is a waste of time if:

- no action is going to be taken for "abnormal" results (what is "abnormal" is often not even considered)
- the data are not going to be used as a baseline post-injury
- the data are not being used as part of a research project.

## OTHER THINGS TO CONSIDER

### Consent

The PHA form should contain a consent section that the athlete signs covering the following points, if appropriate:

- the athlete consents to undergo a health assessment to assess their fitness to safely participate in sport
- the athlete understands that clearance may not be given if any significant medical issues or injuries are discovered
- the athlete certifies that their answers to all PHA questions are true to the best of their knowledge
- the athlete agrees to inform the clinician if their medical situation changes significantly after completion of the PHA
- the athlete consents to the use of data collected as part of the PHA for research purposes, as long as the results do not in any way identify the athlete.

A parent or legal guardian should sign the consent form for athletes under the age of consent (18 years of age in most countries).

### Clearance or restriction from play

A very small percentage of athletes undergoing a PHA will be diagnosed with a medical condition that is associated with an increased risk of sudden cardiac death. In such cases a cardiologist with the appropriate experience should review the athlete. However, the assessment of risk is not a precise science and may differ between physicians.

To make decisions more consistent, guidelines have been produced for participation in sport with different cardiovascular conditions. However, the guidelines differ in places and the decision on whether to allow the athlete to participate should be individualised once all the relevant information is available.[42, 49]

If clearance to participate is not given, the athlete may ask to sign a "risk release" acknowledging that they have been fully informed of the risks and assume the risk of participating against medical advice, but this may not be appropriate in all cases. It is important that documentation of any risk release is completed correctly. Some experts recommend that the athlete and/or parents write in their

own words their understanding of the risks of continued participation to prove that they have been fully informed.

A decision to withhold clearance to participate may be subject to legal challenge. The success of a challenge will depend on the circumstances of the individual case and the local legislation, which varies widely from country to country.

### Who should perform the PHA?

Although some parts of the PHA may be performed by other health professionals—for example, a nurse may take a history and vital signs and a physiotherapist may perform musculoskeletal assessment—the overall responsibility to review the PHA and make recommendations on clearance and follow-up should lie with a medical doctor who has the clinical training to deal with the wide variety of issues that might arise as part of the assessment.

### Pre-employment health assessment

Many professional athletes are required to undergo a medical before their employment contract becomes valid. The principles for creating a template for the health assessment are the same as for any PHA but there are some differences that are worth considering. The biggest difference is the doctor–patient relationship.

In general the person performing the health assessment is the athlete's team physician, with whom the athlete has a normal doctor–patient relationship. When completing a new contract health assessment, the doctor is acting on behalf of a third party (the club/employer). The consent form needs to reflect that the athlete understands this difference and agrees to the doctor providing a report on their ability to play sport to the employer using medical information from the assessment.

Even though the consent form requires athletes to promise to provide honest answers, there is a temptation to be economical with the truth (or even to lie) during a new contract health assessment, especially if the contract is worth a large amount of money. The physician performing the assessment should bear this in mind and, if possible, attempt to see the previous medical records. For some sports, injury information as well as matches and minutes played are freely available on the internet and can be a valuable source of information, although the injury details may not always be accurate.

For high-value contracts, some clubs routinely ask for multiple magnetic resonance imaging (MRI) scans as part of the new contract health assessment (e.g. knees, ankles, groin and lumbar spine in soccer players). The value of this approach is unknown as MRI often picks up asymptomatic findings, such as a chondral defect in a knee that may have little or no practical prognostic value when taken in the context of a one-year contract but can be useful as a baseline when repeating imaging at a later date. Clubs can also use this information to negotiate a clause in the contract to protect themselves against prolonged future time lost from identified abnormalities.

In addition to the usual goals of a standard PHA, the role of the medical team performing a new contract health assessment is to provide the potential employer with an estimated level of risk that any identified medical and/or injury issues might preclude the athlete from being able to perform at their best for the duration of their contract. Some studies show a link between previous injury and future playing ability or length of career, such as the reduced performance of running backs in NFL after ACL reconstruction,[50] or the effects of previous injury history noted at the NFL Combine health assessment on future career length.[51] The Combine study also showed, however, that athlete talent was a big factor that also had to be taken into account.

The prediction of future injury risk is complex and depends on a number of factors in addition to injury history. This was highlighted in a pilot study by our colleagues at the Aspetar Orthopaedic and Sports Medicine Hospital in Qatar (personal communication, unpublished). For this study, 12 experienced sport and exercise physicians were given 26 fictional clinical vignettes of professional footballers with a variety of commonly seen clinical issues in new contract medicals. Based on each vignette the physicians were asked to rate the footballers as high, medium or low risk of not being able to fulfil their contractual obligations (due to injury):

- In 11 of the vignettes, both the high- and low-risk options were chosen.
- For 9 questions, only 6/12 physicians chose the same response.
- For another 5 questions, only 7/12 chose the most common answer.
- No questions had 100% agreement, and for only 2 questions did 11/12 physicians choose the same response.

Some months later the same 12 physicians were asked to consider the same 26 vignettes. On this occasion, they were asked to rate the severity of consequences of an injury occurring (high, medium or low) and the likelihood of this occurring (high, medium or low). Only 6 responded. Once again there was a wide variety of responses:

- 7/26 questions were rated as both high and low risk for likelihood of injury.
- 12/26 cases were rated as both high and low severity should an injury occur.

No follow-up was performed to ascertain why some physicians rated risk as high and others rated it as low given the identical clinical scenarios they assessed.

Once any risk has been conveyed to the potential employer, which is best done verbally so that any questions can be answered, it is up to the employer to decide whether they will offer the athlete a contract. This can be quite a complex decision and involves many different factors such as the depth of the squad in the athlete's chosen position, the athlete's experience and talent, the contract cost and duration, and the sport or position played.

## Insurance medical assessment

Many athletes take out income protection insurance and therefore require a medical certificate to be completed by a doctor. The insurance company usually provides a form with the required template. If the athlete does not have a form, they should be instructed to contact their insurance company to provide one, as different companies have different requirements.

It is important that the form is completed accurately as any incorrect answers can render the insurance void and may place the doctor at risk of legal action if there is any suggestion that there was an attempt to be economical with the truth. If the athlete is putting undue pressure on the team doctor to withhold certain information, the medical might be better performed by an independent doctor.

## Action points from the PHA

Any action points identified as a result of the PHA should be discussed with the athlete and written on the discharge summary supplied to the athlete. This should clearly indicate who is responsible for initiating any action points and when follow-up is required (if possible, a follow-up appointment should be given at the same time). If appropriate, the discharge summary may also be sent to any relevant stakeholders, such as team medical staff or the athlete's personal physician. However, it is important to have the athlete's consent prior to sharing any health information.

For athletes who spend a lot of time travelling and/or are members of several teams, there can be some challenges around distributing the results of the PHA to the various medical teams looking after them to avoid any unnecessary duplication of tests or to refer to when required. There is no one solution that will suit all athletes and this should be dealt with on a case-by-case basis.

## KEY POINTS

- Periodic health assessment (PHA) aims to make participation in sport safer for everyone involved.
- There is no universal template for PHA; it varies based on the athlete, sport, league/organisation, jurisdiction and various other factors.
- There are unique risks for each sport (and positions within some sports), and the clinician should familiarise themselves with the injuries common in the sport with which they work.
- In addition to screening for risk factors and assessing the athlete's current health status, the PHA is a time to build trust and rapport between the clinician and the athlete and to provide the athlete with education.
- Obtaining a detailed history is perhaps the most crucial element of the PHA.

- Screening (e.g. for mental health issues, future injury or unknown injury/illness) is an important element of the PHA. If you are screening for a condition, there should be an action plan for athletes who are identified as at-risk.
- Cardiac screening, particularly ECG, is hotly debated. There are pros and cons to pre-participation ECG and there is no consensus. For cardiac screening, there should be established protocols to respond to a cardiac emergency in all sport settings.
- There are medico-legal considerations in conducting the PHA, particularly when it involves an athlete's contract or insurance.
- There are numerous resources available for clinicians who are implementing a PHA for the first time.

## RECOMMENDED RESOURCES

- American Academy of Pediatrics Pre-participation Physical Evaluation:

AAP PPE

- World Anti-Doping Agency:

WADA code

- Lists of contraindications to sports participation: AHA/ACC Scientific Statement—Eligibility and Disqualification recommendations for Competitive Athletes with Cardiovascular Abnormalities:

AHA/ACC contraindications to sports participation

## REFERENCES

References for this chapter can be found at www.mhprofessional.com/CSM6e

## ADDITIONAL CONTENT

Scan here to access additional resources for this topic and more provided by the authors

## CHAPTER 19

# Diagnosis: history and physical examination

with PAUL BLAZEY

*Listen: the patient is telling you the diagnosis.*

WILLIAM OSLER (1849–1919)

## CHAPTER OUTLINE

Diagnosis isn't limited just to tissue diagnosis
Keys to accurate diagnosis
History
Physical examination
Differential diagnoses

## LEARNING OBJECTIVES

By the end of this chapter you should be able to:

- identify the steps required to construct a clinical diagnosis
- recognise scenarios where an exact pathoanatomical diagnosis is difficult to determine
- apply a biopsychosocial lens to your clinical assessment
- list the qualities of a comprehensive history and physical examination
- consider less obvious contributing factors to sport-related injury and illness.

To launch this chapter on diagnosis, we ask: Is there a difference between a diagnosis of (1) swimmer's shoulder and (2) rotator cuff tendinopathy?

The first diagnosis (swimmer's shoulder) reflects sports medicine practice in the 1980s and 1990s. Alongside labels such as tennis elbow, hockey groin and footballer's ankle, a diagnosis consisted of the name of a sport paired with a commonly injured body part. This was an advance at the time, as few clinicians were aware of conditions that the general public now knows well. The major limitation of this type of label is lack of precision. Each label (e.g. hockey groin) could apply to several pathological entities that may benefit from distinct treatment. Such labels have no place in 21st-century sports and exercise medicine.

What about rotator cuff tendinopathy—is that a valid diagnosis? Accurate pathological diagnosis is important because:

- It supports effective patient education. You can explain the diagnosis, prognosis and expected time lines for recovery. If a patient presents with an acute knee injury, the diagnosis of anterior cruciate ligament (ACL) tear has markedly different implications from a diagnosis of small medial meniscal injury.
- It enables shared decision making. Numerous conditions have similar presentations but differ in best practice treatments. Consider the differences in treatment between lateral ligament ankle sprain and osteochondral fracture of the talus; patellofemoral joint syndrome and meniscal tear; and hamstring tear and hamstring pain referred from the lumbar spine.
- It influences how you rehabilitate the patient. For example, rehabilitation after leg pain due to a posteromedial tibial stress fracture will be more gradual than rehabilitation after similar leg pain due to a calf strain.

## DIAGNOSIS ISN'T LIMITED JUST TO TISSUE DIAGNOSIS

Although accurate tissue diagnosis remains desirable, accurate, specific tissue diagnosis often isn't possible. Consider patients who present with low back pain. Is the tissue diagnosis the facet joint, vertebra, fascia, muscle or disc? In such cases, can magnetic resonance imaging (MRI) provide the holy grail of tissue diagnosis? No, MRI cannot.

You don't need an MRI to make an initial assessment. Your goal should be to assess the various structures that might be contributing to symptoms for pain, tenderness and function.

How treatment affects symptoms and signs immediately during the consultation and over time can also help determine which structure is contributing to the patient's symptoms.

When tissue diagnosis is impossible, you can still guide the patient by assessing any impairments, documenting the patient's level of function and providing reassurance based on epidemiological evidence of clinical outcomes and your prior clinical experience.

Even when tissue diagnosis can be made, important personal and social factors can influence the severity of the patient's symptoms. Contextual factors can cause substantially different symptoms in two patients suffering similar tissue-level ailment. Chapters 10 and 11 highlight how context is key to a patient's experience of pain.[1,2]

In a purely biomedical model, pathology (e.g. disc injury) is used to explain the patient's pain experience. On the other hand, the clinician who considers all contextual factors through a biopsychosocial (BPS) approach will discover that the patient works two jobs, doesn't get enough sleep (a risk factor for back pain) and has tremendous anxiety about making mortgage payments. All of these have the potential to affect the patient's pain experience.

Athletes don't live in a bubble and the expert clinician takes many factors into account—not only tissue pathology. Multifactorial treatment that takes psychosocial factors into account is superior to narrowly focused but appropriate treatment.[3] Psychological and social/sport factors are illustrated in Figure 19.1.

For a TED talk on the BPS model:

 **TED talk on BPS model**

## KEYS TO ACCURATE DIAGNOSIS

Diagnosis relies on an appropriately detailed patient history, a thorough physical examination and, where needed, appropriate investigations.

> **PRACTICE PEARL**
>
> Diagnosis may not be achieved on the first visit—it may become clear after a series of appointments.

For decades, clinical educators have been bemoaning learners' "over-reliance on sophisticated investigations

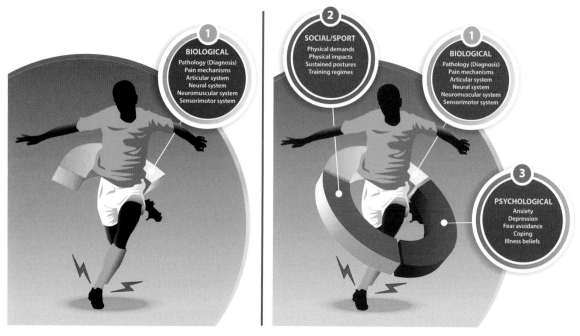

**Figure 19.1** The biomedical (left) and biopsychosocial (right) models of disease

and neglect of clinical skills".[4,5] That's not the case for the *Clinical Sports Medicine* reader but for other learners mastering clinical skills may not be easy.

Keys to accurate diagnosis of patients presenting with musculoskeletal pain include:

- the patient's age
- the mechanism of injury
- possible local causes of the symptoms
- sites that could be referring pain to the site of the symptoms (Chapters 10 and 11)
- biopsychosocial factors (Chapters 10 and 11)
- biomechanics (Chapters 12 and 13) and the relevant kinetic chain (e.g. the back and lower limbs in a shoulder injury in a tennis player)
- other possible causative factors (e.g. metabolic)
- patient expectations and understanding.

## HISTORY

The patient history remains the keystone of accurate diagnosis and will provide the diagnosis in the majority of cases. Here are five tips for taking a history:

- *Allow enough time.* The patient must feel that you have enough time available to allow them to tell their story, otherwise important symptoms will not surface.

In addition to details of the injury, you need time to take a history of the athlete's training program, including details of training workload where this is available. You should explore other possible causes of injury. Diet history may be appropriate (i.e. contributing to stress fracture likelihood). As a minimum, 30 minutes is required to assess a patient with a new injury, but in complex chronic cases up to 1 hour may be necessary in the specialist setting.

- *Be an active listener.* Let the story unravel.[6] Use appropriate body language and focus on the patient, not the medical record or computer screen. Many patients have good body awareness and are generally able to describe their symptoms very well.
- *Get to know the sport.* It is helpful to understand the technical demands of a sport when seeing an athlete, as this engenders patient confidence. More importantly, knowledge of the biomechanics and techniques of a particular sport (Chapter 13) can assist greatly in both making the primary diagnosis and uncovering potential predisposing factors.
- *Discover the exact circumstances of the injury.* The patient history should help you determine the exact context of the injury. The mechanism of injury warrants careful consideration. Most patients can describe in considerable detail the mechanism of an acute injury. In

acute injuries, this is the single most important clue to diagnosis. For example, an inversion injury to the ankle strongly suggests a lateral ligament injury, a valgus strain to the knee may cause a medial collateral ligament injury, and a pivoting injury accompanied by a "pop" in the knee and followed by rapid swelling suggests an ACL injury. In overuse injuries, focus on recent changes in training that may have led to an injury, such as changes in playing surface, equipment or training load.

• *Invite the patient to detail their symptoms.* Common musculoskeletal symptoms include pain, swelling, instability and loss of function. If the consultation occurs some time after the injury, be sure to ask about the symptoms at the time of injury, at the time of your consultation, and how these symptoms have evolved.

## Pain

Pain history has many elements: see Box 19.1.

## Swelling

Immediate swelling following an injury may indicate a severe injury such as a fracture or major ligament tear accompanied by haemarthrosis. Delayed swelling (overnight) after a knee injury is more likely to be associated with a meniscal injury. Record the degree of swelling (mild, moderate or severe) and subsequent changes in the amount of swelling.

## Instability

Any history of giving way or feeling of instability is significant. Try to elicit the exact activity that causes this feeling. For example, in throwing, does the feeling of instability occur in the cocking phase (indicative of anterior shoulder instability) or the follow-through?

## Function

It is important to know whether immediately after the injury happened the athlete was:

• able to continue activity without any problems
• able to continue with some restriction or
• unable to continue.

Note any changes in function over time. When patients present with chronic conditions, or have been receiving treatment already, establish what level of function they have reached. Have they just failed to rehabilitate to the necessary level of function? (See Chapter 28.)

---

**BOX 19.1** Asking the patient about the characteristics of their pain

1. *Location.* Note the exact location of their pain. Detailed knowledge of surface anatomy can be invaluable. If the pain is poorly localised or varies from site to site, consider the possibility of referred pain.

2. *Onset.* Speed of onset helps determine whether the pain is due to an acute or overuse injury. Was the onset of pain associated with a snap, crack, pop, tear or other sensation?

3. *Severity.* Severity may be classified as mild, moderate or severe. A pain score (e.g. numerical rating scale [see Chapter 9]) or specific outcome measure (see Chapter 23) may be useful to gauge severity and monitor improvement. Another very helpful method is to have the patient detail the most important activity for them and rate that with a pain score. Assess the severity of the pain immediately after the injury and how it evolved. Was the patient able to continue the activity?

4. *Irritability.* This refers to the level of activity required to provoke pain and how long the pain subsequently takes to settle. The degree of irritability is especially important because it affects how vigorously the physical examination should be performed and how aggressive the treatment should be.

5. *Nature.* This refers to the quality of the pain. It is important to allow patients to describe the pain in their own words, without any prompting or leading questions. For example, "burning pain" can suggest neural involvement.

6. *Behaviour.* Is the pain constant or intermittent? What is the time course of the pain? Is it worse on waking up or does it worsen during the day? Does it wake the patient at night?

7. *Pain site and distribution.* Does the pain radiate at all? If so, where? Might this pain be a red flag? (See Chapter 22.)

8. *Aggravating factors.* What activity or posture aggravates the pain?

9. *Relieving factors.* Is the pain relieved by rest or the adoption of certain postures? Do certain activities relieve the pain? Is the pain affected by climatic changes (e.g. cold weather)?

10. *Previous treatment.* What was the initial treatment of the injury? Was ice applied? Was firm compression applied? Was the injured part immobilised? If so, for how long? What treatment and rehabilitation have been performed since and what effect did that treatment have on the pain? The latter is particularly important when you are providing a second or subsequent opinion in cases of long-standing problems. What medications are being used?

## History of similar injury

If the athlete has had a similar injury before, record full details of all treatments, their response to each type of treatment and whether they have undertaken any maintenance treatment or exercises following initial rehabilitation. Previous injury is a risk factor for recurrence.[7]

## Other injuries

Past injuries may have contributed to the current injury; for example, an inadequately rehabilitated muscle tear may have led to muscle imbalance and a subsequent overuse injury. Because of the importance of spinal abnormalities as a potential component of pain (Chapters 10 and 11), the patient should always be questioned about spinal symptoms, especially pain and stiffness in the lower back or neck.

Past or present injuries in areas that may at first seem unrelated to the current injury may also be important. For example, a hamstring injury in a throwing athlete can impair the kinetic chain leading to the shoulder, altering throwing biomechanics and thus contributing to a rotator cuff injury.

## General health

Is the patient otherwise healthy? Musculoskeletal symptoms are not always activity related (Chapter 22). Red flags for serious medical conditions masquerading as sports injuries include:

- no specific mechanism of injury
- pain unrelated to activity
- night pain
- associated symptoms and signs such as weight loss, fever, malaise, lymphadenopathy
- poor response to treatment.

Consider asking specifically about diabetes, possible undiagnosed inflammatory conditions (e.g. skin problems of psoriasis, bowel complaints associated with spondyloarthropathies) and familial conditions.

## Work and leisure activities

Work and leisure activities can play a role in both the aetiology and subsequent management of a sports injury. For example, a job that involves continual bending or spending leisure time gardening may aggravate an athlete's low back pain. It is important to know about these activities and to ascertain whether they can be reduced in any way.

## Other health-related factors

Predisposing factors should be considered not only in overuse injuries, but also in medical conditions and acute injuries. An athlete struggling to return to sport after an ACL injury, for example, may have an underlying psychological component. An athlete with an acute hamstring tear may have a history of low back problems or have had an ACL reconstruction using the hamstring tendons as the graft. Injury recurrence can be prevented only by eliminating the underlying cause.

## Training/activity history

For any overuse injury, a comprehensive training history is required. This is best done as a weekly diary, as most athletes train on a weekly cycle. Ask the patient to bring a training diary or activity history to the consultation, or to share data from the mobile apps they use on their phone. Ask about both the quantity and quality of training and any recent changes. Note also the total amount of training (distance or hours, depending on the sport) and training surfaces. Ideally, the patient will have a detailed training history that includes a perception of how hard training was.

Training can be measured as (1) internal load (e.g. as measured by rate of perceived exertion) or (2) external load (e.g. as training volume in distance covered or balls pitched or bowled; see Chapter 15). Continual activity on hard surfaces or a recent change in surface may predispose to injury.

In running sports, pay particular attention to footwear (Chapters 12 and 13). For both training and competition shoes, note the shoe type, age and wear pattern. Record recovery activities such as soft-tissue therapy, spa/sauna and hours/quality of sleep (Chapter 16).

### Equipment

Inappropriate equipment may predispose an athlete to injury (see Chapter 13 for sport-specific tips on equipment and injury prevention, and Chapter 17 for the relationship between equipment and injury prevention). Commonly cited examples of equipment and injury are incorrect bicycle setup and knee pain,[8-10] and racquet changes in tennis.

### Technique

Ask the patient to outline any technique problems that either they or their coach have noted. Faulty technique may contribute to injury. For example, a "wristy" backhand drive may contribute to extensor tendinopathy at the elbow.

### Overtraining

Symptoms such as excessive fatigue, recurrent illness, reduced motivation, persistent soreness and stiffness may point to overtraining as an aetiological factor. The vast majority of athletes will not consider themselves to be overtraining; therefore, it is important to evaluate this using objective data where possible.

## Psychological factors

Injury can be caused or exacerbated by a number of psychological factors that may relate to sport (e.g. pressure of impending competition) or personal or business life. You need to consider this possibility and approach it sensitively. While anxiety or depression may not directly cause a sports injury, it can alter symptoms and affect hormone health (which in turn may influence the patient's recovery).

## Nutrition

Inadequate nutrition can predispose to the overtraining syndrome and may play a role in the development of musculoskeletal injuries. The role of relative energy deficiency in sport (REDs)[11] is described in Chapter 9. Eating disorders may also inhibit healing. For an athlete presenting with excessive tiredness, a full dietary history is essential.

## Drugs: prescription and others

A medication history is essential. Fluoroquinolone antibiotics may be the cause of a patient's tendinopathy, while cold and influenza medications have been associated with arrhythmias. Social drugs and performance-enhancing anabolic steroids may have systemic side effects. Athletes are unlikely to volunteer any information on their use of non-prescription drugs; direct questioning is not only appropriate but reveals your understanding of the world of sport.

### History of exercise-induced anaphylaxis

Exercise-induced anaphylaxis[12] and food-dependent, exercise-induced anaphylaxis[13] are rare but potentially life-threatening clinical syndromes associated with exercise. You should question the patient about allergies.

## The importance of sport to the athlete

The athlete's level of commitment to the sport, which won't necessarily correlate with their expertise, has a bearing on management decisions. Be aware of the athlete's short- and long-term future sporting commitments to schedule appropriate treatment and rehabilitation programs. See also Chapter 4 on shared decision making.

## Differential diagnosis

When you have finished the history, consider the differential diagnoses and the possible aetiological factors. This will help guide your focused physical examination.

## PHYSICAL EXAMINATION

In this section we share a number of general principles that might speed the junior clinician towards a more confident and more effective physical examination. We acknowledge the limitations of both learning the physical examination and teaching it,[5, 14] but in our health discipline it can provide invaluable information.

Even if an MRI is needed for confirmation, it is very reassuring for patients to be given an early accurate clinical diagnosis from a physical examination: "I appreciate you are in pain and we need to get to the bottom of this knee injury but I can assure you that your ACL is intact. That test I did (Lachman) has a perfect end-feel so I know it isn't torn."

On the other hand, if the physical examination indicates that the news is bad, you can begin the process of helping the patient to prepare for that outcome and letting them share their feelings.

### General principles (the what)

#### Develop a routine

Experienced clinicians from all disciplines examine each joint, region or system in a routine manner. The routine enables them to concentrate on the findings rather than thinking what to do next. In *Clinical Sports Medicine 6e: Managing Injuries* we outline a routine for examining each body part. There are many online resources to help you develop your routine; the challenge is knowing which ones to trust—Figure 19.2 shows two high-quality examples.

Because athletes function in the upright position in most sports, don't default to only examining the patient in a supine or prone position. Running sports involve supporting the body on one or other leg most of the time. Simulate this in your examination. Consider starting the examination assessing posture and having the patient perform various stress tests on one leg (e.g. hopping, one-legged squat). As part of your routine, perform exams on both limbs (e.g. ligamentous laxity or muscle tightness). The uninjured side serves as a comparator and is often a good side to begin on to give the patient a feeling for what's going to come on the injured side.

#### Examine joints above and below to identify potential contributing factors

Try to ascertain the cause of the injury. It is not sufficient to examine the painful area only (e.g. the Achilles tendon). Is there a problem with the kinetic chain (a concept discussed in Chapter 9)? Examine joints, muscles and neural structures proximal and distal to the injured area,

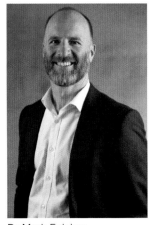

Dr Mark Hutchinson's tips

Dr Mark Fulcher's tips

Dr Mark Fulcher

**Figure 19.2** Dr Mark Hutchinson's tips on how to examine various body parts have stood the test of time. First created with the *Clinical Sports Medicine* team 15 years ago, the free YouTube videos have been viewed more than 10 million times. Dr Mark Fulcher, a New Zealand sport and exercise physician, shares a wealth of clinical knowledge via FIFA's free YouTube channel.

seeking predisposing factors (e.g. limited dorsiflexion of the ankle, tight gastrocnemius–soleus complex, lumbar facet joint dysfunction). A useful tip is to examine all areas that may possibly contribute to the injury before homing in on the site of pain.

### Reproduce the patient's symptoms

Reproduce the patient's symptoms whenever possible. This can be achieved by active and/or passive movements and by palpation either locally or, in the case of referred pain, at the site of referral. This can sometimes be done in the consulting room (e.g. a deep squat) or the patient may be able to show it to you via a video on their phone (e.g. a long jumper taking off or a gymnast performing a backward walkover). You may need to ask the patient to undertake their activity first (run, dance) before you examine them (see functional testing below).

### Assess local tissues

Assess the joints, muscles and neural structures at the site of pain for tenderness, tissue feel and range of motion.

### Assess whether pain may be referred

Assess the joints, muscles and neural structures that may refer to the site of pain (Chapters 10 and 11).

### Assess neural mechanosensitivity

Assess neural mechanosensitivity (Chapters 10 and 11) using one or more neurodynamic tests (see below).

### Assess the spine

Many painful injuries—particularly those that have not responded to routine first-line treatment—have a spinal component to them. Abnormal neural mechanosensitivity can provide a clue to such a component. In lower limb injuries, examine the lumbar spine and the thoracolumbar junction. In upper limb injuries, examine the cervical and upper thoracic spine. Examine for hypomobility of isolated spinal segments as this may contribute to distant symptoms. See the routine for spinal examination below.

### Assess relevant biomechanics

How biomechanical abnormalities can contribute to overuse injuries is discussed in Chapters 12 and 13. Include this examination in your assessment. If your patient is a golfer with back pain, you need to look at their golf swing sequence using clubs. And remember that poor mechanics in the lower limbs may contribute to an upper limb injury (e.g. weak hip stabilisers can lead to overload of the elbow in throwing sports—failure of the kinetic chain).

## The examination routine (how to do it)

### 1. Look

It is important to observe the patient walking into your office or walking off the field of play as well as inspecting the injured area. Note any evidence of deformity, asymmetry, bruising, swelling, skin changes or muscle wasting. Note that a degree of asymmetry might be expected due to one side being dominant, such as the racquet arm in a tennis player.

## 2. Feel

Palpation is a vital component of the physical examination and precise knowledge of anatomy, especially surface anatomy, optimises its value. At times it is essential to determine the exact site of maximal tenderness (e.g. when differentiating between bony tenderness and ligament attachment tenderness after a sprained ankle).

When palpating soft tissues, properties of the soft tissue that need to be assessed include:

- resistance
- muscle spasm
- tenderness.

Palpate carefully and try to visualise the structures being palpated. Commence with the skin, feeling for any changes in temperature or amount of sweating, infection or increased sympathetic activity. When palpating muscle, assess tone, focal areas of thickening or trigger points, muscle length and imbalance.

It is important to palpate not only the precise area of pain (e.g. the supraspinatus tendon attachment), but also the regions proximal and distal to the painful area, such as the muscle belly of the trapezius muscle. Determine whether tenderness is focal or diffuse. This may help differentiate between, for example, a stress fracture (focal tenderness) and periostitis (diffuse tenderness).

To palpate joints correctly, it is important to understand the two different types of movement present at a joint:

- Physiological movements are voluntary movements that patients perform themselves.
- In order to achieve the full range of physiological movements, accessory movements are required. Accessory movements are involuntary, interarticular movements—including glides, rotations and tilts—that occur in both spinal and peripheral joints during normal physiological movements.

Loss of these normal accessory movements may cause pain, altered range or abnormal quality of physiological movements. Palpation of the spinal and peripheral joints is based on these principles. An example of palpation of accessory movements involves posteroanterior pressure over the spinous process of the vertebra, producing a glide between that vertebra and the ones above and below.

## 3. Move

### Range of motion testing (active)

Ask the patient to perform active range of motion exercises without assistance. Look carefully for restriction in the range of motion, pain at a particular point in the range and abnormal patterns of movement. In many conditions, such as shoulder impingement and patellofemoral pain, the pattern of movement is critical to making a correct diagnosis.

If the pain is not reproduced during single plane movements (e.g. flexion or extension), examine combined movements (i.e. movements in two or more planes such as extension combined with lateral flexion of the cervical spine). By combining movements and evaluating symptom response, you can gain additional information to help predict the site of a potential lesion. Other movements, such as repeated, quick or sustained movements, may be required to elicit the patient's pain.

### Range of motion testing (passive)

Passive range of motion testing is used to elicit joint and muscle stiffness. Injury may be the cause of joint stiffness. Alternatively, stiffness may already have been present and predispose to injury by placing excessive stress on other structures (e.g. a stiff ankle joint can predispose to Achilles tendinopathy). Passive range of motion testing should include all directions of movement appropriate to a particular joint and should be compared with normal range and the unaffected side. Overpressure may be used at the end of range to elicit the patient's symptoms.

### Ligament testing

Examine ligaments for laxity and pain. Specific tests have been devised for all the major ligaments of the body. These involve moving the joint to stress a particular ligament. This may cause pain or reveal laxity in the joint. Laxity is graded as 1 (mild), 2 (moderate) or 3 (severe). Pain on stressing the ligament is significant and may indicate, in the absence of laxity, a mild injury or grade 1 ligament sprain. A number of different tests may be used to assess a single ligament; for example, the anterior drawer, Lachman's and pivot shift tests all test ACL laxity.

### Strength testing

Muscles or groups of muscles should be tested for strength and compared with the unaffected side. Muscle weakness may occur as a result of an injury (e.g. secondary to a chronic joint effusion) or may be a predisposing factor towards injury. Muscle strength can be assessed manually or with the use of a hand-held dynamometer.

### Neurodynamic testing

Changes in the normal mechanics, neurophysiology and homeostasis of the nervous system may contribute to pain. Neurodynamic testing is an important part of physical examination that needs to be executed skilfully (requires training) and the findings need to be interpreted thoughtfully (clinical reasoning).

At a superficial level, a beginner might imagine that neurodynamic testing examines restriction of normal mechanics and how this restriction affects the patient's symptoms; however, this is an oversimplification. Strictly speaking, neurodynamic tests use movement to systematically increase tension on the nervous system, which in turn may activate receptors that then lead to hyperalgesia if nerves have heightened nerve mechanosensitivity.

Neurodynamic tests may provoke the patient's presenting symptoms or symptoms such as pins and needles or numbness. The main reliable criteria for a positive test are:

1. at least partial reproduction of symptoms, and
2. positive structural differentiation.

Structural differentiation during a neurodynamic test refers to moving a body part distant to the provoked symptoms to selectively increase neural tension without altering the local surrounding tissues (e.g. muscle, joints). In the slump test shown in Figure 19.3(a), alterations in symptoms with cervical flexion and extension in the slump position can differentiate between neural and non-neural contributors to pain. Similarly, in the upper limb tension test 1 (median nerve) shown in Figure 19.3(b), cervical side-bending (towards the right shoulder) or releasing wrist extension are examples of structural differentiation.[15]

Beyond these main criteria, neurodynamic testing might reveal side-to-side differences in range of motion (e.g. the degree of elbow extension in Figure 19.3b) or resistance. It is less clear how to interpret these due to the large inter-side variation even in healthy people. There are also interindividual range of motion differences for these tests. The assessment of symptom production and resistance may be affected by each step in the neurodynamic test (see Box 19.2).

We underscore that these tests are only a small part of how you assess the nervous system. There are many nerve disorders where neurodynamic tests are completely normal. It is a mistake to perform neurodynamic tests and then "clear" the nervous system if the tests are normal.

The techniques used in neurodynamic tests can also be used as a treatment procedure. This is discussed in Chapter 24.

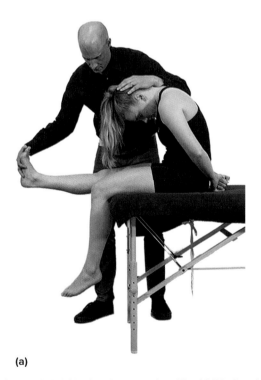

(a)

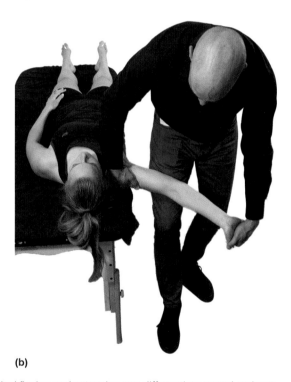

(b)

**Figure 19.3** (a) In the slump test (see Fig. 19.5 in Box 19.1), cervical flexion and extension can differentiate neural and non-neural contributors to pain. (b) Likewise in the upper limb tension test (median nerve) shown fully in Figure 19.7, cervical side bending (towards the right shoulder) or release of wrist extension are ways to different the structures. If those movements reduce the patient's pain, it suggests that neural structures are contributing to the pain.

## BOX 19.2  Neurodynamic tests

Neurodynamic tests use movement to systematically increase neural mechanosensitivity. The tests may provoke the presenting symptoms or symptoms such as pins and needles or numbness. The amount of resistance encountered during the tests is significant, especially when compared with the uninjured side.

Assessment of symptom production and resistance may be affected by each test. This may help indicate the site of the abnormality. The main neurodynamic tests are:

- straight-leg raise (Fig. 19.4)
- slump test (Fig. 19.5)

- neural Thomas test (Fig. 19.6)
- upper limb neurodynamic test (Fig. 19.7) (one of four variations shown).

A summary of these tests is shown in Table 19.1. Neurodynamic tests are non-specific but form an extremely useful part of the examination. Abnormalities of neural mechanosensitivity should lead the clinician to examine possible sites of abnormality, especially the spine. The techniques used in neurodynamic tests can also be used as a treatment procedure. This is discussed in Chapter 24.

**TABLE 19.1  Neurodynamic tests**

| Test | Method | Indications | Normal response | Variations |
|------|--------|-------------|-----------------|------------|
| Straight-leg raise (Fig. 19.4) | • Patient supine<br>• Leg extended<br>• Clinician lifts leg | • Leg pain<br>• Back pain<br>• Headache | • Tightness and/or pain in posterior knee, thigh and calf | • Ankle dorsiflexion<br>• Ankle plantarflexion/ inversion<br>• Hip adduction<br>• Hip medial rotation<br>• Passive neck flexion |
| Slump test (Fig. 19.5) | • Patient sitting<br>• Slumps<br>• Neck flexion<br>• Knee extension<br>• Ankle dorsiflexion<br>• Release neck flexion | • Back pain<br>• Buttock pain<br>• Leg pain | • Upper thoracic pain<br>• Posterior knee pain<br>• Hamstring pain | • Leg abduction (obturator nerve)<br>• Hip adduction<br>• Hip medial rotation<br>• Ankle and foot alterations |
| Neural Thomas test (Fig. 19.6) | • Patient supine<br>• Hip extension<br>• Neck flexion<br>• Knee flexion | • Groin pain<br>• Anterior thigh pain | • Quadriceps pain and/or tightness | • Hip abduction/ adduction<br>• Hip medial/lateral rotation |
| Upper limb neurodynamic test (Fig. 19.7) | • Patient supine towards side of exam table<br>• Cervical contralateral flexion<br>• Shoulder girdle depression<br>• Shoulder abducted to 110° and externally rotated<br>• Forearm supination<br>• Wrist/fingers extended<br>• Elbow extended | • Arm pain<br>• Neck/upper thoracic pain<br>• Headache | • Ache in cubital fossa<br>• Tingling in thumb and fingers | • Forearm pronation<br>• Wrist deviation<br>• Shoulder flexion/ extension<br>• Add straight-leg raise |

*continues*

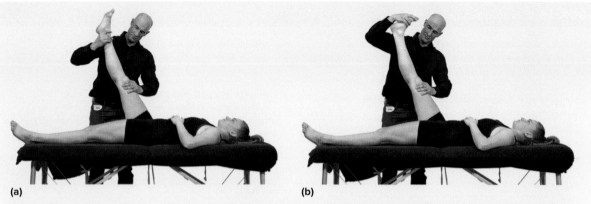

**Figure 19.4** Straight-leg raise. (a) The patient lies supine. The clinician places one hand under the patient's Achilles tendon and the other above the knee, then lifts the leg perpendicular to the bed with the hand above the knee to prevent knee flexion. (b) They then add dorsiflexion of the ankle. Eversion and toe extension may sensitise this test further. The clinician can add other variations (Table 19.1).

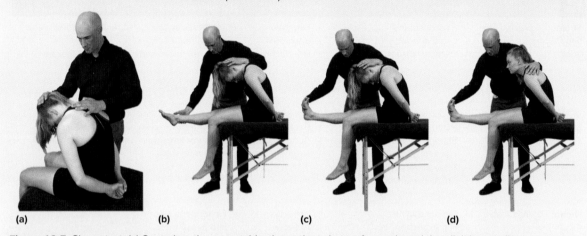

**Figure 19.5** Slump test. (a) Seated on the exam table, the patient slumps forwards and the clinician applies overpressure. The sacrum should remain vertical. The patient puts their chin on their chest and the clinician applies overpressure. (b) The patient actively extends one knee. (c) The patient actively dorsiflexes the ankle and the clinician may apply overpressure. (d) The clinician slowly releases neck flexion. Other variations can be added (Table 19.1).

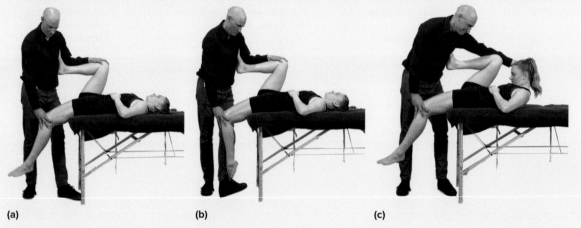

**Figure 19.6** Neural Thomas test. (a) The patient lies supine over the end of the exam table in the Thomas position. (b) The patient flexes their knee. (c) The clinician passively flexes the patient's neck then the patient's knee.

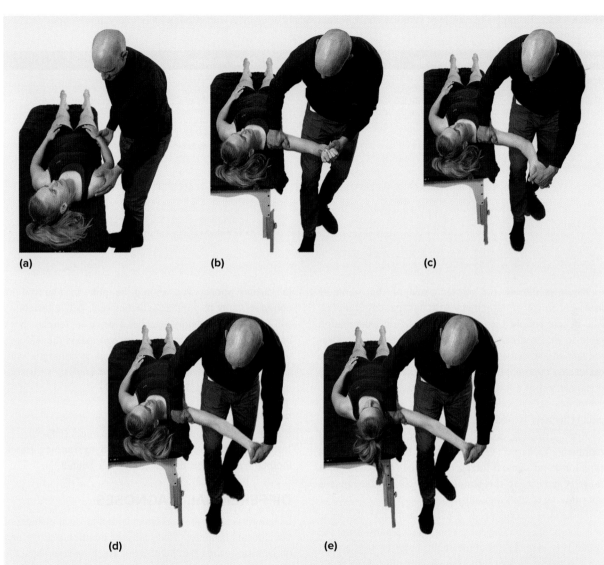

**Figure 19.7** Upper limb neurodynamic test. (a) The patient lies supine close to the edge of the exam table with their neck laterally flexed away from the side to be tested. (b) The clinician uses their hand to depress the patient's shoulder and abducts the arm to approximately 110° with external rotation. (c) The clinician supinates the patient's forearm and extends the patient's wrist and fingers. (d) They then extend the patient's elbow to the point of the onset of symptoms. (e) The patient returns their neck position to neutral and then laterally flexes it towards the side of the test. The clinician looks for changes in symptoms. Other variations can be added (Table 19.1).

## Spinal joint examination

Clinical experience suggests that intervertebral joint stiffness (e.g. hypomobility) can present as pain or injury locally (at the spine) or distally. Examples of upper and lower limb spinal abnormalities are shown in Table 19.2. The pathophysiology underlying these concepts has been discussed in Chapters 10 and 11.

For patients presenting with upper limb pain, examine the cervical and upper thoracic spine. For any patient presenting with lower limb pain, examine the lumbar spine (including the thoracolumbar junction). An abnormal neurodynamic test strongly indicates a spinal component to the pain. However, a negative neurodynamic test does not rule out the possibility of a spinal component.

**TABLE 19.2**    Examples of how joint stiffness can manifest locally or distally, with either pain or injury in the upper and lower limbs

| Presentation | Local findings | Distal findings |
| --- | --- | --- |
| **Upper limb** | | |
| Pain | Hypomobility of C5–C6 joint presents as neck pain | Hypomobility of C5–C6 joint presents as elbow pain |
| Injury | | Hypomobility of C5–C6 joint can predispose to lateral elbow tendinopathy in a tennis player |
| **Lower limb** | | |
| Pain | Hypomobility of L5–S1 joint presents as lumbosacral pain | Hypomobility of L5–S1 joint presents as buttock and hamstring pain |
| Injury | | Hypomobility of L5–S1 joint predisposing to a hamstring tear in a sprinter |

Begin examining the relevant area of the spine by assessing range of movement with the patient standing. The patient should then lie prone on a firm examination table so that you can palpate the vertebrae centrally over the spinous processes and laterally over the facet joints to detect any hypomobility and/or tenderness. Hypomobility or tenderness at a level appropriate to that of the patient's symptoms indicates the site is a possible source of referred pain (Chapters 10 and 11).

After detecting spinal abnormality, perform a trial treatment (Chapter 24) and reassess the patient's symptoms and signs. If there is a change in the pain and/or range of movement, this strongly suggests that the spine is contributing to the symptoms.

Sometimes, palpation of a particular site in the spine will reproduce the patient's symptoms distant from the spine. It is important to understand, however, that even if the symptoms are not reproduced by palpation of the spine, this does not rule out the possibility of a spinal component.

### Biomechanical examination

The role of abnormal biomechanics in the production of injuries, especially overuse injuries, is discussed in Chapters 12 and 13. Because abnormal biomechanics can contribute to any overuse injury, you need to perform a biomechanical examination. As with other components of the physical examination, it is important to develop a routine to assess biomechanical abnormalities.

Faulty technique is a common cause of injury. Faults in technique associated with particular injuries are discussed in Chapter 13. While you cannot be aware of all techniques

in various sports, you should be able to identify the common faults in popular activities (e.g. pelvic instability while running or faulty backhand drive in tennis). Seek biomechanical advice and assistance to assess the athlete's technique from the athlete's coach or a colleague with expertise in the particular area. Video analysis with slow motion or freeze frame may be helpful.

### Equipment

Inappropriate equipment predisposes to injury (Chapter 17). Inspect the athlete's equipment, such as running shoes, football boots, tennis racquet, bicycle or helmet.

## DIFFERENTIAL DIAGNOSES

Diagnosis is iterative—you think about it at various stages of the clinical encounter. That's why we mention it at the end of the history and again here! When you have completed the physical examination, you'll reflect on possible diagnoses and how confident you are about them. If you are certain of the primary diagnosis and of the predisposing factors, you are ready to explain the options as part of shared decision making. Explain what you have deduced and see how the patient feels about that information (Chapter 4).

At other times, you may feel you need more information. Explain to the patient that you feel you have narrowed the options and that you'll discuss the next investigative steps with them. Chapter 20 focuses on imaging. Chapter 21 provides a contemporary view of how to decide among (1) competing diagnoses when things are not clear cut and (2) treatment options when they are numerous (which is often the case in our field).

## KEY POINTS

- Patients and clinicians benefit from accurate, pathoanatomical diagnoses rather than outdated terms like "tennis elbow" or "hockey groin".

- In scenarios where you are unlikely to identify an exact anatomical cause of pain (e.g. low back pain), it is important to rule out red flags, to exclude the diagnoses you can and rely on good clinical skills to create a treatment plan.

- A comprehensive history and physical examination (along with appropriate investigations) are the cornerstone of constructing a clinical diagnosis. Sophisticated tests and expensive medical imaging are not always as valuable as once thought.

- A good medical history requires sufficient time, excellent listening skills, sport-specific knowledge and consideration of the patient's lifestyle, psychological, social and biological contributing factors.

- The history is also a time to enquire about the patient's short- and long-term goals to support a shared-decision making process once the diagnosis is established.

- The physical examination should be informed by the patient's medical history. There are several components of a comprehensive physical examination including palpation, observation, movement assessment, neurodynamic examination and spinal examination.

- The physical examination should incorporate sport-specific movements or activities where appropriate.

- The physical examination should focus on the site of pain or dysfunction reported by the patient, as well as proximal and distal structures that may contribute.

- Always consider possible differential diagnoses and whether additional investigations may inform the diagnosis.

## REFERENCES

References for this chapter can be found at www.mhprofessional.com/CSM6e

## ADDITIONAL CONTENT

 Scan here to access additional resources for this topic and more provided by the authors

# CHAPTER 20

# Diagnosis: imaging

with BRUCE FORSTER

*Imaging by a sports radiologist can improve athlete outcomes when its guided by validated decision rules or sound clinical judgment, but widespread use of imaging can be harmful and waste of health resources.*

CAROLYN BRODERICK (SPORTS AND EXERCISE MEDICINE PHYSICIAN)

*At major games, access to diagnostic imaging is important, but it's the immediate access to high-quality sports radiology expertise that is the real game changer.*

MICHAEL KOEHLE (SPORT PHYSICIAN)

## CHAPTER OUTLINE

Five imaging habits of top clinicians
Conventional radiography
Magnetic resonance imaging
Ultrasound

Computed tomography
Radionuclide bone scanning
Artificial intelligence (AI) in imaging

## LEARNING OBJECTIVES

By the end of this chapter you should be able to:

- discuss the role of imaging in sports medicine diagnosis, including normal variants, age- and sport-related findings
- explain the key concept of "treat the patient, not the image"
- recognise the modalities that involve ionising radiation, and how this affects the choice of imaging tests in patients in different age groups
- differentiate between the typical imaging modalities used in various clinical scenarios in terms of their advantages and disadvantages.

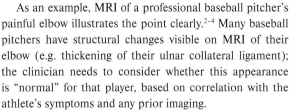

Sports medicine radiology has provided dramatic advances for patients—particularly since the advent of relatively widely available magnetic resonance imaging (MRI) from around 2000 and the more recent advent of bedside and pitchside ultrasound scanning. As well as providing remarkable insight into sports medicine pathologies, superior imaging capability has brought with it new challenges for clinicians: "Yes, that bright signal is abnormal most of the time, but what does that mean in this patient?"

Before we tackle that difficult question, we begin with what we know to be true—the five habits of highly effective clinicians with respect to imaging. Every top sport and exercise clinician is highly skilled at interpreting sports imaging and works closely with top musculoskeletal radiologists to perform at the level that champions expect and that every patient who sees a specialist deserves.[1]

## FIVE IMAGING HABITS OF TOP CLINICIANS

In certain clinical settings, appropriate investigations can confirm or exclude a diagnosis suggested by the history and physical examination. A conventional radiograph can confirm that a cyclist has fractured her clavicle. Computed tomography (CT) with multiplanar reformat and three-dimensional volumetric rendering can provide the precise configuration of that fracture. MRI can rule out a stress fracture in a dancer's foot if there is no sign of abnormal T2 signal on a fat-suppressed imaging sequence.

### PRACTICE PEARL

In many clinical contexts imaging does not identify a single structure that is the source of pain. Imaging the patient with back pain is the historical example used to illustrate that point, but there are many more examples.

As an example, MRI of a professional baseball pitcher's painful elbow illustrates the point clearly.[2-4] Many baseball pitchers have structural changes visible on MRI of their elbow (e.g. thickening of their ulnar collateral ligament); the clinician needs to consider whether this appearance is "normal" for that player, based on correlation with the athlete's symptoms and any prior imaging.

Other very prominent regions where structural changes are often evident on MRI but may not be symptomatic include the tennis player's elbow, the football player's ankle and the fast bowler's lumbar spine. The take-home message is that imaging alone cannot substitute for careful history taking and a comprehensive examination (see Chapter 19). Because diagnosis is complex, the leading clinicians in our field have embraced the following behaviours.

### 1. Understand imaging results

If you work in sports and exercise medicine, we recommend that you learn to interpret imaging yourself. Learn basic imaging anatomy of the musculoskeletal system—it is only a fraction of what radiologists have to know.[5] It is unwise to rely blindly on imaging reports. A competent sport and exercise clinician knows that about 25% of asymptomatic elite jumping athletes have ultrasound appearances of structural change in their patellar tendon (hypoechoic region, Fig. 20.1).[6, 7]

This is critical knowledge as the patient may have no pain there; in fact, the tendon may have been scanned as the asymptomatic knee for comparison with the symptomatic side. Without requisite clinical awareness, the clinician could be guided by the test to a potentially false-positive result (depending on the criteria for "positive", see below). Management must be guided by clinical assessment, not by imaging appearance alone.

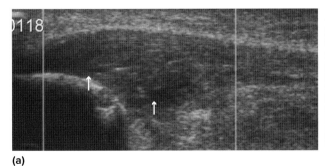

(a)

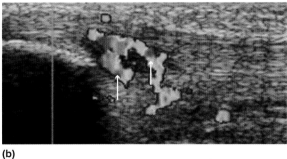

(b)

**Figure 20.1** Variations from "normal" imaging are common among athletes who place great loads on tissue. (a) Greyscale and (b) Doppler ultrasound appearances of the patellar tendon in a volleyball player, demonstrating hypoechoic regions (arrows in a) and hyperaemia (arrows in b). Experienced clinicians appreciate the high prevalence of these findings in asymptomatic players.

- *Timing of imaging tests.* Imaging may be performed too early to detect a pathology. That radiography can be performed too early to detect a stress fracture is widely known and therefore a "negative" result does not exclude this diagnosis (high or moderate negative likelihood ratio, so not good for ruling out that pathology).
- *A "true" finding may be age-related.* For example, triangular fibrocartilage tears of the wrist seen on MRI can be a normal finding, even in a non-athlete, for patients over 50 years of age.[8] Clinical correlation with the patient's symptoms and the physical examination is crucial.
- *The wrong test can give false-positive or false-negative information.* For example, a routine MRI of the shoulder in a 26-year-old baseball pitcher will miss most labral tears, other than those involving the superior labrum (SLAP tears); an MR arthrogram is needed to make the diagnosis. Radiologists are not only image interpreters, they are also consultants who can advise on the choice of imaging tests to best demonstrate pathology. Indeed, the most accurate imaging test for a given musculoskeletal pathology may not necessarily be the most sophisticated or complicated test.
- *Be able to judge the adequacy of the quality of obtained images for diagnostic purposes.* Be alert so as not to draw conclusions from imaging tests that may be incomplete or are limited by image degradations. Also, each imaging test may be specifically obtained to evaluate for one type of pathology but not others. For example, two-view radiographs of the shoulder in internal and external rotation to evaluate for calcific tendinopathy should not be used to exclude glenohumeral dislocation.
- *Intravenous contrast is usually reserved for CT or MRI cases in which the diagnosis of neoplasm or infection is being considered.* It is very important to indicate as such on the requisition if these need to be ruled out.
- *It is important to minimise ionising radiation, especially in children and adults aged under 30 years.* The dose is especially significant in nuclear medicine bone scans, positron emission tomography scans and CT scans (other than those of the distal extremities). If any of these tests are truly indicated, the principle of ALARA (as low as reasonably achievable) with respect to dose should be followed by the imaging department. Note that there is no ionising radiation in MRI or ultrasound, and the dose is negligible in most clinical radiographs.

Why do we share these detailed examples about clinicians needing to understand tests? Because the days of thinking that "imaging reveals X, therefore treatment is Y" are essentially over. Imaging fits into the treatment algorithm and helps update your thinking of the likelihood of a diagnosis (see "Likelihood ratios", Chapter 21). You must understand imaging because it is a tool, not a solution, and far from a panacea.

## 2. Only order imaging that will influence management

It is inappropriate to perform imaging to confirm an already obvious diagnosis, or a diagnosis for which the investigation result will not influence management. Most concussions are diagnosed clinically and do not need brain CT or MRI. Most cases of back pain in sport are not helped by adding low back imaging (radiography, CT or MRI). If an ankle sprain does not appear to have caused a fracture (and there are clinical guidelines to help with the assessment),[9] initial management does not include any imaging.

Players/athletes can put clinicians under pressure to order tests; in theory this should always be resisted. In real life, it can be difficult to resist such pressure in the professional sport setting so we will not pretend that ideal management is always followed. But understanding the usefulness of tests and test metrics (see Chapter 19) as well as normal patterns of imaging in sport (habit 1, above), allows you to have a valuable conversation with the athlete, to make an informed decision (see also Figure 2.1 in Chapter 2). Clinical decision support tools have been shown to reduce low-value imaging.[10] Also see Chapter 4 on shared decision making.

## 3. Explain the imaging to the patient

Give the patient an understanding of the rationale behind each imaging test. An athlete who complains of persistent ankle pain and swelling several months after an ankle sprain may need a radiograph and MRI. If the patient is merely told that radiography is necessary to exclude bony damage, they might become confused when told that the radiograph is normal, but that further investigations are required to exclude bony or osteochondral damage.

Also, be sure to alert patients undergoing a procedure that involves contrast (e.g. MR arthrogram) that there will be an injection, and obtain any history of contrast allergy. It is helpful to provide the patient with resources (either as printed material or as weblinks to videos) explaining the investigation. Follow-up plans should be made explicit in the clinical consultation.

## 4. Provide relevant clinical findings on the requisition

Accurate and complete clinical information on requisition forms helps to avoid imaging and reporting errors and improves diagnostic accuracy. For example, in one study, fracture detection was increased by 60% when location of pain or tenderness was provided in the history.[11] When particular radiographic views are required, they should be specified. If you cannot remember the names of certain views, write that down on the request form—the imaging technologists will generally know them and, if not, the radiologist will.

If there is uncertainty, it is always helpful to call the radiologist in advance to discuss the best way to image a patient. Do not assume that imaging technologists are familiar with the specific views required for sports-related musculoskeletal conditions (e.g. correct anteroposterior, "frog" and Dunn views for hip femoroacetabular impingement, skyline views for patellofemoral joint evaluation, the Bernageau view for shoulder instability). Remember that weight-bearing views are important to assess suspected osteoarthritis at the hip, knee and ankle. "Functional" views (with the patient placing the joint in the position of pain) are useful when you suspect anterior or posterior impingement of the ankle (see Chapter 30 in *Clinical Sports Medicine 6e: Managing Injuries*).

## 5. Develop a close working relationship with members of the imaging department

Optimising communication between colleagues improves the quality of the service.[1] Discuss optimal imaging sequences with imaging technologists and view the images together with radiologists providing clinical input. Regular clinical–radiological rounds (multidisciplinary team rounds) or case presentations should be encouraged. Digital imaging and telemedicine have made this much easier, and such collaboration can also facilitate research, quality assurance initiatives and educational opportunities.

If you develop those habits, you will be well on your way to providing high-value care. We deliberately used the umbrella term "imaging"—now it's time to dive into the pros and cons of the specific imaging modalities. We suggest you read Table 20.1 across in rows—beginning with the modalities you know best. Table 20.2 illustrates how the specific imaging modalities can be used to address nine common clinical scenarios.

**TABLE 20.1**   Key principles about the various imaging modalities that clinicians wished they had known earlier in their careers

| Imaging modality | Utility | Strengths | Weaknesses | Ionising radiation concerns |
|---|---|---|---|---|
| **Radiography (X-ray)** | First-line imaging modality for suspected fracture or bony abnormality; low utility for soft-tissue investigation; fluoroscopy useful in guiding procedures | Inexpensive; available; high specificity for fracture | Low sensitivity for stress fractures and undisplaced fractures | Use with caution in spine and pelvis |
| **Ultrasound** | Increasingly available modality well-suited to image soft tissues like tendon and muscle; useful in guiding procedures | Increasingly available modality well-suited to image soft tissues like tendon and muscle; useful in guiding procedures | Inability to penetrate bone; poor visualisation of cartilage | None |
| **Computed tomography (CT)** | Often used as a follow-up to radiography for suspected bony abnormality* | Better bony detail visualisation than radiography; ability to image in multiple planes | Cost; availability | Highest radiation dose among imaging modalities |
| **Magnetic resonance imaging (MRI)** | Routine first-line imaging modality for soft-tissue abnormality | Excellent soft-tissue visualisation; high sensitivity; ability to image in multiple planes | Cost; availability; poorer bony visualisation | None |
| **Radionuclide bone scan** | Ability to identify areas of bony stress, but largely replaced by MRI technology for sports indications | High sensitivity fo bony stress | Availability; poor specificity | Moderate to high |

*CT also has utility in ruling out intracranial hemorrhage or skull/facial fracture in the athlete with head trauma.

**TABLE 20.2** Pros and cons of various imaging modalities

| Suspicious for ... | Radiography (X-ray) | Ultrasound | Computed tomography (CT) | Magnetic resonance imaging (MRI) |
|---|---|---|---|---|
| Rotator cuff injury | Possible utility if suspicious for calcific tendinopathy | Useful diagnostic tool; preferred for older patients | Not indicated | Preferred diagnostic tool |
| Shoulder/ hip labrum tear | Not indicated | Possible utility if suspicious for paralabral cyst | CT arthrogram has possible utility if MR arthrogram is contraindicated | MR arthrogram is preferred diagnostic tool |
| Hamstring injury | Useful first modality if suspicious for avulsion fracture | Useful diagnostic tool | Possible utility if suspicious for avulsion fracture | Preferred diagnostic tool |
| Meniscus tear | Not indicated | Not indicated | Not indicated | Preferred diagnostic tool |
| ACL tear | Possible utility if suspicious for Segond fracture; avulsion fracture in youth athlete | Not indicated | Not indicated | Preferred diagnostic tool |
| Superficial tendon injury (e.g. ECU, Achilles) | Not indicated | Preferred diagnostic tool | Not indicated | Useful diagnostic tool |
| Superficial ligament injury (e.g. ATFL, elbow UCL) | Not indicated | Useful diagnostic tool | Not indicated | Preferred diagnostic tool |
| Acute fracture | Preferred diagnostic tool | Not indicated | Possible utility if radiograph is negative, but clinical suspicion for fracture remains high | Not indicated |
| Stress fracture | Not indicated | Not indicated | Useful for high-risk stress fractures (femoral neck, tarsal navicular, anterior tibia) | Preferred diagnostic tool |

ATFL, anterior tibiofibular ligament; ECU, extensor carpi ulnaris; UCL, ulnar collateral ligament

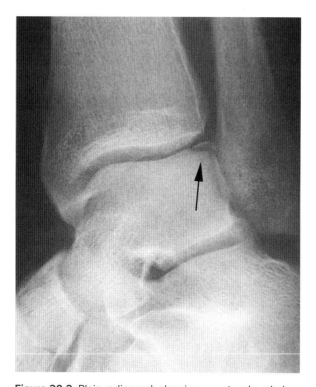

**Figure 20.2** Plain radiograph showing an osteochondral fracture of the lateral talar dome
COURTESY OF IAN "JOCK" ANDERSON

## CONVENTIONAL RADIOGRAPHY

Even in the mid-2020s, radiography provides diagnostic information about bony abnormalities such as fractures, dislocations, dysplasia and calcification (Fig. 20.2), and is highly cost-effective. Correctly positioning the patient is vital for obtaining radiographic images that are meaningfully interpretable. A minimum of two orthogonal views are required to evaluate any bone adequately. Complex joints such as the ankle, wrist or elbow may require additional or specialised views. Weight-bearing views are critical in the assessment of osteoarthritis of the hip, knee and ankle. However, as previously noted, it is important to minimise ionising radiation exposure in younger athletes and therefore oblique views of the lumbar spine ("Scotty dog views"), which have a high effective dose, should be eliminated from clinical practice in favour of MRI detection of spondylolysis in the young athlete.

## MAGNETIC RESONANCE IMAGING

The 2003 Nobel Prize in Medicine was awarded to the inventors of MRI. This imaging method has revolutionised sports and exercise medicine by providing clinicians with remarkably detailed information about structure, especially soft tissues, and helpful information about dynamic pathophysiology.

Because of MRI's unparalleled contrast resolution, commonly injured musculoskeletal tissues such as the menisci in the knee, the labrum in the shoulder and hip, spinal discs and joint surfaces can be visualised non-invasively and without ionising radiation. MRI allows clinicians to appreciate fairly dynamic processes such as bone and cartilage turnover, changes in tendon structure even in the absence of rupture, and recovery of ligament after acute sprain.

The physics that underpins MRI is well beyond the scope of this book. At a most superficial level, MRI relies on the biology that hydrogen protons exist within a tissue sample. Slightly more than one-half of these protons align with the external magnetic field, producing a vector. When a series of radiofrequency pulses are applied to the tissue sample in the magnet, protons release energy, which creates the MR image.

Unparalleled sensitivity to detect deviation in structure from anatomical norms does not, however, equal unparalleled accuracy in diagnosis for the patient (see Chapter 19). Erroneous interpretation of an MRI can have serious clinical consequences. For example, if a 50-year-old person's knee MRI is misinterpreted, a patient who in reality has patellofemoral pain may be inappropriately slated for arthroscopic meniscal surgery (Fig. 20.3).

The price of additional medical data is that the clinician who cares for the patient needs to determine how heavily to weigh the imaging information. Specifically, the clinician must arrive at a post-test probability of a diagnosis based on how much the MRI result (positive or negative) changes the pre-test probability of the diagnosis.

## Specific features and patient benefits of MRI

MRI is a routine part of the medical landscape the world over, although access to MRI for sports and exercise medicine imaging is limited in some regions. The tide is heading powerfully towards greater and greater use of MRI in sports and exercise medicine. Paradoxically, in developed countries too much imaging and overdiagnosis, associated with overtreatment (particularly arthroscopic surgery), has a deleterious effect on health. So, the challenge is to choose imaging with care. Here we review the features of MRI as a tool for clinicians in sports and exercise medicine.

MRI:

- is non-invasive, so it has dramatically reduced the need for diagnostic arthroscopy.
- can provide images in multiple planes. Need a sagittal view of the knee to image the patellar tendon? Sure! A coronal to assess joint surfaces and menisci? No problem!
- does not involve ionising radiation. This is particularly important for two populations: (1) adolescents and (2) professional athletes who may have many clinical encounters and thus need many scans.
- has superb contrast resolution for soft tissues, allowing accurate assessment of most ligaments, tendons and hyaline and fibrocartilage. Note that although bones are also well-assessed, if the clinical concern is one of primarily bony pathology (e.g. preoperative evaluation for a bony Bankart lesion), CT may be more appropriate, bearing in mind radiation dose.
- is ideal to assess patients who have had soft-tissue trauma (e.g. contact injuries) and it complements the use of CT in high-velocity injuries.
- has an emerging role in helping clinicians to evaluate overuse injuries. Anatomy is markedly affected by microtrauma/adaptation to load and this is increasingly being characterised. In the late 1980s, journals commonly carried treatment recommendations from "experts" based on false premises of what was "normal" in athletes.[13] The problem was that "normal" for an elite athlete had not been well documented. The subspecialty of sports radiology and greater experience of musculoskeletal radiologists with sport is addressing that challenge.[1] As with all research, knowledge translation remains a challenge; getting the key messages to the community of clinicians who will apply it is paramount.

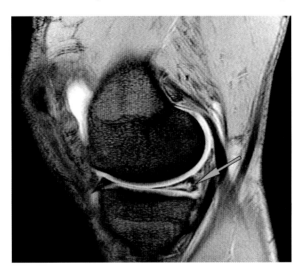

**Figure 20.3** Incidental MRI-detected meniscal pathology occurs in 19% of women aged 50–59 years.[12] The figure shows a horizontal cleavage tear of the posterior horn of the medial meniscus (arrow). Whether or not this MRI-detected lesion is clinically relevant in a patient presenting with knee pain depends on the entire clinical picture, including a detailed history and physical examination findings. The take-home message is that a clinician cannot, and should not, make a diagnosis and decide how to treat the patient solely based on MRI findings.

**BOX 20.1**  What does this MRI tell me? Tips for clinicians

The four most common sequences you will see are outlined below and shown in Figure 20.4.

1. *T1-weighted* provides sharp anatomical detail, shows bone marrow and is good for meniscal pathology (Fig. 20.4a). It lacks the sensitivity to detect soft-tissue injury. MRI signal key: fat = bright; muscle = intermediate; water, tendons and fibrocartilage = all dark.
2. *Proton density-weighted* is good for imaging menisci and ligaments (Fig. 20.4b). MRI signal key: fat = bright or intermediate signal; calcium, tendons and fibrocartilage = all dark; water = intermediate.
3. *T2-weighted* is highly sensitive for most soft-tissue injury, especially tendons. Abnormal tendons have high signal intensity (bright) which contrasts with normal tendons, which have low signal (arrowhead) (Fig. 20.4c). MRI signal key: water = bright; fat = intermediate; muscle, hyaline and fibrocartilage = all dark.
4. *STIR* (short tau inversion recovery) highlights excess water (blue arrow and blue arrowheads) which can occur due to bone stress and bone marrow oedema (shown), joint fluid and soft-tissue pathology. This is the sequence of choice for bone stress injuries or subtle, radiographically occult fractures (Fig. 20.4d). MRI signal key: water = very bright; fat, muscle, menisci = all dark.

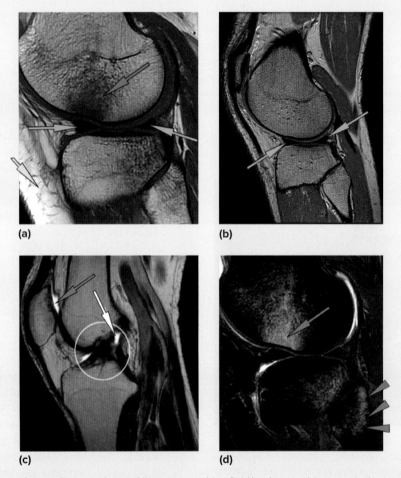

(a)  (b)  (c)  (d)

**Figure 20.4**  Arrows: fat = yellow; tendon and ligament = white; fluid/oedema = blue; menisci = green
(a) T1-weighted image showing bone marrow oedema (also called bone marrow lesion) after full-thickness ACL tear. Arrows to high signal fat (yellow arrow), very low signal normal lateral menisci (green arrows) and low signal oedema (blue arrow). (b) Proton density-weighted image showing normal anterior and posterior horns of the lateral menisci (green arrows). (c) T2-weighted image showing full-thickness ACL tear (white arrow). Note bright joint fluid (blue arrow). (d) STIR image (fat suppressed) showing the same patient as in (a). Bone marrow oedema (high signal, blue arrow) as a result of the acute knee giving way episode and ACL rupture. Note additional bone marrow oedema (high signal, blue arrowheads) in the fibular styloid process as a result of concomitant torn arcuate ligament.

## Difference added by MRI sequences

Spin echo, gradient echo and inversion recovery sequences are the basic categories of sequences used in musculoskeletal imaging. T1-weighted, T2-weighted, proton density-weighted and STIR sequences are often used (Box 20.1, Fig. 20.4). Fat-suppressed fast or turbo spin echo sequences are used in almost every musculoskeletal protocol to demonstrate bone marrow oedema, focal cartilage defects and tendon/ligament pathology with the highest conspicuity. 3D sequences are increasingly used to decrease imaging time and increase spatial resolution.

Zero echo time (ZTE) imaging is a new MRI technique that produces images similar to those obtained with radiography or CT (Fig. 20.5). The ZTE sequence clearly shows many fractures, including stress fractures, that are not as easily identified with other MRI sequences and that are obscured on standard radiography.

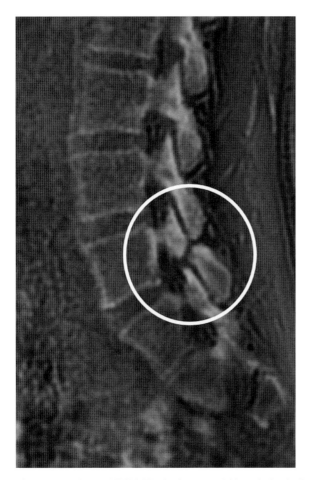

**Figure 20.5** Sagittal ZTE MRI of a 21-year-old female football player with back pain. A right L4 pars interarticularis stress fracture (circled) is conspicuously displayed on the image.
WITH COURTESY OF DR USTUN AYDINGOS

## Other clinical points about MRI

The clinical workhorse for sports MRI is the 1.5T (Tesla) MRI platform. For almost all clinical indications, MRI at this field strength is generally sufficient. The 3T magnets, which are somewhat more expensive to purchase, offer higher spatial resolution and therefore may offer advantages in evaluating small structures, such as tendon pulley injuries in rock climbers (although there are currently no trials to support this). Advanced applications in 3T may prove useful in the future in dedicated cartilage imaging.

The contrast agent for MRI is gadolinium, which has an excellent safety profile, even more so than the safe iodinated contrast agents used in CT. It is used intravenously for musculoskeletal imaging in cases in which tumour or infection are being considered, and in an intra-articular fashion to optimally evaluate fibrocartilage, such as shoulder and hip labra. However, MR arthrography should only be ordered if the patient is a surgical candidate, or is of a suitable age and otherwise appropriate for meniscal or labral repair.

Physiological (or compositional) imaging of cartilage can be performed at 1.5T and 3T, but not accurately at lower field strengths. Special sequences can detect loss of cartilage proteoglycan (T1-rho mapping and dGEMRIC) and collagen degradation (T2 mapping). These techniques hold promise in biochemical, pre-morphological chondral assessment in early osteoarthritis, and for follow-up of interventions (e.g. chondral surgery and, one day, biologics that can block the progression of osteoarthritis). However, currently their clinical role is undefined.

There are a few strict contraindications to MRI (e.g. certain brain aneurysm clips, neurostimulators and cardiac pacemakers among them).

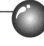

> **PRACTICE PEARL**
>
> Contrary to popular medical opinion, patients with metallic orthopaedic hardware and metallic surgical clips outside the brain, in place for more than 6 weeks, can be safely scanned.

MRI can be overly sensitive to abnormal tissue signals and thus provide false-positive results. In numerous studies involving athletes, MRI revealed structural appearances consistent with significant injury but the athletes were asymptomatic and high functioning.[7,8] This emphasises the need for the appropriate selection of patients for investigation and careful clinical–imaging correlation.[1] As with any medical investigation, diagnostic errors can occur; ideally, images should be read by an experienced musculoskeletal MRI radiologist.

## ULTRASOUND

High-resolution ultrasound scanning with 10–12 MHz probes is ideal for imaging tendons, muscles and other soft tissues without exposing the patient to any radiation.[13] It allows clinical correlation—imaging with the patient reproducing their pain and providing feedback to the radiologist. Other advantages include its dynamic nature (the patient can move the part), compact platform, short examination time and ability to guide therapeutic aspiration or injection under real time.

Ultrasound is the imaging instrument of choice "in clinic",[14, 15] where patients present with injuries of muscle and tendon. Units are affordable in the clinic because the unit cost, installation and service are in the order of 100 times cheaper than MRI. Another advantage of ultrasound is its low carbon footprint.

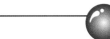

**PRACTICE PEARL**

Ultrasound has been referred to as the sport and exercise clinician's stethoscope and the analogy applies to the portability of ultrasound—small units can be used on the sideline.[16] However, laptop-sized portable units don't have the same image quality as the larger units that are designed to stay in the clinic.

We might consider ultrasound equipment as having three different levels:

1. The most expensive, best-quality equipment would be located at a specialist radiology clinic. The radiologist and team with the full battery of complementary imaging modalities provide the tertiary resource as well as continuing professional education (formal and informal) and research partnerships as appropriate. Advanced features include power/colour Doppler, 3D/4D imaging, harmonic imaging and research tools such as shear-wave elastography.
2. Leading specialised clinical practices often choose to have quality ultrasound imaging capacity at the clinic to assist with speed of diagnosis, for injections with ultrasound imaging and because having ultrasound skills advances clinicians' understanding of anatomy.
3. Portable sideline equipment (laptop scanner shown in Fig. 20.6, and also hand-held units) still provide quality images but the users appreciate the limitation compared with that outlined in point 1.

Disadvantages of ultrasound include it has less graphic images, is operator-dependent with respect to image quality and cannot penetrate tissues to show bone, shoulder/hip

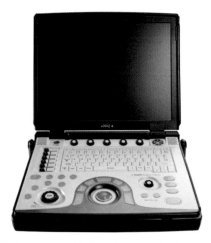

**Figure 20.6** Portable sideline ultrasound unit
COURTESY OF GENERAL ELECTRIC (GE)

labra or anterior cruciate ligaments/menisci. Commonly examined areas are large tendons (e.g. the Achilles and rotator cuff tendons), bursae, and the muscles of the thigh and calf. Ultrasound can also demonstrate muscle tear, haematoma formation or early calcification.

Ultrasound scanning can distinguish complete tendon rupture from other tendon abnormalities (e.g. tendinopathy). As with MRI, ultrasound imaging of asymptomatic athletes can reveal morphological "abnormalities" that do not appear to predict imminent tendon pain (Fig. 20.7).

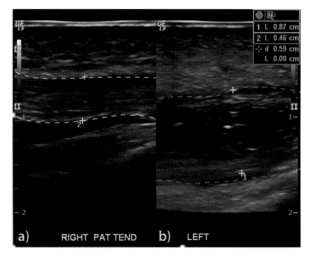

**Figure 20.7** Patellar tendon ultrasound images in the sagittal plane. (a) Tendon is of normal thickness (46 mm between the green lines) and has normal echo texture. (b) "Abnormal" tendon appearance in an athlete who has never had knee pain. The tendon is thickened (87 mm between the red lines) and has abnormal echo texture which reflects abnormal tendon architecture.
COURTESY OF DR BRUCE FORSTER

Real-time ultrasound examination during active movement (dynamic ultrasound) is particularly helpful in the evaluation of shoulder impingement and tendon (e.g. extensor carpi ulnaris) subluxation/dislocation. The use of ultrasound to help guide injection is discussed in Chapter 24.

## The role of colour Doppler

Colour Doppler ultrasound gained popularity in sports medicine for the assessment of tendons in the early 2000s, as it was hoped that abnormal tendon flow detected using the colour Doppler feature would provide a better guide as to whether tendons were painful (see Fig. 20.1b). Longitudinal studies failed to show that colour Doppler ultrasound findings of vascularity predicted changes in symptoms.[17] Also, exercise affects the level of vascularity, which adds a challenge to the clinical utility of this method. This modality is proving useful in certain areas of medicine but has dropped off the "hot topics" list in sports medicine. To return to a theme from early in this chapter, there appears to be no substitute for careful clinical examination and patient monitoring to track patients' current progress and to predict outcomes.

## COMPUTED TOMOGRAPHY

CT scanning (Figs 20.8 and 20.9) allows cross-sectional imaging of soft tissue, calcific deposits and bone. CT scanning is particularly useful in evaluation of the spine, fractures in small bones and fractures in anatomically

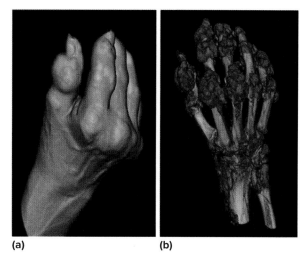

**(a)** **(b)**

**Figure 20.9** A patient with chronic tophaceous gout showing the value of dual-energy CT in detecting monosodium urate. (a) 3D surface-rendered dual-energy CT of a thumb showing prominent tophi. The patient had gout. (Note this is not a photograph of the patient's hand—the image is of a CT reconstruction). (b) 3D reconstruction of the same patient as in (a) showing extensive monosodium urate deposition (red) detected by the dual-energy technology.
COURTESY OF DR SAVVAS NICOLAOU

complex regions, such as the ankle, foot or pelvis. CT scanners provide high-resolution reconstructions of the imaging data in any plane. Remember that CT defines bone

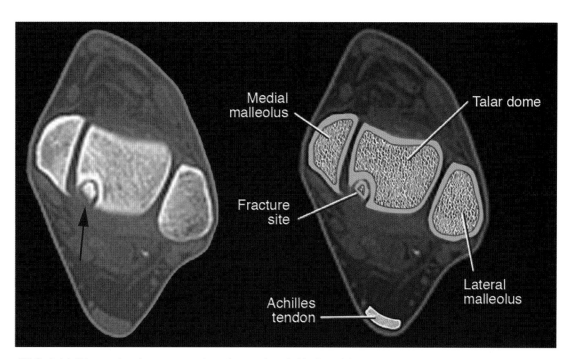

**Figure 20.8** Axial CT scan showing cross-section of osteochondral lesion of the posteromedial talar dome (arrow)

details and can detect small areas of calcification better than MRI can, even though the latter will reveal occult bony abnormalities (Fig. 20.8). Advances in multidetector CT technology enable rapid image acquisition and superb multiplanar reconstruction. Dual-energy CT now allows accurate assessment of monosodium urate deposition to diagnose and follow gout (Fig. 20.9) and shows promise in the assessment of bone marrow oedema in occult fractures. The disadvantage of CT scanning is the significant radiation dose, especially in children. However, the effective dose of CT examinations of the distal extremities (e.g. hand/foot) is trivial, even in younger patients.

## RADIONUCLIDE BONE SCANNING

Radionuclide bone scanning (scintigraphy) has fallen out of favour in sports medicine practice because of the availability of MRI with appropriate pulse sequences (e.g. 3D, T1-weighted) and because of its high radiation dose. MRI provides similar information about bone while adding superior anatomical localisation. Radionuclide bone scans had high sensitivity for stress fractures and low negative likelihood if negative for stress fracture. This meant that they were useful (in their day) for ruling out stress fractures.

Does radionuclide bone scanning still have a role in sports imaging? Very rarely, with the exception of assessment of metastatic disease. Expert and experienced radiologists may use it at times to seek a tibial or a metatarsal stress fracture but it has essentially been superseded by MRI and CT.

Single photon emission computed tomography techniques are also used in sports medicine, particularly in the detection of stress fractures of the pars interarticularis of the lumbar spine, although the correct MRI sequence should be able to detect these changes.

## ARTIFICIAL INTELLIGENCE (AI) IN IMAGING

No discussion of imaging would be complete without reference to AI. Radiology employs sophisticated computer technology perhaps more than any other area of medicine, making AI especially important to consider. The replacement of radiologists by such technology is grossly exaggerated, but AI can assist radiologists with a narrow and defined series of medical imaging tasks. For example, AI is being used to assist with diagnosis of fractures, increase the speed of image acquisition in MRI and manage large data sets.[18] The role of AI in radiology is to complement the clinician, rather than replace them.

Sports radiologists can be supported by AI in several domains, including workflow optimisation, image enhancement, image interpretation, and reporting.[19]

- In terms of optimising workflow, AI may be used to streamline several non-diagnostic tasks, including assistance with scheduling and the requisition process or triaging studies.
- The quality of medical images can be enhanced using AI technology. For example, in cases where orthopaedic hardware may create an artifact on CT images, AI may be able to suppress the noise and create a clearer image.[20]
- One of the clinical (interpretation-related) uses for AI in radiology applies to fracture detection. A 2024 systematic review indicated that AI can detect and classify fractures with relative accuracy.[21] AI may be narrowly used in interpreting images across other areas of radiology (e.g. in tumour identification) but fracture detection is the primary function of AI in sports radiology image interpretation at present.
- AI may have the ability to support radiologists while they are dictating the findings from a medical imaging study and generating their report.

There is huge variability (due to geography, resource limitations, legal issues etc.) in how AI is being used in each of these domains.

Collectively, AI can increase efficiency in some non-clinical areas of sports radiology, improve the quality of medical images themselves, and support radiologists in streamlining their workflow and communicating their findings. Ultimately, if we are successful in each of these areas, patient care will be improved. There are, however, a few important caveats.

First, there are broad concerns in the adoption of AI, including the quality of data on which the technology is trained, its risk of bias, and how to create appropriate policies and procedures around its adoption. Second, it is important to note that some of this technology is still in the pre-clinical exploratory stage, and not yet integrated into routine clinical care. Third, there is the question of the patient's attitude towards, and acceptance of, AI.

Finally, there are issues of medico-legal liability, data security and ethics to be considered when adopting AI into clinical practice. However, it would be foolish to ignore or minimise the importance of understanding the role that AI can play in improving clinical care, as well as its significant limitations.

## KEY POINTS

- Radiologists and radiology technologists are an important part of an athlete's care team when medical imaging becomes necessary.

- Communicating with these medical imaging experts can ensure that an athlete receives the most appropriate test, at the right time, using the most appropriate protocols.

- Each imaging modality has its own strengths and weaknesses; the best test for an athlete is not always the most expensive or sophisticated study.

- For some imaging modalities (e.g. CT and radiography), ionising radiation dose should be considered, especially in young athletes.

- Medical imaging must be considered in the context of a comprehensive history and examination. There are often "abnormal" findings in asymptomatic individuals. Treat the athlete, not the image!

- Don't use medical imaging to confirm an otherwise obvious diagnosis or if the results will not change an athlete's treatment plan. Imaging is explicitly not recommended for some conditions (e.g. chronic non-specific low back pain).

- Even in the mid-2020s, radiography remains the best imaging modality for bony abnormalities. It is also cost-effective and often readily available. CT may be used for more detailed investigation of bony issues.

- Soft tissue is best visualised via MRI or ultrasound. Both are excellent options with strengths and weaknesses. Neither emits ionising radiation, but there are significant differences in accessibility and cost.

## REFERENCES

References for this chapter can be found at www.mhprofessional.com/CSM6e

## ADDITIONAL CONTENT

Scan here to access additional resources for this topic and more provided by the authors

# CHAPTER 21

# Diagnosis: phases of clinical assessment

with GARRETT S. BULLOCK and CHAD E. COOK

*Orthopaedic special tests: Promise so much and deliver so little.*

JEREMY LEWIS (CONSULTANT PHYSIOTHERAPIST AND PROFESSOR)

*The number of studies investigating the diagnostic accuracy of special tests is inversely proportional to the likelihood we will ever be accurate on the diagnosis*

ERIC HEGEDUS (PHYSIOTHERAPIST)

## CHAPTER OUTLINE

Clinical assessment
Phase 1: Gathering clinical data
Phase 2: Making the diagnosis and sharing the prognosis
Phase 3: Choosing the treatment plan

## LEARNING OBJECTIVES

By the end of this chapter you should be able to:

- state the goals of a sports-related clinical assessment
- discuss the three phases of clinical assessment
- list the elements of an intake form, a complete medical history and physical examination
- explain the steps in making a clinical diagnosis
- describe the metrics used to determine the usefulness and accuracy of various diagnostic tests
- outline how the concept of causality applies to choosing clinical treatments.

## CLINICAL ASSESSMENT

All top clinicians agree that clinical assessment is a foundation stone of quality clinical care—and that it is a complex skill. Assessment may occur on the field or in the clinic, and when determining clinical findings, imaging or laboratory tests. The primary goals of clinical assessment are to:

- identify the patient's pathoanatomical diagnosis (what's wrong with me?)
- identify the underlying disease-, pain- or disability-related mechanisms (why did it happen?)
- identify the patient's prognosis, with and without management options (when will I be back?)
- differentiate the data accumulated during the data gathering, diagnosis and prognosis phases for optimal decision making (what are my treatment options?).

Despite the caution about special tests captured in our opening quotes, we believe that in the mid-to-late 2020s medical science has ways to provide patients with an accurate window on both prognosis and treatment. To make our case, we divide clinical assessment into three phases that build on each other to enable you and the patient to make quality management decisions (Table 21.1).

**TABLE 21.1** The three phases of clinical assessment

| Phase 1 | Phase 2 | Phase 3 |
|---|---|---|
| Gather clinical data | Make the diagnosis and share the prognosis | Choose the treatment plan |

## PHASE 1: GATHERING CLINICAL DATA

In phase 1, your goal is to purposefully gather critical information. This will enable you in later phases to make the diagnosis, understand the underlying injury/illness mechanisms and advise on the prognosis.

Elements of phase 1 are discussed in Chapters 19 and 20 and include: (1) using a patient intake form[a] that has a clear purpose; (2) obtaining an appropriate patient history and completing a focused physical examination; (3) gathering both patient-reported and objective outcome measures; and (4) understanding the load/physical demands of the patient and their sport. We review these briefly here:

1. In addition to personal information and consent, the patient intake form should include current health concerns (i.e. the reason for the visit, symptoms, duration of symptoms) and any recent changes in health and lifestyle, hobbies and habit (i.e. diet, exercise, smoking, alcohol consumption, drug use and other relevant lifestyle factors).

2. A comprehensive patient history (discussed in detail in Chapter 19) should include the chief complaint, mechanism of injury, history of the current complaint, degree of severity, past similar or related injuries, current demands and any additional questions that arise after reading the patient intake form.

3. A focused physical examination should incorporate an examination of systems and organs through direct observation, palpation (touch) and other clinical techniques. An examination is essential to evaluate and maintain the patient's health, diagnose medical conditions and provide guidance on prevention and treatment.

   Outcome measures are often used to standardise the clinician's interpretation of the patient's levels of pain, disability or sport-related dysfunction, and should be selected based on their reliability and validity (discussed in detail in Chapter 24).

4. A detailed understanding of the load/physical demands of the athlete and their sport will give greater perspective on how they are compromised for participation in their sport and what options may improve their ability to return without compromise. Load/physical demands refer to the physical stresses and demands placed on the athlete's body during training and competition (see also Chapter 15). These demands vary substantially depending on the type of sport, the level of competition and the athlete's individual training program. Load demands are central to an athlete's recovery program: they will influence the rehabilitation progression, help determine when the athlete is ready to return to sport and provide invaluable data as you aim to reduce the athlete's risk of re-injury.

## PHASE 2: MAKING THE DIAGNOSIS AND SHARING THE PROGNOSIS

The aim of phase 2 is to detail the steps in making a diagnosis. As detailed in Chapter 19, clinical diagnosis is the act or process of identifying and determining the nature of a disease, medical condition or health problem that a patient is experiencing. Diagnoses are made after gathering data from the patient and/or their proxy (phase 1) and through judicious use of physical examination and, if needed, medical testing (i.e. imaging and laboratory work).

Differential diagnosis is a systematic process used to identify the correct diagnosis from a competing set of possible diagnoses. The diagnostic process involves identifying

[a] A patient intake form is a document used by healthcare providers to collect initial information from patients before they receive care or treatment.

or determining the aetiology of a disease or condition by evaluating the patient's history, conducting a physical examination and reviewing laboratory data or diagnostic imaging. Diagnosis also refers to the subsequent descriptive title of that finding. Regardless of treatment environment, most clinicians follow a three-step process to make a diagnosis:

1. *Are the patient's signs and symptoms reflective of a visceral disorder or a serious or potentially life-threatening illness?* (See also Chapter 22 on red flags.) It is critical to identify patients with symptoms that arise from a potentially life-threatening pathology or a non-mechanical disorder (i.e. referred pain).
2. *Where does the patient's pain arise from?* This is confirmed by:
   - ruling out a location
   - ruling in a location but not knowing the tissue-related structure
   - confirming the tissue-related structure that is causing the problem.

   Although it is assumed that clinicians can make an accurate tissue-related diagnosis, differentiating tissue in the low back, shoulder, abdomen and hip is very challenging and it is not uncommon to see clinicians treat these areas without full knowledge of the tissue of origin.
3. *What has gone wrong that would cause the pain experience to develop and persist?* This requires carefully exploring the social, psychosocial and socioeconomic contextual elements. This is outlined in Chapter 1 (the patient), Chapters 10 and 11 (pain) and Chapter 24 (treatment), and given more detailed attention in specific chapters in *Clinical Sports Medicine 6e: Managing Injuries* such as Chapter 6 (neck pain) and Chapter 15 (low back pain).

## How good is the diagnostic test?

Not all clinical tests are equal, so there are standard terms to discuss their value and enable them to be compared with each other to see which is better for the patient. These terms apply broadly to imaging, clinical testing and laboratory testing.

### Reliability

In diagnostic terms, reliability is either the ability of a test to consistently identify a similar finding when retested (e.g. dynamometer testing for strength) or used by a different clinician, or the level of consistent agreement among two or more clinicians when a particular test that requires interpretation is used (e.g. Lachman's test). Reliability is a required characteristic of diagnostic testing and is generally scored between 0 and 1 when evaluating a numerically scored test such as a goniometer, or when assessing agreement among clinicians (with a higher score reflecting greater agreement).

### Sensitivity and specificity

Sensitivity and specificity are internal measures (meaning they are relatively independent of the sample) that are used in two distinct populations:

1. the disease of interest or injured population (sensitivity)
2. a competing disease or non-injured population (specificity).

Let's begin with the textbook descriptions. Sensitivity refers to the percentage of people who test positive for a specific disease among a group of people who have the disease and is generally scored from 0 to 100%. Higher values mean the test is better able to accurately identify those who have the disease of interest. When a sign, test or symptom has a high sensitivity, a negative result rules out the diagnosis (SNOUT). A good example of a test with high sensitivity is an MRI for a bone stress injury—if the scan is negative, the patient is very unlikely to have that injury.

Specificity refers to the percentage of people who test negative for a specific disease among a group of people who do not have the disease and is also scored from 0 to 100%. Tests with higher values are more accurate at identifying those who do not have the disease of interest. When a sign, test or symptom has an extremely high specificity, a positive result tends to rule in the diagnosis (SPIN). An example is a tissue biopsy for a tumour such as a malignant melanoma. If you have a positive test result, you probably have a tumour.

Moving from the textbook to the real world, it's not so easy! Although the acronyms SPIN ("high specificity rules in the diagnosis") and SNOUT ("high sensitivity rules out") are used in clinical practice, remember that most tests are either sensitive or specific, but usually not both.

Unfortunately, both SPIN and SNOUT have limitations because they require at least a moderate level of sensitivity (for SNOUT) or specificity (for SPIN) for use in clinical practice. Otherwise, highly sensitive tests with low specificity may lead to high levels of false negatives, which reduces the utility of the adage. Similarly, highly specific tests with low sensitivity may lead to high levels of false negatives (Fig. 21.1).

### Positive and negative predictive values

Predictive values reflect the clinical setting and are relevant when asking the question, "The clinical screening test is positive. What is the likelihood that this patient truly has the condition?" A positive predictive value is the probability that those with a positive screening test truly have the disease. A negative predictive value is the probability that those with a negative screening test truly don't have the disease.

Like sensitivity and specificity, positive and negative predictive values capture only a portion of the population (Fig. 21.2) and should not be used exclusively in clinical practice because they fail to tell the full story of the test's

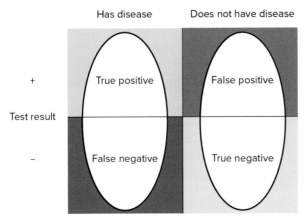

**Figure 21.1** Sensitivity is measured among those individuals who have the disease. A great number of true positives and few false negatives lead to a high sensitivity (left ovoid). Specificity is measured among those who do not have the disease. In this case, a low number of false positives and a high number of true negatives generate a high specificity. Each of these numbers only represents half the diagnostic story.

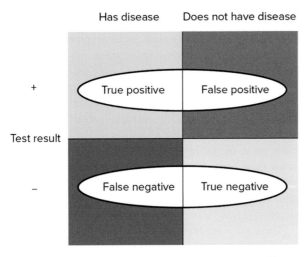

**Figure 21.2** Positive and negative predictive values. These should be used when the clinician is trying to answer the question, "The clinical screening test is positive. What is the likelihood that this patient truly has the condition?"

utility. Positive predictive values include only true positives and false negatives. Negative predictive values include only false positives and true negatives.

### Likelihood ratios

A high positive likelihood ratio (LR+) influences post-test probability with a positive finding. A value of >1 rules in a diagnosis. A low negative likelihood ratio (LR−) influences

post-test probability with a negative finding. A value closer to 0 rules out a condition. Although others have suggested thresholds for independent decision making, likelihood ratios should be evaluated within the context of pre-test prevalence and in each clinical setting.

Both sensitivity and specificity are used to determine positive and negative likelihood ratios. LR+ is calculated using the formula (sensitivity)/(100−specificity), whereas LR− is calculated using the formula (100−sensitivity)/(specificity). In LR+ and LR− the full population of interest, including those with and without the disease of interest, is factored into the decision-making metrics.

Likelihood ratios are the best metric to determine the influence of post-test probability and for clinicians to truly understand the influence of a test on diagnosis accuracy. Likelihood ratios account for the prevalence, give further perspective and allow for adjustments of test values in extreme cases of low or high prevalence. Some consistencies occur regardless of disease of interest.

A higher pre-test probability will always improve the post-test probability. A lower pre-test probability will demand a strong LR+ (to rule in); conversely, a higher pre-test probability will require a lower LR− (to rule out) to notably alter the post-test probability.

In essence, an effective clinician evaluates all the information and places the test findings in context. The term "diagnostic utility" is used when describing a test (clinical, imaging or laboratory) that markedly influences post-test probability (either ruling out the condition or ruling it in) and improves the probability of making a correct pathoanatomical diagnosis of the condition. However, differential diagnosis is an imperfect science, and some diagnoses are extremely difficult to make.

Sadly, many clinicians place too great a value on single testing mechanisms during differential diagnosis. Although one can find "validation" for single clinical, imaging-related or laboratory tests or combinations of tests, it is very rare for tests to have the capacity to differentially diagnose most conditions. A test in isolation cannot support differential diagnosis because a single test cannot discriminate in the absence of additional important information.

---

**PRACTICE PEARL**

Many clinicians overestimate the utility of special tests (e.g. the empty can test for supraspinatus tendon tear, McMurray's test for meniscus tear).[1] They are not "yes/no" tests—a positive test adds some weight to the likelihood of a diagnosis. Experienced clinicians use special tests in context alongside the rest of the clinical assessment.

## Disease mechanisms

By understanding the aetiology (Latin, "science of causes") of a diagnosis or disease, we can further understand the disease mechanisms that underlie the development and progression of a medical condition. Disease mechanisms refer to how specific factors, such as injuries, infections, environmental exposure or lifestyle choices, change the body's function and lead to disease.

Disease mechanisms are commonly multifactorial and involve a cascade of physiological manifestations. For example, peripheral neuropathy involves nerve damage related to impaired blood flow, trauma or infection, which can lead to axonal changes, demyelination and potential immune responses. Understanding underlying disease mechanisms allows you to better tailor treatments (when they exist) that target the disease mechanisms.

The most common forms of sports-related disease mechanisms include musculoskeletal-related phenomena associated with inflammation, sprains, strains, fractures and dislocations. Other disease mechanisms may include brain-related trauma (concussion), overtraining syndromes, cardiac-related phenomena and/or environmental-related challenges such as heat-related illnesses.

## Prognosis

A diagnosis serves as the foundation for establishing a prognosis. Prognosis refers to the likely outcome or course of a diagnosis, with or without treatment, based on the available information about the patient's health status, the natural history of the disease and our understanding of typical responses to treatment. Once you have identified the patient's specific disease or condition (diagnosis), you can use your expert knowledge and clinical judgment to make predictions about how the condition is likely to progress and what the patient can expect in terms of outcomes (prognosis).

Prognosis is useful because it answers the patient's "how long until … ?" questions and "if" they can continue playing in their sport. Prognosis has been promoted as equal in value to diagnosis and may be critical in reducing unnecessary care and costs associated with that care.

Prognostic tests have the capacity to identify patients by categories (or recognisable groups) that are likely to have a specific outcome (good or bad). As with diagnostic tests, prognostic tests require validation to determine their "utility". Some prognostic models have been presented to improve our capacity to determine prognosis for musculoskeletal injuries.[2] This area of research (and clinical transfer) is not as mature as research in diagnostic testing.

Targeting prognosis-related factors[3] in rehabilitation care is a promising way to personalise treatment approaches and optimise clinical outcomes.[4] Variables associated with prognosis for injured individuals can be divided into prognostic factors and treatment-effect modifiers:

- prognostic factors are characteristics that have an association with the natural course of a health condition (i.e. poor coping strategies, high pain intensity, negative recovery expectations)
- treatment-effect modifiers can predict an individual's treatment response (i.e. centralisation of symptoms, socioeconomic status).[5-7]

These individual factors can be integrated into wider prognostic models, thus improving the precision of outcome prediction for an individual patient (see example in phase 3 later in the chapter).[8]

Prognostic models, also known as prediction models, are mathematical models that include multiple predictors that calculate a risk score. Prognostic models include causal and non-causal factors and thus cannot be used to make causal inferences.[9-11] Within the last decade, prediction models have become a burgeoning tool for assessing injury risk in sports and exercise medicine environments but most of these models are poorly developed or not appropriate for clinical use.[12, 13]

Some prognostic models can aid clinicians by helping with what might otherwise prove to be a complex decision.[6] Prognostic models include multiple predictor variables which combine to estimate an individual's risk of a health outcome in the future (prognosis).[14] Individual predictors often have limited prediction performance[15] so multiple predictors should be included in the model.[6] Prognostic models output a forecast of the probability of an outcome occurring in the future, either in a 0 to 1 or 0 to 100 format.

There are many intricacies to developing and validating a prognostic model.[9-11] While it is beyond the scope of this chapter to cover how prognostic models are developed and validated, we introduce here three performance metrics for evaluating them: calibration, discrimination and clinical utility.[9-11]

### Calibration

Calibration is the agreement between a model's predicted risks and what was observed.[16] It should be assessed graphically and through a calibration slope with 95% confidence interval (see Fig. 21.3).[17] Perfect calibration is a slope of 1. As calibration diverges above or below 1, calibration performance is reduced. A calibration slope

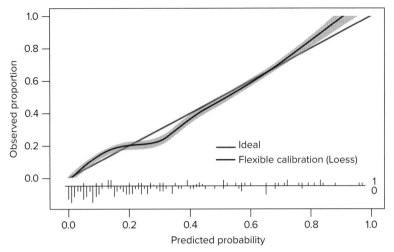

**Figure 21.3** Calibration is the relationship between the predicted and actual probability of an event. Perfect calibration would result in a 45° line. Within this figure, the grey line denotes the calibration of a prediction model, while the red line depicts perfect calibration (i.e. 45° line). Calibration above the red line suggests that risk is underpredicted compared with actual risk, while a calibration curve below the red line suggests that risk prediction is too extreme. In this calibration curve, the grey line goes above and below the red line between 0.0 and 0.4 risk, suggesting that risk may be slightly under- and overpredicted through this range of values. However, these calibration changes are only slight compared with ideal calibration and thus are within acceptable limits. Starting at 0.7 risk, there is a systematic divergence in predicted risk, with the calibration curve going over the ideal calibration red line. This may change risk identification in a patient for risk predicted above 0.7.

of less than 1 suggests that the predicted risks are too extreme. A calibration slope greater than 1 suggests that the predicted risks are not varied enough.

### Discrimination

Discrimination assesses how well model predictions can differentiate between individuals with and without an outcome.[17] Discrimination is assessed through the concordance statistic (*c* statistic) or the equivalent area under the receiver operating characteristic curve (AUC).[18, 19] An AUC of 0.5 means that the model predictions are no better than random chance, whereas an AUC of 1.0 means that the predictions discriminate perfectly.

### Clinical utility

Clinical utility is the usefulness of a model for making clinical decisions and is evaluated through net benefit.[20] Net benefit calculates the benefits and risks of making clinical intervention decisions through risk outputs from the prediction model.[17, 20, 21] Net benefit should be reported in tabular format and through a decision curve.[20] Net benefit tables and decision curves have the added benefit of directly comparing the clinical prediction model with other clinical decisions (or models), such as current evidence-based practice.[20]

To help you understand prognostic models, we provide a brief real-world example in Box 21.1.

---

**BOX 21.1** A prognostic model

A prognostic model was developed by a physical therapy researcher to estimate the risk of sustaining a lower extremity injury over the course of an English Premier League season.[22] A total of 138 events occurred over five seasons. Model performance was poor with a calibration slope of 0.718 (95% CI 0.275 to 1.161) and discrimination of 0.589 (95% CI 0.528 to 0.651).

The researcher hypothesised that poor model performance was related to the inadequate prediction value of the selected predictors. The researcher

recommended that the model should not be externally validated or used in clinical practice.

This highlights how prognostic models do not always add value to clinical practice. In this case, the problem was poor model performance due to data limitations and not methodology. You can use the three performance metrics to decipher which models are high performing and can be considered for use in practice.[10, 11] Even with proper methods and data size, you can see that this particular model should not be used in clinic.

# PHASE 3: CHOOSING THE TREATMENT PLAN

When determining the appropriate intervention for an athlete, consider two items: causal mechanisms and patient-specific elements.

## Causal mechanisms

*Causality*, better known as cause-effect, is the relationship between exposure to a factor (the cause, e.g. smoking) and an outcome/event (the effect, e.g. lung cancer).[23] Within a cause-effect relationship, there can be more than one cause for an individual effect.[24] However, in sports and exercise medicine and in the health professions broadly there is great confusion as to what constitutes a true causal mechanism and how it differs from association or prediction of an outcome.[25] We provide precise definitions of these terms to help you understand the critical differences among causality, association and prediction (see also Fig. 21.4).

*Association* is a statistical relationship between a factor and an outcome/event that has a direction and magnitude.

For example, at the knee, intracondylar notch size (factor) is associated with a greater risk of ACL rupture (outcome). Whether this is casual or not remains unknown.

*Prediction* is the use of mathematical models (i.e. algorithms or equations) that include multiple factors that forecast the risk or probability of a future outcome (prognostic) or current diagnosis.[26] For example, the Framingham Risk Score for coronary artery disease uses seven factors (including age, sex and blood pressure) to calculate a 10-year estimate of the risk of death (Fig. 21.5).

### Causal mechanisms and their supportive constructs

Intervening in associative factors will not change the outcome. For example, ice-cream sales and shark attacks have a very strong positive association. However, stopping ice-cream sales will not affect shark attacks, as the number of people at the beach is the main cause of shark attacks. However, intervening in causal mechanisms will alter the desired outcome. Within sports and exercise medicine, many associations are confused with causes.[25] To work out what is a causal mechanism, there is a three-step process.[27]

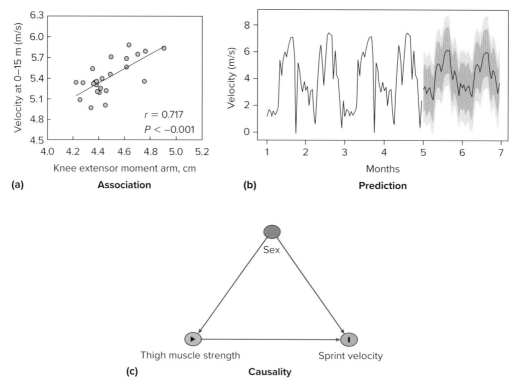

**Figure 21.4** (a) Association. The blue line depicts a regression equation of the association between the variables *x* and *y*—in this case, muscle strength (*x*) and sprint velocity (*y*). The equation describes the direction and magnitude of this relationship. (b) Prediction. The black part of the line depicts the measured sprint velocity over the first 5 months of the season. The blue part of the line is forecasting future events—the next 2 months. (c) Causality. The blue outcome is determining the causal effect of thigh muscle strength on sprint velocity, while blocking the path (i.e. controlling) for sex.

## Framingham Risk Score for Hard Coronary Heart Disease ☆

Estimates 10-year risk of heart attack.

**INSTRUCTIONS**

There are several distinct Framingham risk models. MDCalc uses the 'Hard' coronary Framingham outcomes model, which is intended for use in **non-diabetic** patients age 30-79 years with no prior history of coronary heart disease or intermittent claudication, as it is the most widely applicable to patients without previous cardiac events. See the official Framingham website for additional Framingham risk models.

| When to Use ⌄ | Pearls/Pitfalls ⌄ |
|---|---|

| Age | | years |
|---|---|---|
| Sex | Female | Male |
| Smoker | No | Yes |
| Total cholesterol | | mg/dL ⇆ |
| HDL cholesterol | | mg/dL ⇆ |
| Systolic BP | | mm Hg |
| Blood pressure being treated with medicines | No | Yes |

| When to Use ⌄ | Pearls/Pitfalls ⌄ |
|---|---|

| Age | 63 | years |
|---|---|---|
| Sex | Female | Male |
| Smoker | No | Yes |
| Total cholesterol | 3.9 | mg/dL ⇆ |
| HDL cholesterol | 1.4 | mg/dL ⇆ |
| Systolic BP | 120 | mm Hg |
| Blood pressure being treated with medicines | No | Yes |

**16.2** %
10-year risk of MI or death for this patient

**20** %
Average 10-year risk of MI or death

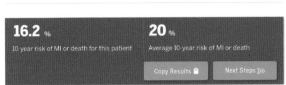
Copy Results 📋 | Next Steps 》》

**Figure 21.5** Framingham Risk Score

Box 21.2 includes a comprehensive clinical example of this process.

1. Step 1 studies are exploratory and establish the potential relationship between factors and outcomes of interest. These studies are cross-sectional or small cohort studies. Imagine a study where the factors include measures of running biomechanics, training load and ligament laxity, and the outcome is whether the person had suffered a sports-related ankle sprain. This design means that if the study authors find a difference between groups in any of the three factors, they need to limit any claims of the relationship to that of "association".

2. Step 2 studies examine the strength and direction of the relationship between a factor and an outcome. These studies are larger prospective cohort studies or small randomised controlled trials. Imagine a study of track and field athletes where key risk factors for bone stress injury (such as calf muscle strength, bone mineral density, calcium intake and energy balance) are measured at baseline and the athletes are followed for 1, 2 and 5 years with a particular focus on stress fracture as the outcome. This type of study reveals the relative importance of those risk factors in predicting future stress fractures.

3. Step 3 studies investigate whether intervening in a factor alters the outcome and assess generalisability across populations.[27] These studies are usually large randomised controlled trials and can also evaluate different populations.

Of course, sport and exercise clinicians are not expected to generate these scientific processes (i.e. undertake potentially large and expensive studies), but they are well-trained to filter and decipher the scientific literature to inform the best treatment for their patients (see Chapter 3 on clinical reasoning). Far too often, clinicians tout cross-sectional association studies (step 1) as if they were "silver bullets" to treat specific sport injuries.

This is flawed clinical reasoning and low-quality patient care. Patient outcomes can only change[25] if you intervene on causal mechanisms; and these can only be discovered using a multi-study scientific process, and clearly defining the strengths and weaknesses of the study design, sample and data.

### Patient-specific elements

Patient-specific elements constitute patient goals (evaluated through shared decision making), the physical demands of the sport, the cost of injury and subsequent return to health, and where the athlete is within their career. These are further detailed in Chapters 1 and 4.

**BOX 21.2** Illustrating the three-step process to identify causal mechanisms

A high-school baseball pitcher (Fig. 21.6) suffered a medial elbow injury during the spring season. They have no history of any arm injury. After examination, the diagnosis was ulnar collateral ligament grade 2 sprain, with a prognosis of expected return in 2 months,[28] and no surgery recommended.

To determine the best interventions for this athlete, the sport and exercise clinician does their due diligence in examining the scientific literature. They find three articles that all identify important factors for medial elbow pitching injuries:

- The first article (step 1) is a cross-sectional study of 100 high-school baseball pitchers. Pitchers with a medial elbow injury demonstrated smaller landing leg ankle dorsiflexion range compared with non-injured pitchers.
- The second article (step 2) is a prospective cohort study of 100 high-school baseball pitchers. Pitchers were uninjured and performing all baseball activities when the study began. Over the course of the season, those pitchers who sustained a medial elbow injury were found to have 20° less trunk rotation (at the start of the study, when this was measured) on their non-dominant side compared with pitchers who did not sustain a medial elbow injury.
- The final article (step 3) was a randomised controlled trial of 100 high-school baseball pitchers. The intervention group was prescribed rotator cuff and forearm strengthening twice a week over the course

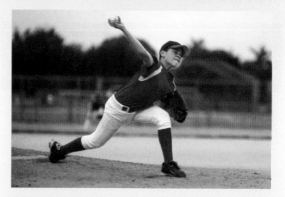

**Figure 21.6** Medial elbow pain is common in high-school baseball pitchers. This box illustrates an approach to finding the most relevant literature to help guide treatment.
ISTOCK/THEPALMER

of the baseball season, comprising 6 exercises, each performed for 3 sets of 10 repetitions. The intervention group had 20% fewer medial elbow injuries than the control group. The randomised controlled trial is evidence of causal factors that reduce medial elbow injuries in high-school baseball pitchers.[29]

Based on this evidence, the clinician prescribed rotator cuff and forearm strengthening exercises for the patient.

## KEY POINTS

- The process of assessing and diagnosing a clinical problem involves collecting and synthesising multiple data sources in a systematic way.

- In phase 1 of clinical assessment, the clinician gathers information about the athlete via an intake form, medical history, physical examination and selected outcome measures.

- In phase 2, the clinician develops a working diagnosis by ruling out red flag conditions, determining the anatomical source of pain and then deciding what has caused the pain.

- A number of tests are available to support the diagnostic process. The clinical value of

each test is subject to its reliability, sensitivity, specificity, likelihood ratio and predictive value.

- Any test must be interpreted in the context of the athlete's medical history and physical examination.

- Prognostic (predictive) models are mathematical models that use numerous predictors to create a risk score for an athlete. The majority of these models are not well-developed and should not be used clinically.

- In phase 3, selecting a treatment/intervention should be based on a number of factors specific to the athlete, their injury and goals. The chosen treatment should also reflect an understanding of the relationship between causal mechanisms and risk of injury.

## REFERENCES

References for this chapter can be found at www.mhprofessional.com/CSM6e

## ADDITIONAL CONTENT

 Scan here to access additional resources for this topic and more provided by the authors

C

## CHAPTER 22

# Red flags

**with CHRISTA JANSE VAN RENSBURG and PAUL D. KIRWAN**

*The week before he was due to fly to the 2023 World Championship, US shot-putter Ryan Crouser woke up with calf pain which he and his team thought was a muscle tear. Understandably, it was treated as such but after 10 days it as investigated and the pain was coming from two blood clots.*

## CHAPTER OUTLINE

What is a red flag?
Three tips to spot red flags
Conditions that often come with red flags

## LEARNING OBJECTIVES

By the end of this chapter you should be able to:

- distinguish between specific and general red flags
- identify elements of a patient history or physical examination that could indicate a red flag
- discuss the ways in which red flags can masquerade as sport-related illness or injury
- memorise clinical checklists (e.g. THINK BROAD, SCREEND'EM) to assist with interpretation of possible red flags.

Some chapters in *Clinical Sports Medicine* relate to topics where clinicians can save lives: this is one of those chapters. Each of the more than 70 clinician authors of this book has recognised red flags (defined below) during their career and made important diagnoses that have allowed patients to avoid severe medical complications.

Sometimes making the diagnosis is not enough—it may be too late to intervene or there is no effective treatment. The aim of this chapter is to share lessons from real-life cases to help you to recognise red flags and thus save one or more lives. Too strong? Not at all—osteosarcoma, deep venous thrombosis, cerebral bleed ... Read on.

## WHAT IS A RED FLAG?

A red flag is a clinical indicator of a possible serious underlying condition.[1] It is the symptoms the patient provides you in the history or signs you elicit during the physical examination (see Chapter 19).

In a sports injury consultation, red flags tend to be specific to the musculoskeletal system: a middle-aged runner complaining of back pain only when lying down in bed (vertebral metastases from breast cancer); a basketball player explaining that his right arm feels "pumped up" as if he were in the middle of a weight-training session, except he hasn't lifted weights for a week (axillary vein thrombosis).

Table 22.1 provides examples of conditions that can mimic others; such mimicry works in both directions. These real-life examples from *Clinical Sports Medicine* authors illustrate where an "obvious" first diagnosis (left column) was incorrect and red flags contributed to the clinician correctly identifying the real culprit (right column).

Physical examination signs that might reflect a sinister pathology include fever (even mild) alongside joint pain, or muscle weakness arising in an otherwise healthy person.

Red flags may also be general—unexplained weight loss or loss of appetite, general malaise and deep fatigue are classic examples. Potentially sinister pathologies may be at the root of those symptoms.

Not every condition discussed in this chapter is life-threatening. You may recognise that the patient has an osteoid osteoma, psoriasis or abnormal thyroid function when that was not what the patient was expecting. These important diagnoses allow the patient to understand their symptoms and begin appropriate treatment.

**TABLE 22.1**  Examples of conditions that can mimic one other

| "Obvious" (but incorrect) diagnosis | Alternative (correct) diagnosis, based on red flags |
| --- | --- |
| Migraine headache | Upper cervical facet joint hypomobility/cervicogenic headache |
| Rotator cuff tendinopathy | Glenohumeral joint instability (in a younger athlete)<br>Acromioclavicular joint osteoarthritis (in an older athlete) |
| Tennis elbow | Cervical disc abnormality |
| Wrist "tendinitis" | Cervical abnormality |
| Hip osteoarthritis | Upper lumbar spine disc degeneration |
| Persistent hamstring strain | Abnormal neuromechanical dynamics |
| Patellofemoral pain/knee osteoarthritis | Referred pain from hip |
| Bucket handle tear of the meniscus | Referred pain from a ruptured L4–5 disc |
| Patellar dislocation | Anterior cruciate ligament rupture |
| Osgood-Schlatter lesion | Osteoid osteoma tibial tuberosity |
| "Shin splints" (periostitis, tendinopathy) | Chronic compartment syndrome or stress fracture |
| Achilles tendinopathy | Posterior impingement<br>Retrocalcaneal bursitis |
| Plantar fasciitis | Medial plantar nerve entrapment |
| Morton's neuroma | Referred pain from an L5–S1 disc prolapse |
| Shoulder pain | Scapular pain caused by rib dysfunction or referred pain from the cervical spine |
| Compartment syndrome | Popliteal artery entrapment syndrome |
| Persistent lateral midfoot pain following sprain | Cuboid subluxation |

## THREE TIPS TO SPOT RED FLAGS

Experienced clinicians suggest that three behaviours will assist you to spot red flags:

1. *Keep an open mind to the possibility that things may not be what they seem (i.e. think broadly).* Avoid the "blink" mindset where you jump to conclusions within 30 seconds. If things seem a little strange at a first consultation, make a note to discuss them later with a more experienced colleague if you feel it's not an emergency.

2. *Take a detailed history and don't skimp on the physical examination.* If you come across any of the following clinical features, be suspicious—all may not be what it seems.

   (a) From the history:
   - constitutional symptoms—fever, night sweats, fatigue, weight loss, myalgias, anorexia ($\pm$ nausea/vomiting)
   - pain out of proportion in severity and/or duration to the history
   - pain more persistent than one would expect ("unremitting")
   - night pain
   - no convincing history of activity-related/sports injury.

   (b) From the physical examination:
   - look—redness, abnormal swelling, abnormal vasculature
   - feel—warm, palpable mass ($\pm$ skin infiltration, ill-defined, etc.), diminished or absent pulse, neurologically compromised
   - move—unexpected weakness.

3. *Be prepared to go back to square one.* Consider alternative conditions when the patient's clinical progress does not fit the pattern you expected. For example, a lingering contusion that should have resolved long ago could represent an underlying blood dyscrasia or tumour of the soft tissue or bone.

## CONDITIONS THAT OFTEN COME WITH RED FLAGS

In the clinic, the red flag comes first—that's what points you to the diagnosis. In a textbook it's more efficient to share a list of conditions first and then tag them with their red flags.

In Table 22.2 we use the acronym THINK BROAD to illustrate some disorders that may present as sports and exercise medicine conditions but that usually reveal at least one red flag. You might find this acronym useful as a reminder of 10 categories of conditions that can trip up even experienced clinicians.

We expand on these categories below and encourage you to go to primary sources to learn more, as this chapter does not discuss management of these conditions. Rather, for example, it is designed to remind you to think of Marfan syndrome if you see a tall, very flexible athlete with visual problems and a family history of sudden cardiac death.

## T: Trauma unrelated to or aggravated by sports conditions

Athletes, particularly recreational athletes, can suffer injuries from work- or hobby-related activities. An office-bound computer worker may develop elbow pain associated with how they use their computer mouse. They may also suffer cervical spondylosis due to incorrect office ergonomics. An activity like mountain biking may then aggravate their neck pain. If you focus on the mountain biking alone, your management plan will not help them as much as finding the associated root cause will.

## H: Hereditary (genetic) disorders

Genetic disorders increase the risk of injury—sometimes catastrophic injury—in athletes. The clinician who considers a broad differential diagnosis based on clinical presentation and history is more likely to consider these genetic diagnoses.

- Ehlers-Danlos syndrome (Fig. 22.1) is a condition of abnormally lax ligaments that increases the risk of ligament injuries including subluxation and frank dislocation.

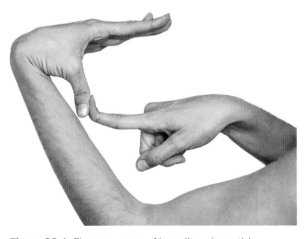

**Figure 22.1** Flagrant cases of hereditary (genetic) conditions are usually diagnosed early in life but there are mild forms of these conditions that go undetected. Excessive ligamentous laxity is a clue to the athlete having Ehlers-Danlos syndrome or a related disorder.
ISTOCK/LUCIA IZQUIERDO

**TABLE 22.2**   The acronym "THINK BROAD" may be useful when you're wondering whether your patient's story is pointing to a red flag

| | The conditions that make up the acronym THINK | | The conditions that make up the acronym BROAD |
|---|---|---|---|
| **T** | **Trauma unrelated to or aggravated by sports participation**<br>*Examples*<br>• Bone, tendon, ligament | **B** | **Blood-related (including vasculature)**<br>*Examples*<br>• Venous thrombosis, artery entrapment, peripheral vascular disease, blood dyscrasia, idiopathic thrombocytopenia, sickle cell trait<br>• Artery entrapment<br>• Peripheral vascular disease<br>• Blood dyscrasia |
| **H** | **Hereditary (genetic)**<br>*Examples*<br>• Marfan syndrome<br>• Haemochromatosis<br>• Haemophilia | **R** | **Referred pain or regional pain syndromes**<br>*Examples*<br>• Referred: aortic aneurysm, eroding peptic ulcer, etc.<br>• Regional pain syndromes: fibromyalgia, chronic regional pain syndrome |
| **I** | **Infective**<br>*Examples*<br>• Osteomyelitis, septic arthritis, shingles, Lyme disease | **O** | **Other (endocrine, granulomatous)**<br>*Examples*<br>• Endocrine: thyroid disease, hyperparathyroidism, hypercalcaemia, hypocalcaemia, diabetes mellitus, Cushing syndrome, acromegaly<br>• Granulomatous: tuberculosis, sarcoidosis |
| **N** | **Neoplastic (benign or malignant)**<br>*Examples*<br>• Bone: osteosarcoma, Ewing sarcoma, osteoid osteoma<br>• Synovium: synovial sarcoma, synovial chondromatosis, pigmented villonodular synovitis<br>• Muscle: rhabdomyosarcoma<br>• Joint fluid: ganglion cyst, Baker cyst | **A** | **Arthritis (rheumatological conditions)**<br>*Examples*<br>• Rheumatoid arthritis<br>• Seronegative arthropathy<br>• Psoriasis |
| **K** | **Keep on thinking and talking to colleagues**<br>*Examples*<br>• If you don't feel comfortable<br>• If the patient's trajectory is not fitting the diagnosis | **D** | **Disorders of muscle**<br>*Examples*<br>• Muscular dystrophy<br>• Inflammatory muscle disorders (polymyositis, dermatomyositis, etc.) |

• Osteogenesis imperfecta increases fracture risk.
• Down syndrome is associated with an underdeveloped odontoid bone (odontoid hypoplasia). The odontoid process contributes to stability when a person rotates their head. Thus, people with Down syndrome have an inherent increased risk of cervical spine injuries.
• Marfan syndrome is associated with sudden cardiac death. Marfan syndrome is an autosomal dominant disorder of fibrillin characterised by musculoskeletal, cardiac and ocular abnormalities.[2,3] Musculoskeletal problems arise as a result of joint hypermobility, ligament laxity, scoliosis or spondylolysis. A quick clinic screen for Marfan includes pectus carinatum/excavatum, an arm span 1.05 times the patient's height, arachnodactyly (excessively long slim fingers), Steinberg/Walker-Murdoch signs of excessive flexibility, dental overcrowding and a high arched palate. Consider referring patients with Marfanoid habitus for echocardiography and ophthalmological opinion as there is a risk of sudden cardiac death or lens dislocation.

Marfan syndrome: signs

• Haemochromatosis is an autosomal recessive disorder that results in iron overload. Patients may present with arthropathy with characteristic involvement of the 2nd and 3rd metacarpophalangeal joints, with hook-shaped osteophytes seen on radiographs. While ferritin levels are raised in patients with haemochromatosis, it is important to remember that ferritin may also be elevated in athletes taking iron supplements or responding to any acute inflammatory illness.[4] Fasting transferrin levels are a clue to diagnosis and the definitive test is for the haemochromatosis gene (*HFE* gene).

## I: Infective

Bone and joint infections can begin slowly and evade the clinician who is inexperienced or rushed. This can have disastrous consequences.

Bone pain in children, or bone pain that is worse at night or with activity should alert you to the possibility of osteomyelitis.[5] Bone infection near a joint may result in a reactive joint effusion. Septic arthritis is rare in a normal joint. However, gonococcal arthritis may occur in a previously normal joint and can cause substantial and permanent joint damage. Consider sexually transmitted infection (i.e. ask about unprotected intercourse).

In arthritic or diabetic joints, or joints that recently underwent arthroscopy, sepsis is much more common. Rapid joint destruction may follow if left untreated.

Even though *Staphylococcus aureus* is the causative organism in more than 50% of cases of acute septic joints, it is imperative that joint aspiration for Gram stain and culture, and blood cultures, be taken before antibiotic treatment begins. One-off or repeated joint lavage may be considered for patients receiving intravenous antibiotic treatment.

The immunocompromised patient may present with chronic septic arthritis; in this situation, tuberculosis or fungal infections should be considered. In suspected cases of septic arthritis, the patient should be admitted to hospital.[6]

Another cause of arthritis is Lyme disease, a common arthropod-borne infection in some countries, including the US and Canada. The number of territories in which this infection can be found is increasing because of climate change. Hallmarks of Lyme disease are erythema migrans, disruption of the electrical conduction of cardiac muscle, the development of neurological abnormalities and episodes of arthritis.

Intermittent episodes of arthritis develop several weeks or months after infection, and despite adequate antibiotic therapy, symptoms persist in 10% of patients with arthritis. The severity of arthritis can range from mild to moderate inflammation of the joints and tendons months after infection to a chronic, debilitating osteoarthropathy complete with destruction of cartilage and erosion of bone within a few years, leading to permanent joint dysfunction.

The diagnosis of Lyme disease is clinical and serological tests should be used to confirm the clinical diagnosis.[7]

## N: Neoplastic (benign or malignant)

Primary malignant tumours of bone and soft tissues are rare, but when they occur, they are most likely to be in the younger age group (second to third decades). Osteosarcoma can present with pain at the distal or proximal end of long bones, more commonly in the lower limbs—the patient

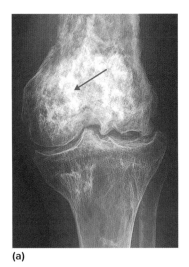 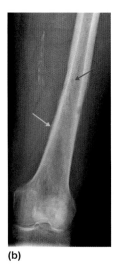

**(a)**                                                    **(b)**

**Figure 22.2** Neoplasia. Radiography is indicated to rule out red flags with persistent bone or joint pain, particularly if it is not associated with activity. (a) PA radiograph shows an osteosarcoma in the distal femur (arrow), characterised by a mixed lytic-sclerotic appearance. (b) Master athlete with a Ewing sarcoma. Note the lytic ("moth-eaten") permeative bone destruction (red arrow) and lamellated periosteal reaction (green arrow)—both signs of an aggressive process.
(B) COURTESY OF DR BRUCE B FORSTER

may complain of "joint pain". Patients often recognise that activity aggravates pain and present to the sports and exercise medicine clinic.

The pathological diagnosis of osteosarcoma depends on detecting tumour-producing bone. A radiograph may reveal a moth-eaten appearance, with new bone formation in the soft tissues and lifting of the periosteum (Fig. 22.2). In young patients, the differential diagnosis includes osteomyelitis.

**PRACTICE PEARL**

Consider the possibility of a tumour in any child or adolescent with unexpected or unremitting bone pain. Radiography is a simple and potentially life-saving investigation.

Also consider a tumour when a patient presents with a mild injury that is not improving or with an atypical finding on radiographs of a fracture. A fracture that occurs with a relatively low energy injury or without an appropriate mechanism of injury is a red flag. A bone tumour may present as progressive pain rather than pain that improves with rest and treatment.

Malignant tumours—particularly breast, thyroid, lung and prostate tumours—may metastasise to bone. Patients may not recognise that a previously treated malignancy could be related to limb pain. Breast cancer may present as shoulder pain.[8] Signs of malignancy include prominent night pain and constitutional symptoms including pain, fever, loss of appetite, weight loss and malaise. In the sports population, patients with metastatic disease are more likely to be older and have more complex medical histories.

Giant cell tumours, aneurysmal bone cysts and unicameral (single) bone cysts (Fig. 22.3) are benign or less aggressive bone tumours that also present with pain and failure to resolve in the time frame expected for a simple contusion or traumatic injury.[9]

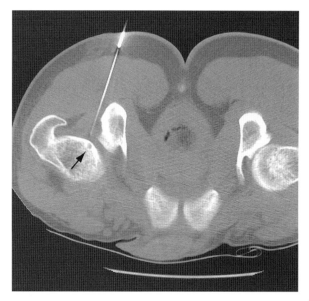

**Figure 22.4** Transverse CT image (cutting through the pelvis at the level of the pubic symphysis anteriorly). The arrow points to an osteoid osteoma in the posterior cortex of the femoral neck. The long bright line coming from the top of the picture is a radiofrequency probe in position for an ablation procedure—to remove the painful benign tumour.

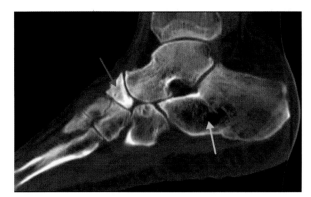

**Figure 22.3** Some cysts are detected incidentally. This CT scan was not requested for heel pain, but revealed an area of lucency (green arrow) commonly seen as a normal variant in the calcaneus. It represents relative lack of trabeculation. This pseudocyst was not the cause of any pain for this patient. Note the avascular necrosis of the navicular (red arrow) as a sequela of a stress fracture.
COURTESY OF DR BRUCE B FORSTER

Osteoid osteoma is a benign bone tumour often presenting as exercise-related bone pain and tenderness and is frequently misdiagnosed as a stress fracture.[10,11] This condition is characterised clinically by the presence of night pain; aspirin may abolish the symptoms. The tumour can occasionally be seen on plain radiographs and has a characteristic appearance on CT scan with a central nidus (Fig. 22.4).

Synovial cell sarcoma frequently involves the larger lower joints, such as the knee and ankle.[12] The patient presents with pain, often at night or with activity, frequently with instability and swelling. They report chronic swelling and pain that does not resolve with standard treatment.

As with synovial sarcoma, synovial chondromatosis and pigmented villonodular synovitis (Fig. 22.5) are benign tumours of the synovium found mainly in the knee, which present with mechanical symptoms, persistent swelling and failure to respond to rest, ice and anti-inflammatory regimens.[13] The term "benign" can be misleading as the

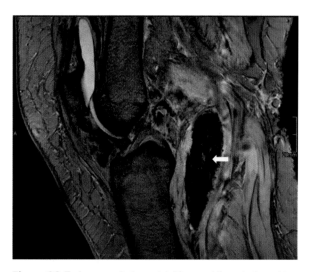

**Figure 22.5** A runner in her mid-40s went from being able to run more than 40 km per week to having severe pain when walking. This sagittal T2*-weighted gradient echo MRI revealed the characteristic black signal of pigmented villonodular synovitis (arrow) when imaged using the susceptibility sequence.
COURTESY OF CHRISTA JANSE VAN RENSBURG

condition itself is not mild—it can be devastating because of the mechanical effects of the nodules and it can greatly limit the patient.

If an athlete reports persistent pain after direct trauma to muscle tissue (contusion), consider the red flag of myositis ossificans. Imaging studies show calcification within the muscle that is not in continuity with the bone itself (Fig. 22.6). Biopsies should be performed cautiously, as there are case reports of the active edge of myositis ossificans being misread as osteosarcoma.[14] Even less typically, trauma may result in a haemorrhage into an indolent, underlying rhabdomyosarcoma. Consider alternative diagnoses in patients with haematomata that are slow to resolve or when the history of trauma does not fit with the clinical signs.

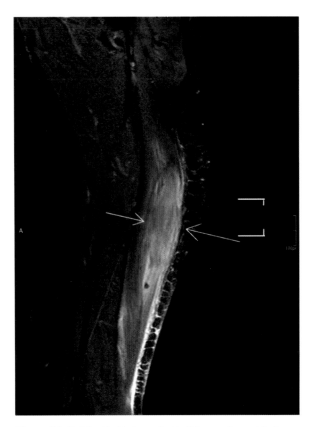

**Figure 22.6** A football player in his 20s was kneed in the hamstring region in a rugby tackle. The hamstring has a region of ossification (arrows)—the classic appearance of myositis ossificans.
COURTESY OF CHRISTA JANSE VAN RENSBURG

The most common benign soft-tissue tumours are ganglion cysts. These cysts are lined by connective tissue, contain mucinous fluid and are found mainly around the wrist, hand, knee and foot. They may be attached to a joint capsule or tendon sheath and may have a connection to the synovial cavity. They are usually asymptomatic but occasionally cause pain and cosmetic deformity (see Chapter 11 in *Clinical Sports Medicine 6e: Managing Injuries*).[15]

However, ganglion cysts may also represent an important clue regarding other underlying, masquerading disease processes such as osteoarthritis or chronic tendinopathy.

## K: Keep on thinking and talking to colleagues

If the condition is not responding to treatment, reconsider the diagnosis. Take time to think (which we appreciate can be hard to find) (Fig. 22.7a). Consider revisiting the athlete's history, re-examining them and referring for appropriate special investigations or an opinion from a colleague (Fig. 22.7b). Consider other options if the clinical picture does not make sense or the special investigations (laboratory results and/or imaging) do not fit the expected diagnosis. This is where the broad clinical team can be invaluable.

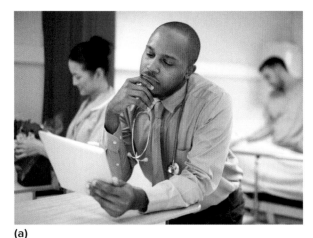

**(a)**

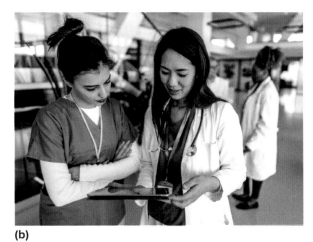

**(b)**

**Figure 22.7** When the patient doesn't seem to be recovering, (a) reflection and (b) referral can prove lifesaving for the patient
(A) ISTOCK/STURTI (B) ISTOCK/PEKIC

## B: Blood-related (including vasculature)

Patients with venous thrombosis or arterial abnormalities may present with limb pain and swelling aggravated by exercise. Calf, femoral or axillary veins are common sites for thrombosis. While a cause may be apparent (e.g. recent surgery or air travel), consider other medical causes such as a thrombophilia (e.g. antiphospholipid syndrome) or deficiencies of protein C, protein S, antithrombin III or factor V Leiden. When athletes with no other risk factors for thrombosis develop a blood clot, a more extensive work-up is necessary. See the following for an example of a suspected "calf tear" turning out to be deep vein thrombosis:

Ryan Crouser: unexplained calf pain

The claudication pain of peripheral vascular disease is most likely to be first noticed with exercise, so patients may present to the clinician. Remember that arteriopathy is more prevalent in patients with diabetes. Specific vascular entrapments include popliteal artery entrapment, which presents as exercise-related calf pain; and external iliac artery endofibrosis (fibrosis on the inside of the vessel) in cyclists (Fig. 22.8), which presents as leg pain and weakness, paraesthesia and numbness, muscle cramping and sometimes swelling of the thigh.[16] In the upper limbs, thoracic outlet syndrome presents as numbness or tingling of the fingers, hand or arm, pallor or cyanosis of the fingers or hand, and a fatigued arm after activity.

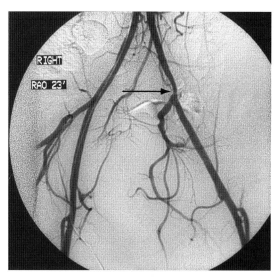

**Figure 22.8** A cyclist presented with left leg cramping and pain as well as inability to run. Angiogram showing common iliac artery stenosis (arrow).

## R: Referred pain or regional pain syndromes

Pain in a specific region can be referred from other areas. It is important to consider referred pain as a potential diagnosis, especially when the pain is poorly localised or does not respond to usual treatment. The most common origins of referred pain are the spine and myofascial trigger points. Referred pain is discussed in Chapter 11. Table 22.3 shows areas of pain due to referred pain from the spine but masquerading as musculoskeletal injuries.

Complex regional pain syndrome type I is a post-traumatic phenomenon characterised by localised pain out of proportion to the injury, vasomotor disturbances, oedema and delayed recovery from injury. We have seen this present as a sprained ankle that doesn't improve.

**TABLE 22.3**   Areas of pain due to referred pain from the spine but masquerading as musculoskeletal pathologies

| Area of pain | Nerve | Alternative diagnosis |
|---|---|---|
| Neck/trapezius | C5 or C6 nerve root | Levator scapula syndrome |
| Scapula | C7 or C8 nerve root | T4 syndrome |
| Posterior shoulder | C8 nerve root | Quadrilateral space syndrome |
| Lateral elbow | Posterior interosseous nerve | Tennis elbow |
| Knee pain | L3 or L4 nerve root | Patellofemoral or iliotibial band pain |
| Buttock | L5 nerve root | Piriformis syndrome |
| Anterolateral shin pain | L5 nerve root | "Shin splints" |
| Hamstring | S1 nerve root | Back-related hamstring pain |
| Ischial tuberosity | S1 nerve root | Ischial bursitis |
| Lateral foot pain | S1 nerve root | Bone stress injury |

The vasomotor disturbances of an extremity manifest as vasodilatation (warmth, redness) or vasoconstriction (coolness, cyanosis, mottling).[17] Early mobilisation, use of motor imagery and avoidance of surgery are important keys to successful management (see also Chapter 11).[18]

Myofascial pain syndromes develop secondary to either acute or overuse trauma. They present as regional pain associated with the presence of one or more active trigger points. You can find more on trigger points in Chapter 9.

Fibromyalgia is a chronic pain syndrome characterised by widespread pain, chronic fatigue, decreased pain threshold, sleep disturbance, psychological distress and characteristic tender points.[19] It is often associated with other symptoms, including irritable bowel syndrome, dyspareunia, headache, irritable bladder, and subjective joint swelling and pain. Fibromyalgia is a diagnosis of exclusion. Although helpful, it cannot be solely diagnosed on the examination finding of 11 of 18 specific tender point sites in a patient with widespread pain.[19, 20]

Chronic fatigue syndrome has many similarities to fibromyalgia and may be the same disease process.[21] It may present as excessive post-exercise muscle soreness but is always associated with extreme fatigue. There is evidence that exercise improves global wellbeing for women with this condition.[22]

Visceral organs can also be the source of referred pain. For example, older athletes may present with back pain unrelated to spondylosis (e.g. dissecting aortic aneurysm, eroding peptic ulcer or pancreatic carcinoma). Rapidly dissecting aortic aneurysm classically presents as sudden, severe chest, back or abdominal pain characterised as ripping or tearing in nature.

## O: Other (endocrine, granulomatous)

Both endocrine disorders and granulomatous diseases such as tuberculosis and sarcoidosis can mimic other conditions.

### Endocrine disorders

Because of the remarkably diverse function of the endocrine system, it is not surprising that some endocrine pathologies present as musculoskeletal conditions and wave red flags.[23] Proximal muscle weakness and fibromyalgia may develop with hypothyroidism. Thyroid acropachy (soft-tissue swelling and periosteal bone changes) results from hyperthyroidism; adhesive capsulitis and painless proximal muscle weakness are also associated with an overactive thyroid.[24]

As a result of the parathyroid gland's role in regulating bone metabolism, hyperparathyroidism may be associated with calcium pyrophosphate deposits in joints. Patients may

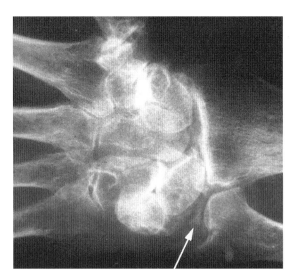

**Figure 22.9** Chondrocalcinosis of the triangular fibrocartilage of the wrist (arrow) in calcium pyrophosphate dehydrate deposition disease

develop acute pseudogout or polyarticular inflammatory arthritis resembling rheumatoid arthritis. Radiographs of the knees or wrists may demonstrate chondrocalcinosis of the menisci or triangular fibrocartilage complex, respectively (Fig. 22.9).

Adhesive capsulitis or septic arthritis may be the first manifestation of diabetes mellitus. Patients with endocrine disorders such as acromegaly may develop premature osteoarthritis or carpal tunnel syndrome.

Patients with hypercalcaemia secondary to malignancy (e.g. of the lung) or other conditions such as hyperparathyroidism can present with bone pain as well as constipation, confusion and renal calculi. A proximal myopathy may develop in patients with primary Cushing syndrome or after corticosteroid use.

When symptoms of myalgia, joint stiffness and swelling do not resolve, a more in-depth laboratory work-up hunting for masqueraders is appropriate and indicated.

### Granulomatous diseases

Granulomatous diseases such as tuberculosis and sarcoidosis have been called "the great mimickers" due to their ability to present in many varied and atypical fashions. They can look like tumours, inflammation, infection or traumatic injuries.

Tuberculosis is a granulomatous mycobacterial infection. Musculoskeletal involvement includes chronic septic arthritis and Pott's spine fracture.

Patients with acute sarcoidosis may present with fevers, a lower limb (commonly) rash and ankle swelling. The rash

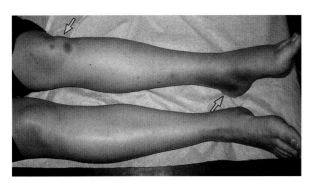

**Figure 22.10** Erythema nodosum (arrows) in acute sarcoidosis
PHOTO COURTESY OF DR RAHEEM B KHERANI

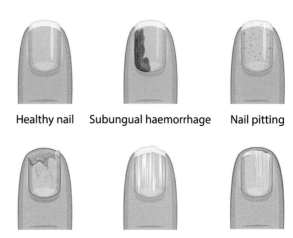

**Figure 22.11** Athletes' nails can be a clue to red flags. Nail psoriasis can present as subungual haemorrhages, nail pitting, onychomadesis (separating of the nail plate from the nail matrix beginning proximally), trachyonychia (rough nails, longitudinal ridges) and onycholysis (separating of the nail plate from the nail matrix beginning distally).
ISTOCK/SCIO21

of erythema nodosum (Fig. 22.10) may be mistaken for cellulitis, and antibiotics have frequently been prescribed in error. The diagnosis is easily made by chest radiograph, which shows changes of bilateral hilar lymphadenopathy. If considering a differential diagnosis of bilateral hilar lymphadenopathy, consider also tuberculosis and lymphoma.

Chronic sarcoidosis is a systemic disorder involving the lungs, central nervous system, skin, eyes and musculoskeletal system. Patients can present with chronic arthropathy together with bone cysts or bone pain due to hypercalcaemia.

## A: Arthritis (rheumatological conditions)

Inflammatory musculoskeletal disorders frequently masquerade as a traumatic or mechanical condition. Common examples include low back pain from ankylosing spondylitis, psoriatic enthesopathy presenting as patellar tendinopathy, and flitting arthritis in early rheumatoid arthritis.[25,26] A detailed description of rheumatological conditions that can present to the sport and exercise clinician is outside the scope of this chapter.

Clues to a systemic inflammatory aetiology include constitutional symptoms, morning stiffness and progressive symptoms despite limiting physical activity. If there is no clear mechanism of injury, consider this red flag. Management includes a more complete work-up including radiographs, MRI and laboratory testing for autoantibodies.

If a patient presents with an acutely swollen knee without a history of precipitant trauma or patellar tendinopathy without overload, be alert to the possibility that this could be inflammatory in origin (Clinical case 22.1). Prominent morning joint or back stiffness, night pain or extra-articular manifestations of rheumatological conditions (e.g. skin rashes, nail abnormalities [Fig. 22.11], bowel disturbances, eye involvement [conjunctivitis, iritis] or urethral discharge) may all provide clues. The screening lab test is acute phase reactants, which are elevated in a positive test.

Inflammation of entheses (e.g. in lateral elbow pain, patellar tendinopathy, insertional Achilles tendinopathy and plantar fasciopathy) is almost universal among those with human leucocyte antigens (HLA) B27-related, seronegative (for rheumatoid factor) arthropathies. Enthesopathy is usually associated with other joint or extra-articular involvement, although a subgroup exists with enthesitis as the sole presentation.[27]

Tendon and joint pain are a common complaint among those involved in sports. It is often easy to attribute such symptoms to the load that tissues are exposed to from sporting activity. However, inflammatory arthritis is common in young adulthood and can present as tendon and/or joint pain. It is not always easy to identify inflammatory arthritis. This explains the long delay from onset of symptoms to diagnosis for many who suffer from spondyloarthropathies. Typical delay to diagnosis can range from 7 to 10 years.

Pain at the enthesis, such as in patellar tendinopathy, lateral elbow tendinopathy, plantar heel pain or insertional Achilles tendinopathy, may be the first sign of an underlying spondyloarthropathy. Patients who seek help are usually focused on their main complaint (e.g. tendon pain) so they won't mention what we know to be associated problems—psoriasis, uveitis, colitis etc. You will need to ask about other symptoms.

Dr Paul Kirwan was the lead developer of a simple tool with an easy to remember acronym—SCREEND'EM

---

**CLINICAL CASE 22.1** Inflammatory arthritis in disguise (by Peter Brukner)

One of my patients, an international cricketer (Fig. 22.12), had suffered from knee pain for a couple of years. He was having difficulty playing and was on a reduced training load. He had also put on some weight. Despite seeing multiple specialists, having numerous investigations and a knee arthroscopy, no one could work out what was wrong with him. After having had symptoms for more than 2 years, a rheumatologist finally diagnosed him with seronegative arthritis—an inflammatory arthritis.

The rheumatologist commenced him on some powerful drugs, methotrexate and prednisolone, which gave him a slight improvement in symptoms. He then began taking etanercept, an even more powerful (and expensive) drug, a tumour necrosis factor blocker. When I first met him, he was self-injecting with etanercept every 2 weeks. He told me that after 10 days his knee would start to hurt and he knew it was time for his next injection.

He approached me about trying a low-carbohydrate, healthy fat diet, primarily to lose some weight. He embraced the diet enthusiastically and strictly and reduced his carbohydrate intake substantially. After 3 weeks he came to me a bit sheepishly and admitted that he had "forgotten" to take his etanercept the previous week as he hadn't had any knee pain. He wanted to know whether he should take it anyway. I suggested he wait to see if he developed any pain.

A year later he was still pain-free and off all medication. Apart from saving $15,000 on medication, he had dropped a few kilograms and was able to complete full training sessions.

Over that year, not only had he gone from being out of the national team to being a key member of it, but he had climbed to be ranked as one of the top 10 batsmen in the

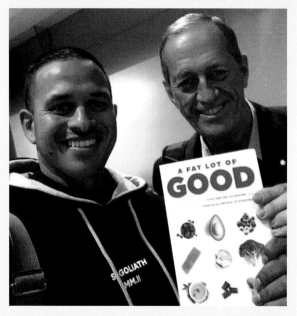

**Figure 22.12** Usman Khawaja and Peter Brukner. When joint pain persists and has no obvious mechanical cause, consider whether it may be a red flag for an inflammatory cause.

world. He is still committed to a low-carbohydrate way of life, as are his wife and children. He remains at the top of his profession and was named ICC Test Cricketer of the Year in 2023, 10 years later.

This case opened my eyes first to how often inflammatory arthritis presents as musculoskeletal pain, and second to the link between diet and inflammation.

---

(Fig. 22.13)—designed to help you to ask about, and look for, specific characteristics that may be features of inflammatory arthritis:

**SCREEND'EM**

**S** Skin, psoriasis, rash; ensure to ask if the patient's parents or siblings have psoriasis

**C** Colitis, Crohn's disease

**R** Relatives/any family history of inflammatory arthritis

**E** Eyes: uveitis, iritis, dry eyes, photosensitivity

**E** Early morning stiffness beyond 30 minutes

**N** Nocturnal pattern, nail changes (Fig. 22.11) and number of joints involved

**D** Dactylitis

**E** Enthesitis

**M** Movement and medication effect

## D: Disorders of muscle

Dermatomyositis and polymyositis are inflammatory connective tissue disorders characterised by proximal limb girdle weakness, often without pain. Dermatomyositis is also associated with a photosensitive skin rash in light-exposed areas (hands and face).

In older adults, dermatomyositis may be associated with malignancy in approximately 50% of cases. The primary malignancy may be readily detectable or occult. In younger adults, weakness may be profound (e.g. unable to rise from the floor), but in the early stages it may manifest only as underperformance in training or competition.

Dermatomyositis and polymyositis may also be associated with other connective tissue disorders such as systemic lupus erythematosus and systemic sclerosis. The muscle abnormality is characterised by elevated creatine

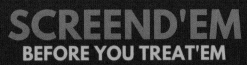

# SCREEND'EM
## BEFORE YOU TREAT'EM
A clinical tool to help identify spondyloarthropathy (SpA)

**SKIN**
6-42% of patients with psoriasis develop psoriatic arthritis.

**COLITIS OR CROHN'S**

Arthritis is one of the most common extra-intestinal manifestations of inflammatory bowel disease. The prevalence of SpA in patients with Crohn's is estimated to be 26% at 6 year follow up.

**RELATIVES**

There is a strong relationship between SpA and HLA-B27 positive patients.

Family members of patients with SpA who are HLA-B27 positive have a 16-fold increase chance of developing ankylosing spondylitis if they are also HLA-B27 positive.

**EYES**

Acute anterior uveitis (AAU) can cause a painful, red eye with photophobia and blurred vision. 40% of patients presenting with idiopathic AAU have undiagnosed SpA. 50% of patients with AAU are HLA-B27 positive and >50% of these have SpA.

**EARLY MORNING STIFFNESS**
Inactivity related stiffness that lasts for more than 30 minutes is suggestive of inflammatory disease.

**NAILS**
Nail lesions occur in 87% of SpA patients and include:
- small depressions in the nail (pitting)
- thickening of the nails
- painless detachment from the nail bed (onchylosis).

**DACTYLITIS**
Sausage like swelling of the digits is a hallmark sign of psoriatic arthritis, occuring in 50% of cases.

**ENTHESITIS**
98% of SpA patients have at least one abnormal enthesis. The most common sites are the Achilles tendon, plantar fascia and patellar tendon.

**MOVEMENT & MEDICATION EFFECT**
SpA patients report improvement with activity but not with rest, and a favourable response to NSAIDs.

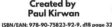
**Created by Paul Kirwan**    @pdkirwan    **THE KNEE RESOURCE**
ISBN/EAN: 978-90-75823-92-9, d18 page 32    designed by freepik.com

kinase levels and electromyographic and muscle biopsy changes. Other important blood tests include inflammatory markers and anti-nuclear factors with extractable nuclear antigen screening.

Endurance athletes may complain of myalgia and fatigue that is out of proportion with their training schedule. The differential diagnosis to explain these symptoms is broad. Mitochondrial myopathies, though uncommon, may present as cramping and muscle pain.[28] Consider myoglobinuria in these patients. Referral to a specialist neurologist for investigations and diagnosis may be necessary.[28]

Regional limb dystrophies such as limb-girdle dystrophy and facio-scapulo-humeral dystrophy may present with proximal limb girdle weakness in young adults. They are also associated with characteristic electromyographic changes. Ultimately, when an athlete complains of muscle fatigue, aches and pains that fail to respond in the time frame expected with the training patterns, a broader differential diagnosis must be considered.

## Red flag thinking with respect to persistent symptoms

Red flags traditionally refer to diagnosis—ensuring that symptoms that appear to have a benign cause are not really the harbingers of a condition with a poor prognosis. Can we use a "red-flag mindset" to address the underlying cause of a condition?

Remember that musculoskeletal symptoms can be the result of repeated activity (e.g. swimming, running)—the sinister pathologies we have been discussing here are important but some are quite rare. If you find the athlete is not responding to what you consider to be high-value care, ask yourself—is there a biomechanical cause that is perpetuating the problem? You might like to refresh your knowledge of the content in Chapters 12 and 13: Chapter 12 covers the important fundamentals of biomechanics and injury; and Chapter 13 provides tips from clinician experts who work in nine common sports, including cycling, baseball and volleyball. Experienced clinicians know what biomechanical clues to look for in their sport—and share them.

**Figure 22.13** SCREEND'EM is an acronym designed to consider specific characteristics that may be features of inflammatory arthritis

Also consider the very simple biomechanical examples in Table 22.4. These examples guide you to specific biomechanical patterns you might see in patients from the sports listed. The purpose of the table is to provide examples (not exhaustive) of how you can look for a cause that underlies the athlete's symptoms—and feel the satisfaction of finding that cause together with the athlete.

**TABLE 22.4** Common biomechanical causes of persistent symptoms

| Symptom | Biomechanical factors that may contribute to the symptom |
| --- | --- |
| Shoulder pain in a volleyball player | Poor scapular stability |
| Shoulder pain in a swimmer | Limited trunk rotation |
| Elbow pain in a throwing athlete | Letting the elbow "hang" because of trunk and lower limb weakness |
| Back pain in a tennis player | Failing to control lumbar hyperextension when serving |
| Anterior knee pain in a runner | Vastus medialis wasting and poor gluteal control of the pelvis (this might best be seen on a video of the athlete running) |
| Shin pain in ballet dancer | "Forcing turnout"—excessive tibial external rotation in an attempt to improve lower leg alignment |
| Patellofemoral pain | Hip weakness |
| Back, neck and shoulder pain | Poor posture, particularly for long periods of time or repetitively |
| Iliotibial band pain | Proximal hip muscle weakness |

## KEY POINTS

- Common signs and symptoms in sport-related illnesses/injuries may occasionally indicate a more serious underlying medical issue. These are red flags.

- To avoid missing a red flag, take a comprehensive history and focused physical examination, and avoid having a narrow focus. Don't rush to a diagnosis.

- In the context of sport, red flags are often specific to the musculoskeletal system (e.g. pain or swelling disproportionate to training load). More general red flags include unexplained weight loss or malaise.

- Remember factors like age when considering possible underlying medical issues. Certain conditions are more often associated with younger individuals (e.g. osteosarcoma) or older adults (e.g. metastatic disease).

- One indication to screen for an underlying medical condition is a disparity between the severity of an injury and the presentation of pain. Pain is a complex phenomenon (see Chapter 11).

- In cases of enthesopathy, always consider inflammatory arthritis as a possible contributing factor.

- When an athlete does not respond to a treatment program as you would expect, consider revisiting the diagnosis and/or screening for underlying medical issues.

- THINK BROAD is a helpful acronym to remember the various conditions that can produce red flag signs and symptoms.

## REFERENCES

References for this chapter can be found at www.mhprofessional.com/CSM6e

## ADDITIONAL CONTENT

 Scan here to access additional resources for this topic and more provided by the authors

C

## CHAPTER 23

# Using PROMs in clinical practice

with LINA HOLM INGELSRUD, ERIN M. MACRI and NATALIE COLLINS

*The patient experience can and should be assessed systematically, consistently and repeatedly over time. All clinicians need to be familiar with the science behind PROMs in general and with a few specific PROMs in their own clinical field.*

TRISH GREENHALGH (PROFESSOR)

*Ask the athlete–instead of us deciding what is good for them.*

PAUL DIEPPE (PROFESSOR EMERITUS)

## CHAPTER OUTLINE

What are PROMs?
Using PROMs to benefit the injured athlete
Choosing which PROM to use
Interpreting the PROM score
Examples of commonly used PROMs
Clinical case

## LEARNING OBJECTIVES

By the end of this chapter you should be able to:

- define PROMs
- discuss how PROMs inform the clinical consultation
- describe the criteria that you should consider when selecting PROMs
- select an appropriate PROM for a given sports-related injury or illness
- interpret the results from PROMs.

## WHAT ARE PROMs?

Think back to a recent consultation with an athlete who had sustained an injury during sport. What was the athlete's main complaint? How did you monitor that problem during treatment? What was the athlete's treatment goal? How did you evaluate whether that goal was reached?

When you are monitoring how treatment is progressing in an athlete who sustained a traumatic knee injury, for example, it is important to evaluate functional performance as well as muscle strength. However, core clinical outcomes also include knee-related pain, other symptoms (e.g. stiffness, instability), cognitive behavioural factors that influence learning and performance, self-reported function, health-related quality of life, and physical activity and sports participation.[1] All of these outcomes can be evaluated using patient-reported outcome measures (PROMs).

Health aspects such as pain, self-perceived functional ability, and health-related quality of life are complex domains that are not directly observable; they are hidden underlying constructs (Fig. 23.1). PROMs[2] can be used to capture the patient's own perception of these domains and their health state.

PROMs measure aspects of health that are of direct importance to the patient. They provide a standardised way to get direct input from the patient about their health condition or experience with an injury. PROMs

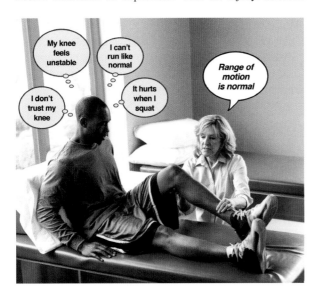

**Figure 23.1** PROMs reflect the patient's own perceptions of their health condition. With PROMs, we can measure those hidden underlying constructs that we cannot directly observe, such as pain and health-related quality of life.
ISTOCK/KALI9

are often composed of several questions that together reflect one underlying domain or construct, or they can be multidimensional and grouped into subscales that each reflect separate domains. A PROM can also be one question: a very simple, commonly used PROM in clinical practice is asking the athlete to rate their pain severity on a scale from 0 to 10—a numerical rating scale.

Specific PROMs can be developed for:

- an injury or a disease, such as the Victorian Institute of Sport Assessment-Gluteal (VISA-G) score[3]
- a patient population, such as the Disablement in the Physically Active scale-mental summary component (DPA-MSC)[4]
- a particular joint or region, such as the Functional Arm Scale for Throwers (FAST).[4]

PROMs can also be generic, providing an overall summary of a health aspect that makes it possible to compare health across different populations.[5] An example of a generic questionnaire is the Short-Form 36 (SF-36). Specific PROMs are often more useful for clinical practice than generic PROMs, because they are more sensitive in capturing changes related to a specific injury or disease.[5]

PROMs can be developed to:

- evaluate
- discriminate
- predict.[6,7]

Many PROMs have been developed to evaluate outcomes and monitor treatment progression in sports and exercise medicine. However, PROMs can also be used for screening purposes, for which they need to have high discriminatory ability; for example, to identify people who have a certain condition or level of severity. A common PROM-based screening tool is the Injury-Psychological Readiness to Return to Sport (I-PRRS) scale.[8] The I-PRRS is recommended in current consensus statements to inform whether an athlete feels ready to return to sport after injury.[9,10] Another tool, the Patient Health Questionnaire-9 (PHQ-9), has proved valuable to screen for depression in collegiate student athletes.[11]

Some PROMs were initially developed to monitor outcomes and then later their discriminative or predictive abilities were evaluated. For example, certain items from the Copenhagen Hip and Groin Outcome Score (HAGOS) were found to be important components to predict the outcome of hip arthroscopy and were subsequently included in a prediction tool.[12] In clinical practice, it is important to select a PROM that has been developed, or later confirmed to be informative, for your intended purpose.

# USING PROMs TO BENEFIT THE INJURED ATHLETE

You can use a specific PROM to:

- obtain a structured overview of the athlete's symptoms before initiating treatment
- communicate with the athlete about their PROM responses regarding specific factors impacted by their injury
- facilitate shared treatment decision making by focusing on aspects that are considered most important to the athlete
- target treatment aims by obtaining insights into the athlete's priorities, preferences and goals
- monitor the athlete's progress after initiating treatment, and evaluate treatment effectiveness during and after treatment
- relate the athlete's health status to a comparable population by comparing the athlete's score with population or reference values for the PROM[13]
- assist with predicting the outcome of a certain treatment choice.

You can use a generic PROM to:

- measure the athlete's overall health (if doing so can inform treatment for your patient).

You can use short and simple questions to evaluate:

- the athlete's current pain at every consultation, such as a numerical rating scale or visual analogue scale for pain at rest or during activity[14]
- whether the athlete considers their current symptom state to be acceptable and satisfactory
- whether the athlete considers the experienced change in a domain as important to them.[1]

## CHOOSING WHICH PROM TO USE

When choosing which PROM to use in a specific clinical setting, there are seven important factors to consider (see also Fig. 23.2).

### Which domain do you intend to measure?

Consider what you intend to measure. A PROM can measure one or more defined domains. Evaluate which domains are most important to your athlete and whether the PROM captures these. To guide this evaluation, published core outcome sets may be helpful.

Core outcome sets were initially developed for research purposes, to address the challenge of comparing different outcome measures used in different clinical trials conducted on the same health condition. Published core outcome sets can inform both research and clinical care. For research, a

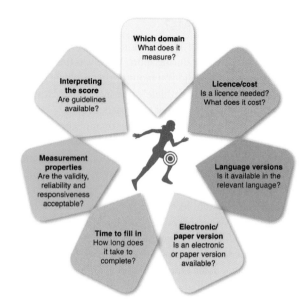

**Figure 23.2** Consider these factors when choosing a PROM to inform clinical practice

core outcome set defines the minimum set of outcomes that should be evaluated in a clinical trial in a specific condition.[15]

From a clinical care perspective, information from core outcome sets can guide which domains are considered most important in a certain context and often specific tools (i.e. PROMs or other measurement tools) to measure those domains.[16] For example, for lateral elbow tendinopathy, the domain *disability* is important, and the Patient-Rated Tennis Elbow Evaluation (PRTEE) is endorsed to evaluate it.[17]

Available core outcome sets and ongoing development work can be searched for in the online database, Core Outcome Measures in Effectiveness Trials:

 Core Outcome Measures in Effectiveness Trials

### Is there a cost/licence requirement?

Some PROMs require a licence to use, while others are free. Check the accessibility of the PROM you are thinking of using on the specific PROM's web page.

### Is the PROM available in the relevant language?

When a PROM has been developed in one country and language, it needs to be translated and validated for use in other languages and cultural contexts. There are strict requirements for the translation process to ensure that the questions in the translated version reflect the same content as the original version. Furthermore, the translated version should possess the same quality of measurement properties.[18] Before selecting a PROM that has been translated, check that it has undergone appropriate cross-cultural validation, and that the measurement properties of the translated version are adequate for use in your target population. You can often find this information on the web page where the translated version is available.

## Is an electronic or paper version available?

In a busy clinical practice, administering PROMs to patients may seem burdensome and disrupt workflow. Even though a PROM may be free to use, the time to administer, review and score it has a cost. There is high agreement between paper-based and electronically derived scores,[19, 20] so the format used depends on what works best in your clinic.

In our experience, integrating the PROM directly into the electronic health records works best if this is available. Having the patient complete the questionnaire on a tablet or touch screen is efficient in clinical practice; it helps ensure complete responses, scoring is automated and you can present the scores visually,[21] which enhances communication with the patient.[22]

It is also worth considering whether the PROM can be completed on the athlete's own device, as this gives them the option to complete the questionnaire at home. This depends on local privacy and confidentiality regulations of course.

## How long does it take to complete?

In daily clinical practice, shorter PROMs may be preferred because they take less time to complete. But it is important to consider the length of the PROM in relation to what information it provides. For example, does it measure the domain(s) of interest? Does it have good measurement properties? If combining several PROMs is necessary to capture all domains of interest, you will need to determine the total number of questions and the time required to complete them in combination.

It is also important to consider how often the PROM will be completed. It may not be relevant or feasible to have an athlete complete a PROM at every appointment. The questionnaire used can be longer as the time interval increases between each administration.

## Is there evidence that the PROM has acceptable measurement properties ("clinimetrics")?

A useful PROM needs to have acceptable measurement properties when tested in the relevant patient population. When selecting PROMs for use in clinical practice, it is important to consider whether the measurement properties have been evaluated in the population of interest. For example, some PROMs were developed for use in adults and have been shown to have acceptable measurement properties for use in adults. However, they may not be appropriate for use in children or adolescents, unless they have undergone additional testing to establish their measurement properties in this population.

Many well-known and well-established PROMs used in sports and exercise medicine, such as the Shoulder Pain and Disability Index (SPADI),[23] the Knee Injury and Osteoarthritis Outcome Score (KOOS)[24] and the Roland-Morris Disability Questionnaire (RMDQ)[25] to evaluate low back pain, were developed more than two decades ago. Since then, the standards for evaluating measurement properties have changed, and in those cases, the PROMs developers should update the psychometric properties of the instrument or researchers should undertake methods studies of the PROMs.

Finding evidence in the original development paper alone is rarely sufficient. Often, additional evaluation of a PROM's measurement properties has been performed, either in the same or other settings, other patient populations, other countries or using newer and refined validation methods, such as item response theory. Therefore, the most recent systematic reviews, or core outcome sets that involve a systematic review, are the best place to get an overview of a PROM's measurement properties.[15, 26]

Whether a PROM is valid is not a yes/no question: a PROM is not inherently either valid or not. We need assurance that measurement properties are sufficient, and that the evidence is of high quality and evaluated in the relevant patient population. As such, a PROM's measurement properties should be demonstrated using rigorous research methodology.

Different nomenclature exists to describe these measurement properties. In this chapter, we follow the COnsensus-based Standards for the selection of health Measurement INstruments (COSMIN) taxonomy.[27] The most important measurement properties to consider when using a PROM to evaluate individual athletes are:[27]

- *validity:* the degree to which the PROM measures the construct(s) it aims to measure
- *reliability:* the degree to which the measurement is free from error
- *responsiveness:* the ability of the PROM to detect change over time in the construct being measured.

### Validity: does it measure what it is supposed to?

It is essential that a PROM measures what we intend it to measure. Consider HAGOS, which was specifically

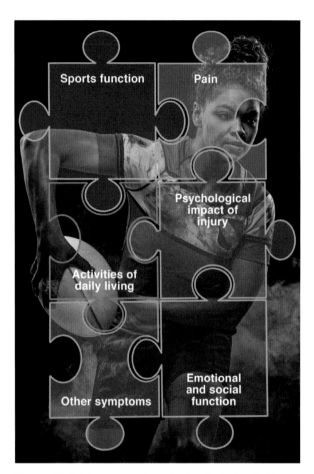

**Figure 23.3** A jigsaw puzzle metaphor illustrates that to get a complete picture of the patient, one or more PROMs may be necessary to capture all relevant domains.
ISTOCK/LORADO

designed for physically active, young to middle-aged individuals with hip and groin pain.[28] It consists of 37 questions grouped into 6 domains: symptoms (7 questions), pain (10 questions), activities of daily living (5 questions), sport and recreation (8 questions), participation in physical activity (2 questions) and hip- and groin-related quality of life (5 questions). Each question has 5 response options scored from 0 to 4, indicating *no* to *extreme* problems. For each domain, a score can be calculated by summing the responses and transforming them to a 0 to 100 scale, indicating *extreme* to *no* hip/groin problems.

How can you ensure that the 8 questions regarding sport and recreation accurately reflect your athlete's experience with sport and recreational functional capability? How do you know that it makes sense to sum the responses to a numerical score? These considerations tap into the aspect of validity.

A PROM that has a high degree of validity makes us more confident that it measures what it is supposed to measure. Several domains can be considered important to athletes when evaluating the impact of an injury on their health, and when monitoring the progress of treatment. Domains such as pain and sports function are common, but the total number of domains included in a PROM varies (Fig. 23.3). A high-quality PROM has clearly described domains so that you can evaluate whether the questions adequately reflect those domains.

## Content validity

First, consider whether the questions adequately cover all aspects of the target domain. This is known as content validity. To ensure high content validity, PROM developers must involve experts during the development phase. A variety of healthcare and content experts may be included, but the most important experts are the patients themselves. For example, when HAGOS was developed, 25 patients contributed to ensure that relevant aspects were covered and that the proposed questions were understandable and formed a comprehensive measure of the domain.[28]

A thorough description of how PROMs are developed is beyond the scope of this book, but it is essential to understand that the process of identifying questions is iteratively performed by conducting literature searches and interviews with experts to identify, formulate, evaluate and select questions.

## Construct validity

Second, consider how well the PROM measures its intended domain(s). This is termed construct validity. A high-quality PROM has the least number of and most informative questions necessary to best reflect the domain (Fig. 23.4). When developing a PROM, questions are selected by performing statistical tests (e.g. factor analysis, item response theory) to identify the questions that best reflect the domain. The tests also identify which questions can be omitted because they are superfluous or redundant.

When questions are combined into a total score, they should reflect a unidimensional construct (i.e. only one domain). If a PROM is not unidimensional, questions relating to two or more domains will be summed into a total score, making it impossible to understand or interpret what the score means for the athlete—which domain is affected, and how. For example, if an athlete has no problems with activities of daily living, but experiences problems with sport, then summing those questions into a total function score will mask the problems with sport-related function.

Hypothesis testing can also be used to determine whether PROM scores reflect the target domain.[18] For example,

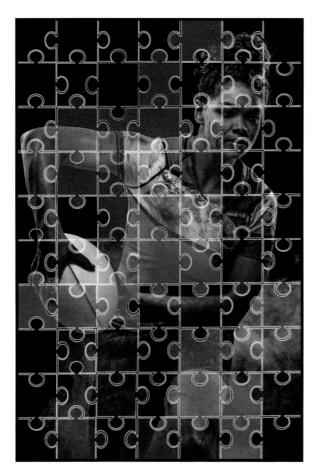

**Figure 23.4** PROMs developers begin with a large number of questions (depicted here by all 70 pieces in the 7 x 10-piece jigsaw). The questions that prove most useful are retained and organised into separate domains. Each domain is depicted by a separate colour, and the discarded questions are represented by uncoloured pieces.
ISTOCK/LORADO

we might hypothesise that a new PROM measuring pain would be highly correlated with another PROM for pain (convergent validation) but would be only moderately correlated with a PROM measuring self-efficacy (divergent validation).

HAGOS is a good example of a PROM that has undergone thorough testing for construct validity. During development, factor analysis was used to explore which questions fitted together best as a summed score and this resulted in 6 separately scored subscales. Hypothesis testing was also performed, confirming the authors' assumptions how the 6 subscales should correlate with other validated health measures.[28]

A revised version of HAGOS was developed later using more advanced statistics (item response theory). The revised version is 7 questions shorter, which improves the score structure. When HAGOS is used to compare results across countries, a conversion table is needed because there are cross-cultural differences in responses to the questions. The HAGOS authors caution that further validity testing of this revised version is needed, for example in women.[29]

### Reliability: what is the degree of measurement error?

All measures are associated with some degree of measurement error. If you were to measure your athlete's muscle strength three times in a row, within half an hour, the results might differ slightly, but you know that your athlete's true muscle strength has not changed. PROMs are no different.

When using a PROM in clinical practice for individual athletes, the degree of measurement error can be quite high. Measurement error is always higher when PROMs are used for individual patients rather than a group of patients (e.g. in a research study) because the degree of measurement error decreases with the number of individuals included—the measurement error averages out.[30] In clinic, you need to be able to trust the measurements you perform, because the results may directly affect a clinical decision. The question is, how large an error is expected around a score, and how do you know whether a change in score exceeds the degree of expected error?

Reliability is evaluated in several ways. For PROMs, we need reassurance that it measures consistently—to what degree can the measurement be reproduced? One statistic that is commonly presented is Cronbach's alpha, which measures internal consistency: how well the questions correlate to each other (Box 23.3 later in the chapter).

### Test-retest reliability

Test-retest reliability is evaluated when the same PROM is filled out by a group of individuals whose condition or health state is assumed stable. A common reliability measure, the intraclass correlation coefficient (ICC), relates the degree of variation between the scores in the sample to the degree of error, and is expressed from 0 (poor reliability) to 1 (perfect reliability). This type of reliability expresses both the agreement between the two measures and how well the questionnaire distinguishes between individuals.

When using a PROM in clinical practice, it is important that its reliability has been tested on a population similar to the athlete's, since the degree of variation between individuals can have a substantial impact on the ICC value.[31] The larger the variation between individuals, the more measurement error can be tolerated. An ICC value can be calculated for any PROM for which a score is expressed on a continuous scale.

Test-retest reliability is considered adequate for use in individual athletes if the ICC is greater than 0.9,[32,33] and adequate for use in groups if it is greater than 0.7.[33,34] The reason that the ICC criterion is stricter for use in individuals is that the degree of measurement error decreases with the number of individuals under study.

## Measurement error

We can also express measurement error in the measurement unit of the specific PROM: the standard error of measurement (SEM). The SEM quantifies measurement error around a score at one point in time and is directly clinically applicable. For example, the KOOS Patellofemoral pain and osteoarthritis subscale (KOOS-PF) score ranges from 0 to 100 (maximum to no disability) and the SEM was reported to be 6.8. Using the SEM, we can calculate a confidence interval around the observed score that gives us an idea of the uncertainty around that score.

When comparing an athlete's PROMs scores over time (the change score) measurement error occurs at both measurements. The minimal detectable change (MDC), also known as the smallest detectable change (SDC), is the change in score needed for us to be relatively sure that the reported change is larger than the measurement error—and thus represents a real change in the athlete's condition. The MDC can be calculated as SEM × 1.65 × √2 (Box 23.1). Again, in research, the MDC for a group of individuals is smaller, since the measurement error decreases with the number of individuals, and is calculated by dividing the MDC by √n.

You might think that the measurement error for KOOS-PF seems quite large. That's true and holds for most PROMs used in sports and exercise medicine when evaluating individual athletes. When the SEM is used to quantify the uncertainty around the score, the error is assumed equal across the whole scale.

Tools that have been evaluated using item response theory have the advantage that measurement error can be evaluated more precisely for each possible score on the scale.[37,38] We may see more use of item response theory to improve the clinical applicability of PROMs in the future.

## Responsiveness: can the PROM detect true change over time?

When we evaluate health improvement or deterioration over time, can we be certain that the change we measure adequately reflects true change in the clinical condition? Let's return to the example of an athlete with patellofemoral pain (Fig. 23.6), where KOOS-PF was used to monitor their response to treatment over time. This athlete, after a period of best-practice treatment, scored 70 points on the KOOS-PF, a 40-point improvement from before treatment commenced. We need assurance that this improvement validly reflects the actual change that has happened.

---

**BOX 23.1** Measurement error: an important "detail" that helps clinicians know whether patients are getting better or staying the same

Figure 23.5 provides the KOOS-PF score of an athlete who scored 30 points before they began receiving treatment for patellofemoral pain.

We can evaluate the uncertainty around that score by calculating a confidence interval. For example, we can be 90% confident that the athlete's true score is in the area between the observed score plus or minus the SEM × 1.65; hence, within the range between 19 and 41 points.[35,36] At some time during treatment, the athlete fills out the questionnaire a second time. The athlete's score improves by 12 points. For KOOS-PF, the MDC was 16.[36] The difference between the two measurements may therefore reflect measurement error, rather than a true change in the athlete's condition.

This example underscores the importance of considering measurement error when using the PROM score to assess changes in the athlete's condition over time. Calculating the degree of uncertainty around the PROM score, when used in individual patients in clinic, helps clarify to what degree you can be certain that the PROM score reflects actual improvement.

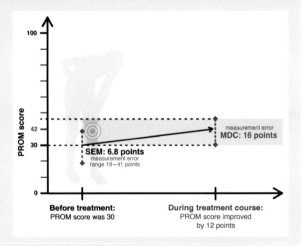

**Figure 23.5** PROMs reliability can be quantified for an individual with the SEM and the MDC. For the KOOS-PF, the reported SEM was 6.8 and the MDC was 16 points.

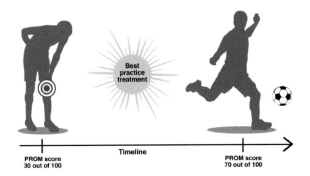

**Figure 23.6** In addition to taking the measurement error into account (Fig. 23.5), we also need assurance that the PROM used to evaluate change over time is responsive, that its score change over time is a valid reflection of the actual change in the domain it measures. Using highly responsive PROMs can help you and the athlete make more informed treatment decisions.

Responsiveness is defined as the validity of change scores. There are different views on how to best evaluate responsiveness. Former custom was to calculate an intervention's effect size, measured with the PROM under study; the PROMs with the highest effect sizes were considered more responsive.[39] However, effect size reflects the intervention effect and not necessarily whether that measured effect is valid.

Within the COSMIN framework, responsiveness is best evaluated using a hypothesis-based approach.[40] For example, KOOS-PF was deemed responsive, based on confirming hypotheses relating to how the change in KOOS-PF scores would correlate with another self-reported evaluation of change over time. Hypotheses can also be based on the expected change in the PROM score following a certain intervention of known effectiveness, or in certain subgroups in the population where a different PROM change score is expected.

## INTERPRETING THE PROM SCORE

Once you have selected a PROM for use with your patient and they have completed the questionnaire, how do you make sense of the score and convert numbers into meaningful information to help guide treatment? This is where the concept of "interpretability" of PROMs comes in. Interpretability refers to "the degree to which one can assign qualitative meaning" to the numerical score derived from completing a PROM.[27]

Clinicians use PROM scores to assist with clinical decision making in three main ways:

1. to evaluate how a patient compares with similar patients or the general population; for example, self-reported health-related quality of life (QOL) in a person following an anterior cruciate ligament (ACL) injury could be compared with known reference values in an ACL population or a general population[41, 42]

2. to screen a patient, such as to identify an athlete whose pain score might be above a certain threshold that indicates their pain may have a neuropathic component, and who therefore may benefit from a different treatment approach[43]

3. to understand how the patient feels about how they are doing; for example, does the patient believe they are getting better, and is that improvement meaningful to the patient?

## Is your athlete feeling better?

A responder threshold that can help answer the third point is known as a minimal important change (MIC). MIC represents the minimum amount of improvement (or worsening) in a PROM score that a patient would perceive as important to them.[44, 45] In the literature, terms similar to this may be used (e.g. minimal clinically important difference, smallest worthwhile change) and different methods are used to calculate MIC, but what most have in common is that in addition to the PROM, patients are asked to complete an "anchor" question.

A typical anchor is a Global Rating of Change (GROC) question, in which the patient evaluates their overall improvement (or worsening) on a Likert scale. The Likert response corresponding to the minimal amount of improvement deemed to be important to the patient is then used to determine the MIC for the PROM change score.

A similar concept can be used to ask the patient if their current status is satisfactory, and the answer to this anchor question can be used to determine the PROM score (an absolute score in this case, not a change score) corresponding to the patient acceptable symptoms state (PASS).[46] This is the PROM score value beyond which the patient considers themselves well. PASS thresholds are being used more frequently as outcomes in clinical trials as patients don't just want to feel "better", they prefer to feel "good".[47]

## PROM scores and interpretation thresholds can aid your conversation

The methods used to determine the interpretability of PROM scores, or changes in PROM scores over time, continue to evolve. There are two key considerations when using known values to assist with interpreting PROM scores for the individual patient:

- Research aimed to determine values for interpreting scores almost ubiquitously does so by evaluating group-level data. Such values are essentially average values meant to represent and summarise a range of scores in a given

**BOX 23.2** Anchor questions that can be used in the clinic to help evaluate an athlete's progress[1,49]

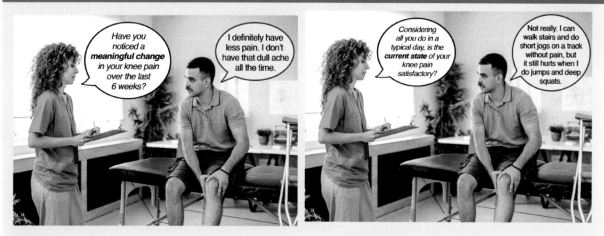

**Figure 23.7** Anchor questions that may be used to help evaluate an athlete's progress
ISTOCK/ENIGMA IMAGES

In these examples, we used knee pain as the outcome of interest. You and the patient may also be interested in their perceived knee function or knee-related quality of life. In such cases you can substitute those outcomes for "knee pain" above (or add questions).

group of patients. MIC values actually vary from person to person, and most individuals won't have an MIC equal to the calculated average. A mean group-derived value may be useful for research purposes but may not inform you of how your patient is doing, because your patient's score is highly contextual and unique to them.

- Published values in the literature differ substantially among different studies, probably due to a combination of differences in study quality, methodological approach and clinical factors like sample demographics, type of intervention or follow-up duration. Group-derived thresholds for MICs and PASS scores differ even when different approaches are applied to identical samples.[48] For example, a systematic review of MIC thresholds in people treated for ACL tears found that MICs for the KOOS pain subscale differed by change scores of more than 20 points on a 100-point scale.[45]

Given the challenges faced with using threshold values like MIC or PASS, you should use these values cautiously. Instead, we recommended that evaluation of your patient's status or progress be individualised. Specifically, you should ask each patient to answer PROMs and anchor questions directly (Box 23.2).

Then, instead of relying on total scores, change scores and published thresholds, use the answers as an entry point for a conversation with the patient. Graphs of scores over time may serve as a useful visual aid for both you and your patient.[50]

To pull together those concepts of measurement properties, change over time and anchor questions, Figure 23.8 illustrates a conversation that you could initiate with the patient whose case was captured in Figures 23.5 and 23.6.

By engaging your patient in a meaningful conversation about their condition and treatment like this you can gain very tailored information about them—and that's a key component of shared decision making.[1,49,51] This type of clinician–patient conversation also avoids the risk of false-negatives or false-positives that could arise if you were to

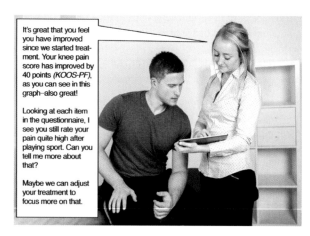

**Figure 23.8** Sample conversation with the patient from Figures 23.5 and 23.6
ISTOCK/LSOPHOTO

rely on a single published MIC or PASS value to assess a patient's status.

These clinical conversations also enrich your understanding of your patient, possibly identifying contextual factors that cannot be captured in a questionnaire—for example, the patient's perception of treatment benefits, the feasibility or convenience of the treatment, their personal preferences, and any risks or harms they may experience.

## EXAMPLES OF COMMONLY USED PROMs

Table 23.1 illustrates some common examples of PROMs that are used across the athletic population to evaluate:

- pain
- function
- health-related quality of life
- psychological impairment.

**TABLE 23.1** Examples of PROMs that are applicable across the athletic population

| To evaluate pain | |
|---|---|
| *Pain Numerical Rating Scale*[52] | |
| Domain and description | A single question about pain intensity within a defined period, or average pain intensity |
| Scoring | The athlete rates their pain level on a numerical scale from 0 (no pain) to 10 (worst imaginable pain) |
| Availability | Freely available |
| **To evaluate function** | |
| *Patient-Specific Functional Scale*[53] | |
| Domain and description | The athlete nominates 3–5 activities that are difficult because of their injury/condition |
| Scoring | The athlete rates the difficulty for each activity on an 11-point scale from 0 (unable to perform activity) to 10 (able to perform activity at same level as before injury or problem) |
| Availability | Freely available |
| **To evaluate health-related quality of life** | |
| *Short Form-36*[54] | |
| Domain and description | 8 domains are covered by 36 questions:<br>• physical functioning<br>• physical role<br>• bodily pain<br>• general health<br>• vitality<br>• social functioning<br>• emotional role<br>• mental health<br>A physical and mental component summary score can be computed |
| Scoring | Responses are summed and transformed to a score from 0 (worst health state) to 100 (best health state); computer scoring algorithms are necessary; norm-based scoring is recommended, which requires a licensed computer scoring algorithm |
| Availability | The original version is freely available from www.rand.org; the most recent version (developed in 1998) requires a licence: www.qualitymetric.com/health-surveys/the-sf-36v2-health-survey |
| *Assessment of Quality of Life-6 Dimensions*[55] | |
| Domain and description | 6 domains are measured by 20 questions:<br>• independent living<br>• mental health<br>• relationships<br>• senses<br>• coping<br>• pain |
| Scoring | Scoring algorithms and an online scoring service are available from www.aqol.com.au; score ranges from −0.04 (health state worse than death) to 0.0 (death) and 1.00 (full health) |
| Availability | Freely available; requires registration for use in studies, but not for clinical practice |

*continues*

**TABLE 23.1**    Examples of PROMs that are applicable across the athletic population (continued)

| To evaluate psychological impairments | |
|---|---|
| **Pain Catastrophising Scale[56]** | |
| Domain and description | A measure of catastrophic thinking related to pain; 3 domains are measured by 13 questions:<br>• rumination<br>• magnification<br>• helplessness |
| Scoring | A total score can be calculated by summing the responses; each question is responded to on a 5-point scale reflecting whether the patient has experienced certain feelings, from 0 (not at all) to 4 (all the time); domain-specific scores can also be calculated |
| Availability | Freely available; requires registration for use in studies, but not for clinical practice: https://eprovide.mapi-trust.org/instruments/pain-catastrophizing-scale |
| **Tampa Scale for Kinesiophobia[57, 58]** | |
| Domain and description | A measure of the athlete's fear of re-injury due to movement; they consider their agreement with 17 statements about their experiences and feelings |
| Scoring | A total score from 17 to 68 can be easily summed from the 4-point response options ranging from 1 (strongly disagree) to 4 (strongly agree); beware that 4 items are reversely scored |
| Availability | Freely available |
| **Injury-Psychological Readiness to Return to Sport** | |
| Domain and description | A measure of the athlete's confidence to return to sport; comprises 6 questions |
| Scoring | For each question, the athlete rates their confidence on a scale ranging from 0 (no confidence) to 100 (utmost confidence), with increments of 10; the 6 scores are summed and divided by 10 to calculate a total score |
| Availability | Available in the original publication[8] |
| **Patient Health Questionnaire-9[59]** | |
| Domain and description | A measure of depression severity; it can be used as an initial tool to screen for depression; the athlete reports to what degree they have felt bothered by 9 different problems on 4-point scale from 0 (not at all) to 3 (nearly every day) |
| Scoring | A total score is calculated by summing the responses to each problem; a score above 5 can reflect some degree of depression |
| Availability | Freely available from www.phqscreeners.com |

# CLINICAL CASE

## CLINICAL CASE 23.1:  Using PROMs to inform clinical practice

Sophia (Fig. 23.9) is a 34-year-old who underwent an ACL reconstruction (hamstring tendon autograft) of her right knee 7 years ago. She returned to social soccer 18 months after surgery. She has recently been experiencing pain and stiffness in her right knee and has stopped playing soccer and running as she fears that this may increase her pain and the damage in her knee.

Her family physician ordered radiographs, which revealed mild to moderate osteoarthritis in her right patellofemoral and tibiofemoral joint compartments.

Sophia was then referred for physiotherapy management.

In addition to performing her usual clinical assessment, Sophia's physiotherapist administered the KOOS to better understand Sophia's knee condition. The KOOS was developed for patients with knee injuries and/or osteoarthritis. It consists of 5 individually scored subscales: pain, symptoms, function in activities of daily living (ADL), function in sport and recreation activities, and knee-related quality of life (QoL).

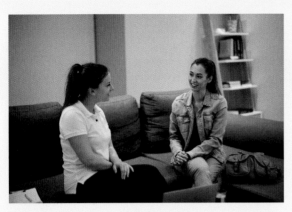

**Figure 23.9** Sophia's physiotherapist used the KOOS to track her progress and flag persisting challenges. She actively discussed these outcomes with Sophia during and after treatment.
ISTOCK/DRAZEN ZIGIC

She also administered the KOOS-PF since it was specifically developed to evaluate patellofemoral knee pain.[36] The SEM for adults with mild osteoarthritis after ACL reconstruction is pain 7.2, symptoms 9.0, ADL 5.2, sport/rec 9.0, QoL 7.4 and PF 6.8. The MDC is pain 16.8, symptoms 21, ADL 12.1, sport/rec 21, QoL 17.3 and PF 15.9.

Figure 23.10(a) shows Sophia's KOOS scores at baseline (at her first physiotherapy session) compared with population-based reference data.[60] Unfortunately, the physiotherapist could not find population reference values for the KOOS-PF. Using the reported SEM values, the physiotherapist calculated that the measurement errors around Sophia's scores before treatment are 66–90 for pain, 53–83 for symptoms, 82–100 for ADL, 0–30 for sport/rec, 13–37 for QoL and 19–41 for PF.

Sophia's baseline scores are well below the population-based reference data for the sport/rec and QoL subscales. These differences exceed the measurement error ranges—so the differences are real. In comparison, the differences in scores for the pain and symptoms subscales are smaller, and the measurement error for the ADL score overlaps with the reference data value. This may be because younger patients who undergo ACL reconstruction are more concerned with sport/recreational function and QoL and it may reflect ceiling effects observed in this population.

The physiotherapist starts a rehabilitation program of lower limb strengthening and neuromuscular control exercises, combined with manual therapy and patella taping to address pain and symptoms. Sophia's KOOS scores after 3 months are shown in Figure 23.10(b). Although her scores are better on the symptoms, ADL

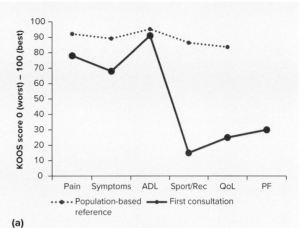

**(a)**

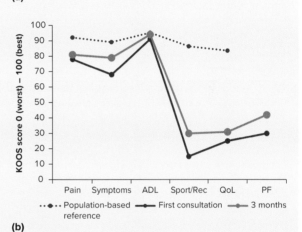

**(b)**

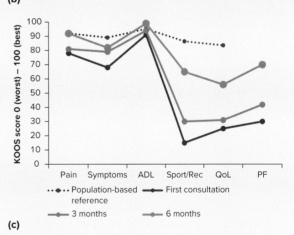

**(c)**

**Figure 23.10** Sophia's KOOS profiles of the 5 subscale scores (and the additional PF subscale) at (a) first consultation, (b) 3 months and (c) 6 months, compared with population-based reference data

*continues*

and sport/rec subscales, the change scores from baseline are within the error of the measure and therefore may not represent real change. Furthermore, while her scores on the pain, symptoms and ADL subscales are approaching population norms, the sport/rec and QoL scores remain substantially lower.

The physiotherapist communicates these results to Sophia and asks about the items with the lowest scores. In addition, she asks Sophia whether she feels that her sports-related function and overall knee-related QoL have improved since they initiated treatment. She also asks Sophia whether she feels that her current functional level and knee-related QoL are satisfactory to her.

Based on these outcomes, the physiotherapist and Sophia decide to integrate some interventions to address QoL into Sophia's rehabilitation program. Specifically, the physiotherapist uses some graded exercises, combined with education, to improve Sophia's confidence in her knee (assessed by KOOS QoL item 3) and reduce any fear-avoidance of potentially damaging activities (KOOS QoL item 2). Sophia continues to progress her strength and neuromuscular exercises, in preparation for return to sport.

From Figure 23.10(c), you can see that after 6 months of physiotherapy intervention Sophia's pain, symptoms and ADL scores are almost identical to population norms. Her sport/rec and QoL scores have also increased by an amount that exceeds the MDC for individuals.

The physiotherapist interprets these findings as representing a true change in Sophia's knee condition, and Sophia reports that she is improving. At the final appointment, the physiotherapist hands over the KOOS profiles to Sophia so that she can refer to those scores if her condition worsens in the future.

---

**BOX 23.3** What does Cronbach's alpha measure?

Cronbach's alpha measures how well the items in a PROM are related to each other. It ranges from 0 to 1, and a value between 0.7 and 0.95 is considered adequate. A value less than 0.7 suggests that questions are not correlated enough, and a value greater than 0.95 suggests that some questions are redundant. If the correlation is 1, all questions give the same information about the domain of interest.

It is important to understand that Cronbach's alpha is not a measure of unidimensionality, and it is only relevant to report it for confirmed unidimensional PROM scales. In fact, Cronbach's alpha is considered to be a measure of reliability, not validity. It gives little information on its own, but is very often reported, probably because it is easily calculated, age-old and a well-known statistic for scientific journals.[38]

---

## KEY POINTS

- Patient-reported outcome measures (PROMs) are tools that you can use to understand a patient's experiences with a disease, an injury or a condition.

- PROMs can be developed for several reasons, including evaluating outcomes and monitoring treatment progression, discriminating between conditions, screening for a condition or level of severity, and predicting outcomes of certain interventions.

- Using PROMs can benefit the athlete in a number of ways, including facilitating a shared decision-making process between the athlete and clinician and guiding return-to-sport decisions.

- There are many PROMs from which to choose. Not all PROMs are created equal, nor is any one given PROM always the best choice for an individual athlete. You should be familiar with the options, the relative strengths and weaknesses of a given PROM, and how to choose the best option for a particular situation.

- Determining the domain of interest (e.g. pain, function) is a key first step, followed by the selection of a core group of outcomes.

- There are practical factors to consider when choosing a PROM, including possible costs, licensing rules, the language that a PROM is available in, and the format (online, written).

- Many PROMs have been studied by methodologists and their measurement properties are reported. The most important among those are reliability, validity and responsiveness.

- Interpreting a PROM means trying to assign qualitative meaning to a quantitative value. This requires you to look beyond just the scores, and think about how these measurements fit into the larger picture of patient care.

## REFERENCES

References for this chapter can be found at www.mhprofessional.com/CSM6e.

## ADDITIONAL CONTENT

Scan here to access additional resources for this topic and more provided by the authors

**C**

# CHAPTER 24

# Treatment of sports injuries

*There's not one size that fits all. You may have relatively the same injuries, but one method of treatment really works well for somebody and that method doesn't work well for somebody else.*

CONAIRE TAUB, VOLLEYBALL, UBC/CANADIAN YOUTH NATIONAL TEAM

## CHAPTER OUTLINE

Overview of Chapters 24–28
Acute injury management
Therapeutic exercise
Manual treatments
Taping
Bracing
Electrophysical agents

Dry needling and acupuncture
Therapeutic medication
Nutraceuticals and nutrition
Autologous blood, blood products and
   cell therapy
And finally ...

## LEARNING OBJECTIVES

By the end of this chapter you should be able to:

- identify the components of musculoskeletal injury treatment and discuss how/why they have evolved
- explain how therapeutic exercise produces changes to different tissue types at a cellular level
- list common treatments for sport-related injuries, explain their proposed mechanism of action and summarise the evidence of their role in high-value care
- articulate the risks and benefits of common treatments for sport-related injuries and list contraindications for their use
- design a multimodal rehabilitation plan that incorporates appropriate and effective treatment strategies.

## OVERVIEW OF CHAPTERS 24–28

This chapter is the first in a group of linked chapters that describe the patient's journey after diagnosis. On this journey, the patient receives some form of treatment (Chapter 24) and education (Chapter 25), and perhaps surgery (Chapter 26), they should be skilfully rehabilitated (Chapter 27) and ultimately they aim to return to sport (Chapter 28). In Box 24.1,

Professor Kieran O'Sullivan shares a lifetime of clinical experience that is relevant to all five chapters.

While the terms "treatment" and "rehabilitation" are often used synonymously, we define treatment as specific clinical interventions aimed at modifying tissue pathology, impairments or symptoms, and rehabilitation as a holistic process aimed at restoring the athlete to their pre-injury function—a part of which means delivering the right treatment at the right time.

---

### BOX 24.1 A cautionary tale
### with **KIERAN O'SULLIVAN**

Before we launch into specific treatments and the evidence that underpins them, we need to share a cautionary tale. Treatment is typically not what a glitzy pharmaceutical video might suggest it is.

Several very important factors that are unrelated to the pathology of a condition can influence treatment outcomes. You will have seen patients who are positive in their outlook and others who seem to live in a world of gloom and doom. You probably suspect that this might affect the outcome of treatment, and evidence indicates that it most certainly does.

A patient's response to treatment is greatly influenced by cognitive (e.g. thoughts, self-efficacy, hypervigilance), psychological (e.g. depression, stress, anxiety, perceived injustice), social (e.g. work, family, financial, cultural, social support, life events) and lifestyle (e.g. poor sleep, sedentary behaviours, physical activity levels, diet, smoking) factors (Fig. 24.1). These systemic factors are widely acknowledged as being key in the onset and maintenance of pain[1–3] among non-sporting populations reporting pain or injury (e.g. chronic low back pain, hip and knee osteoarthritis). Sports and exercise medicine is just beginning to recognise and embrace this undeniably important concept.

Psychosocial, cognitive and lifestyle factors are related to:

- the onset of symptoms[4,5]
- treatment response[6,7]
- return to sport.[8,9]

While these systemic factors are often perceived as being difficult to modify, they are likely to be at least as modifiable as many physical factors (e.g. posture, muscle tightness), which are often the main targets for treatment but do not objectively change as the athlete recovers.[10,11] Successful clinical outcomes after treatments typically considered to be "physical", such as exercise, are often mediated by changes in cognitive and psychological factors.[12] Critically, there is evidence that these systemic factors are related to more traditional physical factors (e.g. fear affects movement patterns and thus can slow an athlete's return to sport).[13,14]

Rather than considering rehabilitation from injury as physical or psychological, rehabilitation is best approached combining these aspects in a manner

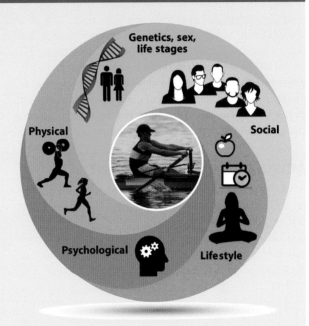

**Figure 24.1** A wide range of factors influence a patient's response to treatment

that matches the individual needs of each athlete. For example, exercise is a core component of injury rehabilitation. Since exercise can enhance a range of systemic factors (e.g. sleep, mood, catastrophising, fear, self-efficacy), there may be occasions when athletes benefit more from the health-enhancing systemic effects of exercise (e.g. it aids relaxation and sleep) than from local loading tissue effects (e.g. an athlete whose pain or injury is not explained by the typical tissue injury model).

In such situations, clearly communicating with the athlete (and their coach) regarding the mechanism of effect of exercise, and the context in which that exercise is completed, is critical. Furthermore, traditional rehabilitation can then evolve to incorporate additional treatment components (e.g. relaxation, cognitive behavioural therapy, sleep hygiene, dietary advice) to influence several of these wellness factors as required for the athlete.

This chapter provides essential background for the treatments detailed in *Clinical Sports Medicine 6e: Managing Injuries.* Evidence for treatment effectiveness is continually changing. However, remember that our profession remains as much an art as a science. Level 1 evidence is not always available and the decision whether to use a certain treatment is also influenced by your experience and professional training and the patient's expectations. Critically, you should have a solid understanding of the theoretic rationale for the treatments you provide, as well as up-to-date knowledge of the evidence of their effectiveness and potential side effects.

The effect of each treatment should be evaluated by objectively comparing symptoms and signs before and after the treatment, and at the next visit. Functional testing and patient-reported outcome measures (PROMs; see Chapter 23) should also be used regularly throughout to monitor and guide treatment. This enables you to choose the most appropriate mode of treatment for the specific injury and individual. In presentations that fail to improve, this also allows you to change modalities or pursue further investigations.

## ACUTE INJURY MANAGEMENT

Acute soft-tissue injury causes an immediate inflammatory response that manifests clinically as pain, redness, swelling and loss of function. Inflammation is an essential process that initiates tissue regeneration and repair. However, excessive bleeding and oedema can delay recovery and may cause secondary ischaemic damage to nearby tissues.[15] The goal of acute soft-tissue injury management is therefore to prevent excessive bleeding and oedema, reduce pain, promote faster return to function and reduce risk of re-injury.

The principles of acute soft-tissue injury management are based largely on expert opinion and laboratory studies (level 4–5 evidence), and there are few randomised controlled trials (RCTs) upon which to base recommendations.[16, 17] Traditionally, treatment of soft-tissue injuries is guided by one of the most commonly known acronyms in sports and exercise medicine: PRICE (Protection, Rest, Ice, Compression and Elevation).[18]

Various authors have proposed modifications of this classic acronym, such as POLICE (Protection, Optimal Loading, Ice, Compression and Elevation)[19] and PEACE & LOVE (Protection, Elevation, Avoid anti-inflammatory medication, Compression, Education & Load, Optimism, Vascularisation, Exercise),[20] the latter coined in consideration of the role of ice (cryotherapy) and routine use of anti-inflammatory medications in acute soft-tissue injury management. We consider the management of acute soft-tissue injury below using the POLICE acronym.

## Protection

A brief period of complete immobilisation is necessary for the initial protection of injured tissue and to help reduce pain-related movement of the injury site, reduce the size of the haematoma and thus minimise the size of the connective tissue scar.[21] During this period, you may consider the use of casts, splints, slings or rigid braces to protect the injured body part, as well as crutches for severe lower-limb injuries.

Although protection is important in the period immediately following trauma, prolonged immobilisation has a detrimental effect on healing in a range of musculoskeletal soft tissues, including ligament, tendon and muscle.[21-24] Immobilisation also affects surrounding structures, leading to skeletal muscle atrophy and loss of strength, as well as joint stiffness, osteopenia and potentially long-term degenerative changes in articular cartilage.

It is therefore important that soft tissues remain completely unloaded for as short a period as possible. This will vary depending on the extent and nature of the injury and the tissue involved. For most muscle injuries, 2 days is sufficient before the forming scar has adequate tensile strength to withstand gentle stress.[25] Severe ligament sprains (grades 2 and 3) may require up to 10 days of immobilisation before the patient can begin controlled loading.[26, 27]

A number of systematic reviews with meta-analyses have demonstrated the advantage of early functional treatment of soft-tissue injuries:

- Jones and Amendola included nine studies involving 920 participants to compare immobilisation with early functional treatment for acute ankle sprain.[28] They reported that functional treatment allows earlier return to sport and work, while there was no substantial difference concerning ankle instability and re-injury rate, although studies seem to favour early functional treatment.
- Kerkhoffs and colleagues included 22 studies involving 2157 participants to analyse immobilisation as a treatment for acute ankle sprain.[29] They found that functional treatment has better results considering time to return to pre-injury activities, swelling reduction, joint stiffness, and subjective and objective joint instability. They did not find any differences for recurrence or pain.
- Kemler and colleagues included nine studies involving 1250 patients to compare braces with other functional treatment types for acute ankle sprain.[30] They found no differences concerning time to return to pre-injury activities, time to reduce symptoms, re-injury and joint instability rates, but it seems that braces have better functional outcomes using the Foot and Ankle Outcome Score (FAOS) and the Karlsson scoring scale.

## Optimal loading

Optimal loading replaces rest from the classic PRICE acronym due to concerns that rest may encourage an overly conservative approach that fails to harness the benefits of early tissue loading through exercise.[19, 31, 32] In comparison with immobilisation, early loading promotes strength, morphology and function of regenerating tissue as well as maintaining the wider (non-injured) neuromusculoskeletal system.[19, 33] For example, early mobilisation of lateral ankle sprains improves subjective function and patient satisfaction, reduces swelling and accelerates return to activity, work and sports participation (level 1 evidence).[34, 35]

Basic science studies support early loading compared with immobilisation for a range of soft-tissue injuries.[21-24] For example, early mobilisation of skeletal muscle injuries improves capillarisation and muscle fibre regeneration, and leads to a more parallel orientation of the regenerating myofibres compared with immobilisation (Fig. 24.2[36]). Muscle injuries demonstrate persisting weakness when treated with prolonged immobilisation (Fig. 24.3).[21]

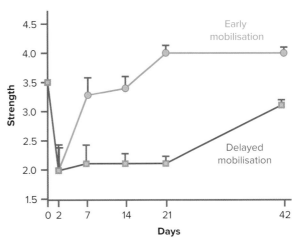

**Figure 24.3** Strength improvements in rat skeletal muscle injuries treated with a progressive exercise protocol after 2 days of immobilisation (shown in green) and in injuries treated with the same protocol after 21 days of immobilisation (shown in red). Note that strength did not naturally return during the immobilisation period.
Source: Adapted from Järvinen TA, Järvinen M, Kalimo H. Regeneration of injured skeletal muscle after the injury. *Muscles Ligaments Tendons J* 2014;3(4):337–45.

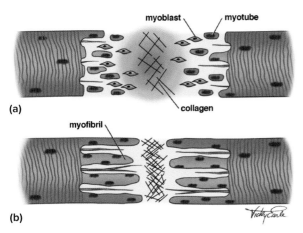

**(a)**

**(b)**

**Figure 24.2** Muscle injury treated with (a) immobilisation and (b) early mobilisation
Source: Adapted from Järvinen TA, Järvinen M, Kalimo H. Regeneration of injured skeletal muscle after the injury. *Muscles Ligaments Tendons J* 2014;3(4):337–45.

A major challenge facing clinicians is to determine the "optimal" soft-tissue loading for each individual at each phase of healing. This should be driven by the tissue type and pathological presentation, as well as the tissue adaptation required; for example, increased tensile strength, collagen reorganisation, increased muscle–tendon unit stiffness or neural reorganisation.[31]

You need to consider a range of variables when attempting to achieve optimal loading, such as the type, magnitude, duration, frequency, intensity and direction of load. Manipulation of these variables will not only affect local tissue healing processes, but also stimulate central nervous system adaptations, leading to improved motor learning and movement efficiency.

Variable loading offers several benefits:

- small variations in the magnitude, direction and rate of loading may shield injured tissues, at least somewhat, from overload
- it may provide a more potent stimulus to mechanotransduction because the mechanoreceptors can't just accommodate to a steady signal (accommodating to a monotonous signal is referred to as the receptors getting "deaf" to the signal)
- variable tensile, compressive and torsional forces may create a stronger biological scaffold.[31]

The characteristics of optimal and suboptimal loading are outlined in Table 24.1.

## Ice

Ice (or other forms of cryotherapy) is one of the most common treatment modalities used in the initial management of acute musculoskeletal injuries.[16] Cryotherapy aims to decrease oedema through vasoconstriction and reduce secondary hypoxic injury by lowering the metabolic demand of injured tissues.[16, 21] Local analgesia is thought to occur when the skin temperature drops below 15°C because of decreasing nerve conduction velocity.[37, 38]

**TABLE 24.1** Characteristics of optimal and suboptimal loading

| Optimal loading | Suboptimal loading |
| --- | --- |
| Directed to appropriate tissues | Non-specific generalised loading |
| Loading through functional ranges | Loading through limited ranges of movement |
| Appropriate blend of compressive, tensile and shear loading | Loading exclusively in a single manner |
| Variability in magnitude, direction, duration and intensity | Constant, unidirectional load |
| Include neural overload | Minimal neural stimulus |
| Tailored to individual characteristics | Generic, non-individualised |
| Functional | Non-functional, isolated segmental loading |

Source: Glasgow P, Phillips N, Bleakley C. Optimal loading: key variables and mechanisms. *Br J Sports Med* 2015;49(5):278–9. Reproduced with permission.

Laboratory studies show that cooling injured tissue to between 5°C and 15°C reduces cellular metabolism, white blood cell activity, necrosis and apoptosis.[15, 39] However, this amount of cooling is difficult to achieve in practice, with human studies showing that intensive cooling leads to tissue temperatures of between 21°C and 25°C. The actual metabolic effects of cryotherapy may therefore be questionable, particularly for deep injuries or for patients with higher levels of adipose tissue.[39]

Nevertheless, the analgesic effects of cryotherapy are well established and icing remains a part of most current acute injury management guidelines.[40] Ice is typically applied for 20 minutes every 2–4 hours for the first 48–72 hours following injury. Intermittent application—for example, 10 minutes on, 10 minutes off—may enhance analgesia and reduce the risk of adverse reactions such as skin burns and nerve damage.[37, 40]

Ice should not be applied where local tissue circulation is impaired (e.g. in Raynaud's phenomenon or peripheral vascular disease), or to patients who suffer from a cold allergy. As ice can impair muscle strength and proprioception, it should be used cautiously during competition.[41]

Although there are many commercial cryotherapy products available, in most situations a plastic or cloth bag containing crushed ice and water remains the modality of choice.[42] A wet towel should be placed between the ice pack and the skin. Cryotherapy modalities are summarised in Table 24.2.

Despite the longstanding popularity of applying ice in sports injury management, the evidence for its use in humans is limited. Guillot and colleagues were able to show a positive impact of ice application on inflammatory cytokines in osteoarthritis.[43, 44] However, others argue that traditional cold therapy in the early phases of soft-tissue injury has limited value[45] or should be discontinued in the management of soft-tissue injuries.[20] In a classic systematic review of 22 studies and almost 1500 participants,[16] there was marginal evidence that cryotherapy was effective for

ankle sprains when it was added to exercises during the early stages of injury. From those studies, the authors could not extract a common message about how long cryotherapy should be applied or which method of delivery was best.

Consequently, the acronym PEACE & LOVE has emerged.[20] While ice application (cryotherapy) for acute injury management is still frequently used pitchside for sporting contact and non-contact injuries, it has more recently been transferred to form part of a periodised recovery approach to facilitate performance.[46]

## Compression

Compression is often used following acute soft-tissue injury to increase pressure gradients in the venous and lymphatic systems, thereby counteracting oedema. Combining compression with ice may also help reduce tissue temperatures (Fig. 24.4).[47] Although a number of specific products are commercially available, such as cold compression wraps and devices, a standard elastic bandage is a cheap, versatile and effective solution. Compression can be

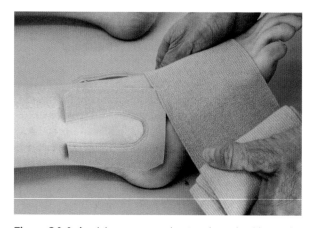

**Figure 24.4** Applying compression to a lateral ankle sprain: horseshoe-shaped foam around the ankle malleolus may help distribute compression pressures more evenly

**TABLE 24.2**　Cryotherapy modalities used to treat sports injuries

| Modality | Description | Special concerns | Surface temperature | Duration | Exercise during application | Expense |
|---|---|---|---|---|---|---|
| Crushed ice bags | Crushed ice moulds easily to body parts | Apply a towel between the bag and skin to avoid ice burn, nerve damage or frostbite | 0°C (32°F) | 10–20 min | No | Inexpensive |
| Reusable cold packs | Durable plastic packs containing silica gel that are available in many sizes and shapes | Apply a towel between the bag and skin to avoid nerve damage or frostbite | ≤15°C (59°F) | 20–30 min | No | Inexpensive |
| Endothermal cold packs | Packets are squeezed or crushed to activate; convenient for emergency use | Single use only | 20°C (68°F) | 15–20 min | No | Expensive |
| Vapocoolant sprays | Easily portable therapy for regional myofascial pain syndrome, acute injuries, pain relief, and in rehabilitation with spray and stretch techniques | Intermittently spray the area for <6 sec to avoid frostbite | Varies depending on duration of treatment | Multiple brief sprays | Spray <6 sec and stretch to increase range of motion | Expensive |
| Ice water immersion | An athlete's body part is submerged in cold water | Carries the most risk of hypersensitivity reactions; restrict amount of extremity immersion | 0°C (32°F) | 5–10 min | Allows motion of the extremity during treatment | Inexpensive |
| Ice massage | Used to produce analgesia: freeze water in a foam cup, then peel back cup to expose the ice; massage area as often as needed | Apply for short intervals to avoid frostbite; avoid excess pressure | 0°C (32°F) | 5–10 min | Can allow supervised, gentle, stretching during analgesia | Inexpensive |
| Refrigerant inflatable bladders | When cold and compression are needed | Avoid excess compression | 10–25°C (50–77°F) | Depends on temperature | No | Expensive |
| Thermal cooling blankets | To provide constant temperature, such as after surgery | Scrutinise temperature settings | 10–25°C (50–77°F) | Depends on temperature | No | Expensive |
| Contrast baths | Transition treatment between cold and heat for a subacute injury, sympathetic mediated pain, stiff joints | Do not use in acute setting due to potential to increase blood flow | Hot bath 40.5°C (105°F) Cold bath 15.5°C (60°F) | 4 min hot, 1 min cold | Allows motion of the extremity during treatment | Inexpensive |

C

focused on certain tissues by applying ice packs underneath the elastic bandage. Similarly, pressure peaks around bony prominences can be avoided by applying foam or other material to fill gaps.

The external mechanical pressure is thought to increase the hydrostatic pressure of the interstitial fluid, thereby forcing fluid from the injury site towards the capillaries, lymph vessels or tissue spaces away from the traumatised area. Smaller external forces may achieve this effect; many standard protocols recommend pressures between 15 and 35 mmHg. Despite a lack of consensus on the optimal compression pressure, there is some evidence that high pressures (>80 mmHg) are ineffective.[48]

Bandaging should start just distal to the injury site, with each layer of bandage overlapping the underlying layer by one-half. It should extend to at least a hand's breadth proximal to the injury margin.

### Elevation

The rationale for elevation in the treatment of soft-tissue injuries stems from the fundamental principles of physiology and traumatology. Elevation of an injured extremity above the level of the heart decreases hydrostatic pressure and subsequently reduces the accumulation of interstitial fluid.[25] Elevation can be achieved by using a sling for upper-limb injuries and by resting lower limbs on a chair. It is important to ensure that the lower limb is above the level of the pelvis. A graduated return to standing after elevation is likely to minimise rebound swelling and discomfort.[40]

### Do no HARM

In the 72 hours following injury, HARMful factors should be avoided:

- H: Heat and heat rubs—heat may increase bleeding at the injured site. Avoid hot baths, showers, saunas, heat packs and heat rubs.
- A: Alcohol—moderate consumption of alcohol after eccentric-based leg exercises significantly increases the loss of dynamic and static quadricep strength.[49] Alcohol may mask pain and the severity of injury and therefore increase the risk of re-injury.[50] To minimise exercise-related loss in muscle function and to accelerate recovery, avoid alcohol post-injury.
- R: Running/moderate activity—running or any form of moderate activity can cause further damage at the injury site.
- M: Massage/vigorous soft-tissue therapy—vigorous massage should be avoided especially in the first 24–48 hours. It could cause further bleeding and swelling.

## THERAPEUTIC EXERCISE

The substantial health benefits of regular physical activity are undisputed.[51, 52]

WHO physical activity recommendations

In this chapter, we focus on how the exercises that clinicians prescribe (treatment) promote tissue healing and pain relief (e.g. how hamstring exercises promote hamstring healing and function). In each edition of *Clinical Sports Medicine* we have reported more and more evidence that exercise has no peer in treating sports injuries: now RCTs, systematic reviews and meta-analyses, as well as network meta-analyses and more, tell clinicians, "Prescribe exercise— you won't regret it!"

Below we review the two primary benefits of therapeutic exercise:

1. stimulating tissue repair and remodelling, including how mechanotherapy relates to different tissues in the musculoskeletal system
2. exercise-induced hypoalgesia (pain relief).

### Turning exercise into repair and remodelling: mechanotherapy

We imagine that every reader has exercised to improve their musculoskeletal function. Most clinicians will have personal and/or professional experience of performing or prescribing exercises for treatment and recovery from musculoskeletal injury, for instance: wrist exercises to regain movement and strength after fracture immobilisation; shoulder exercises to facilitate function and repair following a rotator cuff strain; or knee injury rehabilitation to return to sport and mitigate the risk of future osteoarthritis. You and your patients will have benefitted from mechanotherapy— perhaps unknowingly.

#### What is mechanotherapy?

Mechanotherapy relates to a term you may have come across in some physiology/biomechanics courses— mechanotransduction. Mechanotransduction is the physiological process whereby mechanical stress caused by exercise or physical activity applies forces to tissue and is converted into biochemical signals that drive the cells, and thus tissue, to change (adapt/heal). Mechanotransduction is critical all over the body—it is essential for hearing, balance, touch and even dilation of blood vessels.

An overview of mechanobiology

Box 24.2 summarises the process by which mechanotransduction converts mechanical stress into biochemical signals in cells.

A range of studies have shown (or implied) a potential for mechanotherapy to promote healing of muscle, tendon, ligament, cartilage, intervertebral disc and bone.[54] The key to successful clinical application of mechanotherapy is to find the correct dosage (and thus progression of exercises).

In some cases, such as patellar and Achilles tendinopathy, literature exists to guide exercise prescription. "Research-proven" treatment regimens, such as tendon training protocols (Chapters 24 and 29 in *Managing Injuries*) have considerable clinical popularity and are often applied to a variety of other injury types. However, we warn against taking a one-size-fits-all approach. You should follow general training principles of progressive overload, periodisation and specificity (Chapter 14) and individualise exercise prescription according to each patient's functional capacity, sport-specific demands and treatment response.

In the following sections, we review some of the evidence for the mechanisms of how mechanotherapy works for muscle, tendon, articular cartilage and bone.

### Muscle

Muscle offers one of the best opportunities to exploit and study the effects of mechanotherapy, as muscle is highly responsive to changes in loading. Increasing load on muscle leads to the immediate, local upregulation of mechano growth factor, which in turn stimulates muscle hypertrophy via activation of satellite cells.[55] Satellite cells bring genetic material and cellular machinery to the tissue that is adapting to the exercise load. In the early 2020s William Roman and colleagues proved that muscle also had intracellular repair mechanisms that didn't rely on satellite cells.[56]

If athletes have a fracture or undergo surgery that results in them needing to rest a body part (immobilisation or greatly reduced muscle load) for some weeks, mechanotransduction causes catabolism of tissue—the tissue rapidly adapts to the reduced load and removes physiologically unnecessary extracellular matrix (in this case, muscle tissue). Loading improves the alignment of regenerating myotubes (multi-nucleated muscle cells), promotes faster and more complete regeneration, and limits atrophy of surrounding myotubes.[57]

### Tendon

Tendon is a dynamic, mechanoresponsive tissue. Increased load upregulates insulin-like growth factor I (IGF-I) which is associated with cellular proliferation and matrix remodelling within the tendon.[58] However, in addition to IGF-I other growth factors and cytokines are also likely to play a role.[59]

Human tendons subjected to mechanical loading programs increase in stiffness and cross-sectional area. However, the extent of tissue adaptation depends on the applied loading parameters. High-intensity muscle contractions (70–90% of maximum) are necessary to increase tendon stiffness,[60] and interventions longer than 12 weeks are necessary to achieve optimal adaptations.[61, 62] The mechanical, material and morphological properties of tendons respond similarly to high-intensity loading programs involving eccentric, concentric–eccentric and isometric muscle contractions. However, plyometric training may not lead to optimal adaptations.[63]

### Articular cartilage

Like other musculoskeletal tissues, articular cartilage is populated by mechanosensitive cells (chondrocytes), which signal load and cause cell changes. Immobilisation leads to cartilage atrophy and loss of stiffness, whereas cartilage subjected to high loads has a higher proteoglycan content and higher cell volume, and is stiffer.[64]

Advances in magnetic resonance imaging (MRI), in particular the ability to estimate cartilage glycosaminoglycan content, have improved our understanding of loading on human articular cartilage. In one study a 16-week moderate loading program increased the glycosaminoglycan content of articular cartilage among patients at high risk of developing tibiofemoral osteoarthritis.[65] However, vigorous loading programs have provided mixed results: some led to improved cartilage quality among people with and without osteoarthritic changes, whereas others were detrimental in people with pre-existing bone marrow lesions.[65]

### Bone

Mechanotransduction is very well described in human bone. Appropriate loading of osteocytes, the primary mechanosensors, activates a number of extracellular and intracellular signalling pathways which stimulate osteoblasts to proliferate and form new bone.[66] However, both insufficient (deloading) and excessive loading of bone stimulate osteoclast activity, which leads to a loss of bone tissue.

## BOX 24.2 Mechanotherapy: how cells respond to exercise loading

When you prescribe exercise to a patient, the exercise applies load to tissue and thus cells (Fig. 24.5). If a patient has pathology in the midportion of the Achilles tendon, consider how exercise (i.e. loading) promotes tendon repair. (The illustrations simplify very complex multi-step biological processes.)

Figure 24.5a depicts the patient performing a heel-drop. Figure 24.5b illustrates the abnormal tendon collagen fibrils (pale camel colour, not the characteristic golden reflectivity of healthy tendon fibrils under polarised light).

Figures 24.5c and d depict the network of tenocytes (specialised fibroblasts that maintain tendon) and one cell highlighting the integrin switches that contribute to the exercise load (message) being converted to a

biochemical signal. This signal activates the nucleus to move into a synthesis phase (gene expression).

Figure 25.4e shows new procollagen synthesis by ribosomes attached to the rough endoplasmic reticulum. Procollagen, the building block of collagen fibrils, is extruded from the tenocyte (right side of Fig. 25.4e) so that it can embed in the repairing collagen fibril (Fig. 24.5f). In Figure 24.5f, repaired collagen fibrils are depicted as more golden (more normal).

Contrast Figure 24.5f (repaired) with Figure 24.5b (symptomatic, pathological). Note that tissue does not need to return to pristine condition to be pain-free and to function well. Think of an element of scar tissue as being a normal part of the repair process (some camel-coloured fibrils in Fig. 24.5f).

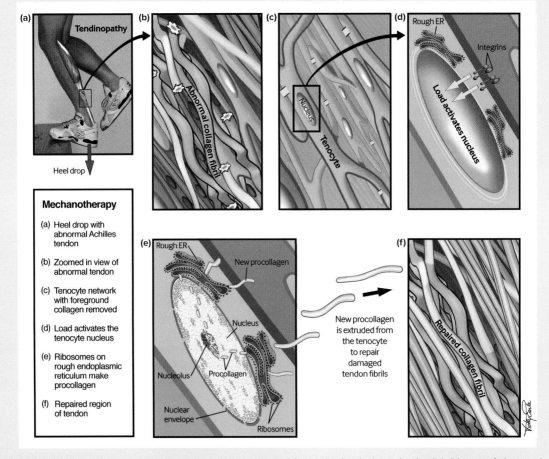

**Mechanotherapy**

(a) Heel drop with abnormal Achilles tendon

(b) Zoomed in view of abnormal tendon

(c) Tenocyte network with foreground collagen removed

(d) Load activates the tenocyte nucleus

(e) Ribosomes on rough endoplasmic reticulum make procollagen

(f) Repaired region of tendon

**Figure 24.5** Mechanotherapy—key tissue and cellular anatomy: (a) exercise loads tissue (and cells), (b) area of abnormal collagen fibrils with tenocytes (green) in the background, (c) foreground fibrils removed to show the complex tenocyte network connected by gap junctions (light-green bridges between tenocytes) and a box around one nucleus, (d) one cell focus—load activates the cell nucleus (gene expression), (e) the activated nucleus produces mRNA (not shown) for procollagen synthesis by ribosomes on the rough endoplasmic reticulum (ER) and (f) the extruded new procollagen fibrils contribute to tissue repair/ remodelling.

Mechanotransduction can be exploited to improve fracture healing, through active load bearing (e.g. partial weight-bearing mobilisation), pneumatic compression or electrophysical agents.[67] There are no definitive guidelines on the amount of loading required to optimise bone formation, particularly as many factors influence each case, such as the loading type, the site and size of the fracture, and the patient's age and hormonal status. However, dynamically applied loads are more effective than static loads in stimulating bone remodelling.

### PRACTICE PEARL

Therapeutic exercises are the heart of high-value care of musculoskeletal conditions.

## Exercise-induced hypoalgesia

Several different forms of exercise, including aerobic exercise, isometric muscle contractions and traditional resistance training, have been suggested as a means of reducing musculoskeletal pain, a phenomenon known as exercise-induced hypoalgesia. Isometric exercises are widely used for conditions such as tendinopathies to reduce pain.

The evidence to support these exercise interventions is mixed. Three different types of patients have been studied: "normal patients" (i.e. those without pain), patients with a specific musculoskeletal pathology (e.g. tendinopathy) and those with more generalised musculoskeletal pain (e.g. fibromyalgia).

There is a large body of evidence demonstrating that in healthy adults, exercise attenuates experimentally induced pain.[68] This is achieved by elevating pain thresholds and pain tolerance, as well as by reducing pain intensities during and after exercise.[69, 70]

Exercise-induced hypoalgesia is likely to be caused by a combination of factors, including the release of endogenous opioids and non-opioid substances affecting pain perception such as endocannabinoids, serotonin and norepinephrine (noradrenaline),[71] as well as activation of spinal or supraspinal mechanisms of pain inhibition.[72] Different exercise parameters may alter the predominant mechanism.[69, 71-74]

A 2016 study of athletes with patellar tendinopathy found that five 45-second isometric contractions at 70% of maximal voluntary contraction with 2 minutes of rest between contractions significantly reduced pain for at least 45 minutes after exercise.[75] Based on these findings, isometric training became part of the early management of tendinopathy.

More recently a number of systematic reviews have failed to show a positive effect of isometric exercise on pain reduction in those with local musculoskeletal pain,[76] tendinopathies,[77] patellar tendinopathy,[78] plantar fasciopathy[79] and knee osteoarthritis.[80] In contrast, two systematic reviews have confirmed a positive effect of aerobic exercise on pain reduction in patients with musculoskeletal pain.[81, 82] Resistance exercise was also beneficial in this group.[81] Further high-quality research is needed to determine the precise role of exercise in pain management in acute and chronic musculoskeletal injuries and conditions.

We now consider two examples of therapeutic exercise you are likely to encounter in practice.

## Altering biomechanics: motor-control training
### with PAUL BLAZEY

Exercise prescription is used to stimulate repair and remodelling of injured tissues (through mechanotherapy), but clinicians also prescribe therapeutic exercise to influence the way a patient moves their body. We often refer to this as "neuromuscular" or "motor-control" training.

Clinicians usually prescribe motor-control training in an attempt to:

- *directly or indirectly unload injured or sensitised tissue to reduce pain and/or symptoms.* For example, overhead athletes with rotator cuff tendinopathy may be prescribed scapular retraction and upward rotation exercises to reduce posterior impingement of their cuff tendons during throwing. Patients with patellofemoral pain may be encouraged to adopt a forefoot strike during running. This reduces stress on the front of the knee by transferring more of the joint forces to the lower leg (Achilles–calf complex).
- *reduce the risk of injury or re-injury by improving strength, balance, coordination and/or sensorimotor control.* For example, neuromuscular warm-up exercises are included in many injury prevention programs (e.g. the FIFA 11+ program). Patients recovering from anterior cruciate ligament (ACL) injury are also prescribed a wide range of neuromuscular exercises throughout the entire rehabilitation process.

Prescription of motor-control exercises is based on a belief that an ideal movement pattern (or range of patterns) exists. For example, motor-control training to reduce dynamic knee valgus in the frontal plane can reduce pain and improve function for people suffering from patellofemoral pain.[83] However, the results of programs

C

that focus solely on motor control for knee osteoarthritis and people recovering after ACL injury are inconclusive.[83] There is scepticism and in some instances outright rejection of the need to improve motor-control of scapular mechanics, lumbar flexion when performing a lift, or foot and ankle pronation during running.[84-86]

Motor control exercises should always be part of a multi-component rehabilitation program. Where the evidence for a relationship between motor-control exercises and less pain or better function is inconclusive, you and your patient may still agree to trial a motor-control program because the exercise prescription may also improve the athlete's strength or power, and promote tissue remodelling and repair. Trying to improve an athlete's movement pattern and their resiliency to move the way they currently do (through strength and conditioning) may offer mutually exclusive benefits for a patient dealing with an overuse injury related to load (e.g. tendon-related pain).

The absence of evidence to support changing many common movement patterns means that there are often no definitive guidelines for the dosage of motor-control training. However, neuromuscular "perturbation" programs performed 3 times per week for 3–4 weeks have been shown to alter motor-control patterns in uninjured[87] and ACL-injured athletes,[88] and to improve ACL rehabilitation outcomes.[89]

Similarly, training programs aiming to improve neuromuscular control during standing, cutting, jumping and landing have been shown to prevent knee injuries in female handball and football players when performed for 15 minutes, 3 times per week (Chapter 17).[90] As for all types of skill acquisition, regular high-quality practice is necessary to learn and engrain new motor patterns (through neural plasticity).

Motor-control training programs should target specific deficits identified during the clinical assessment. Complex movements should be broken down into separate components before the whole task is re-trained. As pain (or the distraction caused by pain) may interfere with the normal neuroplastic changes that occur with skill training,[91] motor-control training should be performed once the athlete is pain-free.

You have the option to use internal or external cues to help athletes to alter their motor-control or movement patterns. Both have utility but internal cues may work better in novices or those struggling to adopt new or altered movements.

Examples of external cues include using audiovisual aids or instructing a patient to "push through the floor" or "hit a mark on the wall"; internal cues include instructing an athlete to adopt a "mid-foot" landing pattern or advising them to "keep their chest up". Regardless of the form

of cueing, feedback should be provided on the athlete's performance so that it can be corrected ideally in real time or at least immediately following the exercise (e.g. using video analysis).

Understanding the relationship between sport-specific biomechanics and injury (Chapter 13) will help identify movements that may form part of a motor-control retraining program for athletes in different contexts and for rehabilitating specific conditions.

### PRACTICE PEARL

Effective motor-control training programs focus on movement quality and are sport-specific. Athletes should be supported to understand what they are trying to achieve and why it is important.

## Blood flow restriction
### with FARAZ DAMJI

Blood flow restriction is another popular form of therapeutic exercise intervention. Blood flow restriction training is a form of rehabilitation that combines lower load exercise with controlled vascular occlusion (Fig. 24.6). A pneumatic cuff is applied to the proximal upper/lower limb to reduce arterial inflow and completely occlude venous outflow during exercise. With respect to comparable non-occluded exercise, blood flow restriction exercise generates an environment with relatively greater anaerobic demands that sets the stage for recruitment of a greater number of motor units, type II fast-twitch muscle fibres, and muscle groups proximal to the level of occlusion.[92]

As a result, blood flow restriction promotes the development of skeletal muscle mass and function (hypertrophy and strength gains) via a synergistic response to metabolic stress and mechanical tension.[93] Mechanistically, important changes include increased release of anabolic hormones (growth hormone, insulin-like growth factor), down regulation of myostatin, activation of myogenic stem cells (satellite cells), muscle cell swelling causing an anabolic reaction, and enhanced cell signalling pathways (mTORC1) (Fig. 24.7).[94]

Beyond increases in skeletal muscle cross-sectional area and strength, there is growing evidence that blood flow restriction improves muscular endurance and cardiovascular fitness, reduces bone loss and attenuates pain.[95, 96] However, it does not replace high-load resistance training, the most successful means of stimulating increases in muscle strength and hypertrophy.

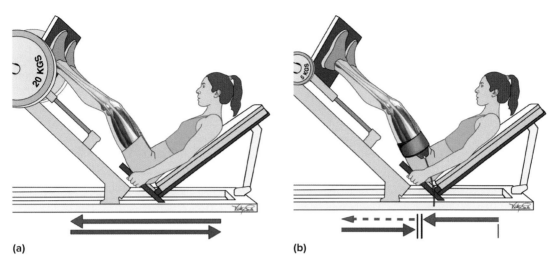

(a)          (b)

**Figure 24.6** Comparing the effect of the same exercise without (a) and with (b) a cuff to restrict blood flow. Note that the 5-kg weight being pushed in the right image (b) is much lighter to reflect real-life rehabilitation settings that use lighter weights, such as after ACL surgery. The solid blue and red lines indicate full flow in veins and arteries. In (b), venous blood is prevented from returning to the right side of the heart.

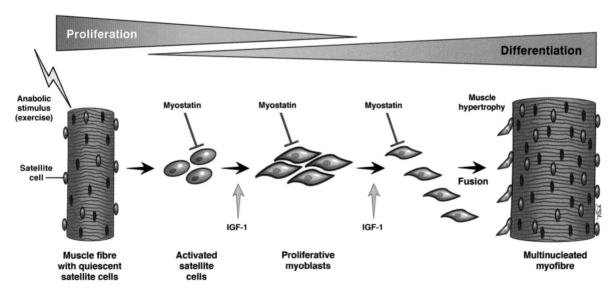

**Figure 24.7** When blood flow is restricted during exercise (a known anabolic stimulus for skeletal muscles) at a relatively low load, it produces additional metabolic stress mimicking the response to training with higher resistance. An anabolic cascade ensues, resulting in myogenesis.

## What it is used for

Blood flow restriction is designed for people who could benefit from resistance training but cannot tolerate high loads. It is most commonly used with athletes rehabilitating after injury who are advised to avoid high-load resistance training. It may also be used in postoperative patients to attenuate muscle atrophy and loss of strength during an extended period of immobility.

## Clinical tips: how to do it right

The most common and well-studied form of blood flow restriction is with resistance exercise.[97] For the best results, patients should use 20–40% of their one repetition maximum for the specified exercise, with 15–30 repetitions per set and 30–60-second rest intervals. Cuff pressure should be set between 40% and 80% of limb occlusion pressure; continuous rather than intermittent pressure will maximise the stress for adaptation. The exact cuff pressure depends on the cuff width and material, limb size and underlying soft tissue.

A tourniquet device is recommended such that the amount of blood flow occlusion can be closely calibrated and monitored. Two to three sessions per week are generally sufficient, but accelerated regimens of training 1–2 times daily (if resources allow) may be reasonable in the early rehabilitation phase following an injury or surgical intervention.

Blood flow restriction can similarly be applied with aerobic exercise like walking or cycling, with limited evidence of improved aerobic capacity including $VO_2$.[98] The study of blood flow restriction with passive application (i.e. in the absence of exercise) is more limited, yet represents a potential solution for the prevention of muscle atrophy in hospitalised individuals.

## Safety considerations

Paraesthesia, bruising, pain, discomfort, delayed-onset muscle soreness, fainting and dizziness are side effects that may be experienced during routine use. Rhabdomyolysis is a rare serious adverse effect that has been reported from inappropriate blood flow restriction training.[99] Early studies cited an increased risk of thromboembolic events but the risk appears to be low.[100] Potential contraindications to consider are vascular disease, obesity, diabetes, sickle cell trait/disease, malignancy, severe hypertension and a history of deep vein thrombosis.[101]

# MANUAL TREATMENTS
## with BENHAM LIAGHAT

In this section, we refer to "hands-on" treatment, including techniques targeting joints (mobilisation and manipulation), soft tissues (massage/myofascial release techniques) and nerves (neurodynamic techniques). There is a substantial body of evidence demonstrating the immediate effects of manual treatments, such as altered pain sensation, muscle activation and joint range of motion.[102-107] However, these effects are unlikely to be maintained over an extended time period, or to change the natural history of a disorder. Therefore, you should regard manual treatments as an adjunct to addressing the underlying causes of injury.

Rather than adhering strictly to the conventional concept of hands-on treatment as a passive therapeutic approach, a more nuanced approach focuses on empowering the athlete to actively engage and mobilise the injured area. This approach transforms the treatment into a patient-activating strategy towards achieving functional goals.

Manual treatments are typically directed at specific tissues or structures identified as being abnormal on physical examination, such as stiff joints, tight muscles or restricted nerves (Chapter 15). Traditionally, the rationale for using manual treatments is their proposed local biomechanical and physiological effects; for example, to reduce joint stiffness, increase intramuscular temperature and circulation, or break up adhesions in nerves or connective tissue. However, the following factors suggest that local tissue changes are unlikely to explain the clinical benefits of manual treatments:

- spinal manipulations are only associated with transient increase in joint mobility; there is no evidence of lasting changes in mobility[108] or joint position[109]
- there is conflicting evidence[110, 111] that massage affects passive or active muscle stiffness, and the effect on global range of motion and skeletal muscle blood flow is marginal[112]
- clinical methods for assessing joint position, joint translation and soft-tissue qualities have poor reliability;[113-116] different clinicians are therefore unlikely to agree on which structures require treatment.

The effect of manual treatments may be distant from the area treated. For example, treatment of the thoracic and cervical spine may affect lateral elbow pain (Chapter 25).[117, 118]

The actual mechanism of manual treatments is thought to be a complex neurophysiological response from the peripheral and central nervous systems, initiated by a local biomechanical stimulus.[113] Mechanical stimulation of afferent neurons located in skin, joints and skeletal muscle can activate a number of responses, such as pain inhibition[102, 119-121] and neuromuscular inhibition or facilitation.[118, 122-124]

Manual treatments also have autonomic,[125-127] endocrine,[128, 129] immunological[130] and psychological effects,[131] which may further explain their potential clinical efficacy. Based on current understanding of the potential mechanisms of manual treatments, we propose that you offer sensible and evidence-based explanations about the rationale for using manual treatments in sports (Box 24.3).

## Joint techniques: mobilisation and manipulation

There are a number of different philosophical approaches to manual treatment of joints, such as Cyriax, Kaltenborn, Maitland, McKenzie and Mulligan.[132-134] Each differs in its approach to patient assessment and in its justification for treatment selection. The Cyriax and Kaltenborn approaches, for example, base their examination and treatment selection on arthrokinematic and biomechanical theories such as capsular patterns, coupled motions and concave–convex rules. In contrast, the Maitland, McKenzie and Mulligan approaches place more emphasis on patient response during assessment and treatment (symptom provocation and resolution) rather than rigid biomechanical theories.[136] Irrespective of the clinical reasoning paradigm, though, the most common manual techniques applied to joints are mobilisation and manipulation.

Mobilisation involves rhythmic, low-velocity, oscillatory movement techniques applied to spinal or peripheral joints. They are usually passive techniques performed within the patient's tolerance and may involve physiological joint motion (movements that patients could perform themselves) and/or accessory motions (movements that patients cannot actively control, such as distraction, compression, sliding, spinning and rolling).

The aim of mobilisation is often to restore full, pain-free range of motion to a joint found to be stiff or painful on clinical examination. Treatment parameters such as the location, direction and magnitude of applied force, and the duration of loading, will vary based on patient presentation, clinical examination findings and response to treatment. Although mobilisation is a continuum, and an art of clinical practice, it can be helpful for the learner to think of the continuum as having grades which overlap with each other. Australian professor Geoffrey Maitland outlined four grades:[134]

- I: Small amplitude movement at the beginning of range
- II: Large amplitude movement within the free range but not moving into any resistance or stiffness
- III: Large amplitude movement up to the limit of range
- IV: Small amplitude movement at the limit of range.

In most cases, you will use the first two grades to reduce pain and irritability (e.g. cervical spine mobilisation in cervicogenic headache). Grades III and IV are used to stretch the joint capsule and passive tissues to increase range of motion (e.g. as part of the progression to full range of movement after a joint has been immobilised).

Amplitude is not the only dimension of a mobilisation of course. A mobilisation has direction, rhythm and duration. As a clinician, you will decide whether you are using pain or range of motion as your outcome of choice and your guide to if and when to progress the extent of mobilisation that you will use. Physiopedia provides valuable links on this topic.[135]

Mobilisation may be combined with active movements (Fig. 24.8), and in some cases patients may be able to perform mobilisation themselves (Fig. 24.9).

Joint manipulation involves high-velocity thrust techniques exerted at the end of joint range, using either a long or a short lever arm. Long-lever techniques move many joints simultaneously, such as rotatory manipulations of the cervical spine. Short-lever techniques involve a low-amplitude thrust aimed at a specific joint or spinal segment. This is achieved through careful positioning of the patient, using arthrokinematic principles to isolate movement in the target joint and "lock" surrounding joints.

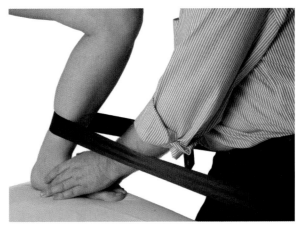

**Figure 24.8** Mobilisation with movement technique for ankle dorsiflexion

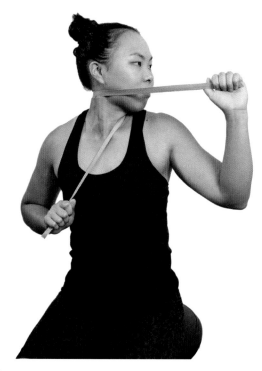

**Figure 24.9** Self-mobilisation of cervical rotation

"clinically relevant" site is superior to manipulation applied at a supposedly "not clinically relevant" site for individuals with spinal pain.[137] This lack of support warrants further research to determine the underlying mechanisms.

Manipulation is usually associated with an audible "pop" sound, which is thought to be caused by an event called cavitation (Fig. 24.10). This refers to the formation of bubbles (or cavities) within synovial fluid due to reductions in hydrostatic joint pressure. Cavitation is traditionally viewed as the sign of a successful manipulation.[138] However, there is no association between an audible pop and the clinical outcomes of spinal manipulation techniques.[139-142]

### Safety of manipulation techniques

Manipulation has been associated with a variety of adverse effects, ranging from minor short-term reactions such as headache, stiffness and local discomfort, to rare severe catastrophic events including stroke and death. Minor reactions can be surprisingly common, with one study finding that more than 60% of patients experienced a mild adverse reaction in the 24 hours after receiving spinal manipulation.[143] While the vast majority of side effects are benign self-limiting problems, you should inform your patients of their likelihood prior to treatment.

Fortunately, severe injuries caused by spinal manipulation are extremely rare. While the actual risk is unknown, estimates range from 1 in 50,000 manipulations to 1 in 5 million.[143] The majority of catastrophic injuries caused by cervical spine manipulation are due to the

Manipulation differs from mobilisation due to the velocity of the technique; patients can theoretically prevent the movement during mobilisation but with manipulation they cannot. Recent evidence on spinal manipulation does not support the idea that manipulation applied at a supposedly

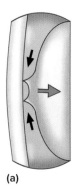
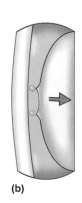
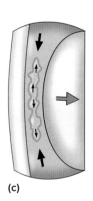
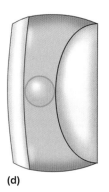
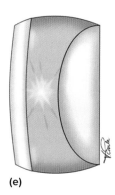

(a)  (b)  (c)  (d)  (e)

**Figure 24.10** The principle of cavitation explains the audible popping sound made during joint manipulation. (a) During separation of the joint surfaces, the outer regions of the circular contact zone become pointed. This deformation occurs because at high speeds, the central region of the contact zone separates before the outer region moves, creating a circular rim. (b) Joint surfaces snap back at the circular rim where the cavity initially forms, forming small bubbles. (c) Small bubbles collect to form a single large bubble. (d) The newly formed spherical bubble reaches its maximum size. (e) Because of its instability, the single bubble pops to form a "cloud" of many smaller bubbles (demonstrable by radiography as a radiolucent region), which later shrink as the gas and vapour dissolve.
Source: Adapted from Evans DW. Mechanisms and effects of spinal high-velocity, low-amplitude thrust manipulation: previous theories. *J Manipulative Physiol Ther* 2002;25(4):251–62.

proximity of the vertebral artery to the lateral vertebral joints. However, thoracic and lumbar spine manipulation may also cause serious injury, such as rib fractures and cauda equina syndrome.[144-147]

Manipulation should be performed only by practitioners with formal training in manipulative skills. Cervical artery function should be tested prior to manipulation of the cervical spine (Chapter 23), and short-lever techniques should be used in preference to long-lever techniques.

You should be aware of the contraindications to the use of mobilisation and manipulation techniques (Table 24.3).[136]

**TABLE 24.3** Absolute and relative contraindications for mobilisation and manipulation techniques

| Absolute contraindications of mobilisation—high risk of a deleterious consequence | | |
|---|---|---|
| | **Mobilisation** | **Manipulation** |
| Malignancy or tumour in the targeted region | × | × |
| Cauda equina lesion producing bladder or bowel disturbance | × | × |
| Fractures | × | × |
| Local bony infection (e.g. osteomyelitis, tuberculosis) | × | × |
| Systemic disturbance | × | × |
| Rheumatoid collagen necrosis | × | × |
| Unstable upper cervical spine | × | × |
| Signs of coronary or vertebral artery dysfunction | × | × |
| Practitioner lack of ability | — | × |
| Spondylolisthesis (symptomatic) | — | × |
| Gross foraminal encroachment | — | × |
| Joint fusions | — | × |
| Psychogenic disorders | — | × |
| Relative contraindications of mobilisation—possibility of deleterious consequences | | |
| | **Mobilisation** | **Manipulation** |
| Active inflammatory conditions | × | × |
| Significant segmental stiffness | × | × |
| Systemic diseases | × | × |
| Neurological deterioration | × | × |
| Irritability | × | × |
| Osteoporosis | × | × |
| Condition worsening with present treatment | × | × |
| Acute radiculopathy | × | × |
| History and examination do not add up | × | × |
| Use of oral contraceptives (cervical spine) | × | × |
| Long-term corticosteroid use (cervical spine) | × | × |
| Blood clotting disorder | × | × |
| Patient does not consent | × | × |
| Immediately postpartum | — | × |
| Children/adolescents with open epiphyseal plates | — | × |
| Pregnancy (last trimester) | — | × |

x, contraindicated; –, no contraindication

## Neural mobilisation techniques

### with ANNINA SCHMID

Changes of the normal mechanics, neurophysiology and homeostasis of the nervous system may contribute to pain. The term "neurodynamics" is used to describe the biomechanical, physiological and structural dysfunction of the nervous system.[148] Assessment[149] of neural mechanosensitivity using neurodynamic tests is described in Chapter 19.

The nervous system needs to adapt to mechanical loads. It can do this through elongation, sliding, cross-section change, angulation and compression.[148] However, when the nervous system cannot cope under loads, this can lead to ischaemia, hypoxia, neural oedema and fibrosis, as well as changes to axon and myelin integrity—all of which can alter neurodynamics.[148] This change in neurodynamics may contribute to the patient's symptoms and signs in certain injuries. If these abnormalities are not addressed, complete recovery as indicated by full pain-free range of motion may not occur.

Neurodynamic mobilisation techniques are widely used in the treatment of musculoskeletal pain. Human and animal studies have shown that neurodynamic mobilisation reduces intraneural oedema, improves intraneural fluid dispersion, reduces thermal and mechanical hyperalgesia, promotes axonal and myelin regeneration and reverses immune responses following a nerve injury.[150, 151]

One neurodynamic mobilisation technique is treatment of the interface (e.g. joint mobilisation or soft-tissue techniques targeted at the narrow anatomical spaces through which nerves travel). Two other techniques are neural sliders and tensioners:[152]

- A sliding technique is one in which joints are moved so that neural tissue elongation at a given joint is simultaneously relieved by neural tissue shortening at another joint.
- A tensioning technique is one in which there is either a displacement of both neural tissue endings in opposite directions, or the displacement of one of the endings in a tensioned direction while the other remains fixed.

A commonly used example for each technique is shown in Figure 24.11. The most commonly used techniques include slump mobilisation for low back pain and lower leg pain, and cervical lateral glides for upper limb pain.[153–155]

What determines how you use these techniques? Sliding techniques allow for more nerve excursion while minimising strain. It is hypothesised that sliders allow movement to be presented to the brain in different ways, disengaging learned expectations of pain. Larger amplitude movements may decrease fear of movement and may help with remapping altered representations. This has not yet been proven in studies.

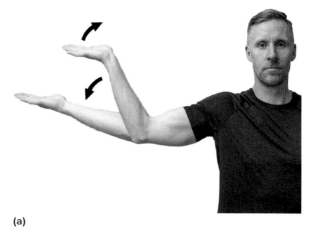

(a)

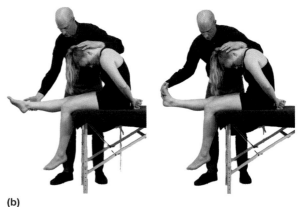

(b)

**Figure 24.11** Neural mobilisation exercises. (a) Slider. The waiter exercise slides the medial nerve. The patient begins in elbow flexion. They then extend the elbow (tending to elongate the median nerve), at the same time flexing the wrist (tending to shorten the median nerve). (b) Gentle tensioner. The patient sits on the bench as illustrated and one leg is extended and the ankle is dorsiflexed.

Tensioning techniques appear to improve pressure pain thresholds and disperse intraneural oedema.[156] As with most clinical treatment techniques, if there is insufficient loading, the technique can be ineffective, while too much loading can also be detrimental. Therefore, your selection of the appropriate treatment technique should be based on a careful assessment of the individual, including the severity of the condition and your assessment of irritability. Careful clinical monitoring following treatment is important.[149]

An umbrella review of 10 systematic reviews that included 133 RCTs showed neurodynamic mobilisation reduced pain and improved function for people with musculoskeletal conditions as well as improving neural mechanosensitivity for asymptomatic people. Although neurodynamic mobilisation was effective, there were insufficient data regarding key parameters of the treatment, such as the duration and frequency of the sessions and the total intervention time. In addition, only the immediate, not the medium- and long-term, effects of the interventions were reported.[157]

## Soft-tissue therapy

### with ROB GRANTER

Soft-tissue therapy is a broad term encompassing types of massage (Box 24.4). For many years, massage has been used to treat many different medical conditions as well as to help people relieve stress from their everyday lives.

---

**BOX 24.4** Types of soft-tissue therapy

Broadly, there are two main types of massage:

- Regular massage is an umbrella term for massage modalities that include relaxation and stress-relief techniques, muscle tension removal, and methods for improving circulation, energy and mental alertness (e.g. Shiatsu massage and Swedish massage).
- Massage therapy focuses on helping to treat various pain and medical conditions. Other terms used to describe this type of massage are therapeutic massage, remedial massage, sports massage and myotherapy. A category of massage therapy is lymphatic drainage massage, also known as manual lymphatic drainage, which is characterised by gentle, long strokes along the skin to increase the movement of lymph through the body.

---

Soft-tissue therapy is traditionally directed at subjective clinical examination findings such as reduced quantity and quality of joint movement, skeletal muscles with increased tone, soft-tissue thickening or muscles containing taut, sensitive bands that may refer pain in distinct patterns, often referred to as myofascial trigger points (Chapter 9).

### Treatment position

For successful soft-tissue therapy, place the target tissue in a position of either tension or laxity. Treating soft tissue in an elongated position can make focal sites of abnormality more easily palpable and may enhance referral patterns from myofascial trigger points. Treating in a position of laxity enhances the ability to access and assess deeper layers of soft tissue.

### Sustained myofascial tension

Sustained myofascial tension is described as applying a tensile force with your thumb, braced digits or forearm (Fig. 24.12) to an assessed site of fascial thickening or reduced fascial glide in the direction of greatest restriction,

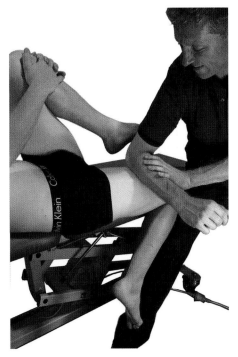

**Figure 24.12** Sustained myofascial tension

or in the direction of elongation necessary for normal function. Tension is developed in the tissue by applying compression to the fascial layer, then moving your thumb, braced digit or forearm through the target tissue to impart a shear force. Greater shear force can be imparted using passive through-range movement or active movement in the direction of assessed restriction in conjunction with the local tissue contact.

### Digital ischaemic pressure

Digital ischaemic pressure describes the application of force perpendicular to the skin towards the centre of a muscle to evoke a temporary ischaemic reaction. The aim is to stimulate the mechanoreceptors within muscle and fascia to reduce resting muscle tone, to provide an analgesic response in soft tissue by eliciting a release of pain-mediating substances, and to deactivate symptomatic trigger points that may optimise muscle activation patterns.[158] You can apply pressure using your thumb (Fig. 24.13a) or elbow (Fig. 24.13b) or a hand-held device such as a T-shaped bar.

### Friction

Friction massage is applied selectively to a localised area palpated as an abnormal tissue thickening; for example, due to excessive intramuscular scar formation following acute muscle injury. It is essential to assess pain and restrictions

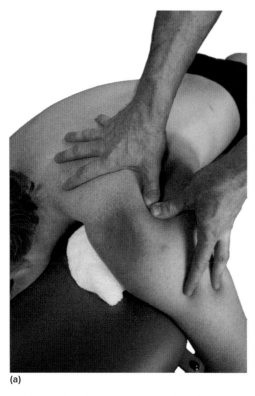
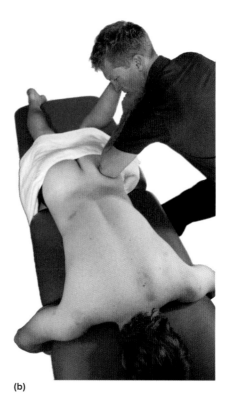

(a)                                                              (b)

**Figure 24.13** (a) Applying digital pressure to the infraspinatus trigger point using the clinician's thumb. (b) Applying digital pressure to the gluteus medius trigger point using the clinician's elbow.

in muscle length and/or neural mobility before, during and at the end of each treatment session to monitor its effectiveness.

You should apply sufficient pressure so that your finger/ thumb and the patient's skin move as one, and the friction must work deeply enough and be of sufficient sweep to impart a friction movement to the target tissue. The friction is normally applied at 90° (perpendicular) or 45° to the target structure, and must be applied at a level that maintains contact with the target tissue and is within the patient's pain tolerance.

It is vital to ensure that the region being treated is totally relaxed. Pressure should be increased gradually to reach the required treatment level within the patient's pain tolerance. Ice can be applied to the region post-treatment in a position of pain-free stretch for 5–10 minutes, particularly for the initial application, to minimise post-treatment tenderness.

### Lymphatic drainage

Lymphatic drainage is a gentle massage treatment to stimulate the circulation of lymph fluid around the body. This helps to speed up the removal of wastes and toxins.

Lymphatic drainage can also be used to help people who have had damage to their lymphatic system following surgery or trauma or due to developmental disorders.

A 2009 systematic review[159] of the effect of lymphatic drainage in sports medicine suggested that manual lymphatic drainage techniques may be efficacious in the resolution of raised serum enzyme levels associated with acute structural skeletal muscle cell damage as well as in the reduction of oedema following fracture of the distal radius and acute ankle sprain. However, there is currently insufficient evidence to establish clinical practice guidelines for the use of lymphatic drainage in rehabilitating athletic injuries.

### Depth of treatment

A number of scales have been developed to describe the depth of massage. The most widely used scale was developed by Tracy Walton in 2002.[160]

Walton massage therapy pressure scale

## Combination treatment

If soft-tissue techniques are aimed at restoring joint range of motion and function, they can be followed by static, contract/relax or dynamic stretching to facilitate the effect.

## Lubricants

For many soft-tissue techniques you need to apply a lubricant to the patient's skin to aid both patient comfort and your ability to palpate the tissue for sore spots or abnormalities. Ensure that you use a sufficient amount of lubricant, particularly when palpating areas with large amounts of hair, as irritation of hair follicles may result in contact dermatitis.

With techniques such as sustained myofascial tension and ischaemic pressure, skin contact should be maximal so no lubricant is required, and as there are fewer repetitive movements, there is less risk of irritation to hair follicles.

## Vacuum cupping

Vacuum cupping, a therapy used in many traditional medicine systems, has become popular among professional athletes. It is based on a sucking traction of the skin and hypodermis: a cupping glass is applied to a predefined area and negative pressure (compared to atmospheric pressure) is generated mechanically (pumping) or thermally (cooling heated air), withdrawing the trapped air from under the cup.[161] This results in reddening and warming of the area due to increased perfusion.

In dry cupping, negative pressure is applied on an intact skin surface, whereas in wet cupping the skin under the cup is pricked with a needle, so the cupping is accompanied by a slight bleeding. Pulsating or pulsatile cupping uses a mechanical device that generates a pulsating/pulsatile vacuum with a pump.[162]

The exact mechanism of action of cupping is unclear but it may promote skin's blood flow, change skin's biomechanical properties, increase pain thresholds, improve local anaerobic metabolism, reduce inflammation and modulate cellular mechanisms of the immune system.[163]

Three recent systematic reviews[164-166] all suggest that there is low to moderate evidence that cupping is effective in the reduction of pain, especially chronic neck pain and non-specific low back pain, and improving function. However, the evidence is of low quality and the two trials comparing cupping with sham cupping did not show any significant difference.[162, 167]

The risks of dry cupping appear to be low. Typical side effects such as haematoma under the cupping area are minor and transient, but it is contraindicated with the use of anticoagulants and disorders with increased risk of bleeding.[165]

## Self-treatment

Athletes may use spiky balls, tennis balls or foam rollers for self-treatment of soft tissues (Fig. 24.14).[168] A number of studies have found that this leads to a short-term increase in range of motion, without any detriment in sports performance.[169-172]

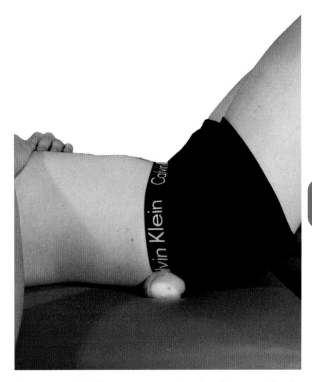

**Figure 24.14** Self-treatment: treating the gluteus medius in a lying position with a tennis ball

Self-treatment can be undertaken daily, or as warm-up for or recovery from sports participation. Typically, it involves applying force to the identified site with sustained pressure until perceived tone/tension reduces and pain or referred symptoms resolve. Functional re-assessment should be carried out after an initial trial period, for example 1–2 minutes, to ensure that positive changes are occurring. As initial presenting symptoms, soft-tissue characteristics and patient responses vary, dosage time and repetitions should be individualised to achieve optimal results. Self-treatment should not cause excessive or lasting pain that adversely affects training or increases symptoms.

## Evidence of effectiveness

A systematic review found limited evidence of the effectiveness of soft-tissue therapy in the management of musculoskeletal disorders and injuries in the upper and lower extremities.[173] The review identified six studies with low risk of bias that investigated clinical massage, localised relaxation massage and movement re-education for the management of persistent lateral elbow pain, subacromial impingement, carpal tunnel syndrome and plantar heel pain.

The evidence suggested that clinical massage (myofascial release) and movement re-education (muscle energy technique) may benefit patients with persistent lateral elbow pain, in contrast to a previous systematic review which did not show any benefit.[174] Clinical massage was not effective for managing subacromial impingement. Relaxation massage (self-massage to the hand/forearm with the intent to relax muscles, move body fluids and reduce pain) combined with multimodal care may provide short-term benefits to patients with persistent carpal tunnel syndrome.

For plantar heel pain related to a gastrocnemius strain, the evidence suggests that clinical massage (manual trigger point therapy) may provide minimal added benefit when combined with a self-stretching protocol. However, clinical massage (myofascial release) to the gastrocnemius, soleus and plantar fascia was effective in improving foot function in patients with plantar heel pain. No high-quality studies were found examining the effectiveness of soft-tissue therapy for other musculoskeletal disorders or injuries of the lower extremity.

## TAPING

Taping was the third most-used intervention at the London 2012 Olympic Games polyclinic,[175] reflecting its popularity as a treatment modality and injury prevention intervention. However, research into both the mechanisms and effects of taping is limited and marked by heterogeneous results,[176, 177] making it difficult to draw firm evidence-based conclusions on its benefits and application.

### Proposed mechanisms of taping

Taping is proposed to have a range of effects depending on the application method and type of tape used. Traditionally, clinicians have applied rigid strapping tape in an attempt to restrict patients' range of motion or to alter their anatomical alignment; for example, to realign the patella within the femoral trochlea (Fig. 24.15).[178] Flexible cloth tape, often referred to as kinesiology tape, has also gained in popularity.

Taping appears to have a range of neurophysiological effects:

- Cutaneous stimulation by tape may inhibit afferent nociceptive signals at the spinal level (pain-gate theory).[179]

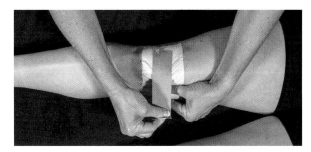

**Figure 24.15** Taping is often used to relieve patellofemoral pain

- Applying tape alters brain activity in a variety of areas, including the motor cortex, sensory cortex, thalamus, basal ganglia and cerebellum.[180] This may have a wide range of effects, including improved proprioception[181] and motor coordination, and explain how taping influences factors such as muscle activation timing[182] and concentric/eccentric control.[183]
- Restricting the range and amplitude of joint motion may enable increased reaction time of surrounding musculature during high-velocity activities.[176, 183-185]
- Patients' conscious and subconscious expectations of the effects of taping may relieve pain (i.e. placebo effect).[179] Once thought to be a purely psychological phenomenon, it is now considered to be at least partly caused by the secretion of endogenous opioids in response to treatment.[74]

However, the proposed mechanisms remain largely speculative. For example, tape intended to limit range of motion loosens after 10–30 minutes,[186, 187] and recent systematic reviews disagree on whether patellofemoral joint taping influences vastus medialis obliquus onset timing and knee extensor moments.[182, 188] Research in this area is ongoing.

### Evidence of effectiveness

Although taping is used for a wide range of conditions, high-level evidence of its efficacy is scant. The available evidence is of varying quality—one of the main challenges when studying taping is the inability to blind patients or practitioners.[182, 189]

#### Patellofemoral pain

A number of systematic reviews have investigated the use of patellar realignment taping (often referred to as McConnell taping—see Chapter 24 in *Managing Injuries*) in patients with patellofemoral pain syndrome.[182, 189, 190] Although results are conflicting, there is moderate evidence that taping provides an immediate reduction in pain,[182, 190] particularly when an individualised taping technique is used.[182] However, its benefit seems to be limited to the short term, and prolonged use is not supported. The effect of kinesiology tape (Box 24.5) on patellofemoral pain remains unclear; one randomised crossover trial found that McConnell and kinesiology taping were equally effective in immediately reducing pain,[191] whereas two RCTs found kinesiology tape was ineffective in reducing pain.[192, 193]

### Ankle sprains

Several studies have suggested that taping can prevent ankle sprains.[197-199] Ankle sprains are associated with a high rate of recurrence and the use of taping or bracing to prevent recurrence is common. The risk of re-injury is increased sevenfold in the year following an initial sprain.[200] Taping reduced the recurrence rate by 71% in a classic 1973 study.[198]

### Other conditions

There is some evidence that taping may be effective in treating pain and strength deficits associated with lateral epicondylalgia,[201] de Quervain tenosynovitis,[202] plantar fasciopathy pain[179, 203, 204] and shoulder pain.[179, 194, 205] However, many of these studies are of low quality with a moderate to high risk of publication bias.

## Practical considerations

In practice, taping is applied across a far wider range of conditions than there exists evidence for, and it should be considered just as much an art as a science.[200] You should consider not only the available literature, but also the diagnosis, scenario (e.g. competition, acute management, rehabilitation) and patient's preference and expectations.

Much like any exercise program should be progressive, the use of taping should be gradually reduced over time.[26] When taping is successful in alleviating a chronic condition such as patellofemoral pain, you should plan to wean the patient off the use of tape to avoid creating a dependence on a passive treatment. Following an acute injury, taping may provide immediate pain relief and restrict excessive movement.[206] Controlled stress (optimal loading) can then be facilitated by gradually reducing the amount of support taping provides over subsequent days and weeks.

> **PRACTICE PEARL**
>
> For long-term application of tape, consider teaching the athlete to tape themselves. This will increase the sense of control over their own management, decrease dependency on you and save valuable time in a busy treatment clinic.

---

**BOX 24.5** Kinesiology tape: valuable tool for athletes or fashion statement?

Kinesiology tape has gained considerable popularity, as demonstrated by the large number of athletes using it at the Olympic Games and other major sporting events (Fig. 24.16). The approach was developed in Japan in the 1970s and is claimed to permit unrestricted range of movement while supporting the fascia, muscles and joints.[194]

Kinesiology tape has been proposed to improve pain and blood flow via dermal lifting, which decreases the pressure on cutaneous nerve receptors and capillaries, decreasing nociceptive input and increasing afferent feedback.[194] However, these effects last less than 24 hours and may be trivial, and the actual benefits for injured athletes are yet to be established in high-quality studies.[195]

The use of kinesiology tape remains controversial among clinicians, with some even claiming it may provide a psychological crutch for athletes.[196]

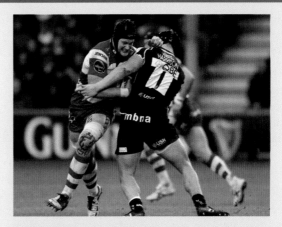

**Figure 24.16** Kinesiology tape comprises elastic cotton with an acrylic adhesive, historically marketed for enhanced proprioceptive feedback
IMAGE COURTESY OF ROCKTAPE UK

To protect the patient's skin from irritation, apply hypoallergenic tape under rigid sports tape. This is particularly important when tape containing zinc oxide is used for a longer duration. In some situations, such as prophylactic ankle taping, pre-wrap may be applied under the tape. This does not alter the amount of motion restriction, the time to maximum range or the velocity of range;[185] however, it may reduce the cutaneous stimulus.

> **PRACTICE PEARL**
>
> Where possible, introduce new taping techniques to athletes in a controlled environment prior to competition.

Despite the limited and conflicting evidence base, taping continues to play an important role in clinical sports and exercise medicine practice. You should consider the available literature, retain a healthy scepticism towards commercial claims and trends, and take a trial-and-error approach. Clinical experience and athlete preference should not be discredited.

## BRACING

Bracing can be used in both prevention and rehabilitation. In rehabilitative bracing, the prime focus is to allow a protected joint range of motion after injury or surgery. Depending on the desired restriction of range of motion the brace can be soft or rigid. Braces are made from a variety of materials, from cloth with associated Velcro straps or laces to thermoplastic materials.

Braces are commonly used in the treatment of:

- wrist sprains or overuse injuries
- lateral elbow pain
- scoliosis
- knee ligament injuries (e.g. ACL)
- fractures of the lower leg or foot
- stress fractures (e.g. navicular, medial malleolus)
- Achilles tendon rupture
- severe ankle sprains/instability.

One of the most common types of brace is the moon boot, also called the controlled ankle movement walker (Fig. 24.17), used to protect the joints of the lower leg after surgery or severe injury. It can be a rigid brace for complete immobilisation of the joint or allow restricted movement. Many boots can be adjusted over the rehabilitation period to allow a gradual increase in range of motion.

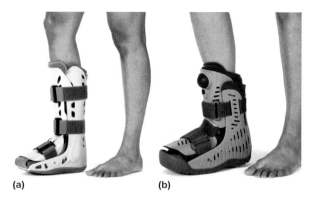

(a)          (b)

**Figure 24.17** The moon boot or controlled action motion walker may be (a) tall or (b) short in length. The boot is adjustable, reusable and completely removable.
PHOTOGRAPHER YOHAN KIM. IMAGES COURTESY OF PARIS EVERYBODY (VANCOUVER, CANADA).

## Ankle braces

There is limited evidence for the effectiveness of ankle bracing after an ankle sprain. A 2019 review found no significant differences between semi-rigid or posterior rigid supports and tape or bandages with regards to pain, range of motion, function or return to sport or work. There was some evidence that patients treated with semi-rigid or posterior rigid supports had a significantly higher "benefit score" than those treated with tape or bandages (Fig 24.18).[207]

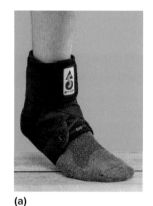 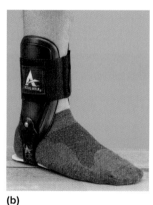

(a)          (b)

**Figure 24.18** Ankle braces: (a) Evo lace-up ankle brace with stays and (b) Active Ankle rigid brace with stirrups
PHOTOGRAPHER RYLAND HAGGIS. IMAGES TAKEN WITH THE SUPPORT OF PARIS EVERYBODY (VANCOUVER, CANADA).

An earlier RCT conducted to evaluate the effectiveness of combined bracing and neuromuscular training, or bracing alone, against the use of neuromuscular training on recurrences of ankle sprain after usual care, found that bracing was superior to neuromuscular training in reducing the incidence but not the severity of self-reported recurrent ankle sprains after usual care.[208]

A multicentre randomised trial that studied 584 participants with severe ankle sprains demonstrated that patients who received a below-knee cast for 10 days had a more rapid recovery than those who had a tubular compression bandage, Air-Stirrup brace or walking boot. The researchers concluded that, contrary to popular clinical opinion, a short period of immobilisation was the most effective strategy for promoting rapid recovery. Patients best achieved this by wearing a below-knee cast.[209]

For prevention of recurrent ankle sprain, there is moderate quality evidence that ankle braces are effective.[210] There are a wide variety of ankle braces that provide varying degrees of restriction of range of motion.

## Knee braces

Braces for treating knee injuries range from simple sleeve braces to unloader braces and functional braces. For knee osteoarthritis, the most common braces are a simple knee sleeve (Fig. 24.19a) and an unloader brace. A Cochrane review, originally published in 2005 and updated in 2015,[211] identified five RCTs, with sample sizes ranging from 33 to 117 patients. The trials compared a type of brace for knee osteoarthritis to no treatment or to another treatment such as restricted activity, patient education, exercise, pharmacological treatment and orthoses, or surgery. The evidence was of low quality, and when data from the trials were combined, people who used a knee brace saw little or no change in knee pain and function, and in their quality of life.

Clinically, an adjustable hinged knee brace (Fig. 24.19b) is commonly used in the treatment of moderate or severe medial collateral ligament injuries and post knee meniscus surgical repair. The brace is set to a specific range of motion—for instance, 30–90° of knee flexion—and prevents full knee extension and limits stress on the healing ligament. A hinged brace allows the patient to commence early weight-bearing exercises. The degree of available knee movement can gradually be increased as rehabilitation progresses.

Bracing after ACL injury as part of non-surgical management or after surgical reconstruction of the ACL is debated. There is considerable variation in protocols between different countries. The effectiveness of postoperative functional bracing following ACL reconstruction remains elusive. Functional bracing may have some effects on in-vivo knee kinematics and may protect the graft after ACL reconstruction without sacrificing function, range of motion or proprioception. Whether routine functional bracing reduces re-injury after ACL reconstruction is still unclear.[212] Some knee surgeons recommend wearing an extension brace at all times (except for exercise) until quadriceps control is regained after ACL reconstruction.

A specific brace, sometimes known as a "Jack", is often used when treating posterior cruciate ligament injuries. The brace provides a dynamic anterior-directed force to hold the tibia in a neutral position and prevent posterior sagging.[213] Figure 24.19(d) illustrates how the brace helps avoid the posterior drawer position during knee flexion and extension. The force set through the hinge is adjusted to the size and mass of the patient's leg and is appropriate for patients who choose either non-surgical or surgical treatment. The ligament is secured over the entire knee range of motion and functional rehabilitation can take place without risking instability of the knee—avoiding extensive immobilisation and supporting early return to daily activities. The Jack brace is worn throughout the rehabilitation period.

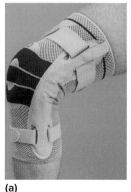 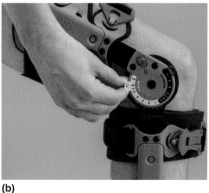 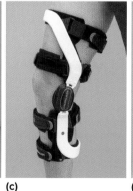 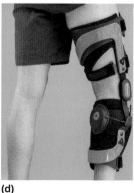

(a)  (b)  (c)  (d)

**Figure 24.19** Braces used in the treatment of knee injuries: (a) Bauerfeind Genutrain S Hinged Knee Sleeve, (b) Ossur Rebound Post-Op, acute injury and post-op adjustable range of motion brace, (c) Donjoy Defiance Pro, ACL deficient or post-reconstruction hinged knee brace and (d) Ossur Rebound PCL, dynamic custom knee brace for non-surgical treatment or for post-operative support of a reconstructed posterior cruciate ligament.
PHOTOGRAPHER RYLAND HAGGIS; BRACES COURTESY OF PARIS EVERYBODY (VANCOUVER, CANADA).

# ELECTROPHYSICAL AGENTS
## with DALE FORSDYK and ADAM GLEDHILL

Electrophysical agents (i.e. electrotherapy) have a long history as therapeutic agents but in the light of contemporary person-centred approaches to care, their use has been critiqued and their popularity may be waning in favour of active treatments (e.g. exercise therapy). Nevertheless, agents such as ultrasound and neuromuscular stimulation are still prevalent in clinical practice, and there are claims that newer modalities such as extracorporeal shockwave therapy can promote tissue healing.

The decision to use electrophysical agents will be influenced by contextual factors such as time and resource availability, patient expectations, the effectiveness of other treatments, contraindicative presentations and your own experience. If you use electrophysical agents, make sure that you adhere to prescription parameters to apply the recommended dose for treatment-specific effects. Experienced clinicians very rarely (if ever) use electrophysical agents in isolation.

### PRACTICE PEARL

If electrotherapy is used, it should be as an adjunct to other forms of treatment including exercise, advice and education.

Box 24.6 provides strategies that may maximise the potential therapeutic effects of electrophysical agents through increased patient engagement.

### BOX 24.6 Tips to consider if using electrophysical agents

1. Be realistic—balanced—when discussing the relative benefits of electrotherapy with the patient. This will contribute to their education and understanding.
2. Where electrotherapy can be safely self-administered, encourage the patient to do so (e.g. ultrasound at the wrist). This can help them to feel a greater sense of control over their symptoms and elicit their own therapeutic effects, rather than the electrotherapy creating a sense of dependency on you to "fix" them.
3. Provide a balanced rationale for the use of electrotherapy, help the patient to understand the risks and benefits, and involve the patient in the decision to use it or not.
4. Leading clinicians strive to keep patients from becoming dependent on passive treatments (e.g. electrotherapy); they promote active rehabilitation strategies, advice and education.

## Therapeutic ultrasound

Therapeutic ultrasound was a cornerstone of soft-tissue treatment in the 1980s.[214] Typically, the prescription algorithm for therapeutic ultrasound considers the chronicity of the injury and the depth and size of the lesion. The biological rationale for its use relates to proposed thermal and non-thermal effects:

- thermal effects include increased tissue temperature, local blood flow, tissue metabolism, fluid dynamics in the tissue and collagen extensibility
- non-thermal effects include stimulation of fibroblast activity, mast cell degranulation, growth factor activation and angiogenesis achieved through mechanisms of ultrasonic cavitation, gas body activation and mechanical tissue stress.

These potentially beneficial effects have primarily been demonstrated in vitro[214, 215] and are commonly cited to justify the clinical use of therapeutic ultrasound to treat a wide variety of musculoskeletal conditions. The goal is that ultrasound will reduce pain, inflammation and oedema, and improve scar-tissue remodelling, tissue extensibility and soft-tissue healing.[216, 217] Treatment is traditionally directed towards collagen-rich tissues such as ligaments, tendons, fascia, joint capsules and scar tissue, which absorb the greatest amount of energy compared with tissue with high-water and low-protein content (e.g. cartilage).[215, 217]

Despite these proposed benefits, there is little high-quality evidence to support its clinical efficacy.[218-223] This lack of high-quality research evidence supporting therapeutic ultrasound for traumatic, overuse and degenerative musculoskeletal conditions is a pertinent consideration for clinicians.[217] The most common side effect is superficial burns to the skin, which may occasionally occur if used for long periods. This can be avoided by continual movement of the ultrasound wand.

### Ultrasound as a stimulator of bone repair

Ultrasound has been increasingly used in the treatment of acute bone fractures. Meta-analyses suggest that daily administration of low-intensity pulsed ultrasound (LIPUS) can accelerate the healing of fractures by approximately 35%.[224-226]

LIPUS appears to be most effective for conservatively managed diaphyseal fractures, reducing the time to clinical union by approximately 18 days.[226] The evidence is strongest for upper limb fractures, but conflicting for metaphyseal and operatively managed acute fractures.[224, 226]

It is typically applied for 20 minutes every day, which may be an excessive treatment regimen for many patients.

However, in elite sports a faster return to training and competition may be important. LIPUS may also be valuable in cases that fail conservative management (non-union) after bone-graft surgery is performed.[224]

Few studies have investigated LIPUS for the treatment of stress fractures; however, the available results are not encouraging[227,228] and it cannot currently be recommended for this purpose. Similarly, there is currently no evidence that it is effective for accelerating healing of soft-tissue injuries.

## Transcutaneous electrical nerve stimulation

Transcutaneous electrical nerve stimulation (TENS) delivers biphasic electrical current using electrodes applied to the skin.[229] Its clinical application is typically determined by the chronicity of injury (e.g. acute vs chronic pain). There are several mechanisms by which TENS can provide symptomatic relief of pain, including inhibiting the excitability of central nociceptive transmission neurons, stimulating opioid and noradrenergic receptors at the site of application, and opioid, serotonin and muscarinic receptors in the spinal cord and brainstem.[230]

Although there is no evidence that TENS improves long-term outcomes,[231] it may play an adjunct role in pain management in certain patient groups. In a 2022 systematic review and meta-analysis of 381 RCTs (24,532 participants), TENS reduced both acute and chronic pain intensity during and immediately after treatment compared with placebo, and pharmacological and non-pharmacological treatments[232] used as part of standard care.

TENS can provide short-term pain relief for patients with spinal cord injuries,[233,234] postoperative and procedural pain[232], lumbar disc disease,[235] and chronic neck and lower back pain.[236] There is little evidence to support its use for knee osteoarthritis[229,237] and it is not widely used in the athletic population. It can, however, be used in combination with exercise therapy and medication.[233,238] Although in most cases TENS can be safely self-administered, potential adverse effects may include mild erythema and itching underneath the electrodes.[232,238]

## Neuromuscular stimulators

Neuromuscular electrical stimulation is purported to have a range of effects on healthy athletes, including enhanced post-exercise recovery, improved sports performance and reduced muscle soreness. However, commercial claims regarding its benefits for athletes often exceed the existing evidence.[239] In a clinical setting, a neuromuscular stimulator may be valuable to maintain muscle strength after a major injury requiring a period of limited loading or immobilisation (e.g. ACL rupture) (Fig. 24.20).[240]

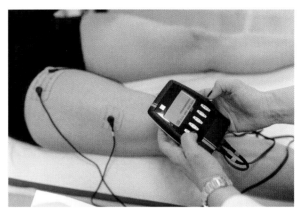

**Figure 24.20** Neuromuscular stimulator
ISTOCK/ZORANM

Traditionally, it has been thought that neuromuscular electrical stimulation improves muscle performance because it reverses the normal motor unit recruitment order, preferentially activating larger motor units composed primarily of fast-twitch fibres.[241] However, this theory has been challenged by Dr Elanna Arhos and others who found that the normal clinical methods for applying neuromuscular electrical stimulation cause random, non-selective motor unit activation.[242,243] Nevertheless, there is high-level evidence that combining neuromuscular electrical stimulation with traditional exercise training is more effective than training alone in improving quadriceps strength following ACL reconstruction.[240,244]

The decision to use neuromuscular electrical stimulation in rehabilitation depends on a number of factors, but there is now a relatively consistent trend in the data in favour of advocating for early and frequent implementation post-injury or surgery.[243]

Effective therapeutic intensity may be uncomfortable, so providing a clear rationale and patient education around its use may increase adherence to the treatment modality.[245,246] We emphasise that, for many patients, traditional strength training is highly effective for rehabilitation. However, a subset of patients experience persistent weakness following major joint injury due to arthrogenic muscle inhibition.[247] In this group, neuromuscular electrical stimulation combined with progressively heavier strength training may get the patient over a hump.[248] Given the strength of evidence surrounding neuromuscular electrical stimulation, Dr Arhos and others contend that it should be part of standard rehabilitation post-injury or surgery.[243]

The recommended parameters to enhance muscle strengthening in rehabilitation are shown in Table 24.4.[242,243,249,250]

**TABLE 24.4**   Recommended treatment parameters to maximise muscle strength gains using neuromuscular electrical stimulation

| Treatment parameter | Details |
| --- | --- |
| Stimulation intensity | The intensity should be as high as the patient can tolerate, and at least 50% of maximal voluntary contraction |
| Pulse frequency | High-frequency stimulation (50–80 Hz) leads to higher force production, smoother contractions and greater muscle fatigue; frequencies over 80 Hz may be more painful |
| Pulse duration (width) | A longer pulse duration (up to 600 μs) maximises force production for a given stimulation intensity; the currently recommended duration is 200–400 μs |
| Training regimen | 3–10 s on-time followed by 10–40 s recovery; 10–15 min per session |
| Program parameters | 1–3 sessions per week for 4–6 weeks |

## Interferential stimulation

Interferential stimulation has a long history in sports therapy and remains widely used in some areas of the world.[251,252] Recommended treatments are based on the chronicity of injury (e.g. acute, sub-acute, chronic). The scientific rationale is that the interference of two medium-frequency currents passed through the tissues causes analgesic effects. The analgesic effect may be due to stimulation of cutaneous receptors that inhibit C-fibre nociceptive transmission,[253] motor stimulation increasing the removal of pain-inducing substances[254] and the release of endogenous opioids.[255]

Based on a review including 35 trials (19 of which were selected for meta-analysis), interferential current alone, or added to other interventions, is not more effective than comparative treatments (e.g. laser, cryotherapy) in relieving musculoskeletal pain.[256] The pain-relieving effects of interferential stimulation are transient and there is little high-quality evidence produced with athletic populations. Evidence from non-athletic populations, however, suggests that it has no adverse effects and can be recommended as a treatment for knee osteoarthritis given its benefits on pain and self-reported function.[257]

## Laser

Low-level laser therapy is a non-invasive treatment in which non-thermal laser irradiation is applied to the site of pain using light generated by high-intensity electrical stimulation. It modulates cell and tissue physiology to obtain therapeutic effects,[258] including promotion of tissue repair,[259,260] and inflammatory effects,[261,262] potentially providing pain relief in common musculoskeletal disorders.[258,263,264]

Prescription of this modality is based on the type of injury (e.g. body area and thickness of tissue) and should adhere to World Association for Photobiomodulation Therapy (WALT) guidelines, the efficacy of which is supported in a systematic review and meta-analysis of 18 studies investigating adult patients with musculoskeletal disorders.[265]

 WALT guidelines

Low-level laser therapy may relieve pain following acute sports injury,[266] and it may reduce pain and improve function in patients with rotator cuff tendinopathy, both as a standalone treatment and when used in combination with therapeutic exercise.[267] It may also improve outcomes for patients with chronic midportion Achilles tendinopathy when combined with an eccentric loading program (Chapter 29 in *Managing Injuries*).[268]

Although there is some evidence that low-level laser therapy is effective in certain conditions, there is little knowledge of dose response and no consensus on the treatment parameters for specific pathologies. Further research using large, homogenous samples of similar pathologies would clarify its efficacy in sports injury management.[266]

## Electromagnetic therapy

Low-frequency pulsed electromagnetic field therapy is purported to have a wide range of local cellular and systemic effects on numerous tissues. However, not all therapeutic effects are empirically supported. Its use is recommended in wound care,[269,270] and there is some evidence supporting short-term benefit in the treatment of certain sports injuries and conditions.[271-273] Long-term benefits are not well-established.[272,273]

Its main clinical applications include delayed union or non-union fractures, osteoarthritis, osteoporosis, osteonecrosis and tendon disorders.[274] In the case of osteoarthritis there is growing evidence to suggest that it has a beneficial effect on pain, stiffness and self-reported physical function.[275, 276]

Laboratory studies suggest that it may be valuable in the treatment of tendon, bone and cartilage pathology.[277-280] For example, when applied to human tendon cells, it may cause cellular proliferation, tendon-specific gene expression and the release of growth factors and pro- and anti-inflammatory cytokines.[279, 280] Similarly, when applied to articular hyaline cartilage, it can stimulate chondrocyte proliferation, proteoglycans and extra-cellular matrix (e.g. TGF-$\beta$).[277]

A possible mechanism is that the pulses impact tissue transmembrane receptors to modulate the action of proinflammatory mediators and stimulate growth factors for tissue repair.[274] As with other electrophysical agents there are limited adverse effects, although repeated long-term use requires further investigation.

### Extracorporeal shockwave therapy
#### with VASILEIOS KORAKAKIS

Extracorporeal shockwaves were first used in medicine in 1980 to break up kidney stones.[281, 282] Subsequent animal research on extracorporeal shockwave therapy demonstrated dose-dependent destructive (high-energy) and regenerative (lower-energy) effects on a range of tissues, including bone and tendon.[283, 284] Since then, extracorporeal shockwave therapy has been used extensively in clinical practice to treat superficial musculoskeletal conditions (Fig. 24.21) such as shoulder tendinopathy, subacromial pain, lateral elbow tendinopathy, greater trochanteric pain syndrome, patellar and Achilles tendinopathy, and plantar heel pain.

Despite extensive use of the modality, the scientific evidence is not strong in terms of both quality and certainty. Even though level 1 and 2 studies are available for data pooling and meta-analyses, you should interpret the results

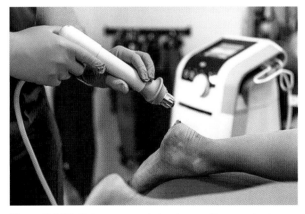

**Figure 24.21** Extracorporeal shockwave therapy device
ISTOCK/PUHIMEC

of systematic reviews with caution given the relative paucity of high-quality data available and the significant clinical heterogeneity. This is because the studies are often marked by methodological flaws, biases and low reporting quality.[285] Be aware of inconsistent reporting of the type of shockwave used (extracorporeal, radial, focused), the intensity (high, medium, low) and the method of application (focal, local, area of pain distribution).

The development of core outcome sets to be used in trials of musculoskeletal conditions would significantly facilitate the ability of reviewers to synthesise the available evidence and inform clinical practice (Box 24.7).

## DRY NEEDLING AND ACUPUNCTURE

The terms "acupuncture" and "dry needling" are often used interchangeably to describe treatments using thin monofilament needles without injectate.[295] However, acupuncture denotes the use of the modality within a traditional Chinese medicine paradigm using needles to unblock the flow of vital energy (qi) along meridians or channels,[296] whereas dry needling implies the use of a modern biomedical paradigm.

Myofascial trigger points, an often overlooked cause of pain found in myofascial pain syndrome, are hyperirritable spots within the muscles that cause pain and dysfunction.[297, 298] The relationship between myofascial trigger points and acupuncture points has been explored for more than 50 years.[299] Travell and Simon's manual on myofascial trigger points discusses the possible correlation,[300] establishing a historical relationship between them.

A 2022 review found that "the 255 most common trigger points illustrated in the first edition of the *Trigger Point Manual* are fundamentally similar to classical acupuncture points".[301] Moreover, a three-part study reported an anatomical correlation of 93.3%.[302]

The physiological effects of acupuncture and dry needling are identical,[303] despite the differences in language and the models used. The clinical mechanisms are identical, regardless of the cultural or linguistic paradigm used.

### Dry needling

Although the mechanism of action of dry needling remains unclear, it is widely acknowledged that it involves the interplay of multiple biochemicals on the sarcomeres of the muscle tissue and their impact on the neural pathways and the sodium–potassium pump, leading to alterations in muscular polarisation.

Dry needling encompasses stimulation of neural, muscular and connective tissues, as well as myofascial trigger points. Trigger point techniques often aim to produce

## BOX 24.7 Extracorporeal shockwave therapy

Consider the following key messages about extracorporeal shockwave therapy in clinical practice:

- Based on the currently available low- to moderate-certainty evidence,[285] there are limited clinically important benefits for patients with rotator-cuff disease with or without calcific deposits. Significant clinical diversity and treatment protocols render unsafe any definitive conclusions of a dose-related effect.
- For the broad diagnosis of subacromial shoulder conditions,[286] there is moderate-certainty evidence for the comparative effects of exercise only on function. Nevertheless, the evidence (mostly low certainty) suggests 5 passive treatments (acupuncture, manual therapy, exercise plus manual therapy, laser therapy and microcurrent TENS) as having a high probability of being most effective (short term) for pain and function.
- For passive treatment modalities in patients with a frozen shoulder,[287] low quality and certainty evidence (with an effect that rarely exceeds the minimal clinically important difference) suggests that extracorporeal shockwave therapy and laser therapy may reduce pain and improve function, while ultrasound therapy does not demonstrate a clinically significant effect. The significant heterogeneity and low quality of evidence suggest that extracorporeal shockwave therapy, laser and ultrasound cannot be recommended for the treatment of frozen shoulder.
- In lateral elbow tendinopathy,[288] the evidence (low to moderate certainty) indicates no clinical benefits of extracorporeal shockwave therapy compared with sham interventions or corticosteroid injections; however, extracorporeal shockwave therapy outperforms other passive treatment modalities such as laser and ultrasound.
- In patients with greater trochanteric pain syndrome,[289, 290] platelet-rich plasma injections and extracorporeal shockwave therapy, and/or structured exercise led to significantly better outcomes (pain scores and function, respectively) when compared with a placebo or no treatment at the very short- to short-term follow up (1–3 months). Caution should be taken in the clinical interpretation and inferences of these findings, as improvements from baseline for most interventions evaluated (including placebo and no treatment) reached the minimal clinically important difference.
- Using extracorporeal shockwave therapy for the treatment of patellar tendinopathy appears to provide limited clinical benefits.[291] The available evidence indicates minimal or no effect on pain and function (VISA-P) at follow-up when compared with other interventions,[292] while moderate evidence suggests that extracorporeal shockwave therapy has no additive effect when used in combination with eccentric exercise for both pain and function (VISA-P).[290]
- For patients with Achilles tendinopathy, consistent evidence suggests that any adjuncts administered as a monotherapy or in addition to exercise (including extracorporeal shockwave therapy) are no more effective than exercise alone.[290, 293]
- Patients with plantar heel pain who do not optimally improve with taping, stretching and individualised education may be offered extracorporeal shockwave therapy (moderate-certainty evidence), followed by custom orthoses.[294]

a local muscular twitch response, thought to be caused by stimulation of a spinal reflex loop. This has been linked to an immediate reduction in extracellular neurotransmitter concentration in muscle tissue surrounding a trigger point,[304] and a twitch response is anecdotally associated with an improved treatment effect.[305]

There is a vast amount of research on the effects of dry needling and acupuncture. However, interpretation of the literature is complicated by the wide variety of conditions treated, differing underlying treatment paradigms (traditional Chinese medicine versus a modern biomedical model[306]), as well as a large variation in treatment protocols and methodological quality. It is particularly difficult to blind patients and clinicians in RCTs, which is problematic as needling is associated with a potent placebo effect.

Nevertheless, a substantial body of level 1 evidence suggests that needling is more effective than placebo or sham treatments for a range of musculoskeletal conditions including chronic lower back, neck[307] and shoulder pain; chronic muscular pain; acute myofascial pain;[308] orofacial pain;[309] headache; lateral elbow pain;[307] hip pain;[310] and knee osteoarthritis.[306, 311-315]

The majority of high-quality studies seem to indicate that dry needling is effective for reducing pain and tenderness in multiple body regions, including the head, trunk and upper and lower extremities. Lack of consistency among the articles regarding patient recruitment, protocol, methodology and outcome measures limits our ability to draw strong conclusions from the data. Nevertheless, an emerging body of evidence exists to suggest that multiple body regions may benefit from dry needling for pain reduction, improved function and improved range of motion.[316]

However, a recent trial involving 116 participants failed to show any added benefit of combining dry needling with a guideline-based physical therapy treatment program consisting of exercise and manual therapy on pain and disability for people with chronic neck pain. The study demonstrated a small, not clinically meaningful, reduction in average neck pain intensity at a month post-randomisation, but not at 3 and 6 months. There was no improvement in disability.[317]

The most commonly used dry needling technique involves inserting the needle into focal trigger points within a palpable taut band and leaving it in place for a few minutes. There is no clear consensus on the time left in situ—some authors have suggested time ranges from 10 to 30 minutes.[134] This will vary according to the patient's experience with dry needling, as well as their emotional and physiological responses and the degree of presenting symptoms.

Some clinicians apply electrical stimulation to the inserted needles. However, there are no clear guidelines for treatment parameters and no evidence that electrostimulation improves the treatment effect.

Alternatively, the needle can be inserted into the muscle and repeatedly moved in and out (such that it still remains in the sub-dermal region), trying to find specific points that reproduce the patient's local or referred pain, or produce a "twitch" response. Initially, the needle may be "grasped" by the muscle, followed by a gradual relaxation.

Clinicians can apply needles to a number of trigger points during each treatment session. Usually, pain relief lasts 3–4 days after the first session and may be longer following subsequent sessions. Up to 3–4 treatments may be required to eliminate a trigger point, but no single trigger point should be needled more than twice in a week.

Various research studies have compared dry needling with injection of local anaesthetic and various other substances. There is some evidence that dry needling can be just as effective.[318, 319]

### Risks of adverse effects

The most common adverse effect associated with dry needling is soreness in the first 24 hours post-treatment.[307] Application of heat and stretching exercises may minimise this.[320] Aggressive treatment should be avoided until the patient's reaction to dry needling is known. Two studies reported that bleeding (16%), bruising (7.7%), and pain during/after treatment (5.9%) were the most prevalent adverse effects after dry needling.[321] A rare major adverse effect is a pneumothorax: extreme care should be taken while needling the thoracic muscles.

High-quality needles, which are sharper and thinner, may reduce pain during and after treatment. If there is excessive resistance to needle removal, the needle should be removed more slowly.

For patients unfamiliar with or apprehensive about dry needling, it is possible to induce an episode of vasovagal syncope. The risk of this occurring can be minimised by careful patient selection—it is especially important to identify those with needle phobias. The patient's response should be closely monitored during treatment, with constant communication to ensure patient comfort. If at any stage the patient becomes distressed, needles should be removed.

Contraindications to dry needling include bleeding disorders, active infection, blood-borne diseases, allergy to metal, unstable epilepsy and the third trimester of pregnancy.

## Acupuncture

Traditional Chinese acupuncture is based on the theory that illness results from imbalances in energy flow (qi) and fine needles are inserted at specific points on the body to correct these imbalances and restore harmony. Acupuncture interventions are thought to achieve their effect by stimulating acupuncture points (i.e. meridian and non-meridian points) with or without penetration of the skin. The proposed mechanisms of action suggest that stimulating acupuncture points increases endomorphin-1, beta endorphin, encephalin and serotonin levels in the plasma and brain tissue, and causes analgesia, sedation and recovery in motor functions.

Acupuncture has been used in the treatment of sports injuries for hundreds of years yet there is a paucity of high-quality evidence regarding its effectiveness. A few systematic reviews show limited evidence in support of its use.

Yaun showed low-quality evidence that acupuncture has a moderate effect (approximately a 12-point pain reduction on the VAS 100 mm) on relieving pain associated with musculoskeletal disorders. Acupuncture was more effective than sham acupuncture at relieving pain caused by chronic neck pain (high-level evidence), shoulder pain (high), chronic low back pain (moderate), myofascial pain (moderate) and osteoarthritis (low).[322]

One study[323] found that acupuncture was more effective than a placebo for lateral elbow pain in the short term but not in the long term. A more recent study[324] reported that acupuncture was superior to sham acupuncture and conventional therapy (i.e. prednisolone injection, triamcinolone acetonide, lidocaine [lignocaine] injection, oral administration of meloxicam tablets) for lateral elbow pain. However, these conclusions were based on small studies.

A systematic review concluded that traditional acupuncture may be beneficial for carpal tunnel syndrome and Achilles tendinopathy, but not for upper extremity pain and patellofemoral syndrome.[325] Another systematic review of case reports suggested that acupuncture can help relieve short-term pain and promote recovery from dysfunction. Acupuncture has been used as a non-invasive and conservative modality for managing sports injuries such as lateral meniscus rupture, femoral acetabular impingement, ganglion cysts and sports hernia.

There is some evidence of the effectiveness of acupuncture but it is not conclusive. There is a significant placebo effect—as evidenced in studies that used sham acupuncture. The outcome of treatment may depend on the skill and experience of the clinician.

## THERAPEUTIC MEDICATION
### with DANIEL FRIEDMAN and JAMES O'DONOVAN

Therapeutic medication can be helpful in the management of acute and overuse musculoskeletal injuries by alleviating pain, modulating inflammation and augmenting recovery. You should strategically use therapeutic medication to support the particular goals of different management phases with the overall management plan in mind.

Doctors prescribing medications should be fully aware of the current anti-doping regulations for the athlete's sport. These regulations are updated annually by the World Anti-Doping Agency (WADA) and can be found on the WADA website. Clinicians and athletes should regularly check the Global Drug Reference Online (Global DRO) for information about the prohibited status of specific medications in and out of competition based on the current WADA Prohibited List. The Global DRO provides information about therapeutic medications sold in Australia, Canada, Japan, New Zealand, Switzerland, the UK and the US. It also has reference links for other nationalities.

 WADA

 Global DRO

### Analgesics

Analgesics are used to relieve and modulate pain and are often prescribed in the acute phase after injury to reduce pain in conjunction with ice, compression, elevation and splinting or immobilisation. Analgesia may also facilitate early movement, although the medical team should decide the optimal initial load based on the diagnosis. In addition, analgesics may have a role in other management phases to treat central pain sensitisation or to facilitate desired movements in rehabilitation. For more about pain sensitisation, see Chapter 10.

### Paracetamol

Paracetamol (acetaminophen) has an analgesic, antipyretic and potentially anti-inflammatory effect, although it should not be considered an anti-inflammatory medication. Its multidirectional mechanism of action includes inhibition of cyclooxygenase (COX) and action on the endocannabinoid system and serotonergic pathways.[326]

Immediate-release paracetamol can be given as 1000 mg every 4–6 hours to a maximum daily dose of 4 g in adults and children over 12 years of age. Modified-release paracetamol can be given as 1330 mg every 6–8 hours, with a maximum daily dose of 3990 mg. At these doses, paracetamol is usually well tolerated and can be an excellent choice in acute and sub-acute sports injuries. Soluble paracetamol is more quickly absorbed and may be an effective choice for athletes who need a quicker onset of analgesia. At higher doses, paracetamol is hepatotoxic and it may be fatal in overdose.

### Codeine

Codeine is a prodrug that is metabolised by the liver to morphine. As a weak opioid, codeine acts centrally through agonism of opioid receptors. Doctors may consider prescribing codeine and codeine-containing combination analgesics (e.g. codeine combined with paracetamol) in the initial management of an acute painful injury but will be cautious prescribing longer term codeine (and other opioids) due to the risk of addiction, nausea, dizziness and constipation. Interestingly, some individuals lack the enzyme needed to metabolise codeine effectively and so gain limited pain relief while still experiencing all of codeine's adverse effects.[327]

### Tramadol

Tramadol is an opioid and serotonin-noradrenaline (norepinephrine) reuptake inhibitor commonly used to treat moderate to severe acute and persistent pain. Its dual mechanism of action produces a different analgesic effect compared with codeine, with potentially less risk of respiratory depression or addiction than stronger opioids. Tramadol is associated with less constipation but increased nausea, sedation and dizziness, as well as specific risks of serotonin toxicity and reduced seizure threshold.[328]

Recently, there have been concerns that tramadol is being abused by athletes across multiple sports to reduce exertional pain and enable greater work rates. To prevent this potential performance advantage, WADA included tramadol on the 2024 Prohibited List of Substances and Methods.[329]

---

**PRACTICE PEARL**

Prolonged opioid misuse has the potential to lead to dependence, overdose and death.

---

### Emergency analgesia

In severe acute injury, more potent analgesia may be required, often administered using routes with rapid absorption. Be familiar with the medications' indications, methods of administration, and risks. Medication may be administered through inhalation such as methoxyflurane (Penthrox®) or Entonox®, or intravenously, such as morphine or ketamine.

## Non-steroidal anti-inflammatory drugs

Non-steroidal anti-inflammatory drugs (NSAIDs) have analgesic and anti-inflammatory properties. The term "non-steroidal" is used to distinguish these drugs from corticosteroids, which also produce anti-inflammatory effects. NSAIDs inhibit the COX system. COX has a key role in the inflammatory cascade that occurs at the site of acute injury. It converts arachidonic acid to prostaglandins and thromboxane, which are key mediators of inflammation.[330] There are two cyclooxygenase iso-enzymes with different physiological roles:

- COX-1 is associated with maintenance of the gastric mucosa, and COX-1 inhibition with traditional NSAIDs can result in gastritis and ulceration.

- Selective COX-2 inhibitors have been available since 1999 with similar efficacy, but fewer gastrointestinal side effects.

The most commonly prescribed NSAIDs include aspirin, ibuprofen, diclofenac and naproxen, and the COX-2 selective NSAIDs, celecoxib and meloxicam. The normally recommended dosage and frequency of administration varies between the different drugs (Table 24.5).

### Topical NSAIDs

Topical anti-inflammatory preparations are available in creams, gels, sprays and prolonged-release patches. These are effective delivery methods for superficial injuries, with less risk of side effects than orally administered NSAIDs.[331] Overnight patches or wraps (e.g. diclofenac) may be particularly useful in limiting early morning stiffness that may be associated with excessive inflammation.

There is high-level evidence that topical NSAIDs are effective in relieving pain associated with acute musculoskeletal injuries such as sprains, strains and contusions,[331,332] as well as with osteoarthritis.[333] Some of the pain relief they provide can be explained by a powerful placebo effect, which may be greater with topical NSAID administration than with oral administration.

### NSAID use in sport

NSAIDs are widely used in competitive sport, with more than one-third of all athletes at Olympic Games,[334] half of all players at Soccer World Cups[335] and one-quarter of athletes in international track and field athletics[336] reporting in-competition NSAID use. They are commonly used in the treatment of injuries, but both elite and non-elite athletes also take them prior to competition to reduce discomfort from potential future injury or post-exercise soreness.[337-339]

**TABLE 24.5** Commonly used NSAIDs

| Drug | Some trade names | Usual dose (mg) | Half-life | Daily dose |
|---|---|---|---|---|
| Acetylsalicylic acid (ASA) | Aspirin® | 650 | 30 mins | 3–4 |
| Celecoxib | Celebrex® | 100–200 | 11–12 hours | 1–2 |
| Diclofenac | Voltaren® Voltarol® | 25–50 | 1–2 hours | 2–3 |
| Ibuprofen | Brufen® Motrin® Advil® | 400 | 1–2.5 hours | 3–4 |
| Meloxicam | Mobic® | 7.5–15 | 20 hours | 1 |
| Naproxen | Naprosyn Anaprox® | 250–1000 | 12–15 hours | 1–2 |

This practice should be discouraged, as there is no evidence of a reduction in delayed-onset muscle soreness or improved performance with prophylactic NSAIDs. However, player perception and the placebo effect can make behaviour change challenging for team clinicians. Regular NSAID use causes significant health risks for the cardiovascular, renal and gastrointestinal systems. You should educate your athletes about these risks and seek safer alternatives, perhaps from nutraceutical products.

### NSAID use in the treatment of musculoskeletal injuries

NSAIDs are usually an excellent choice in the short-term treatment of inflammatory conditions, such as bursitis or synovitis. However, the impact of NSAIDs on cellular metabolism and the tissues of the musculoskeletal system should be considered by athletes and clinicians using these medications in the treatment or prevention of injury. With this knowledge, NSAIDs may be prescribed for particular injuries or in stages of healing determined by the overall goals of the rehabilitation and management phase.

### NSAIDs and muscle

At a cellular level, NSAIDs probably have a negative effect on both muscle healing following injury and muscle hypertrophy after athletic training.[340] NSAIDs can inhibit protein synthesis[341] and reduce satellite cell activation, which is an essential step in muscle repair and regeneration.[342, 343] Inhibition of protein synthesis after resistance exercise may be limited to COX-1 NSAIDs, as selective COX-2 inhibitors do not limit protein synthesis.[344]

As stated above, NSAIDs are often used by athletes in the treatment and prevention of delayed-onset muscle soreness, but the literature demonstrates very little evidence for a positive effect. NSAIDs have been recommended for use in deep muscle contusions at risk of developing myositis ossificans.[345] Regular indomethacin for more than 7 days is widely used by clinicians for this condition.

NSAIDs are not effective in the treatment of acute muscle tears and cannot be routinely recommended.[346, 347] They may have a short-term role to modulate an excessive early inflammatory response, but as this phase is necessary for appropriate muscle satellite cell activation and initiation of regeneration, their use at this time may be detrimental to overall muscle repair.

### NSAIDs and tendon

In cellular and animal-model studies of tendon tearing or surgical repair, NSAIDs reduce tenocyte proliferation and collagen formation, and therefore limit tendon healing.

However, in clinical studies of acute reactive tendinopathy, NSAIDs may facilitate short-term improvements in pain.[348] One small study also demonstrated improvements in leg stiffness and tendon function following treatment with a COX-2 inhibitor.[349]

It has been suggested that NSAIDs may be useful in acute tendon overload despite (or perhaps because of) the potential negative effects on tenocyte activation.[350] However, you should remember that NSAIDs blunt exercise-induced collagen synthesis within tendon tissue.[351] Therefore, the prescribing of NSAIDs should, as with all medication, be considered within the overall treatment goals of the rehabilitation phase.

Ibuprofen and naproxen inhibit the expression of key ground substance proteins responsible for tendon swelling in in-vitro tendon preparations.[352] Ibuprofen has historically been favoured as a treatment for tendon pathology as it does not have a detrimental effect on ultimate tendon repair, although these findings have come predominantly from rodent models.[353, 354] The relevance of rodent studies for human tendinopathy is often questioned,[355] as they typically investigate healing of previously healthy, completely lacerated tendons.

### NSAIDs and ligament

NSAIDs have a negative impact on collagen formation, fibroblast proliferation and healing in animal models of ligament injury.[356-359] Clinical studies of ligament injuries also do not support their use. One study of patients who underwent ACL reconstruction found increased joint laxity at 6 weeks in the NSAID-treated group compared with the group that had not been prescribed NSAIDs.[360] Another study demonstrated similar analgesic efficacy for paracetamol and NSAIDs (diclofenac) following acute ankle ligament injuries, but found increased oedema at day 3 in the NSAID group.[361]

### NSAIDs and bone

Prostaglandins have an important role in bone metabolism, simulating both osteoblasts and osteoclasts.[362] Numerous animal studies have reported a delay in bone healing with NSAID treatment.[363] COX-2 inhibition has the most negative impact due to inhibition of endochondral ossification.[364-366] Although high-quality clinical studies are lacking, a number of studies suggest a delay in bone healing with NSAID use.[367, 368] In one study, NSAID prescription was associated with a 2.9-fold increase in stress fracture risk within the total Army population. The risk was more than 5-fold greater in soldiers prescribed NSAIDs during basic training.[369]

**PRACTICE PEARL**

NSAIDs are a risk factor for delayed fracture healing.

### Adverse effects of NSAIDs

NSAIDs adversely affect the gastrointestinal, cardiovascular and renal systems, and susceptibility to adverse effects increases with prolonged use and patient age.[370] The most common adverse effects are epigastric pain, nausea and reflux. The risk of experiencing these dyspeptic adverse effects can be lowered by using the minimum effective dose, taking the medication with food, using gastroprotective formulations or concomitantly using proton pump inhibitors (such as omeprazole or pantoprazole) or H2-receptor antagonists (such as ranitidine). Occult gastrointestinal bleeding may contribute to iron depletion so you should enquire about NSAID self-prescribing in athletes with iron deficiency.

**PRACTICE PEARL**

Consider co-administration of proton-pump inhibitors with NSAIDs to reduce NSAID-induced gastrointestinal adverse effects such as ulceration.

Selective COX-2 inhibitors with fewer gastrointestinal side effects are available. In 2004, a number of COX-2 inhibitors (valdecoxib and rofecoxib) were taken off the market, as they were specifically associated with a higher rate of adverse vascular events. COX-2 inhibitors, and some non-selective NSAIDs such as diclofenac, are associated with an increased risk of thrombotic events, and are contraindicated in ischaemic heart and cerebrovascular disease. They should be used with caution in patients with risk factors for cardiovascular events.

Aspirin and other NSAIDs can induce bronchospasm and, in rare cases, this reaction can lead to death in aspirin-sensitive asthmatics. This reaction is generally referred to as aspirin-induced asthma. The reported incidence varies widely affecting between 8% and 20% of adult asthmatics. The incidence is increased in asthmatics who also have chronic rhinitis or a history of nasal polyps. Aspirin-induced asthma is most likely to be encountered in the third or fourth decade of life, although rarely it may occur in childhood.[371]

## Medications for neuropathic pain and central sensitisation

Neuropathic pain is defined as pain arising from a lesion or disease affecting the somatosensory nervous system (Chapter 11).[372,373] It is often characterised clinically by amplified pain responses following noxious or non-noxious stimuli and may be present in combination with true nociceptive pain arising from tissue damage. In patients with neuropathic pain, both peripheral and central neural sensitising mechanisms may be present.

Central sensitisation is defined as "an amplification of neural signalling within the central nervous system that elicits pain sensitivity".[374] It is an important feature of a number of musculoskeletal presentations, including shoulder pain, lateral elbow pain and patellar tendinopathy.[375,376]

Management of neuropathic pain or central sensitisation in musculoskeletal injury should involve a number of interdisciplinary elements as discussed in Chapter 11 and may incorporate therapeutic medication. In addition to the analgesic medication previously discussed, a number of other pharmaceuticals may have a therapeutic role. However, although these medications have demonstrated efficacy in RCTs and meta-analyses, there are no clear predictors of treatment success in patients with neuropathic pain. The therapeutic approach is therefore usually a stepwise trial approach to identify which medications provide the greatest pain relief with the fewest side effects, alongside non-pharmacological measures.

### Tricyclic antidepressants

Tricyclic antidepressants inhibit serotonin and noradrenaline (norepinephrine) neurotransmitter reuptake and block sodium channels. Nortriptyline is most widely used and is the active metabolite of amitriptyline. It is recommended in UK, European, US and Australian guidelines for the treatment of neuropathic pain, although not as a first-line treatment.[377] A starting dose of 10–25 mg is usually prescribed at night to avoid sedative effects during the day. A Cochrane review concluded that there was little evidence to support the use of nortriptyline in neuropathic pain, particularly when compared with duloxetine and pregabalin.[377]

### Serotonin reuptake inhibitors

Duloxetine is a serotonin reuptake inhibitor with moderate to strong evidence for efficacy in the treatment of neuropathic pain.[378,379] A starting dose of 30 mg is often increased to an efficacious treatment dose of 60 mg. Similar to other medications for neuropathic pain, fatigue and difficulty sleeping may be a side effect.

C

### Gabapentin and pregabalin

Gabapentin and pregabalin are gamma-aminobutyric acid analogues that bind to calcium channels on afferent nociceptors and subsequently reduce neurotransmitter release. Pregabalin has a half-life of around 6 hours.[380] The starting dose of pregabalin is usually 75 mg twice daily and this may be titrated to a total daily dose of 300 mg over the course of a week. The most common adverse effect of these medications is fatigue or a mild sedative effect, and they are often not appropriate to take before training sessions. Gabapentin is also available in an extended-release preparation that may be more effective for neuropathic pain but is more likely to impact on the athlete's training program.

### Local anaesthetic patches

Topical lidocaine (lignocaine) patches have demonstrated positive effects in short-term studies on neuropathic pain[378] and may be helpful as a second-line treatment, although the quality of the evidence is weak.

## Counterirritants

Counterirritants produce a superficial irritation in one location that is intended to augment the sensation of irritation in another. The irritation produced is most commonly a result of chemical stimulation of thermal receptors in the skin, which creates a sensation of heat or cold. Topical heat rubs are often used by athletes and mainly act as counterirritants.

Their mechanism of action is probably related to their effect on transient receptor potential channels. These channels are sensitive to heat and initiate a local inflammatory response. Prolonged activation of the nociceptors may lead to a depletion of local neurotransmitters, which may result in a reduction in pain and nociceptor transmission from the site of the more longstanding injury. Counterirritants such as capsaicin or camphor may therefore have a use as mild analgesia before activity, but also potentially in a chronic musculoskeletal injury that demonstrates increased neural sensitisation or elements of neuropathic pain.[378]

## Local anaesthetic injections

Local anaesthetic injections may be used:

- in the treatment of musculoskeletal injury to reduce pain or facilitate movement (Box 24.8)
- on competition day to enable athletes to participate in sport despite injury
- in conjunction with a corticosteroid injection to reduce needle pain.

Local anaesthetics cause a reversible block to conduction along nerve fibres by inhibiting sodium channels, particularly in small neurons. There is a wide variation in speed of onset, duration of action and potency. Lidocaine (lignocaine) and bupivacaine are the most commonly used preparations for musculoskeletal injection. Lidocaine

---

**BOX 24.8** Injection therapy: should injections be performed under ultrasound guidance?

There is high-quality evidence that ultrasound-guided injections (Fig. 24.22) are more accurate than landmark-guided injections;[381] and limited-quality evidence that ultrasound-guided injections are more effective than landmark-guided injections, particularly in large joints, subacromial bursal injections,[382] carpal tunnel and inflamed joints.[383]

Interpretation of research in this area is challenging, as corticosteroid injections are most often studied. Not only might these be an inappropriate therapeutic choice for the particular pathology,[384, 385] but corticosteroid injections have known systemic effects that may affect outcome measures. It is also reasonable to assume that with the development of injectable therapeutic agents without systemic effects, such as hyaluronic acid, these would be unlikely to demonstrate maximal therapeutic efficacy unless accurately positioned. Therefore, if you regularly perform musculoskeletal injections, we recommend that you undertake training in ultrasonography and perform injection therapy under ultrasound guidance.

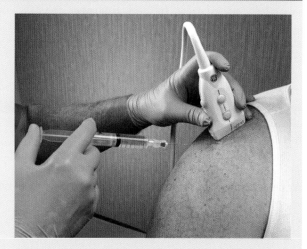

**Figure 24.22** Ultrasound-guided injection; ultrasound training is invaluable for clinicians
USED WITH PERMISSION OF GE HEALTHCARE

(lignocaine) 1% is a quick-acting local anaesthetic that is effectively absorbed from mucous membranes. The duration of anaesthesia is usually 60–120 minutes. Bupivacaine has a slower onset, taking up to 30 minutes for effect, and a longer duration of action, lasting for several hours.

### Local anaesthetics in competition

Anaesthetic injections are sometimes used to enable participation in elite sport in the presence of acromioclavicular joint injuries; finger, rib and sternal injuries; and iliac crest haematomas.[386] We do not recommend intra-articular injections in weight-bearing joints or injecting around tendons of the lower limb, due to the significant risk of further injury to these structures.

### Local anaesthetics in routine musculoskeletal injections

Clinicians traditionally use local anaesthetics in most musculoskeletal injection protocols to reduce the pain of the procedure. However, as local anaesthetics are myotoxic,[387] chondrotoxic[388] and tendon toxic,[389,390] you should reconsider use of local anaesthesia during routine injection protocols.

## Hyaluronic acid

Chondrocytes and synovial cells produce hyaluronic acid, which is the major constituent of synovial fluid and a component of the extracellular matrix of cartilage. Hyaluronic acid is a natural glycosaminoglycan that helps maintains the structural integrity of cartilage and assists with joint mobility and shock absorption. The concentration and molecular weight of hyaluronic acid decreases in osteoarthritic joints.[391] It can also modulate the inflammatory response through inhibition of pro-inflammatory factors, such as arachidonic acid and interleukin-1 (IL-1), which have a degradative effect on the cartilage matrix.

Hyaluronic injection may be useful in the treatment of chondropathy and may reduce pain for a short period due to an anti-inflammatory effect. However, it is generally most effective in the medium and long term,[392] probably through its stimulation of synovial cells to synthesise endogenous hyaluronic acid.

A meta-analysis comparing hyaluronic acid injections with corticosteroid injections suggested greater pain relief following corticosteroid at 2 weeks but not at 4 weeks, and greater benefit of hyaluronic acid at 8–26 weeks.[393] For knee osteoarthritis, there is a lack of high-level evidence demonstrating clinically relevant benefits compared with placebo intra-articular injections.[394] The perceived benefit for the patient should also be weighed against cost and the potential for pain flare-ups.

### Hyaluronic acid in tendons

Hyaluronic acid has been used in the field of hand surgery for several years to provide surface lubrication and enhance postoperative tendon mobility. Hyaluronic acid is a fundamental component of tendon tissue and is thought to help maintain tendon architecture and elasticity. The effect of hyaluronic acid has been studied in various animal models, both in vitro and in vivo. In these models, direct tendon injection of hyaluronic acid maintains tendon structure, decreases the peripheral inflammatory response and promotes healing.

In humans, hyaluronic acid has been studied in various tendinopathies, including rotator cuff, Achilles and patellar. Some initial studies appear promising, but many questions remain unanswered regarding the importance of different hyaluronic acid molecular weights and its metabolism.[395] No high-level evidence currently exists to support hyaluronic acid as a therapeutic approach for tendinopathy.

## Corticosteroids

Corticosteroids are strong anti-inflammatory agents that reduce vascular permeability and leucocyte activation and block inflammatory mediators. The proposed aim of corticosteroid injection is to reduce pain and inflammation to facilitate normal movement and allow therapeutic exercise. However, significant detrimental effects are associated with corticosteroid injection. Therefore, you should consider its use carefully in each case with specific regard to the current evidence, injured tissue and the stage and goals of rehabilitation.

Peritendinous injection of corticosteroids is generally not recommended. Corticosteroids inhibit collagen synthesis and are detrimental to tendon healing. Biopsy studies have demonstrated an increase in the glutamate N-methyl-D-aspartate receptor following corticosteroid injection.[396] This receptor has been associated with chronic pain and tendinopathy.

Studies have demonstrated negative medium- and long-term outcomes from corticosteroid injection around elbow common extensor origin tendinopathy ("tennis elbow"), even compared with a "wait and see" approach.[384] However, there is no doubt that it can provide effective pain relief in the short term and, in certain cases after informed discussions with the athlete and coach, this may be the main priority.

Corticosteroid injection may be of value in inflammatory bursitis with healthy local tendon tissue. However, even in apparently isolated retrocalcaneal bursitis, caution is advised in elite athletes who place high demands on their Achilles tendons.

Intra-articular injection of corticosteroid for joint disease will reduce synovial inflammation and catabolic enzymes that are probably implicated in cartilage breakdown. However, cartilage matrix degradation and reduction in elasticity have been observed following intra-articular injection of corticosteroid into weight-bearing joints.

Corticosteroids are known to be toxic to chondrocytes,[397, 398] particularly if combined with local anaesthetic, and repeated injections may limit cartilage repair and regeneration. The injection of corticosteroid followed by a quick return to running is thought to be more detrimental to the articular cartilage. Injection directed into the inflamed synovial tissue rather than the joint fluid may limit negative impact on the cartilage.

In summary, corticosteroid injection into weight-bearing joints should be approached with caution and considered only in the presence of severe inflammation. There may be a more appropriate and effective role for corticosteroid injection into smaller, non-weight-bearing joints or spinal, facet joints or epidural injections.

### Other adverse effects of corticosteroids

There are other side effects that should be considered and discussed with the patient. Corticosteroid injection may commonly result in skin depigmentation, which may be permanent. Fat atrophy is also a possible effect, particularly in superficial injections. The risk can be minimised by accurate ultrasound-guided needle placement and avoiding steroid placement along the needle track during withdrawal.

Intra-articular injection may result in pericapsular calcification and severe adverse effects such as avascular necrosis, usually following several injections within a short time frame. Joint infection is another significant serious adverse effect so appropriate sterilisation measures with a good injection technique are essential. The presence of an overlying skin infection is a contraindication to injection.

Symptoms are often exacerbated for several days after an injection, so patients should have a short period of rest and modify athletic activity, depending on the joint or location.

### Choice of corticosteroid

The most commonly used corticosteroids are triamcinolone, betamethasone, methylprednisolone, hydrocortisone and dexamethasone. They each have a different duration of action and solubility that should be considered when choosing an appropriate steroid for injection.

Triamcinolone and methylprednisolone are hydrophobic preparations and therefore form microcrystalline suspensions. As a result, they should have a longer duration of action than hydrophilic preparations such as dexamethasone or hydrocortisone, which have a quicker onset of action but reduced duration of effect. Betamethasone, also long acting, is the most potent of these steroids (Table 24.6).

**TABLE 24.6** Potency of common corticosteroids used for injections

| Equivalent dose | Steroid |
|---|---|
| 1.2 mg | Betamethasone (long acting) |
| 1.5 mg | Dexamethasone (long acting) |
| 8 mg | Methylprednisolone (intermediate acting) |
| 8 mg | Triamcinolone (intermediate acting) |
| 40 mg | Hydrocortisone (short acting) |
| 50 mg | Cortisone (short acting) |

According to current guidelines in the US, triamcinolone and methylprednisolone should be avoided in spinal injections due to the risk of inadvertent arterial puncture and subsequent particulate injection with severe vascular consequences. The debate on particulate versus non-particulate spinal injections continues, but there is some evidence to suggest that non-particulate steroids, such as dexamethasone, have an equivalent effect. Therefore, it may be prudent to choose this form of steroid for spinal injections.[399, 400]

The dose and volume of corticosteroid will vary depending on the joint or structure injected. Generally speaking, the dose should decrease as the size of the targeted structure decreases, to allow for space to inject against increasing pressure as the space fills. Many clinicians mix a corticosteroid with a local anaesthetic such as lidocaine (lignocaine) or ropivacaine to provide feedback with accurate anatomical placement of the injection, decrease the propensity of the corticosteroid to cause atrophy and decrease the chance of a local irritant effect of the glucocorticoid. When mixing, you should always weigh up the benefits with the risk of local anaesthetic chondrotoxicity.

## Other medications

### Traumeel

Traumeel® is a herbal preparation of arnica, belladonna, calendula, heparin and echinacea that is reported to have an antioxidant and anti-inflammatory action. Some clinicians inject it in the treatment of muscle injuries[401] and it is also available as a topical anti-inflammatory. Topical application of Traumeel has been demonstrated to be as efficacious as topical diclofenac for pain relief in low-grade acute ankle ligament injuries.[402] There are no clinical studies that evaluate its efficacy in the treatment of muscle injuries.

### Actovegin

Actovegin® is a deproteinated ultrafiltrate of calf serum produced in Austria, a bovine spongiform encephalopathy-free country,[403] and licensed in Europe, China and Russia. It is reported to contain trace elements, amino acids, electrolytes, and carbohydrate and fat metabolites. The active ingredients have still not been identified. In-vitro studies demonstrate that Actovegin may improve the efficacy of energy balance in cells in post-ischaemic metabolic events,[404] by reducing the level of reactive oxygen species and improving intrinsic mitochondrial respiratory capacity in injured muscle fibres.[405] Conflicting opinion and debate on Actovegin as a therapeutic and ergogenic aid continues given the lack of quality clinical evidence to support its use in muscle injury.[406]

### Sclerosant

Early studies reported positive effects of sclerosing injections of polidocanol to areas of neovascularisation, just outside the Achilles tendon.[407,408] However, subsequent studies have not demonstrated positive effects[409,410] and currently it is not widely used in clinical practice.

### Prolotherapy

Prolotherapy is a collective term for the injection of an irritant, usually hyperosmolar dextrose, in the treatment of chronic painful musculoskeletal conditions.[411] The mechanisms of action are not fully understood, but it is claimed that prolotherapy stimulates inflammation and growth factor release, initiates a proliferative response and results in desensitisation through a denervating effect. Stimulation of key growth factors through dextrose prolotherapy for ligamentous laxity and painful tendons could be an inexpensive method of growth stimulation, but there is conflicting evidence regarding its efficacy.[411-413]

A systematic review favoured the use of hypertonic dextrose injection in reducing lateral elbow pain intensity and improving function compared with active controls at 12 weeks post-enrolment.[414]

### Mechanical and high-volume injections

The pain and pathological processes involved in tendinopathy are not fully understood. Some theories suggest that tendon adherence to the adjacent fat pad or neurovascular in-growth from the fat pad is implicated in the pain and pathogenesis of Achilles and patellar tendinopathy. An injection protocol that infiltrates a high volume (up to 40 mL) of normal saline (with a small amount of local anaesthetic, hydrocortisone or aprotinin) to the interface between the tendon and the fat pad has been described.[415-417] While small prospective studies[418,419] have demonstrated positive effects, further high-quality studies are needed.

### Sleep medication, including melatonin

Good restorative sleep is essential for all athletes. It enables tissue adaptation and recovery, as well as improved performance (Chapter 16). Lack of sleep is associated with greater injury risk and can impair performance.[420]

During injury rehabilitation, sleep can be disrupted due to pain and anxiety. For the injured athlete, good-quality sleep is essential for many reasons, but particularly to enable optimal protein synthesis, for soft-tissue healing and strengthening, and neuromotor learning to achieve the biomechanical or skill re-education required during rehabilitation. The sleep strategy for an athlete in rehabilitation is a broad remit for the multidisciplinary team, but medication may have a useful short-term role.

Temazepam is a short acting benzodiazepine with little "hangover" effect, although tolerance can develop quickly. Diazepam is a long-acting benzodiazepine that also reduces muscle spasm and can be of use if this is also a therapeutic goal, most commonly in the treatment of acute low back pain with muscle spasm. Non-benzodiazepine hypnotics, such as zolpidem or zopiclone, have a short duration of action without hangover effects.

The use of sleep medication should be carefully documented in the patient's notes, particularly if there are a number of team physicians. Generally, short-acting hypnotics are the most appropriate for athletes with sleep disturbance associated with acute injury. These will assist with sleep onset and not have a sedative effect the following day.

Patients may develop drug dependence, as with the use of any prescribed medication. Benzodiazepines, antidepressants, antihistamines and anxiolytics all have the potential for abuse and dependence, as well as risks of daytime sleepiness and cognitive impairment. Sleep-walking and sleep-driving have been reported on occasion.

> **PRACTICE PEARL**
>
> Clinicians and athletes should always be aware of the dangers involved with the abuse of sleep medications. When prescribing sleep medication, always warn the patient about interactions with other drugs, including alcohol, which if taken in combination, can cause enhanced central nervous system depression and have catastrophic consequences.

Melatonin supplements, historically used for circadian rhythm disorders, have rapidly increased in popularity.[421] Melatonin is generally considered safe with few adverse effects and low risk of dependence. The hormone helps individuals to fall asleep, but not necessarily stay asleep.[422] In some countries, melatonin is available over the counter (and in very large doses), while in many it is a prescription-only medication.

Timed melatonin can assist sleep latency in athletes suffering from jetlag.[423] Doses range from 0.3 mg to greater than 10 mg. As with all medications, start low, go slow.

### Quinolone antibiotics

Quinolone antibiotics (e.g. ciprofloxacin, ofloxacin) should not be prescribed to athletes unless there is no suitable antibiotic alternative. There is clear evidence linking quinolones with both acute tendon rupture and increased lifetime risk of tendon disease.[424, 425]

### Bisphosphonates

Bisphosphonates inhibit osteoclastic function and therefore increase bone mass. They have been used for many years in the treatment of osteoporosis and decrease fracture risk in this population. The use of bisphosphonates in the prevention or treatment of stress fractures and one-off intravenous injections to reduce bone pain from pubic bone stress (osteitis pubis)[426] in athletes has been proposed.

One study found that bisphosphonates had no effect on stress fracture prevention in military recruits.[427] In stress fracture treatment, a small study suggested bisphosphonates could result in accelerated and safe return to sport.[428]

However, there are several significant concerns regarding the rationale for and use of bisphosphonate treatment in athletes. Bisphosphonates have a half-life of 1–10 years, limit normal microdamage repair and suppress bone remodelling. This may be detrimental to an athlete in the long term, after recovery from the current injury, as normal bone remodelling is essential for adaptation and resilience to normal athletic training.

Short- and long-term use in an elderly osteoporotic population has demonstrated an increased risk of fatigue fractures.[429,430] High-quality studies of the short- and long-term impact of bisphosphonate prescription in athletes are required.

The safety of bisphosphonates in women who may subsequently become pregnant has not been established. In animals, bisphosphonates can cross the placenta and affect foetal bone mineralisation. While there have been no case reports of teratogenic effects in humans, it would seem prudent to avoid the use of bisphosphonates in female athletes.

In addition to these potential adverse effects, there are side effects that should be recognised. Nausea, arthralgia and myalgia for 48 hours after intravenous treatment are common. Oral bisphosphonates can induce oesophageal inflammation and erosion. Osteonecrosis of the jaw has also been reported, usually in patients over 60 years of age with significant dental pathology. However, this risk should be discussed and a dental examination performed prior to bisphosphonate administration.

## NUTRACEUTICALS AND NUTRITION

Dietary supplements and herbal products—often collectively referred to as nutraceuticals—may be used as adjuncts in the treatment of sports injuries. A growing range of nutraceuticals are being studied and recommended to athletes, some ahead of the research curve. As with all interventions, you should weigh the potential benefits against the cost and adverse effects, especially when there may be limited evidence of effect.

### Glucosamine, chondroitin and omega-3 fatty acids

Glucosamine has been advocated as a treatment for cartilage injury. The availability of glucosamine is a rate-limiting step in proteoglycan production.[431] Proteoglycans are large complex molecules that provide elasticity and integrity to cartilage tissue. Numerous basic science studies provide evidence for the important role of glucosamine in supporting joint health. In addition to its role in proteoglycan production, it may also have an anti-inflammatory role and limit chondrocyte apoptosis.

However, despite the promising mechanism of action, there have been conflicting results from randomised trials exploring the effects of glucosamine for patients with osteoarthritis. Meta-analyses have found a negligible effect for symptomatic relief in osteoarthritis, but it may have function-modifying effects in people with knee osteoarthritis when taken for more than 6 months.[432] Compared with placebo, glucosamine may also help stiffness associated with osteoarthritis.[433]

European and international guidelines recommend glucosamine supplementation to treat osteoarthritis at a daily oral dose of 1500 mg. However, high-quality evidence syntheses do not justify its use.[434]

Chondroitin sulphate is a natural glycosaminoglycan and an important component of the extracellular matrix in cartilage. Similar to glucosamine, its use has been recommended in the treatment of inflammatory arthropathy including osteoarthritis and chondropathy.[435] While some analysis of studies suggests chondroitin (alone or in combination with glucosamine) may be better than placebo in improving pain in people with osteoarthritis,[436] there is conflicting evidence suggesting that its symptomatic benefit is minimal at best.[437]

The role of glucosamine and chondroitin in the synthesis of large proteoglycans, such as aggrecan, has led some clinicians to consider their use in patients with tendinopathy.[350] However, early tendon overload is characterised by tendon swelling and aggrecan production,[438] so further increase in large molecule proteoglycan synthesis may be detrimental. Thus it may be appropriate to avoid the use of glucosamine and chondroitin in early, reactive tendinopathy.

Omega-3 polyunsaturated fatty acids have been used as dietary supplements in musculoskeletal injuries, particularly joint injuries, due to their anti-inflammatory and antioxidant effects. Reactive oxygen species are increased in arthritis and associated with cartilage degradation. Some low-level evidence suggests that omega-3 fatty acids may be helpful in reducing morning stiffness in patients with osteoarthritis.[439]

## Vitamin D

Vitamin D is a hormone with a wide range of important physiological effects for health and athletic performance. It has an essential role in the maintenance of muscle strength and mass, particularly for type II muscle fibres and in optimal bone health. Correction of vitamin D deficiency can improve muscle strength and reduce the risk of stress fractures.[440, 441] Vitamin D deficiency is prevalent in elite athletes, and screening and treatment of deficiency are recommended.[442]

## Polyphenols

Green tea and other polyphenol-rich foods such as dark cherry juice may have an important future role in the management of musculoskeletal injuries. Some basic science and animal studies demonstrate a positive impact on tendon and cartilage healing.[443, 444] Catechins, the major active component of green tea, may help healthy joints and skeletal muscle,[445] but further clinical studies are required to determine their clinical impact, as well as the impact of other polyphenol supplements.

## Turmeric

Turmeric, also known as curcumin (the bioactive component), has been used for centuries as a staple spice in many countries, as well as a traditional treatment in Chinese and Ayurvedic medicine.[446] Its range of anti-inflammatory, antioxidant and antimicrobial properties[446] has led to growing interest in using turmeric as an alternative to NSAIDs in different forms of arthritis and as an analgesic agent. A 2016 systematic review of RCTs found that 8–12 weeks of standardised turmeric extract (typically 1000 mg/day of curcumin) may reduce pain and inflammation-related symptoms from knee osteoarthritis, and even result in similar improvements in symptoms as ibuprofen and diclofenac.[447]

## Cannabinoids

Recent and increasing general legalisation of cannabis in different countries has sparked interest in using cannabis-based compounds in musculoskeletal medicine. The cannabis plant contains more than 450 different compounds, with more than 100 classified as cannabinoids that have an effect on cannabinoid receptors in the body. The two most researched cannabinoids are delta 9-tetrahydrocannabinol (THC, the main psychoactive component) and cannabidiol (CBD).

Current available evidence does not demonstrate that any cannabinoids or cannabis products, at a defined dose, reduce pain intensity in any studied musculoskeletal condition. The RCT evidence base for using cannabinoids is of low quality, and there is no high-level evidence to inform the practice of using THC or CBD to treat pain, disability, emotional distress or sleep.[448] To date, the US Food and Drug Administration has approved only highly purified CBD for the treatment of epilepsy.[449] Interestingly, CBD may enhance bone health and metabolism, while THC has an inhibitory effect and may delay bone healing.[450]

Cannabis is listed as Prohibited In-Competition under class S8: Cannabinoids on WADA's Prohibited List. Medicinal cannabis must be accessed through a legal prescription and the prescribing clinician must apply for a Therapeutic Use Exemption for that athlete. WADA no longer lists CBD as a prohibited substance, recognising that it is not psychoactive. However, many cannabinoid products contain a mix of THC and CBD, so any athlete consuming cannabis (or hemp in food products or protein supplementation) must be aware of the risk of contamination.

## Collagen

Collagen is the main structural protein in the extracellular matrix of different connective tissues and is the most abundant protein in the body, constituting up to 35% of body protein content.[451] More than 90% of this collagen is type 1.[452] Collagen is produced by fibroblasts and is made up of amino acids (mostly glycine, proline and hydroxyproline) bound together to form a triple helix of elongated fibrils known as a collagen helix, which provides structure and support to various body tissues (e.g. tendons by weight are up to 80% collagen).[453]

Hydrolysed collagen and collagen peptide formulas are available in pill or powder form, usually derived from pigs, cows or fish, each with differing amino acid content. However, interestingly, there may not be any difference in the plasma availability of amino acids after consumption of collagen from different animal sources.[454] Collagen is commonly combined with vitamin C, thought to be necessary in the synthesis of collagen.

Research on collagen peptides and gelatine products has mainly explored the effect that supplementation may have on bone and joint health,[455, 456] as well as in tendinopathy. In osteoarthritis, it may reduce subjective stiffness, but it has not been found to have an effect on pain or functional limitation.[457] Small-scale studies suggest that collagen supplementation may boost tendon cross-sectional area and have variable effects on tendon stiffness.[458, 459] Exercise is necessary to boost collagen uptake and production, so studies often assess collagen's impact on tendons when combined with resistance programs, which also positively impact tendon health.

When consumed orally, collagen is broken down into amino acids, which are then distributed wherever the body most needs protein. Positive effects from collagen may only be seen if an athlete is consuming sufficient protein for their exercise demands. In general, research into the clinical effects of collagen and more high-quality studies are needed to determine optimal formulations, doses and treatment protocols.

## Nutrition

Adequate total energy intake and appropriate dietary intake are the main nutritional strategies during rehabilitation for injured athletes, along with intake of supplements that have the potential to help.[460] Athletes recovering from injury must be wary of falling into the trap of drastically reducing their energy intake due to their reduced exercise load and as a result becoming susceptible to inadequate intake of essential nutrients.

Increasing protein intake during recovery is one of the first strategies in reducing muscle loss and accelerating the healing process during the injury period.[461] Protein intake should be increased to prevent both muscle loss and anabolic resistance to protein during immobilisation after injury.[462] Increasing protein intake from the recommended 0.8 g/kg/day to 2.3 g/kg/day reduces muscle loss in states of negative energy balance.[463] However, one study showed that increasing protein intake to 1.6 g/kg/day for women on bed rest for 60 days did not prevent muscle loss, whereas a combination of aerobic and resistance exercises prevented muscle loss.[464]

There is limited evidence to support the use of supplements such as creatine, collagen, anti-oxidants (e.g. vitamins C, D and E), gelatine, omega-3 supplements such as fish oil, polyphenols, flavonoids and branched chain amino acids in promoting healing following an injury.[465]

While the inflammatory process is an essential part of the healing response, excessive acute inflammation and chronic low-grade inflammation play an important role in musculoskeletal injury as well as chronic disease. Foods such as sugars and processed carbohydrates, and omega-6 polyunsaturated fats such as seed oils, are considered pro-inflammatory. In certain individuals, dairy products and foods containing gluten, lectins, oxalates, phytates and histamines are also inflammatory. In contrast, foods rich in omega-3 such as oily fish (e.g. salmon, mackerel, sardines), seeds (e.g. hemp and chia) and nuts (e.g. walnuts), and to a lesser extent pasture-raised and omega-3-enriched eggs, as well as meat and dairy products from grass-fed animals, are anti-inflammatory.

There is some evidence that changing from a standard low-fat, high-carbohydrate diet to a low-carbohydrate or ketogenic diet has beneficial effects on osteoarthritis.[466, 467] The incidence of tendinopathy and tendon tears is increased in those with type 2 diabetes, which is not surprising given that glucose is inflammatory in nature. Increased blood glucose levels in the pre-diabetic range are also associated with tendon damage.[468]

The role of diet in promoting recovery from injury is probably underappreciated. Avoiding pro-inflammatory foods and promoting anti-inflammatory foods is likely to enhance recovery and should be included as part of the treatment regimen.

## AUTOLOGOUS BLOOD, BLOOD PRODUCTS AND CELL THERAPY

Autologous blood, blood products such as platelet-rich plasma, and cell therapy are increasingly being used by clinicians in the area of musculoskeletal medicine known as regenerative medicine. These autologous products secrete many growth factors that have the potential to influence the healing of bone, cartilage, ligament, tendon and muscle injuries. This is based on laboratory studies showing increased cell proliferation and collagen synthesis, a reduction in inflammation and stimulation of a well-ordered angiogenesis.[469]

### Autologous blood injections

The main rationale behind treatment with autologous blood injections is the presence of various growth factors in blood with a potential healing effect. Blood is usually drawn from the patient's arm vein and injected directly into the injured tissue. The amount of blood injected depends on the location and type of injury, but 3 mL or 6 mL is most common.[470]

The procedure is used mainly in tendinopathies, despite a lack of evidence of efficacy.[471] Initial randomised trials show efficacy of autologous blood injections in comparison with corticosteroid injections,[472-474] but not compared with placebo or standard physical therapy.[475, 476]

### Platelet-rich plasma

Platelet-rich plasma is the product derived when autologous whole blood is centrifuged to separate out a preparation with a very high platelet content. The preparation is rich in plasmatic and platelet α-granule derived growth factors, as well as many thousands of other substances.[372] Platelets contain a host of physiologically active substances including locally active growth factors such as platelet-derived growth factor, transforming growth factor, platelet factor interleukin, platelet-derived angiogenesis factor, vascular endothelial growth factor, epidermal growth factor, insulin-like growth factor and fibronectin.

Compared with an autologous blood injection, a larger amount of blood is withdrawn for the preparation of a platelet-rich plasma injection. The blood is placed into a tube, which in turn is placed in a centrifuge that spins about 3000 times a minute, with the length of time depending on the protocol. The platelets separate from the other blood components and can be aspirated for injection. Many different versions of platelet-rich plasma are described, each depending on the duration, force and number of spins. Several sub-classifications have been made, which can serve as a basis for evaluation of efficacy in clinical studies.[477]

Platelet-rich plasma is used by many clinicians primarily in the treatment of tendinopathies at the lateral elbow, rotator cuff, patella or Achilles, and secondly in the management of osteoarthritis (e.g. knee or ankle). Currently, there is limited evidence to support its use.

Early trials comparing platelet-rich plasma with corticosteroid injection were encouraging,[478] but subsequent trials using appropriate placebo injection therapies such as normal saline have been unconvincing. Systematic reviews of the use of platelet-rich plasma in lateral elbow pain,[479] rotator cuff injuries,[480,481] frozen shoulder,[481] patellar tendinopathy,[482] Achilles tendinopathy,[483] plantar fasciopathy[484] and following knee surgery such as ACL reconstruction[485] and meniscal repair[486] have generally failed to show a positive clinical effect.

Many systematic reviews and meta-analyses have found positive results for platelet-rich plasma in relieving pain and improving function in knee osteoarthritis. Platelet-rich plasma with an activation method such as calcium chloride or thrombin is suggested to be more effective than platelet-rich plasma without for knee osteoarthritis.[487] However, more high-quality randomised studies with a low risk of bias are needed for this indication.[488]

## Mesenchymal stem cells

Mesenchymal stem cells are found throughout the adult body. Several different tissue sources have been explored including bone marrow, adipose tissue, synovial fluid, dental tissue, skin and foreskin, salivary glands and perinatal tissues, but the best source remains unclear.

Traditionally, bone marrow has been the common source, but adipose tissue yields a larger number of mesenchymal

stem cells and eases their harvest. Human umbilical cord perivascular cells are a rich source of mesenchymal stem cells, are closer to an embryonic cell lineage and show increased differentiation capacity. The source of mesenchymal stem cells depends on the ease of harvest and the differentiation capacity towards a given tissue.[489]

The use of mesenchymal stem cell therapy for articular cartilage regeneration through direct tissue growth, differentiation and inflammation modulation in the treatment of osteoarthritis is promising. The cells migrate to injured sites, inhibit pro-inflammatory pathways and promote tissue repair by releasing paracrine signals and differentiating into specialised chondrocytes.

Multiple clinical trials have demonstrated a significant improvement in both pain and joint function, inflammatory cell reduction within a joint and articular cartilage growth, as well as patient safety. However, high-quality evidence supporting this beneficial role is lacking due to the limited number of studies, small populations tested and use of various derivatives.

Two meta-analyses showed that compared with existing treatments for knee osteoarthritis, mesenchymal stem cells were found to be safe and may reduce pain and improve articular function.[490,491] The safety of the therapy has long been discussed and confirmed by numerous clinical trials. No significant adverse complications have been reported in any of the reviewed literature and all studies indicated that mesenchymal stem cell injections in the knee are safe.[490]

Mesenchymal stem cell therapy has been proposed as a good candidate for tendon healing due to its potential ability to promote proliferation of adipose-derived stem cells and tenogenic differentiation. However, research evidence has been conflicting and there are currently insufficient high-quality studies to provide an evidence basis for its use.[492-495]

## Research versus clinical experience

Blood products, particularly platelet-rich plasma, are widely used by many experienced clinicians who are convinced of their efficacy. For more than 20 years, research has largely failed to support the clinicians' experiences. There may well be a substantial placebo effect.

We appreciate that many variables can influence the effectiveness of injection treatment in musculoskeletal disorders. In the case of autologous blood, blood products and cell therapy, the exact constitution of the product might influence the treatment outcome. There is considerable variation in the product used and no widely accepted standard.

The number of injections and the interval between the injections in the case of multiple injections also probably influences clinical outcomes. Some clinicians advocate 2 or 3 platelet-rich plasma injections at weekly or fortnightly intervals, while others use a single treatment. A period of rest of 48–72 hours for the affected body part following injection is advocated by some clinicians and this may be a key factor in those clinicians believing that they see good outcomes.

Ultrasound guidance can be helpful for improving delivery of these products to the injury site, but in superficial injuries or in the presence of clear anatomical landmarks, this is not always necessary.

Further research is needed to determine whether these products are effective for some conditions. If they are proven effective, research would aim to discover the factors that make up blood or cell-derived products, the ideal number of treatments and how frequently treatment is required.[496]

## AND FINALLY …

This chapter has introduced you to the fundamentals of treating musculoskeletal injuries. From this foundation, you can hone your knowledge and skills and create specific treatments taking the patient very much into account. And of course, *Clinical Sorts Medicine: Managing Injuries* provides suggestions as to which treatments are best for specific injuries from head to toe.

We leave you with an infographic summary of a systematic review[497] that suggests 11 factors might constitute best-practice care of musculoskeletal conditions (Fig. 24.23). What do you think of them? How will they hold up as the tide of evidence rolls in?

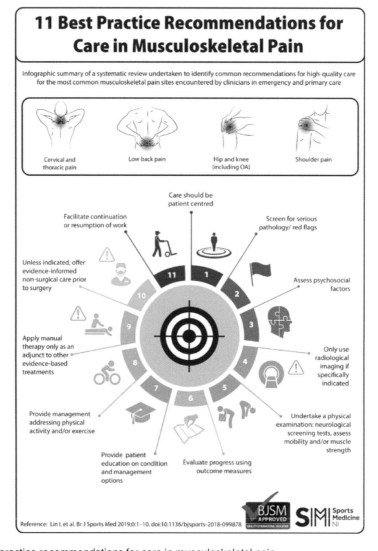

**Figure 24.23** 11 best-practice recommendations for care in musculoskeletal pain
Source: Lin I, Wiles L, Waller R, et al. What does best practice care for musculoskeletal pain look like? Eleven consistent recommendations from high-quality clinical practice guidelines: systematic review. *Br J Sports Med* 2020;54:79–86.

## KEY POINTS

- Rehabilitation is a holistic process aimed at returning an athlete to their pre-injury level of performance. Rehabilitation is composed of various treatments, aimed at addressing a specific issue.

- Treatment of acute musculoskeletal injury is an evolving science. We have progressed from PRICE to POLICE and PEACE & LOVE, reflecting the importance of early mobilisation and optimal loading.

- An initial period of immobilisation helps minimise tissue damage after acute injury. This period should be as short as possible, as early mobilisation and optimal loading shorten the overall length of rehabilitation.

- Certain treatments and behaviours should be avoided in the early window after injury, including applying heat, consuming alcohol and overloading the tissues.

- The cornerstone of a successful injury rehabilitation plan is active therapeutic exercise. The process of mechanotransduction explains how stress applied to the body (bone, tendon, muscle, cartilage) results in tissue strengthening and regeneration.

- Many treatments are used in the rehabilitation of sport-related injuries. Broadly speaking, these should complement a core, comprehensive exercise-based program. Few treatments are as effective in isolation as they are when paired with good exercise prescription.

- Blood flow restriction may be used in individuals who would benefit from resistance training but cannot sustain heavy loads. There are important contraindications to its use.

- Manual therapies can be an effective adjunct to an exercise-based rehabilitation plan. The mechanism of their action is not well understood and the benefits tend to be short-lived.

- Joint mobilisation may be performed by the clinician with appropriate training or self-administered by an athlete who has been educated on proper technique. Generally, the goal is to improve range of motion.

- Joint manipulation may be used by trained clinicians to improve joint mobility. Improvements tend to be transient and hard to quantify. There is a long list of contraindications to performing joint manipulation and special care should be taken at the cervical spine.

- Soft-tissue therapy, in its various forms, is a common treatment used by athletes. The type of massage chosen should be specific to the clinical goal. Evidence supports its use for some musculoskeletal conditions, but not all. Massage paired with exercise-based therapies may increase its effectiveness.

- Taping and bracing are among the most widely used treatments in sport. The overall goal is typically to restrict an athlete's range of motion, but there may be neurophysiological effects as well. Evidence of its effectiveness is unclear and conflicting, so a trial-and-error approach should be considered.

- Electrophysical agents are commonly seen in highly resourced sports injury settings. Few are as effective when used alone as they are when paired with high-quality exercise.

- You should be able to explain the proposed mechanism of action for any electrophysical agent that you use and to communicate the realistic expected benefits, the significant limitations and any relevant contraindications.

- Where an athlete can administer an electrophysical treatment themselves, encourage them to do so. This can help provide a sense of control over their treatment.

- The evidence for most electrophysical agents is of varying quality, is generally conflicting and sometimes fails to demonstrate effects superior to a placebo. Low-intensity pulsed ultrasound for the treatment of acute fracture has the best available evidence to support its effectiveness.

C

- The evidence for any treatment's effectiveness tends to be condition specific. Because a modality works for one condition does not mean that it is effective at treating a seemingly similar condition.

- Dry needling and acupuncture share similar physiological principles but have important contextual and cultural differences. There is generally good evidence to support the use of both treatments for a list of common musculoskeletal conditions.

- Medications are commonly dispensed for a range of sport-related injuries and illnesses. Medication should be dispensed according to the clinician's scope of practice, in accordance with legal restrictions and banned substance lists.

- Commonly used medications, including those available over the counter, can carry significant risks. For example, the prophylactic use of NSAIDs prior to training/exercise should be discouraged.

- There is some evidence to support the use of nutraceuticals and supplements in an athletic population. There are also many supplements with no evidence of effect. Nutraceutical and supplement use should be considered in the wider context of an athlete's diet.

- The use of autologous blood products is becoming popular among high-performance athletes. There is some evidence to support the use of platelet-rich plasma and mesenchymal stem cells for a narrow list of musculoskeletal conditions. However, high-quality evidence of their effectiveness often fails to show effects superior to a placebo.

- In any rehabilitation program, treatments should be selected in a shared decision-making process with the athlete, who has been educated about the risks, benefits, effectiveness and contraindications of each treatment.

## REFERENCES

References for this chapter can be found at www.mhprofessional.com/CSM6e

## ADDITIONAL CONTENT

 Scan here to access additional resources for this topic and more provided by the authors

## CHAPTER 25

# Athlete education

with PAUL BLAZEY, ANTHONY GOFF and JEREMY LEWIS

*Injuries are our best teachers.*

SCOTT JUREK (US ULTRAMARATHON RUNNER)

## CHAPTER OUTLINE

Why educate the athlete?

Theories, models and frameworks relevant to athlete education

Common topics covered in education programs

Preparing successful education sessions for athletes

Using external learning resources: choose wisely

Evaluating the success of your education

When your education program isn't working

## LEARNING OBJECTIVES

By the end of this chapter you should be able to:

- explain the purpose of athlete education
- identify relevant frameworks, theories and models used to structure athlete education
- assess an athlete's needs to inform the education you intend to provide
- construct an athlete education session that is patient-centred and individualised
- evaluate the impact of your athlete education session.

## WHY EDUCATE THE ATHLETE?

Although this chapter is titled "athlete education" it could also be titled "athlete communication". The chapter complements Chapter 4 and touches on aspects covered in Chapter 2.

Much of what we discuss is based on what practitioners (and others outside the healthcare environment) have role-modelled to us and what we have observed as best practice with athletes and patients across many settings. What we know is that when an athlete is injured or seeks care from the healthcare team, education is essential to help them to make sense of their situation, identify their prognosis, understand management options and/or facilitate behaviour change.

Athlete education sessions, often delivered casually as part of a conversation (Fig. 25.1), will undoubtedly focus on myriad related topics, all of which are important and relevant. Topics need to be provided and presented in a time frame, format and environment that is appropriate for the individual athlete. This includes considering the multitude of psychosocial and contextual factors relevant to the individual, their support team and possibly their future career.

Education following an injury will probably include open and honest discussion of any potential harms associated with healthcare interventions (diagnostic and treatment), intended benefits of an intervention, required rehabilitation commitments, potential restrictions from training and competition, as well as anticipated time frames and expected outcomes. Examples of common questions that support athlete education are given in Box 25.1.

---

**BOX 25.1** Examples of common questions that may need to be addressed as part of an education program

**Practitioner to athlete**
- What is it like living with these symptoms?
- What are your concerns?
- What are your immediate and longer-term needs?
- What (if anything) have you been told about your symptoms?

**Athlete to practitioner**
- Why am I hurting?
- What diagnostic test or treatment do you suggest?
- When do you think I will get better?
- How will I/we stop it from happening again in the future?

---

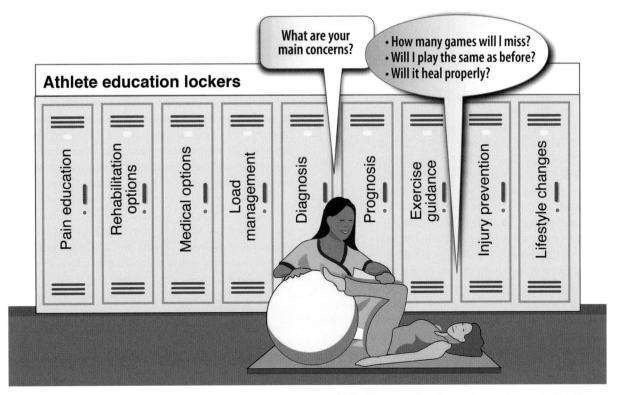

**Figure 25.1** Common concerns raised by an athlete may require multiple different education topics, as designated by the lockers in this image
ARTWORK BY VICKY EARLE. PHOTO CONTRIBUTOR: ISTOCK/ELENA ISTOMINA; ISTOCK/UNITONEVECTO

When provided appropriately and with a "consistent voice" across healthcare providers and all forms of media, education may facilitate a strong non-judgmental therapeutic alliance between the athlete and the healthcare team. The mutual and bi-directional nature of the trust (i.e. athlete to healthcare team, healthcare team to athlete) is paramount to support behavioural change, if required, as part of the agreed management plan. However, education provided poorly or inconsistently may lead to confusion, a breakdown of trust and/or poor engagement with the management plan.[1]

Patient education for non-athletes focuses on health behaviours such as smoking cessation, diet and nutrition, hydration, sleep, reducing anxiety, myth busting, reducing sedentary behaviours, how to deal with unhealthy stress, how safely to increase physical activity, and how to maintain goals when they have been reached. Other important topics include how to manage relapses in symptoms, behavioural change interventions and when to seek care.

These educational priorities are also relevant for many athletes—for instance, avoiding sedentary behaviour in the off-season (especially where load management is a consideration), being consistent with diet and nutrition for health (and performance), and managing sleep when travelling for competition across multiple time zones.

It should be noted that the narrow focus of education as simply "providing information" (e.g. to help an athlete understand surgical versus non-surgical treatment options) does not encompass how practitioners provide education in practice. Practitioners often engage in education discussions to address other aspects of the athlete's beliefs or behaviours, such as their emotive reaction to an injury, or environmental factors that may contribute to the risk of re-injury or illness. Indeed, addressing psychosocial factors has been identified as an important consideration for elite athletes recovering from or learning to manage their low back pain.[1]

The majority of the research literature on patient education includes education within a multi-modal management plan, so we don't know how the education is being provided, or by whom. It is also difficult to emulate contextual factors in the delivery of education as they may be tied to the practitioner's personality, attitudes and beliefs. Therefore, the effect of education as an intervention is often shrouded in mystery as a result of combining it with other interventions and the inability to remove the education component from all of the contextual factors that surround it.

Including education as part of a multi-modal management plan obscures what it is about the education that affects the patient's overall care. This confusion makes it difficult to decide between the many different education topics, as we don't know whether certain types of information or discussions between athlete and practitioner

promote better outcomes. Figure 25.1 illustrates some of the potential "athlete education lockers" that you may need to go to in your athlete education sessions to address different aspects of their care.

What we know (implicitly) is that education is vital to provide context to the rehabilitation process. Athlete education, for instance, is an essential component of shared decision making during the return-to-sport process (see Chapter 28). Also, despite the complexity of factors that affect education for the athlete, and the uncertainty over what information has the biggest impact, education programs are often included in guideline-based care (e.g. Achilles tendinopathy guidelines), and education is consistently one of the most recommended interventions across all musculoskeletal conditions.[2-4]

Although we draw from research and experience with patient education, this chapter focuses on "athlete education". We address the different context in which athlete education takes place compared with a traditional healthcare environment. We therefore refer to "athlete education" for the remainder of this chapter.

## THEORIES, MODELS AND FRAMEWORKS RELEVANT TO ATHLETE EDUCATION

Athletes are the experts on their own health and the experience of their condition. Practitioners, on the other hand, are skilled at directing athletes towards resources they may not have considered or highlighting aspects of their illness/injury recovery or prevention that they may be unaware of. Understanding the theoretical concepts or constructs that an education program may target will help you to decide what education topics will carry the greatest impact. This is where theoretical knowledge can support the practical application of an athlete education program.

The following three models and theories are based on general healthcare contexts and may require some modification for sports and exercise medicine. They serve to provide an overview of who, why and potentially what to target when you choose to educate an athlete as part of their health and/or recovery journey.

### Health belief model

The health belief model attempts to identify symptomatic patients who are the most ready to benefit from education.[5] It comprises six questions:

1. What is the patient's perception of the severity of their illness or injury?
2. What is the patient's perception of their susceptibility to an illness or injury?

3. Does the patient believe the costs/potential adverse effects of treatment outweigh the consequences of their injury or illness?

4. Does the patient report any barriers that would stop them engaging in treatment?

5. Is there a physical and/or emotional cost to treatment?

6. Does the patient have information cues that support action towards treating the injury or illness (e.g. family supportive of treatment, teammates with stories of positive outcomes)?

Addressing relevant combinations of these questions would commonly form the basis of an education program. For example, a football player who has suffered a previous hamstring injury is more susceptible to a subsequent hamstring injury.[6] Therefore, it may be necessary to assess the player's perception of their recovery and provide education on the cost/benefit of undergoing a prehabilitation program (e.g. taking additional time to perform eccentric-loading exercises). The information provided should be reinforced periodically.

Reinforcement of the benefits of prehabilitation (via an educational approach) may be particularly important. One-off education sessions are unlikely to promote long-term behaviour change (i.e. adherence to an exercise-based intervention). Anecdotal evidence suggests that players find it easier to engage in team-based approaches. Therefore, involving teammates or family members in the education process, or having teammates also demonstrate the desired new behaviour, can increase the chances of the educational approach being successful (e.g. sustained improvement of a healthy behaviour).

### Self-efficacy theory

Self-efficacy theory is based on the work of eminent psychologist Albert Bandura (1925–2021). Self-efficacy is defined as a person's belief in their ability to control their actions and the events in their life. High self-efficacy often results in strong and confident athletes. However, an injury or illness may affect an athlete's short- or long-term self-efficacy in performing their specific sport-related activities, and as such, self-efficacy support is an important consideration for athlete education programs.

Self-efficacy may play an important role in an athlete's readiness to return to sport post injury, and the use of healing imagery—delivered as part of an education program—has been recommended to improve self-efficacy in rehabilitating athletes.[7]

### Locus of control

It is vital that you encourage athletes to feel in control of their situation. Locus of control theory is a psychological concept that refers to an individual's belief about the main causes of events in their life. It is the degree to which people believe that they, as opposed to external forces, have control over the outcome of life events. The theory is based on the belief that individuals can make choices that affect their health outcomes. Locus of control has been adapted to the health setting with the rationale that encouraging an internal locus of control is important in supporting self-care and self-management.[8]

Some researchers have speculated that a strong internal locus of control may be associated with superior sporting performance,[9, 10] but the jury is still out. However, encouraging athletes to develop an internal locus of control by providing knowledge, reassurance and support to address barriers to their return to sport may help them with their rehabilitation journey.

## Using the Theoretical Domains Framework to design an education program

To design an effective education program, you should identify gaps in the athlete's understanding of their condition. You should also discuss behaviours that may need to change to prevent injury or improve performance. The Theoretical Domains Framework was developed as a tool to design and facilitate practitioner behaviour change interventions, but it has also been used to understand an individual's behaviour and inform appropriate interventions.[11, 12]

The Theoretical Domains Framework contains 84 constructs covering various cognitive, affective, social and environmental factors—grouped into 14 overarching domains. Table 25.1 shows a simplified version of these 14 domains, with examples of how to apply constructs to education in sports and exercise medicine.[13]

The context in Table 25.1 suggests that there is considerable overlap between what we traditionally consider a therapeutic intervention (e.g. training for skill development) and what we believe constitutes an "education intervention". All interventions require education to support their implementation.

While it is important to understand all 14 domains, it is far more common that clinical interactions focus on one or two of these domains within a single session. Providing information related to a condition and its treatment (the knowledge domain) is likely to underpin early clinical encounters with an athlete. However, consistent re-evaluation of goals (what the athlete wants) and intentions (what they plan to do), and maintenance of their confidence and optimism, are likely to require ongoing evaluation and small amounts of education throughout the rehabilitation process.

**C**

**TABLE 25.1**  Adapted version of the 2012 Theoretical Domains Framework and how clinicians can put it into practice

| Domain | Domain made relevant to the sports and exercise clinical context | Examples of constructs from the Theoretical Domains Framework | Examples of how clinicians can apply the framework with athletes |
|---|---|---|---|
| **Knowledge** | Knowledge | • Knowledge of the task environment | Provide knowledge on injury or illness, prognosis, rehabilitation, etc. |
| **Skills** | Skills | • Skill development<br>• Practice<br>• Ability | Establish what skills are needed to rehabilitate or to avoid future injury (e.g. working on developing new movement patterns) |
| **Social or professional role and identity** | Professional identity | • Professional identity<br>• Leadership | Support the athlete to stay part of the team during the rehabilitation process |
| **Beliefs about capabilities** | Confidence | • Self-confidence<br>• Perceived competence<br>• Self-efficacy | Provide reassurance, emotional intelligence and support to identify where current capabilities are |
| **Beliefs about consequences** | Risk tolerance | • Outcome expectancies<br>• Anticipated regret | Provide reassurance, emotional intelligence and support to identify real (not imagined) risks about consequences (e.g. return to sport) |
| **Emotion** | Emotion | • Fear<br>• Anxiety and/or depression<br>• Stress | Deliver education to address stress related to playing pressure, pressure to perform, etc. |
| **Optimism** | Optimism | • Optimism<br>• Pessimism | Try to provide an optimistic outlook when an injury occurs; see the positives and the negatives—to provide balance |
| **Reinforcement** | Competitive edge | • Rewards<br>• Incentives | Add an element of competition into rehabilitation, to provide added motivation |
| **Intentions** | Intentions (what I plan to do) | • Stability of intentions | Assess whether the athlete is ready to change, and whether they feel that they're ready for rehabilitation or to try to change behaviours like their sleep pattern |
| **Goals** | Goals (what I want) | • Goal/target setting<br>• Action planning<br>• Prioritisation | Set short- and long-term goals to help track the rehabilitation journey and set out what a shared vision of success will look like |
| **Memory, attention and decision processes** | Decision making | • Decision making<br>• Attention control | As the athlete proceeds through rehabilitation, determine whether they need to include more neurocognitive processes to simulate game-play[13] |
| **Environmental context and resources** | Performance environment | • Organisational culture/climate<br>• Barriers and facilitators to change | Consider anything that can help prevent the athlete from being re-injured; return the athlete to a safe space physically and emotionally to perform at their best |
| **Social influences** | Influencers | • Social norms and/or comparisons and/or support<br>• Group conformity<br>• Power | Bring in teammates, family, coaches and other support staff to help provide a unified educational message |
| **Behavioural regulation** | Habits | • Self-monitoring<br>• Habit breaking | Provide ways to monitor health, (e.g. was nutrition or sleep a factor in the injury process?); use automated data processes (e.g. wearable technology) to support and reinforce the health education process |

Figure 25.2 demonstrates how education targets may change in importance over the course of the rehabilitation journey.

It is important to be flexible in your approach and the topics you cover at any given time. An excessive focus on the knowledge domain when the athlete has an emotional need will lead to frustration for both you and the athlete.

**PRACTICE PEARL**

The Theoretical Domains Framework may be used by the healthcare team to spotlight potential areas where an athlete may benefit from an education program.

## Using the COM-B model to choose a target with your education program

While the Theoretical Domains Framework includes a comprehensive list of domains and constructs that you may wish to target with an education program, it doesn't help determine what that education program should include for each athlete. One model to help you decide what will benefit an athlete most is the COM-B model (capability, opportunity, motivation and behaviour). This model has been suggested as a guide to improve long-term health behaviours in the general population.[14]

When using the COM-B model with an athlete, taking a history (Chapter 19) will help you to determine whether their concerns relate to one of the three key areas in the model.

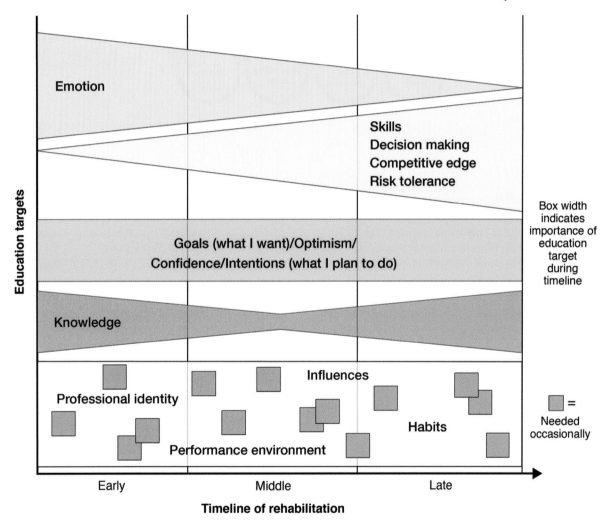

**Figure 25.2** Education targets may change in importance over the course of an athlete's rehabilitation journey: this will vary depending on the athlete and the context

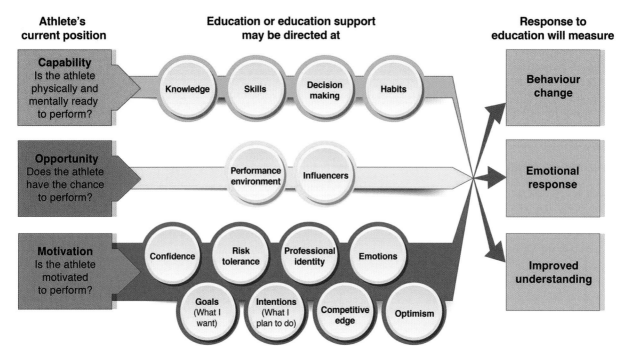

**Figure 25.3** Using the COM-B model to decide which of the 14 constructs from the Theoretical Domains Framework is most relevant to the athlete's educational needs

For example, if the athlete is concerned that they won't return to their previous level of performance, this would indicate that they have a possible "motivation" concern (Fig. 25.3).

You may tailor an education intervention to target the athlete's emotive response, as well as potentially affect a change in their confidence. For example, you may look to pair your education (the knowledge you provide) with an optimistic outlook and begin adding more skills-based training in the rehabilitation process to address their fears about their capability. This one example touches on many of the different educational domains.

To help conceptualise the process and how these models fit together, see Figure 25.3 and Box 25.2.

## Keeping it simple

Assessing an athlete's educational needs in this way might sound complex, but in reality you already take many of these actions in your practice. Making the process and targets of athlete education conscious may support you to proactively consider the educational options available. This may also help you to understand why providing an educational topic might succeed or fail (both considered later in this chapter). The education (information) you currently provide or discuss with an athlete may remain similar, but

you may become more conscious of the additional benefits of education, such as an athlete demonstrating improved confidence or self-efficacy, or reporting a reduction in negative emotions such as fear or anger.

Understanding the theories, models and frameworks outlined can provide you with a starting point for identifying which concepts you wish to target with your education. The theories and model at the start of the chapter relate to psychological aspects of the athlete's understanding. The Theoretical Domains Framework provides a long list of cognitive, affective, social and environmental factors you can look to impact. Finally, the COM-B model provides insight on how to identify potential priorities from this long list of targets.

## COMMON TOPICS COVERED IN EDUCATION PROGRAMS

Arguably, the best answer to the question "Which topic should I focus my education session on?" is "Let the athlete tell you what they want to know". Clinical consultations require active listening when interviewing an athlete. This will give you the ability to assess the athlete's current understanding with regards to their injury, what it means in terms of time out of play, what rehabilitation might look like and how they can stop the injury/illness happening again.

**BOX 25.2**  Using frameworks to select the most pertinent target for an athlete education program

### Example 1

An athlete sustained a grade II hamstring muscle injury (classified using MRI and the British Athletics muscle injury classification). They were given the diagnosis and recommended to follow POLICE (see Chapter 8) for 1 week. They are now presenting for their first rehabilitation session with the team physiotherapist after having a few days off.

**Practitioner:** "Hi, how were your days off and how are you feeling?"

**Athlete:** "Good thanks, it was nice to get a few days with the family. Except for walking upstairs, I don't feel any pain now. I want to get back to playing with the team."

*Analysis*

The athlete has a desire to get back to playing as soon as possible; this speaks to their goals ("I want to") and their confidence (self-efficacy is high). This suggests that the motivation element of COM-B is covered. However, they may not be aware of the prognosis that it could take 4–6 weeks to recover (a knowledge or capability gap). Given the potential gap between expectations and reality, it may be useful to engage their teammates to reinforce your messages about the expected time for recovery (using their experiences) and to add positivity about them returning to their previous level of play (both motivation and opportunity—through influencers, optimism and competitive edge).

### Example 2

An athlete has completed their return-to-sport battery of tests following an ACL reconstruction. They have been working with the rehabilitation team for 12 months, have taken part in full-contact training, and the healthcare and coaching team thinks they are ready to play in a practice match.

**Practitioner:** "The coaching team think you're ready to play in a match situation. You've passed all your medical tests. How would you feel about playing 20 minutes in a match?"

**Athlete:** "To be honest, I don't feel ready. I'm not convinced I've done enough to prevent the injury happening again."

*Analysis*

Return-to-sport uncertainty is normal. It is clear the athlete has the capability at this stage (based on objective testing, tissue healing times and their return to training) and is being offered an opportunity. However, this is an example of a gap in motivation. The athlete's confidence, risk tolerance and emotions are all potential targets of the education program. You may decide to use the results of objective testing as the basis for an education session that describes the low risk of returning to the performance environment and enhances the athlete's self-efficacy.

---

Just like the rehabilitation plan, an education plan should be developed in collaboration with the athlete.

The list of topics an athlete may require information on is extensive, and therefore listing every topic is beyond the scope of this chapter. As we outlined at the start of this chapter, education interventions need to touch on potential harms associated with healthcare interventions (diagnostic and treatment), intended benefits of an intervention, required rehabilitation commitments, potential restrictions from training and competition, as well as anticipated time frames and expected outcomes. Many chapters in this book (and in *Clinical Sports Medicine 6e: Managing Injuries*) touch on the knowledge domain aspects that will support you to educate an athlete on topics related to diagnosis, prognosis and injury prevention.

To provide guidance, below we highlight common key topics to cover in a sports and exercise medicine context, along with the essential information that should be provided (or where you can find out more in other chapters of this textbook).

Note, if your professional scope does not cover providing education on any of these topics (e.g. providing medication

advice as a physiotherapist in many jurisdictions), it is useful to develop links with fellow professionals who can support your athletes as part of a holistic treatment plan.

### PRACTICE PEARL

Speak with "one consistent voice". If you work as part of a rehabilitation team, align your education programs so that team members reinforce the same key messages.

## Pain and other symptoms

Pain and other symptoms are commonly among the most disconcerting aspects of any injury or illness, and have the potential to disrupt an athlete's training, performance and personal life. Chapters 10 and 11 discuss the experience (perception and sensation) of pain and provide essential information that may be used to support you with delivering this key educational need.

Common questions voiced by athletes that your education program will need to address include:

- What is causing this pain?
- Why does my knee keep giving way?
- How long is the pain likely to last?
- Is it okay to train with some pain?
- Does pain mean something is damaged?
- What do I do during a flare-up of my symptoms?

## Load management

Understanding the athlete's context is vital to providing quality information on this topic. For instance, load management for a distance runner will differ considerably from load management for a throwing athlete (e.g. a baseball pitcher).

Load management concepts that an athlete may benefit from understanding include:

- load versus tissue capacity and how this differs between individuals
- *internal load* (the relative biological stress–physiological or psychological–placed on an athlete during training and competition) and *external load* (any external stimulus applied to the athlete, such as laps swum in the pool, balls bowled in cricket), and how an understanding of these concepts may enhance training design/provision
- measuring load relevant to their performance goals and sport (e.g. amateur versus professional environments, running versus climbing sports).

For more detailed analysis of the concepts in load management, refer to Chapter 15.

## Lifestyle factors

Common lifestyle factors may be broken down into various sub-categories such as sleep, nutrition, stress management and physical activity, as well as smoking, alcohol consumption and other substance use. It is unlikely that one practitioner will be able to speak to all of these topics, but having awareness of them and being able to provide consistent messaging to athletes about how they influence health and performance is important, as is knowing where to refer athletes if they need more in-depth help.

Key questions to identify lifestyle factors for an education program might include:

- Do you have any concerns (stressors) outside of the team environment that could be affecting your health or performance?
- Do you follow a specific diet, or dietary pattern?
- Are you struggling with stomach (gastrointestinal) concerns when participating in training or competition?

- Do you struggle to fall asleep? Do you still feel tired after waking up in the morning?
- Do you have any concerns about your alcohol intake?
- Have you tried to quit smoking?

## Exercise prescription

The reason for prescribing exercise requires explanation. Focus on educating the athlete why exercise will be beneficial to their rehabilitation. Ensure that they understand how to perform each exercise and the expected response (e.g. whether it may be painful during or after exercise and how to decide whether this is acceptable or not).

Exercise should be prescribed using the American College of Sports Medicine Guidance for Frequency, Intensity, Time, Type, Volume and Progression (FITT-VP).[15] This supports athletes with a plan of when and how much they need to do to complete their exercise program. Try to consider barriers and facilitators to engaging with the exercise plan and tailor the program to the athlete's environment (e.g. do they have time restrictions which dictate that certain exercises may be paramount?). If you are working with athletes while travelling, the usual equipment for heavy resistance training may not be available, so you need to be aware of alternative (if inferior) options, such as long-hold isometrics that generate greater time under tension for the muscle.

Exercise prescription is discussed further in Chapter 27 and in *Managing Injuries*.

## Injury prevention (primary and secondary)

Many excellent education resources exist to support the teaching of injury prevention programs. You may be aware of *FIFA 11+* for football and apps such as *Get Set–Train Smarter* produced by the International Olympic Committee. These may be adapted to the athlete's participation level: there is a *FIFA 11+ Kids* and the *Get Set* prevention exercises can be adapted to specific sports. Injury prevention education programs for youths are recommended to improve lifelong healthy behaviours.[16, 17]

For more knowledge of preventing injury, see Chapter 17.

> **PRACTICE PEARL**
>
> Implement education in youth development programs. Knowledge of healthy lifestyle options, load management principles and the benefits of recovery may support life-long suitable choices that extend beyond an athlete's sporting career.

## PREPARING SUCCESSFUL EDUCATION SESSIONS FOR ATHLETES

Education may be delivered as a brief intervention, such as a short conversation. It may also take the form of an extensive course of material aimed at increasing the athlete's health literacy—defined as the ability to obtain, read, understand and use healthcare information to make appropriate health decisions and follow instructions for treatment. The size of the intervention (number of resources, time dedicated, etc.) should reflect the importance of the desired change to the athlete's overall health, their current position (i.e. whether they are far away from the necessary change or have made steps to change already) and the resources available.

One model for helping you to organise and carry out education programs is known as ASSURE (Fig. 25.4).[18]

The ASSURE model provides one way of structuring the education process, but most successful education programs share some common principles that you can use to increase your chances of success.

Here we outline 12 education principles for you to consider.

### 1. Make your aims and objectives specific

Your aims and objectives can be framed by two questions:

1. *Am I trying to help the athlete make a choice (e.g. whether to undergo a diagnostic procedure or invasive therapy)?* Providing the athlete with choices may involve a greater focus on facts associated with such choices. For instance, choosing a specific therapy may be associated with a high chance of success and thus this should be included in the education provided. Or your education may specifically aim to address cognitive (knowledge) gaps that support the athlete to make an informed decision.

2. *Am I trying to change a negative behaviour (e.g. non-compliance with an individualised prevention program or poor sleep hygiene)?* Changing behaviour is much more likely to require the cultivation of trust, empathy and the creation of a safe space for the athlete. Thus, your education may specifically target affective domains (e.g. attitudes and feelings towards injury prevention practices).

### 2. Communicate positively and clearly

Consider the impact of your words on the athlete's perceptions of their injury or illness. Contemporary recommendations reinforce the need to move away from impairment-based narratives to participatory-focused communication and education (Fig. 25.5).[19] Positive and participatory-focused education has great potential to positively influence an athlete's motivation and self-efficacy.[1] Conversely, a small negative comment from a trusted practitioner may lead to spiralling mental and/or physical health in an athlete.

Avoid using medical jargon, as technical terms only disguise the message you want to convey. Speak in plain language and check that the athlete has understood your explanations. Using the teach back method (asking the athlete to explain what you have said back to you) may be more illuminating than simply asking "Do you understand?".[20]

The impact of your language extends to the written communication and media sources you share with athletes. Ensure that any supplementary media supports your education messaging and is easy to understand for the athlete (see below for tips on evaluating the quality of education sources).

### 3. Communicate a consistent message

There is no better way to lose an athlete's trust than to give mixed messages within the clinical team or the wider

**A** **Analyse the learner.**
In the sports and exercise medicine context this is most likely to occur while receiving the patient's history, using self-efficacy questions.

**S** **State the objectives.**
Objectives may target cognitive (knowledge), affective (attitudes, feelings and/or emotions) or psychomotor (behaviour or biomechanical) changes.

**S** **Select instructional methods and materials.**
Identify reputable sources and evaluate them for appropriateness in the athlete's context.

**U** **Use instructional methods and materials.**
Use trustworthy materials to support learning.

**R** **Require learner performance.**
Assess changes to whichever cognitive, affective or psychomotor area the education was designed to target.

**E** **Evaluate/revise the teaching plan.**
Based on the learner performance, decide whether any changes are required to the education or whether reinforcement of the messages may be needed.

**Figure 25.4** The ASSURE model is an instructional design model that can help you develop more effective training programs with integrated technology

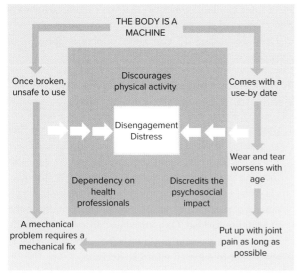

**(a) Impairment-based talk**

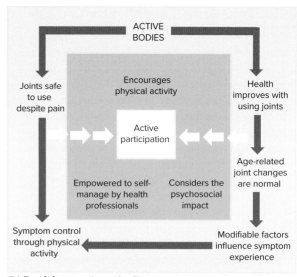

**(b) Participatory-based talk**

**Figure 25.5** Framing education using activity-based rather than impairment-based language
Source: Bunzli S, Taylor NF, O'Brien P, et al. Broken machines or active bodies? Part 2. How people talk about osteoarthritis and why clinicians need to change the conversation. *J Orthop Sports Phys Ther* 2023;53(6):325–30

support team (including health messages being delivered by the coaching staff). Try to ensure that the messages an athlete receives on health-related matters provide a "consistent voice" from everyone on the support team. If it makes sense to do so, include the athlete's family members when you provide education to ensure that changes are easy to make at home. This helps the athlete and those who support them to understand why changes are required so that they are more likely to support those changes.

## 4. Use facts, metaphors and stories

Facts alone do not support people to change their minds, or their behaviours.[19] Fact-driven education programs can be athlete-centred if facts are delivered within the athlete's individual context; that is, framed under the "What does this mean for me?" narrative. Factual education should not be a chance for you to demonstrate what you know— keep all the information relevant to the athlete and their scenario. Ensure that you provide enough information for the athlete to weigh the benefits and costs of undertaking a certain treatment or rehabilitation protocol and make an informed choice. To contribute to a successful intervention (e.g. behaviour change), education needs to be linked to the athlete's own context.

Education programs that aim to drive change in the athlete's behaviour should have a greater focus on the athlete's story. Using the athlete's story (context, such

as family, stage of their career) enables you to weave information on why a change is necessary into a narrative that will fit with the athlete's career or life. It will help the athlete to make sense of how to use that information. Making information personal is far more likely to engender change.

## 5. Demonstrate empathy/emotional intelligence to build trust

"Seek first to understand, then be understood."[22] Understanding the athlete's concerns about their injury or illness from their perspective (including how it may affect their future performance) and being able to demonstrate true "care" for their overall wellbeing is paramount if you want to build trust and/or change behaviour. Showing that you're invested in the athlete's wellbeing will help to develop the therapeutic alliance (Box 25.3).

The best way of doing this is to engage in active listening to fully understand the athlete's position and concerns. Being open and honest about your own knowledge limitations and any grey areas (e.g. where there may not be one "correct" solution for their situation) are also important in building trust with an athlete. If you are struggling to gain an athlete's trust, consider involving other members of the team (e.g. coaches, team captain and other athletes who have gone through the same experience) who already have the athlete's trust to help deliver the education program or focus on key messages.

**BOX 25.3** Developing the therapeutic alliance

The success of athlete education programs isn't just about "what" education we provide for athletes. It is also about the process of building trust and "how" we educate them. Some of how we educate is inevitably tied to our own personality, attitudes and beliefs. All injuries have the potential to induce fear, catastrophising, vigilance, anxiety and worry. Therefore, the ability to provide education in a reassuring and empathetic manner is an underappreciated but vital skill in athlete education sessions.

Demonstrating empathy by understanding the athlete's story and providing education specific to the athlete's context has the potential to promote greater engagement in the rehabilitation process. Empathy facilitates the development of a strong therapeutic alliance and a partnership of mutual trust between the practitioner and athlete. Providing education in a way that demonstrates you understand the athlete's story from "their" perspective (i.e. not from a biomedical reasoning perspective) will help to support, reassure, validate and empower the athlete.

Reassurance can be offered by: (1) addressing fears of underlying pathology; and (2) helping athletes to understand that pain does not always equal tissue damage. Anxiety may also be reduced simply by having an honest discussion about the athlete's prognosis and providing steps to mitigate any risks on the road to recovery.

While we know that empathy is a vital ingredient, unfortunately we cannot point to a specific resource that will make you a more empathetic or emotionally intelligent practitioner. Courses that try to teach healthcare practitioners empathy often fail, and empathy measured via the Jefferson Scale of Empathy has often been seen to drop over the course of healthcare education and training.[21]

Becoming emotionally intelligent means being able to identify, understand and control how your emotions influence an education session (or the clinical encounter generally). To support your ability to demonstrate emotional intelligence, we recommend that you attempt to understand the athlete's lived experience of their injury or illness and what they found helpful (or unhelpful) in a clinical consultation. In training this may be supported through using case studies, role-playing and self-reflection. Seeking out mentors who role-model empathy in the clinical environment can also be helpful.[22]

Measuring your own level of empathy using tools such as the Empathy Quotient may help you to understand your own ability to demonstrate empathy and may be the first step to developing more empathetic and emotionally intelligent education sessions.

Empathy Quotient

Note: There are many different tools available that propose to measure empathy. The Empathy Quotient is one of the best researched, but psychometric tests indicate all have limited validity. Apply insights you gain from using such tests cautiously.[23]

## 6. Have a conversation, don't "deliver an intervention"

Despite how we have framed athlete education in the chapter—that is, as a program or an intervention—it is not something we do to people, but rather something we collaborate on together to make meaning. While your goal is to educate athletes to enhance their health, the best way to achieve a positive result is through open dialogue. This will help the athlete to relax and will help you to understand the athlete's position (which in turn helps you to craft the story).

## 7. Avoid giving too much information at once

Consider how much of a lecture you would retain when you were a student. Research suggests that people best retain information delivered in the first 15 minutes of a lecture.[24] This is true even for engaged and willing learners (which may not be true of all athletes). It is important to consider the athlete's starting point: is this the first time you've spoken? Have they demonstrated prior knowledge of the topic? How experienced are they and have they undergone multiple rehabilitation processes in the past?

If you aim to explain facts, prescribe an exercise program and weave in the rationale for making change in one session, you are asking too much of yourself and the athlete. Split your education into manageable chunks and allow time for reflection. Then repeat key messages to reinforce learning on subsequent days, weeks and even months later.

## 8. Consider the setting

Athlete education sessions may be team-focused or individual-focused. Using a larger team-based environment to develop healthy behaviours (e.g. participation in daily injury prevention routines) may be beneficial, as the education program can be reinforced by watching more experienced team member's role-model good behaviours.

To build trust, demonstrate empathy and provide individual information. Do this in a private environment where the athlete feels "safe" to share their concerns or vulnerabilities away from other team members. This may mean moving out of the usual treatment room environment if multiple athletes often congregate there.

## 9. Learn about the sport, team and individual's culture

Culture includes the language, customs, beliefs, traditions and other ways of communicating in any given sport. This may differ with every athlete or team environment in which you work. If you're working with an athlete for the first time, you may want to wait before attempting to provide a great deal of education—not only to allow time to build trust with them, but also to gain greater awareness of their culture. This may help you to share educational material in a way that better fits their cultural background. In some instances, it may be appropriate for you to "educate yourself" about different customs and cultures within the team to create a culturally safe space for athletes. However, never comply with cultural norms if they are in any way inappropriate. Be aware of the link between team culture and interpersonal violence (formerly referred to as harassment and abuse). Remember your professional commitment to ethical conduct.

## 10. Include a range of resources to reinforce learning

You may use different forms of media during and after a consultation to reinforce information delivered verbally. Ask the athlete whether they prefer to learn through apps, podcasts, videos, diagrams, handouts or simply a follow-up email with key points from the education program. It's likely that a combination of these will work better than one method alone. If you regularly deliver information on a topic (e.g. load management for athletes), keep some trusted sources as go-to items to share.

> **PRACTICE PEARL**
>
> Consider making your own resources on common messages that you provide to athletes, as this ensures consistency and accuracy.

## 11. Be available for follow-up

It would be unusual for a single education session to provide everything an athlete needs to understand and make an informed decision or change a behaviour. Encourage the athlete to ask questions and provide time after the initial session for the athlete to assimilate the information. Set a follow-up time to discuss any questions and provide clarity. Curiosity on the part of the athlete should be encouraged and is a sign of successful engagement with the education material. However, take care not to be seen as an "on call" source of information 24/7. To avoid this, plan and diarise specific times for follow-up discussions.

## 12. Be self-aware

As well as being conscious of your language, you also need to be aware of your mood, behaviours, beliefs, biases and knowledge—all of these have the potential to positively or negatively affect the outcome of the education provided. For example, a stressed mood or behaviours such as being disengaged during the athlete's story telling will affect your ability to demonstrate empathy and build a strong therapeutic alliance.

Furthermore, your beliefs about individuals have the potential to distort the education you provide. For example, sport-specific stereotypes regarding the physical or mental differences between playing positions (e.g. goalkeepers versus outfield players) or types of athlete (e.g. sprinters versus long-distance runners), or more general stereotypes relating to an individual's age, gender, weight or race/ethnicity can affect the education you provide.

Finally, you need to be aware of your biases and knowledge limitations when providing education to an athlete. It is important that the education you provide is honest and objective in nature. If you feel that certain topics are outside your expertise or scope, ask other members of the multidisciplinary healthcare team to facilitate the education on those topics.

## USING EXTERNAL LEARNING RESOURCES: CHOOSE WISELY

External learning resources are information sources that you didn't produce yourself—they include information sheets, posters, graphics, videos, mobile apps, websites, social media and virtual reality games. While we encourage you to consider the plethora of those resources, be aware that commonly used platforms may contain a lot of misinformation. Social media in particular is prone to influencer-based information (based on algorithms) rather than evidence-based practice [25,26]

Using artificial intelligence (AI) to produce education resources has the potential to be extremely useful for generating individualised information, but we are in the early stages of AI use and the knowledge that such tools can be inaccurate means they should be used cautiously until their efficacy has been proven.[27,28] You should vet any sources of information you use or stick to well-recognised programs/trusted sources.

Evaluating a resource can be time-consuming and is often best done before seeing an athlete face to face. Remember that the most reputable sources of knowledge-based information (e.g. peer-reviewed journals) do not always have athlete-friendly resources available for all given topics. One exception is the series "Perspectives for patients" published by the *Journal of Orthopaedic and Sports Physical Therapy.* Trusted sources such as the International Olympic Committee's app *Get Set—Train Smarter*(Fig. 25.6)[28] or government-backed health websites may be useful if you are pushed for time, but again may not provide you with athlete-specific data useful for the individual in front of you.

IOC *Get Set—Train Smarter* app

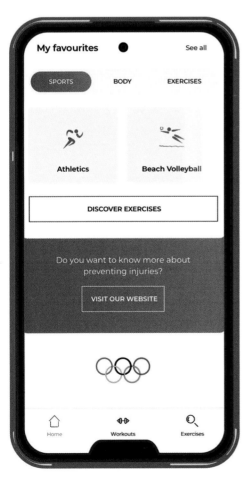

**Figure 25.6** The *Get Set—Train Smarter* app produced by the International Olympic Committee
Source: Reproduced with permission from International Olympic Committee.

The following tools were not created for the sports and exercise medicine context but they provide a template for you to evaluate the quality of information you provide.

## DISCERN tool

DISCERN differentiates between high- and low-quality information sources of consumer health information.[28] The tool is useful for:

- individual consumers making decisions about treatment
- health information providers as a screening tool
- authors and producers of written consumer health information as a checklist
- health professionals to improve communication and shared decision-making skills.

If the information you are vetting is about treatment options, you can use all 3 sections and use scoring scales; if you are using the tool to assess resources, skip section 2 and use your clinical judgment of the questions about reliability and overall quality of the information to decide whether it should be shared with your athletes.

The DISCERN questionnaire provides users a way to assess the quality of consumer health information

## The Patient Education Materials Assessment Tool

An option for those with more time is the detailed framework recommended by the Patient Education Materials Assessment Tool (PEMAT). PEMAT was designed to evaluate and ensure that resources have high understandability and actionability for those they intend to serve.[29]

There are two versions, one for printable materials (24 scoring items) and one for audiovisual materials (17 scoring items). You are asked to rate an education resource against questions such as "The material makes its purpose completely evident" with a score of 0 = disagree, 1 = agree or N/A for not applicable.

Final scores for understandability and actionability are given out of 100. Interpretation often requires comparison with another resource, and the tool works particularly well when trying to decide which is better between two options. There is no cut-off score indicating an "acceptable" level of either understandability or actionability.

Patient Education Materials Assessment Tool (PEMAT)

# EVALUATING THE SUCCESS OF YOUR EDUCATION

The ultimate measure of success for all rehabilitation programs is to have a happy, healthy and well-performing athlete. To objectively measure success, it is best to develop collaborative goals with the athlete. Education-based goals should be broken down into smaller components to establish whether you are achieving each element. Kirkpatrick and colleagues suggested 4 levels at which to evaluate the effectiveness of your education program; these often evolve along a set timeline (Table 25.2).[30]

## Strategies to measure success

The most immediate and obvious form of evaluation is simply to ask the athlete whether they have understood the information provided and field any further questions they may have. However, before you do this, try to observe their body language for cues that they have agreed, disagreed or been indifferent to what you have said. By asking them, "How do you feel about what was said?", you can assess not only their understanding, but also their affective response, which opens up more opportunities to address potential misunderstandings or to help them verbalise any underlying emotive responses such as anxiety.

A common strategy to assess learning is to ask the athlete to repeat the information provided in their own words. You might ask them, "How would you describe your injury/health problem to your partner or friend?" or "What is your interpretation of what I've just told you?" This enables you to immediately evaluate whether any correction or follow-up is required during the intervention. Immediate retention of information should be strong, but after 24 hours >50% may be forgotten, increasing to >90% at 7 days post receiving new information.[23] Hence, follow-up and repetition are important.

Depending on the type of education program delivered it may be necessary to use other forms of feedback such as direct observation or physical performance testing. These strategies can be used to evaluate performance during and after the education program has been delivered. If the intervention is designed to affect performance outside of the immediate environment, you might also consider getting feedback from other staff members (e.g. the coaching team) or from family.

Perhaps the most unwanted form of measurement is via a critical incident such as re-injury or a new injury sustained during the rehabilitation and return-to-sport process. This is most likely to re-set or set-back the clock to earlier parts of the education process, inviting you to again start with reassurance, knowledge and motivation-based education programs.

Long-term monitoring may help you to evaluate whether the athlete has successfully integrated the new information. For instance, education on training load monitoring may reduce spikes in an athlete's training plan and better adherence to measures of internal load (such as completing subject mood scores before training each day).

Critical incidents, adherence to daily monitoring tools and physiological data captured at multiple time points can all add to your evaluation of whether an education program has been a long-term success.

**TABLE 25.2** Evaluating the success of your education program

| Level | When to assess | Questions to ask the athlete or yourself |
|---|---|---|
| **Reaction** | During or immediately after the intervention | Did the athlete like it? <br> Were they engaged? <br> Did they find it useful? |
| **Learning** | Days to weeks after the intervention | Can the athlete explain the education back to you? <br> Does the athlete feel more confident about the subject? <br> Have the athlete's emotions changed? (i.e. do they feel reassured?) |
| **Behaviour** | Weeks to months after the intervention | Has the athlete changed behaviour (e.g. are they doing their prehabilitation exercises)? <br> Is the athlete completing daily health screening tools? |
| **Results** | Months to a year after the intervention | Has the athlete had any further injuries? <br> Have physiological markers changed? (e.g. improved heart-rate variability scores) <br> Has sleep hygiene, quality and quantity improved? |

Source: Andreev I. The Kirkpatrick model. Available from: https://www.valamis.com/hub/kirkpatrick-model.

## WHEN YOUR EDUCATION PROGRAM ISN'T WORKING

Inevitably, not all education programs meet their targets. The ability to retain information is finite, so simply repeating or reiterating information may be enough in the short term to enact greater changes at the learning and/or behavioural level.

If an athlete's negative reaction to an education program is immediate (e.g. disengagement or indifference demonstrated verbally or non-verbally), the next step may be to address attitudes or beliefs that prevent the athlete from engaging in more health-promoting behaviours.

The questions in Table 25.2 will help you to evaluate your success, but guidelines for obtaining and giving feedback can also be useful. Obtaining constructive feedback relates largely to developing your therapeutic alliance with the athlete (or mutual trust), as discussed in Box 25.3. Be prepared to listen more and educate less. Consider using open-ended questions (e.g. "Tell me more about why you feel you aren't ready to play") to solicit more of what the athlete needs and delay what you had planned to deliver for another time. Avoid using an argumentative approach, and present alternatives so that the athlete can choose if the education being presented has nuanced options (such as when choosing between rehabilitation options).

Ultimately, not all athletes will be ready to receive the information you may want to provide. If this is the case, you can consider whether another person is better placed to provide the education, or wait until you feel the athlete is in a better position to change their beliefs or behaviours (review again capability, motivation, opportunity).

## KEY POINTS

- In an athlete-centred framework, you should provide education to allow athletes to form their own opinions and decisions about their care.

- Athlete education is more than just providing facts and figures. It requires placing important information into the context of the athlete's life and injury/illness experience.

- Several theories, models and frameworks—largely from the field of psychology—can help construct the athlete education program.

- You may be asked to provide education across a range of fields. Building a network of colleagues who can fill in gaps is important—you are unlikely to possess all the knowledge an athlete may require.

- When providing athletes with external education resources, be sure to vet their accuracy.

- Engage in self-reflection to determine how your mood, behaviours, beliefs and biases can influence your education efforts with athletes.

- Providing too much information at once can reduce the likelihood that an athlete will retain the information. Like other kinds of education, repetition and reinforcement are helpful.

- Evaluating the effectiveness of athlete education will allow you to identify what worked, and what didn't. This will modify your approach to treating that athlete; it will also help you to improve your future practice.

## REFERENCES

References for this chapter can be found at www.mhprofessional.com/CSM6e

## ADDITIONAL CONTENT

Scan here to access additional resources for this topic and more provided by the authors

## CHAPTER 26

# Surgery in sports and exercise medicine

with **MARK R. HUTCHINSON**

*At 18 I was warned I'd never play again. Then a surgeon saved my football career.*

WES FOGDEN (ENGLISH PROFESSIONAL FOOTBALLER)

## CHAPTER OUTLINE

Identifying surgical candidates
A surgical approach to two current controversies
Communication for better surgical outcomes
Common surgeries in sports and exercise medicine
Post-surgical complications
Return-to-sport decisions post-surgery

## LEARNING OBJECTIVES

By the end of this chapter you should be able to:

- identify athletes most likely to have positive outcomes with surgical intervention
- list various factors that the clinician and athlete should consider in making decisions about non-surgical (e.g. rehabilitation) versus surgical treatment
- discuss the areas of surgical treatment for sports injuries where there is debate or a lack of consensus
- explain the concept of a "weak link" in the post-operative athlete and how it influences their healing and rehabilitation progression
- identify various post-surgical complications and discuss how they should be addressed
- describe the various domains of readiness in return to sport and how they influence an athlete's trajectory.

While a large majority of sports-related injuries can and should be treated non-operatively, many others, due to the nature of the injury or due to a failure to respond to non-operative approaches, may require surgical intervention to allow the athlete the best opportunity to return to full sports participation and success. To achieve the optimal outcomes for the patient, it is critically important to:

- be able to identify patients who would most benefit from a surgical approach
- be aware of when non-operative protocols have failed or plateaued
- recognise the injury patterns that are best treated with surgery
- optimise communication between surgeon and therapist during post-operative rehabilitation and when targeting a safe timeline for return to sport.

Patient selection is about picking the right patient for the right operation. The key is to always be patient-centric. When we all move in the same direction with the patient's best interests in mind, the patient will always benefit.

## IDENTIFYING SURGICAL CANDIDATES

At times, identifying which athletes require surgery is obvious: open wounds need to be washed out and closed; displaced fractures and avulsions require reduction often associated with fixation; and complete injuries of the extensor mechanism of the knee (patellar tendon ruptures, quadriceps tendon tears, displaced patella fractures) require repair, otherwise the athlete will permanently lose the ability to extend their knee. In contrast, some pathologies may have various treatment options ranging from rest and therapy to minimalist interventions and injections to open and arthroscopic surgery.

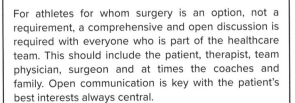

**PRACTICE PEARL**

For athletes for whom surgery is an option, not a requirement, a comprehensive and open discussion is required with everyone who is part of the healthcare team. This should include the patient, therapist, team physician, surgeon and at times the coaches and family. Open communication is key with the patient's best interests always central.

The patient needs to be fully educated to make an informed decision. They should be made aware of all treatment options (non-operative and operative) and their associated risks and benefits. The surgical pathway will always introduce additional risk factors including issues related to anaesthesia, infection, blood clots, surgical techniques or implants that are not present with non-operative pathways. Some non-operative approaches may also not be risk-free. When non-operative pathways fail, the athlete may have lost precious time regarding return to sport when their primary goal was the fastest return to sport possible. Eleven factors that often contribute to shared decision making about surgery are listed in Box 26.1.

> **BOX 26.1** Should I have surgery? Factors to consider when making a shared decision
>
> Patients who are considering surgery will be able to make an informed decision if they understand:
>
> - all non-operative treatments options
> - how long it will take to respond to non-operative treatment measured by return to sport
> - time lost if non-surgical management fails, and the patient eventually undergoes surgery
> - the effort and pain associated with following a non-operative pathway
> - success rates and outcomes for each non-operative treatment based on return to sport
> - failure rates of non-operative treatments based on conversion to surgical options
> - all surgical technique options (minimally invasive, arthroscopic and open)
> - how long it will take to respond to surgical treatment measured by return to sport
> - the effort and pain associated with following a surgical pathway
> - success and failure rates and outcomes for each surgical technique based on return to sport both from the literature and from that particular surgeon's experience
> - general and specific risks of the surgery being considered including infection, blood clots, anaesthesia, iatrogenic injury and failure compared with other surgical options and non-surgical options.

To gather this information, the patient may seek out a variety of sources including their surgeon, therapist, trainer, coach, other players, the internet and personal past experience. The patient will value each source based on their own measure of confidence.

As a clinician, it is important that you are a source of high-quality evidence. You have the benefit of experience and academic knowledge to be able to sift through personal anecdotes or to assess the quality of evidence on the internet. You should strive to be knowledgeable but also be aware of what you don't know. If you are the superspecialist in an area, you will know the literature very well. If you have a broad practice, you can't know everything and a knowledgeable patient may know the literature better than you do. That's not a failing on your part. In the current healthcare landscape, athletes commonly seek second or third opinions, and opinions about surgery are often sought from sport and exercise physicians due to their perceived objectivity.

You need not "convince" them of your opinion, but rather should help them to understand the training and experience on which such recommendations are based and then allow them to make the best-informed decision from their perspective. You should base your recommendations on high-quality evidence, present the data honestly to the patient, and avoid being critical of healthcare providers whose opinions may differ from yours. An important part of shared decision making is that the risk of a poor outcome, which can occur even in the best of hands, is known and the patient has a chance to consider it.

The indications for surgery are complex and depend on myriad factors including:

- the anatomical structure injured
- the actual pathological injury pattern
- the techniques, materials and procedures available to treat the injury (with the inherent risks, strengths and time to recovery for each)
- the demands of the sport and return to sport
- the athlete's willingness to take on both the post-operative rehabilitation and the surgical risk.

A summary of conditions treated by surgery is shown in Table 26.1.

**TABLE 26.1    Most common sports-related problems with surgical treatment by anatomical location**

| Problem | Treatment options |
| --- | --- |
| **Shoulder, common** | |
| Impingement/bursitis | Soft tissue vs bony decompression/distal clavicle excision |
| Instability/labral tears/SLAP tears | Debridement vs repair vs biceps tenodesis |
| Cuff tears | Debridement vs repair vs augmentation |
| **Shoulder, less common** | |
| Fractures/dislocations | Non-op vs open reduction and internal fixation (ORIF) |
| Clavicle/AC joint/SC joint injuries | Non-op vs repair/ORIF |
| **Elbow, common** | |
| Ulnar collateral ligament injuries | Non-op vs injection vs reconstruction in throwers |
| Lateral tendinopathy | Non-op vs debridement vs debridement + repair |
| Osteochondritis dissecans | Non-op vs debridement vs cartilage reconstruction |
| **Elbow, less common** | |
| Biceps/triceps rupture | Surgical repair various techniques |
| Fracture/dislocations | Non-op vs ORIF |
| Avulsions in skeletally immature | Non-op vs ORIF |
| **Wrist and hand, common** | |
| Finger and metacarpal fractures | Non-op vs ORIF if displaced/rotated |
| Scaphoid fracture | Non-op vs early ORIF |
| Flexor/extensor tendon injury | Surgical repair |
| Triangular fibrocartilage complex injury | Non-op vs debridement vs repair |
| **Wrist and hand, less common** | |
| Distal radius/ulna fracture/dislocation | Reduction ± ORIF |
| Nerve entrapment/carpal tunnel | Non-op vs decompression |
| Tendinitis/synovitis | Non-op vs surgery (if resistant) |
| **Hip/pelvis, common** | |
| Femoral acetabular impingement | Non-op vs debridement vs debride and repair |
| Trochanteric bursitis | Non-op vs rarely debridement |
| Femoral neck stress fracture | Surgery for high-risk variants |
| Sports hernia | Non-op vs general surgery for repair |

| Problem | Treatment options |
| --- | --- |
| **Hip/pelvis, less common** | |
| Fracture/dislocation | Non-op vs open reduction and fixation |
| Snapping hip | Non-op vs surgical release |
| Avascular necrosis or osteochondritis dissecans | Non-op vs core decompression |
| **Knee, common** | |
| Meniscus tears | Debridement vs repair |
| ACL surgery | Reconstruction for high-demand patients |
| Patellar tendinopathy | Non-op (common) vs debridement (rare) |
| Patellar instability | Non-op vs reconstruction for 1st time or recurrence |
| **Knee, less common** | |
| Extensor mechanism rupture | Surgical repair |
| Posterior cruciate ligament injury | Reconstruction for high grade or instability |
| Multi-ligament knee | Reconstruction for most |
| Chondroplasty or cartilage restoration | Non-op trial first vs cartilage restoration |
| Tibial plateau fracture | ORIF if displaced |
| **Ankle/leg/foot, common** | |
| Ankle fracture/syndesmosis injury | Non-op (rare) vs ORIF |
| 5th metatarsal fracture (Jones) | Non-op vs ORIF in high risk, high demand |
| Exertional compartment syndrome | Non-op option vs fascial release if resistant |
| Achilles tendon rupture | Non-op vs repair/augmentation |
| **Ankle/leg/foot, less common** | |
| Tibial stress fracture | Non-op vs rodding if resistant |
| Tibia/fibula fracture | ORIF if displaced |
| Acute compartment syndrome | Surgical decompression |
| Midfoot and hindfoot fractures | ORIF if displaced |
| Peroneal tendon subluxation | Surgical stabilisation if recurrent |
| **Spine/centra (cervical/thoracic/lumbar), less common** | |
| Cervical disc disease | Non-op vs injection vs discectomy |
| Thoracic outlet syndrome | Non-op vs decompression |
| Lumbar disc disease | Non-op vs injection vs discectomy |
| Spondylolysis | Non-op vs fusion |

Non-op, non-operative; ORIF, open reduction and internal fixation

## A SURGICAL APPROACH TO TWO CURRENT CONTROVERSIES

### Knee injuries

Anterior cruciate ligament (ACL) tears have one of the highest associations with surgery for all musculoskeletal athletic injuries with an incidence rate of 8 per 100,000 athlete exposures. They also have the lowest rate of return to sport.[1] More than 100,000 ACL surgeries occur each year in the US.[2]

Injuries to the meniscus leading to surgery are also common in sport. In one study, 1082 meniscal injuries were reported during 21,088,365 athlete exposures for an overall injury rate of 5.1 per 100,000 athlete exposures (Fig. 26.1). The overall rate of injury was higher in competition (11.9) than in practice (2.7) (RR = 4.4; 95% CI 3.9-5.0); 12/19 sports showed significantly higher injury rates in competition compared with practice. Of all injuries, 68.0% occurred in boys, yet among the gender-comparable sports of soccer, basketball, track and field, lacrosse and baseball/softball, injury rates were higher for girls than for boys (5.5 and 2.5, respectively, RR = 2.2; 95% CI 1.8-2.7). Contact injuries were the most common mechanism (55.9%). Surgery was performed for the majority of injuries (63.8%)

421

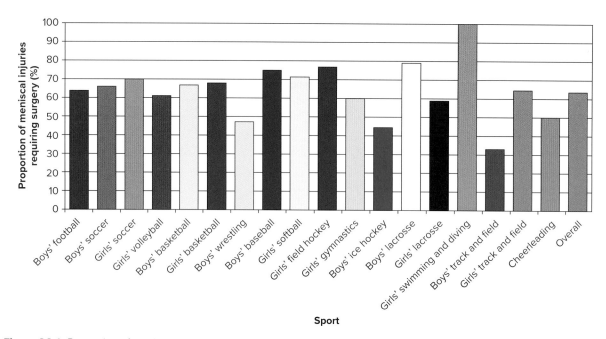

**Figure 26.1** Proportion of meniscal injuries requiring surgery, by sport
Source: Mitchell J, Graham W, Best TM, et al. Epidemiology of meniscal injuries in US high school athletes between 2007 and 2013. *Knee Surg Sports Traumatol Arthrosc* 2016 Mar;24(3):715–22.

and 54.0% of athletes had associated intra-articular knee pathology.[3]

A well-informed patient should be aware of any current controversies regarding how various healthcare providers might approach their injury or current trends in the field that might alter their choices and options. A study based on reported surgical case logs to the American Board of Orthopaedic Surgery in 2003[4] revealed that 4 of the top 10 surgical procedures submitted for review were sports medicine procedures (meniscectomy, knee debridement, subacromial decompression and ACL reconstruction). Since that time, the literature has challenged the absolute surgical indication for various procedures, with surgical treatment of degenerative meniscus tears being a particular area of focus.

### Management of degenerative menisci

In a recent panel of 20 experts, there was considerable disagreement on when to operate:[5] 70% of panellists agreed that neither physical therapy nor surgery are superior to one another, noting that the current literature should be viewed with caution. For diagnosis, most agreed that radiographs (i.e. weight-bearing) should be performed as part of the initial work-up. There was a lack of consensus on when to perform MRI, but the British Association for Surgery of the Knee recommends obtaining an MRI if a treatable tear is suspected.

According to panellists, the physical examination findings most suggestive of a meniscal tear were a history of gradual onset of activity-related pain, joint line tenderness, lack of full extension and localised joint tenderness in the absence of radiographic osteoarthritis. Only half of the panellists agreed that true mechanical symptoms (locking, catching, etc.) were an indication for surgery. Importantly, 90% agreed that initial treatment should be non-surgical and 100% agreed that patients with persistent pain or effusion despite appropriate treatment (>3 months) should have surgery.

There was consensus that repairable lesions should always be repaired regardless of the patient's activity level, with peripheral longitudinal tears being the most amenable to repair. Meniscus repair has similarly low rates of complications compared with partial meniscectomy.[6] There is considerable discord on whether or not to address chondral defects intraoperatively.

### Management of ACL injuries

There is considerable debate regarding the relative merits of surgical versus non-surgical management strategies for acute ACL injuries. Unfortunately, there is a lack of systematic reviews comparing non-operative and operative treatment for high-performing athletes with an acute ACL injury.

Most competitive athletes playing high-risk (i.e. pivoting) sports undergo early ACL reconstruction.[7] There is a trend towards non-operative treatment as first-line treatment for ACL injuries in the large majority of the population who do not have high-intensity and frequent twisting and cutting demand or those who have not proven to be recurrently unstable. In most instances, return to pivoting sports post-surgery occurs within 1 year[8] but not sooner than 6–9 months. While there is one case report of a high-level soccer player treated non-operatively after ACL injury who returned to sport just 8 weeks following initial injury,[9] in general the timing of rehabilitation and return to activities following non-operative management of an ACL rupture should be individualised.

## Surgery for shoulder instability?

There is a lack of consensus in the current literature on the best approaches for managing glenohumeral instability, especially in throwing athletes or for athletes with first-time shoulder dislocations.

### Management of shoulder instability in overhead athletes

Arguello and colleagues suggest that for overhead athletes with any form of glenohumeral instability (anterior, posterior or multidirectional), initiating a comprehensive non-operative treatment regimen should be the first course of action.[10] This consists of physical therapy with the primary goals of restoring motion, improving strength, reducing pain, eliminating the sensation of apprehension and optimising the dynamic stability of the shoulder through strengthening the rotator cuff and scapular musculature.

Non-operative treatment of anterior shoulder instability is associated with relatively poor outcomes.[11] For example, at a median 17-year follow-up, 37.5% experienced recurrent instability, 58.4% had recurrent pain and 12.2% had symptomatic osteoarthritis development. Risk factors for poor non-operative outcomes include increased pain and the number of instability events at initial presentation.[11]

Surgical repair/reconstruction should be considered in the setting of severe bone loss, fracture, significant concurrent shoulder pathology (i.e. full-thickness rotator cuff tear) or when non-operative treatment fails. The repair/reconstruction is commonly achieved through an arthroscopic labral repair with minimal inclusion of the capsule but may occur with open surgical techniques as indicated.

According to the Anterior Shoulder Instability International Consensus Group, indications for non-operative

management include "low risk of recurrence, absence of glenoid bone loss, timing in-season to allow for return to sport, and age <14 or >30 years old".[10] For throwers with anterior shoulder instability undergoing stabilisation surgery, return-to-sport rates were between 63.6% and 71.4%, which was slightly lower than the rates in non-overhead athletes (80.5%). Median Western Ontario Shoulder Instability Index (WOSI) scores were also comparable but slightly higher for non-overhead athletes compared with throwers.

### Management of posterior shoulder instability

Management of posterior shoulder instability has also been a topic of debate within the sports and exercise medicine community. Operative management has shown significant benefits to patients suffering from traumatic instability and those with more severe pathology (i.e. concomitant reverse Hill-Sachs and/or reverse bony Bankart lesions).[12]

A systematic review and meta-analysis showed that patients treated with arthroscopic posterior stabilisation had low rates of recurrent instability (8%), low rates of revision procedures (8%), low rates of persistent pain (12%), excellent subjective stability (91%) and return to preinjury level of play as high as 68%.[13, 14] More specifically, arthroscopic stabilisation procedures using suture anchors led to fewer recurrences and revisions than anchorless repairs in patients engaging in rigorous physical activity. Patients treated arthroscopically also have superior outcomes compared with patients treated with open procedures when examining stability, recurrence of instability, patient satisfaction, return to sport and return to sport at their previous level.[13]

Physical therapy regimens have recently garnered popularity as an alternative to operative management. One study reported significantly improved Oxford Shoulder Instability scores (OSIS) and WOSI scores following a rehabilitation program for patients with atraumatic posterior shoulder instability.[15]

A different study comparing non-operative management and operative management for posterior shoulder instability showed that surgery led to a more significant reduction in pain than non-operative treatment.[12] However, patients treated non-operatively reported a low rate of recurrent instability (8%) and lower rates of progression to symptomatic arthritis than surgically managed patients (8% vs 17%).[12]

Arthroscopic stabilisation and physical therapy display comparable outcomes for patients with posterior shoulder instability. Thus, a patient-centred "goals of care" discussion may act as an important guide for management.

C

# COMMUNICATION FOR BETTER SURGICAL OUTCOMES

Excellent communication is key to success in achieving a patient's expectations. Once a patient has elected to proceed with surgery, it is important that they have a realistic expectation of what their post-operative course will look like and how long it will take to return to their expected level of function. Those needs and goals should be carefully clarified by the various members of the healthcare team. Does the athlete hope to return to a pain-free, functional lifestyle; low-level recreational activities; competitive sport; or their previous level of competition and success? Do they understand the intensity of effort that it will take to achieve those goals?

One advantage of the athlete having a history of the same or a similar injury (such as a contralateral ACL injury) is that they will have a very good idea of what lies in front of them regarding the rehabilitation process, pain and effort. For those athletes without such an experience, extra time should be taken to make them aware of what lies ahead of them.

Most of the time when an athlete realistically understands the hurdles in front of them, it makes it easier for them to take on the rehabilitation challenge. Another helpful strategy is to introduce the athlete to another athlete with the same injury who has either overcome the injury or is in a more advanced stage along the rehabilitation pathway. Such information assists the athlete in being mentally ready to face the challenges ahead.

## The weak link

While the goal of most surgical repairs and reconstructions is to attain immediate strength of construct to tolerate range of motion and loading, every surgery will have a "weak link" that should guide the pace of post-operative recovery. It is important that the weak link is communicated by the surgeon to the therapist and used as a guide to post-operative rehabilitation to avoid complications.

- For a simple arthroscopy and tissue debridement, the weak links are only the portals and small wounds. These should not limit rehabilitation to any significant degree and should enable an aggressive approach to rehabilitation.
- For a fracture being fixed with a plate and screws, the weak link is the quality of the bone and how strong the screws are engaged into the bone. If the surgeon perceives softer bone or poorer quality fixation, rehabilitation will have to be slowed down and restricted to limit the risk of failure.
- For soft-tissue fixation such as ligament and labral repairs, the weak link is how well the suture holds onto

the soft tissue and the strength of the anchor into bone. If the surgeon senses that the tissues are not holding the suture ideally or that the anchors did not solidly deploy in bone, the pace of rehabilitation, including loading and range of motion, may need to be limited.

If at any time the rehabilitation stress overloads the strength of repair beyond the strength of the construct, the surgery and repair will fail.

## Timeline

Another area of communication between the surgeon and the therapist relates to the timeline of when loads can be safely applied. At time zero, the strength of the weak link is often dependent on the strength of the actual surgical construct or repair. How strong is the suture within the tissue? How strong is the anchor or screw in the bone? How strong is the skin suture? As time passes, the repaired tissues will gain strength, which partially offsets the weak link of the initial construct. During that time frame, the restrictions of rehabilitation are usually modified and advanced based on the maturing strength of the surgical repair/reconstruction.

> **PRACTICE PEARL**
>
> The timing of progress needs to account for the pace of healing, the strength of the construct, the goal of early and full motion, the value of loading, the pace and quality of tissue healing, and the goals of the patient regarding return to sport.

Most commonly, this is communicated between the surgeon and therapist based on predefined protocols that break down the stages of rehabilitation into phases:

- The first few weeks focuses on immediate post-operative recovery and wound care.
- The next several weeks target regaining motion within the restrictions provided by the surgeon and usually include early muscle activation. Once the underlying healing or strength of construction allows, muscle strengthening and early functional activities are initiated.
- The final stage of rehabilitation targets advanced functional activities, agility, coordination and sport-specific training with the goal of return to sport.

The timing of each phase must account not only for the patient's response to the rehabilitation challenges but also a respect for the underlying strength of the healing construct. The rate of progression of the rehabilitation program is best guided by subjective as well as objective measures, such as tests of range, strength, balance and agility. History has shown that while accelerated rehabilitation programs can return athletes to sport at a faster pace, this can come at an increased risk of recurrent injury or failure. Throughout the rehabilitation process, open communication should include assessment of patient's goals and perception of status, therapist assessment of progress and skills, and the surgeon's awareness and guidelines regarding healing strength of the healing construct.

## COMMON SURGERIES IN SPORTS AND EXERCISE MEDICINE

### Shoulder instability

Shoulder stabilisation surgery can be performed using open or arthroscopic techniques. Repair entails reattachment of the torn labrum or capsule back to its original position on the glenoid with suture anchors (Fig. 26.2). In cases with bone loss related to a large Hill-Sach's lesion (a dent in the back of the humeral head) or a significant bony glenoid defect, bone augmentation may be necessary using bone graft or bone transfers fixed with screws.

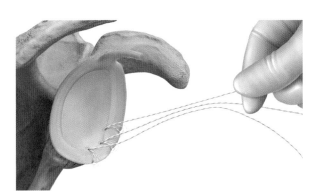

**Figure 26.2** Sutures in place after arthroscopic Bankart repair. The previously torn labrum is now reattached to the bony glenoid.
IMAGE PROVIDED COURTESY OF ARTHREX INC.

### *Weak links*

The quality of the labrum and capsule to hold stitches, the quality of the bone to hold screws and anchors, the strength of the suture and suture knots, the size of bone deficiency and the need to augment with grafting.

### *Critical communication between therapist and surgeon*

1. Is the construct strong enough to allow immediate full range of motion? If not, what are the restrictions and for how long?
2. Is the construct strong enough to allow immediate active motor function against resistance?
3. Were there associated injuries such as glenoid or humeral bone deficiency that will alter the rehabilitation program? Was a bone augmentation procedure performed that would delay rehabilitation or limit extremes of motion?

## Shoulder impingement and cuff injuries

While modern-day cuff and impingement surgery can be performed with open techniques, most surgeries are performed arthroscopically via three to four portals that provide access and visualisation within the shoulder joint and subacromial space. Simple debridement and bursectomy is accomplished with an arthroscopic shaver and leads to minimal restrictions with rehabilitation. When the rotator cuff is torn, it is repaired with 2–4 suture anchors with heavy-duty suture attached. The sutures are secured with knot tying, self-tying knots or anchors (Fig. 26.3).

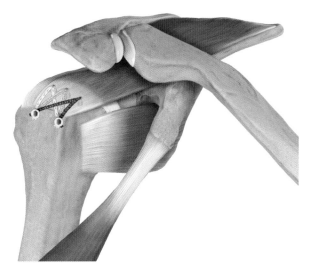

**Figure 26.3** Rotator cuff repair uses 2–4 suture anchors with heavy-duty suture attached
IMAGE PROVIDED COURTESY OF ARTHREX INC.

### *Weak links*

The quality of cuff tissue to hold sutures, the quality of the bone to hold the suture anchor, the strength of the sutures, the quality or strength of knot tying or the suture securing technique.

*Critical communication between therapist and surgeon*

1. Is the construct strong enough to allow immediate full range of motion? If not, what are the restrictions and for how long?
2. Is the construct strong enough to allow immediate active motor function against resistance?
3. Were there associated procedures such as biceps tenodesis, labral repairs or distal clavicle resection that will alter the rehabilitation program?

## Elbow ulnar collateral ligament tear

Reconstruction or repair of the ulnar collateral ligament of the elbow is most commonly required in overhead-throwing athletes but may also be required in gymnasts and upper extremity weight-bearing athletes. The surgery is performed via an open incision with careful identification of the origin and insertion point of the native ulnar collateral ligament.

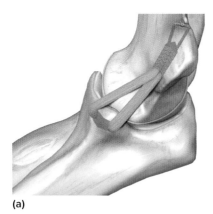

**(a)**

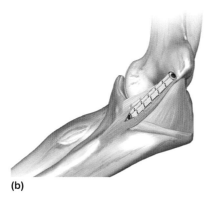

**(b)**

**Figure 26.4** Ulnar collateral ligament elbow reconstruction (a) with docking technique and (b) with internal brace augmentation. In the docking technique, the surgeon loops a single continuous graft through converging ulna bone tunnels and docks the sutured graft ends through two humeral tunnels.

IMAGES PROVIDED COURTESY OF ARTHREX INC.

Most surgeons split the muscle tissue to gain access but some detach and reattach the muscle tissues. Bone tunnels are placed and a new ligament from either autogenous or allograft sources is secured into the tunnel sockets with sutures, buttons or anchors (Fig. 26.4).

*Weak links*

The quality of the tissue graft, suture grasping of soft-tissue graft, the quality of the bone to hold the suture anchor, the strength of the suture knot or suture security with anchor.

*Critical communication between therapist and surgeon*

1. Is the construct strong enough to allow immediate full range of motion? If not, what are the restrictions and for how long?
2. Is the construct strong enough to allow immediate active motor function against resistance?
3. Was the flexor attachment detached and will that alter the rehabilitation program? Was the ulnar nerve transferred? Are there any concerns or restrictions related to harvest site morbidity from palmaris graft or hamstring graft?

## Distal biceps brachii rupture

Failure to recognise and repair complete ruptures of the distal biceps can lead to significant loss of flexion and supination strength at the elbow. Surgical repair is accomplished through either a two-incision or a single anterior incision approach, each having its own risks and benefits. The distal biceps is mobilised and heavy-duty suture is placed in a locking fashion into the distal stump. The end of the tendon is repaired into a bone socket at the radial tuberosity and locked into place with suture knots, interference screws, anchors or buttons (Fig. 26.5).

*Weak links*

The quality of the biceps tissue, the locking suture technique into tendon, the strength of sutures, the quality of bone, the strength of the anchor/button/screw/suture construct in the radial tuberosity, the size of the bone tunnel in the radial tuberosity.

*Critical communication between therapist and surgeon*

1. Is the construct strong enough to allow immediate full range of motion? If not, what are the restrictions and for how long?
2. Is the construct strong enough to allow immediate active motor function against resistance?

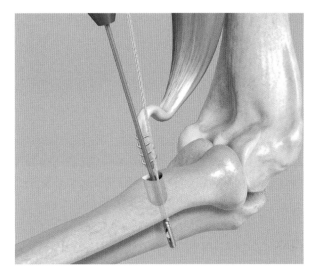

**Figure 26.5** This intra operative illustration shows the distal biceps tendon sutured to a "biceps button", which is passed through a bone tunnel in the radius to anchor the tendon. To complete fixation (not shown), a tendon screw is inserted into the bone tunnel to secure the tendon in the radial tuberosity.
IMAGE PROVIDED COURTESY OF ARTHREX INC.

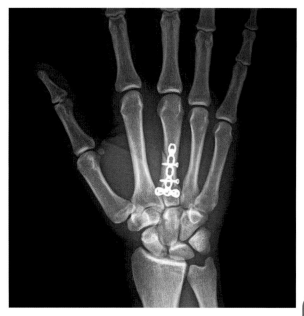

**Figure 26.6** Radiograph of an oblique metacarpal fracture fixed with mini-fragment plate and two screws
ISTOCK/HIPHOTOS35

## Finger and hand fractures

There are numerous technical approaches to finger and hand fractures based on fracture pattern, equipment available and surgeon preference. In general, displaced, rotated and intra-articular fractures require surgical repair. Techniques include percutaneous pinning, mini-fragment plates and screws (Fig. 26.6), and intramedullary fixation. The goal is always a stable fixation with anatomical reduction, which will allow early range of motion to minimise the risk of stiffness.

### Weak links

The complexity of the fracture pattern, the stability and strength of the fixation construct, the quality of the bone tissue, associated injuries to ligaments or tendons.

### Critical communication between therapist and surgeon

1. Is the construct strong enough to allow immediate full range of motion? If not, what are the restrictions and for how long?
2. Is the construct strong enough to allow immediate active motor function against resistance?
3. Can we move the wrist and adjacent fingers?

## Flexor/extensor finger tendon injury

Tendon injuries can occur either mid-substance or at their insertion. Surgical repair is performed by locking sutures into the tendon end with either end-to-end repair of the opposite torn end of the tendon (Fig. 26.7) or anchor or pull-through sutures repaired back to the insertion site. Certain areas of the flexor tendon have reduced circulation, which may compromise repair, or have to transverse the series of pulleys, which may lead to impingement or stiffness.

### Weak links

The strength of the soft-tissue grasp in locking the suture into the tendon, the strength of the sutures, the strength of the suture anchor, the strength of repair of any pulley that was damaged in the surgical approach.

### Critical communication between therapist and surgeon

1. Is the construct strong enough to allow immediate full range of motion? If not, what are the restrictions and for how long?
2. Was a pulley repaired that will lead to restrictions of range of motion?
3. Is the construct strong enough to allow immediate active motor function against resistance?
4. Can we move the wrist and adjacent fingers?

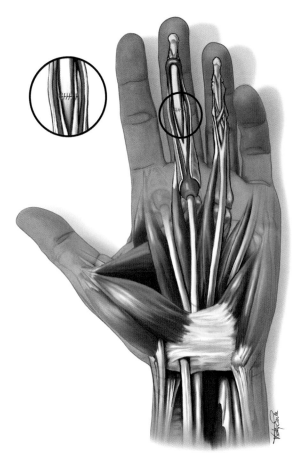

**Figure 26.7** Flexor tendon repair

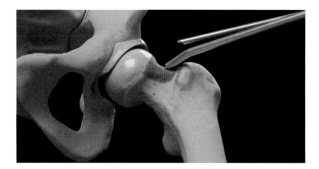

**Figure 26.8** Debridement of cam morphology in a patient with femoroacetabular impingement syndrome
IMAGE PROVIDED COURTESY OF ARTHREX INC.

## Femoroacetabular impingement syndrome (FAI syndrome)

Surgery for femoroacetabular impingement syndrome is most commonly performed arthroscopically and ranges from debridement of labral tissue or cartilage with or without bony decompression to surgical repair or reconstruction of the labrum with sutures and anchors (Fig. 26.8).

### Weak links

For simple debridement: the only restrictions are related to the arthroscopic portals' capsulotomy. For surgical repair and reconstruction: the quality of labral tissue, the strength of the suture, the strength of the suture security by knot-tying or anchor, and the strength of the anchor in bone.

### Critical communication between therapist and surgeon

1. Was a labral repair or reconstruction performed? If yes, what are restrictions to motion and weight-bearing?
2. Is the strength of repair construct as it relates to tissue quality and suture security enough to allow early range of motion?
3. Was a capsulotomy performed, which will require protected range of motion on extremes?
4. Was a cartilage procedure like microfracture performed, which will alter the weight-bearing status?

## ACL injuries

ACL reconstruction is a day surgical procedure performed with arthroscopic assistance. The ligament is routinely rebuilt using one of several graft choices, ranging from donated tissue to autologous hamstring or quadriceps soft-tissue grafts to mid-third patella tendon with bone plugs at the proximal and distal ends. Bone tunnels/sockets are placed within the articular notch at the site of the native ACL footprint, and the graft of choice is then placed into the tunnels and fixed with interference screws, cross pins, or sutures and buttons (Fig. 26.9).

### Weak links

The quality and choice of graft, the strength and quality of the fixation choice, any associated injuries (e.g. meniscus injuries, cartilage injury or concomitant ligament injury) that might limit rehabilitation.

### Critical communication between therapist and surgeon

1. Is the construct strong enough to allow immediate full range of motion? If not, what are the restrictions and for how long?

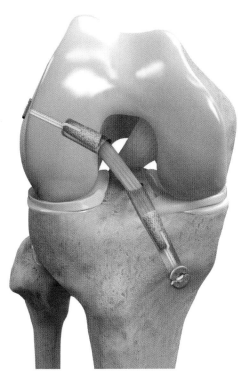

**Figure 26.9** ACL reconstruction showing a graft fixed with a low-profile implant that maintains graft tension
IMAGE PROVIDED COURTESY OF ARTHREX INC.

2. If a knee brace has been prescribed, what angle should the brace be locked in initially, and what is the progression to full extension?
3. Is the construct strong enough to allow immediate full weight-bearing? Was cartilage restoration or meniscus repair performed, which would limit immediate full weight-bearing? How long before commencing weight-bearing?
4. Were there associated injuries (meniscus, cartilage, concomitant ligaments) that will alter the rehabilitation program?
5. Will the choice of graft alter the pace of rehabilitation?

## Meniscus injuries

Meniscus injuries in the athletic population can range from small or degenerative tears where a non-operative treatment can be attempted to large peripheral, vertical bucket-handle tears or meniscus root tears that lead to significant pain and dysfunction and are treated with surgical repair to attain the best long-term outcome (Fig. 26.10). Symptomatic small degenerative tears can be treated with partial

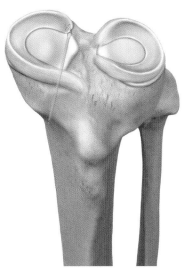

**Figure 26.10** Meniscus root repair is performed to treat meniscal root avulsion. The root is fixed directly to the tibia.
IMAGE PROVIDED COURTESY OF ARTHREX INC.

meniscectomy, which will allow a speedy rehabilitation with no restrictions. Bucket-handle tears, large peripheral vertical tears, root tears and ramp lesions are treated with surgical repair. Repair is performed with arthroscopic assistance placing sutures across the tear with an inside-out, outside-in or all-inside technique and the repair is secured with knot tying, self-tying knots or anchors.

### Weak links

The quality of meniscus tissue and pattern of meniscus tear, the pattern of repair including the number of sutures used, strength of sutures and knots, or strength of sutures and anchors. The repair is also at risk if the knee is unstable with associated ligament injuries.

### Critical communication between therapist and surgeon

1. Was repair, partial meniscectomy or total meniscectomy (rare) performed?
2. If repair, is the construct strong enough to allow immediate full range of motion? If not, what are the restrictions and for how long? If a partial meniscectomy was performed, what is the residual meniscal volume?
3. Is the construct strong enough to allow immediate full weight-bearing? If not, for which functional activities can the patient partially bear weight with the knee in extension? When can full-impact and pivoting activities resume?

4. Were there associated ligament injuries that will alter the rehabilitation program and increase the risk of repair failure?

5. Does the choice of repair technique alter the pace of rehabilitation or introduce restrictions?

## Extensor mechanism injuries of the knee

The extensor mechanism of the knee is made up of the quadriceps tendon and its insertion onto the patella; the patella; and the patellar tendon and its origin on the patella and its insertion onto the tibial tubercle. An intact extensor mechanism is essential for knee extension, normal ambulation and activities of daily living. Therefore, complete tearing at any level requires surgical repair. For injuries of the patellar tendon or quadriceps tendon off the bone, heavy-duty locking sutures are used to grasp the tendon tissue, with the free suture end used to re-attach the tendon tissue to bone with anchors or pull-through sutures (Fig. 26.11). For mid-substance injuries, heavy-duty locking sutures are used to grasp each end of the torn tendon and tied together to reapproximate the tendon ends.

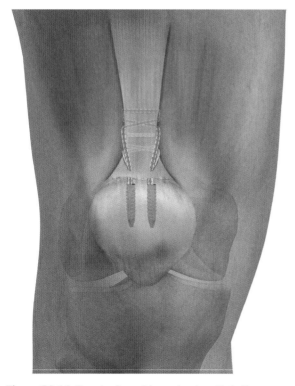

**Figure 26.11** Repair of quadriceps tendon. Note the patellar tendon is deliberately absent so that the illustration focuses on the previously torn quadriceps tendon.
IMAGE PROVIDED COURTESY OF ARTHREX INC.

### Weak links

The strength of the heavy-duty sutures, the quality of the tendon tissue and the ability of the locking suture to grasp it, the strength of knot security or the suture anchor security into bone, injury pattern (a mid-substance tendon injury is a weaker repair than an injury off the bone). If an avulsion or fracture occurred, the strength and quality of bone fixation is the weak link.

### Critical communication between therapist and surgeon

1. Is the construct strong enough to allow immediate full range of motion? If not, what are the restrictions and for how long?
2. Is the construct strong enough to allow immediate full weight-bearing? Can they bear weight with the knee locked in full extension? If not, how long before commencing weight-bearing?
3. Can they begin isometric strengthening?
4. Was the injury mid-substance or directly off the bone?
5. Was any tissue augmentation performed that would suggest a poorer quality native tissue?

## Hyaline cartilage injuries

The treatment of hyaline cartilage injuries depends on numerous factors including the patient's age, limb alignment, joint stability, associated injuries such as meniscus, and the site (weight-bearing or non-weight-bearing, retropatellar or tibiofemoral), size and depth of the lesion. For isolated injuries amenable to surgical intervention, such as displaced osteochondral fractures and isolated full-thickness lesions in young active patients, cartilage repair or restoration is reasonable. Techniques range from marrow stimulation (in which the subchondral bone is drilled to release pluripotential cells) to cartilage restoration (Fig. 26.12) and regrowth, and osteochondral transplantation.

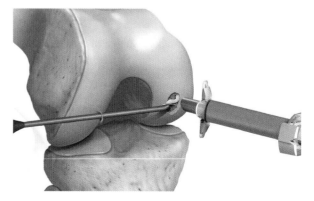

**Figure 26.12** Cartilage restoration with Biocartilage
IMAGE PROVIDED COURTESY OF ARTHREX INC.

### Weak links

How well hyaline cartilage restorative tissue (marrow cells or hyaline cartilage cells) adheres to subchondral bone, the security of the osteochondral plug within a socket, the timeline until maturation of cartilage tissue, the quality of closure of the surgical approach for open techniques.

### Critical communication between therapist and surgeon

1. Is the cartilage restoration procedure stable enough to allow weight-bearing?
2. Is cartilage restoration or repair tissue stable enough to allow early range of motion?
3. Were associated procedures such as osteotomy performed that will delay recovery?
4. What is the timeline for healing of the procedure performed?

## Patellar instability

Surgical treatment of recurrent patellar instability depends on several factors including the presence or absence of generalised ligamentous laxity, the direction of instability, the overall alignment of the lower extremity, and the shape of the patella and trochlear groove. For uncomplicated lateral patellar instability, the most common procedure is a reconstruction of the medial patellofemoral ligament with soft-tissue grafts that are attached to the superomedial aspect of the patella with sutures or anchors, with the opposite end of the grafts locked into a bone tunnel posterior to the medial epicondyle with either a bioabsorbable screw or suture (Fig. 26.13). For more complex instability-associated alignment or bony abnormalities, osteotomies fixed with screws may be required to correct the alignment.

### Weak links

The strength of the suture material, the strength of locking suture grasp of soft-tissue graft, the quality and choice of graft, the strength and quality of fixation choice onto the patella and into the medial condyle, the strength of the screw fixation and the timing to bone healing if osteotomy is required.

### Critical communication between therapist and surgeon

1. Is the construct strong enough to allow immediate full range of motion? If not, what are the restrictions and for how long?

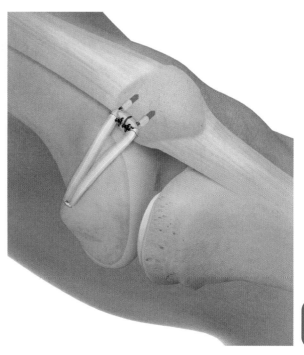

**Figure 26.13** Medial patellofemoral ligament reconstruction is indicated in certain patients (see text) who have recurrent patellar dislocation.
IMAGE PROVIDED COURTESY OF ARTHREX INC.

2. Is range of motion possible with either bracing or taping?
3. Is the construct strong enough to allow immediate full weight-bearing? Can they bear weight with the knee locked in full extension? If not, how long before commencing weight-bearing?
4. Can they begin isometric strengthening?
5. Was an osteotomy performed that will require delay in rehabilitation to allow for bone healing?

## Fractures about the knee (tibial plateau, distal femur) and ankle

Displaced fractures about the knee, including those of the distal femur, proximal tibial plateau and patella, create significant dysfunction and in general require open reduction and internal fixation (Fig. 26.14a). The specific choice of implants will depend on which bone is involved, the complexity of the fracture pattern and the demands of the patient. The surgical goal is to create a stable construct that will allow early motion while maintaining alignment during the healing phase of the bone. After a surgical incision and approach, the surgeon will reduce the fracture as close as anatomically possible and then place pins,

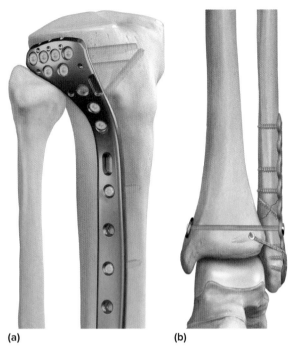

(a)                                    (b)

**Figure 26.14** Lower limb fracture repair: (a) proximal tibia fracture, (b) ankle fracture with syndesmotic repair (see implant crossing from the medial tibia to the lateral fibula and the reconstructed anteroinferior tibiofibular ligament, AITFL).
IMAGES PROVIDED COURTESY OF ARTHREX INC.

intramedullary rods or plates and screws to maintain the reduction (Fig. 26.14b).

### Weak links

The fracture pattern such as comminution, fracture location such as intra-articular, quality of the bone to accept screws and fixation devices, and strength of the actual implant.

### Critical communication between therapist and surgeon

1. Is the construct strong enough to allow immediate full passive range of motion? If not, what are the restrictions and for how long?
2. Can active range of motion be allowed? Can they begin isometric strengthening? Is the construct strong enough to allow resisted motor strengthening?
3. Was the injury intra-articular?
4. Is the construct strong enough to allow immediate full weight-bearing? Can they bear weight with the knee locked in full extension? If not, how long before commencing weight-bearing?
5. Were there any associated injuries to ligaments, tendons or meniscus that require a modification in the timing and type of rehabilitation?

## Achilles tendon conditions

The decision to address an acute Achilles tendon rupture with operative or non-operative treatment is controversial. When surgery is chosen, it can be performed with percutaneous or open surgical techniques. The basic concept is to use heavy-duty sutures to grasp hold of the proximal and distal ends of the torn tendon and then tie the ends together to reapproximate the torn ends as close to anatomical length as possible.

In some cases, surgery is indicated for insertional tendinopathy which can be associated with a large bony protuberance of the calcaneum—Haglund's deformity. Figure 26.15 shows the post-operative view after the deformity has been removed with a microsagittal saw and osteotome.

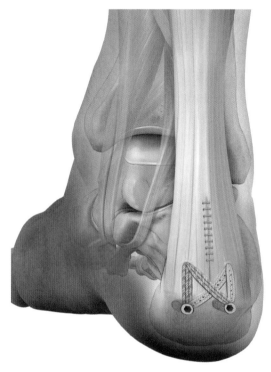

**Figure 26.15** Haglund's deformity surgery. It is difficult to approach the posterior calcaneum surgically without damaging the Achilles tendon. This is the post-operative view after the tendon has been split to permit access to the calcaneum. This illustration is *not* related to Achilles tendon rupture.
IMAGE PROVIDED COURTESY OF ARTHREX INC.

### Weak links

The quality of the tissue, the strength of the sutures, the strength of the suture grasping of soft tissue, the strength of the suture knot or anchor. For open techniques, another weak link is the quality of skin reapproximation, since this surgery carries an elevated risk of wound problems or dehiscence.

### Critical communication between therapist and surgeon

1. Is the construct strong enough to allow immediate full passive range of motion? Will they need a boot or splint for protection? What are the specific restrictions for range of motion and for how long?

2. Can active range of motion be allowed? If so, within what limits? Can they begin isometric strengthening? Is the construct strong enough to allow resisted motor strengthening?

3. Is the construct strong enough to allow immediate full weight-bearing? In the boot? If not, how long before commencing weight-bearing?

4. Were there any associated injuries to ligaments, tendons or bone that require a modification in the timing and types of rehabilitation?

## POST-SURGICAL COMPLICATIONS

Having an awareness of peri-operative and post-operative surgical complications is important for patients to make knowledgeable decisions when considering surgical options, but it is also critically important for the entire healthcare team, to enable early recognition and optimal treatment. Each procedure has unique risks related to its inherent weak links and surgical approach. Every member of the healthcare team—but especially the clinicians who serve as first contacts such as nurses, physiotherapists and athletic trainers—should be observant and willing to raise any concerns with the treating surgeon.

Immediate post-operative concerns include bleeding and compartment syndrome. If the post-operative dressing is soaked, the first response should be to apply pressure and a fresh dressing. If the second dressing is also soaked, notify the surgeon urgently as the patient may need to return to surgery to stop the bleeding. Swelling around the surgical site may represent an underlying progressive haematoma. Most respond to compressive bandaging and ice. Repeated neurovascular assessments are essential to assure that circulation and pulses are maintained.

Compartment syndrome occurs when bleeding and swelling progress within a fixed fascial compartment. As blood fills the compartment, the intracompartmental pressure can rise and cause blood vessels to collapse, leading to tissue ischaemia and pain. If left untreated, this can result in tissue death. Clinically the patient will present with swelling, tense fascial compartments and pain beyond what you would expect from the procedure itself. Pain with passive movement of the muscles within the compartment is suggestive of compartment syndrome. Loss of sensation or motor function, paralysis or pulselessness are seen only late in the presentation. Surgical decompression of compartment syndrome is required and the surgeon should be notified urgently or the patient sent immediately to the emergency room.

Infection and blood clots are complications that tend to present 2–3 days or more after the surgical procedure. Inspection of the skin around the wound may reveal redness, swelling or warmth. The wound may demonstrate dehiscence or purulent drainage. The patient may have fever. Early recognition is important. The therapist should communicate directly with the surgeon to share their concerns. If messages are left through a second party or via electronic means, the therapist should follow up to ensure that the message was received so that the athlete can be expedited for treatment of the infection.

Post-surgical deep venous thrombosis is a complication that requires a high degree of suspicion to recognise. Early recognition can be life-saving. The most common presentation is lower extremity swelling with posterior calf pain or pain in the popliteal fossa associated with lower extremity surgery. The athlete may have a palpable cord in the posterior calf or pain with passive extension of the ankle but some present with minimal pain and only persistent swelling. Diagnosis is usually confirmed with a venous Doppler study.

## RETURN-TO-SPORT DECISIONS POST-SURGERY

Return-to-sport decisions must be individualised based on the specific anatomy of the injury, the routine timeline of physiological healing of the injured or reconstructed tissue, the athlete's ability to rehabilitate and return to the full functional capacity demanded by their sport and, perhaps most importantly, the athlete's confidence and psychological readiness to return to sport.

One issue commonly encountered by sport and exercise clinicians is the pressure created by coaches, team administration or the press who assume that quick post-surgical recovery reflects higher quality care, a better surgeon or a better healthcare team. This can create a scenario in which the athlete returns to sport prematurely with a concomitant greater risk of re-injury.

A wise clinician will quote the best evidence available regarding return to sport and will be cautious about pushing for a speedy recovery based on an image perceived by outside parties, remaining patient-centric regarding safe and timely return to sport. Each athlete is unique and their return-to-sport timeline will be based on their anatomical/ physiological, functional and psychological readiness. Injury and its ensuing uncertainties may place tremendous stress on the athlete. The pressure may be intrinsic or extrinsic, and may lead to mental health issues surfacing during the recovery phase. You should be on the lookout for the signs and symptoms of an athlete's deteriorating mental health.

## Anatomical/physiological readiness

Anatomical and physiological readiness is based on the type of tissues that were injured or reconstructed, the strength of the tissues and the surgical construct, and the time it takes the tissues and healing construct to mature to a level that can withstand the loads of motion, weight-bearing, muscle strength, exercise loading and sport-specific skills.

For bones and non-displaced fractures, bridging callous and early healing commonly occur by 6 weeks (slightly shorter for hands and the skeletally immature; slightly longer for the elderly). Although the strength of bone healing at 6 weeks may allow weight-bearing, it is only 50% of the ultimate strength of healing that will be achieved over time. Thus, precautions may be necessary for an additional 6 weeks.

For surgically repaired fractures, intramedullary bone fixation may allow for earlier weight-bearing than plate fixation due to the strength of the surgical construct. In either case, the goal at the time of surgery is to create a strong enough construct to enable early range of motion and avoid stiffness. Unrestricted activities are usually allowed by 3-6 months[16] when physical examination reveals no pain and therefore clinical healing, and radiographic imaging demonstrates good bony healing and alignment.

For soft-tissue injuries and repairs, return to sport depends on the type of tissue. The timing and quality of healing for muscle and tendon injuries varies depending on the location of injury and whether it is muscle belly, muscle tendon junction, intra-tendinous or insertional (see Chapter 8). Avulsion injuries heal in a time frame that mirrors a bone injury.

Muscle tissue will not hold a suture with the same strength as a tendon injury, which may lead to delay in early range of motion depending on the quality of tissue repair. Modern-day, high-strength sutures are, in general, no longer the weakest link of a suture repair. Rather, the weakest link is the quality of its ability to grab tissue or anchor into bone. Remember, the purpose of a tendon is to connect the contracting muscle to its bony insertion and it is designed to absorb a dynamic tension load. Assuming good strength of repair, early range of motion will prevent stiffness.

Soft-tissue healing for a complete tendon rupture is at 30-50% strength at 6 weeks and gradually increases over

several months.[17] By 3-4 months, repair strength is generally strong enough to take progressive loads for a gradual return-to-sport program.

Like tendons, the purpose of ligaments is to absorb in-line tension loads. Ligaments are designed to maintain alignment of bone structures. When avulsed, surgery is usually a direct repair with anchors, with the goal to have a strong enough construct to allow early range of motion. Direct repairs of mid-substance injuries may require additional protection with internal bracing or augmentation since the quality and strength of repair is less than avulsion repair or reconstruction with tunnels.

The timing of return to sport after knee reconstruction should include an assessment of how long a graft takes to incorporate (allograft takes longer), the strength of the initial construct (to allow early range of motion or weight-bearing), and graft and tissue maturation over time. For autograft ACL reconstruction, the construct is considered to be about 50% at 2 months and 80% at 4-6 months, with continued gradual maturation over the next 1-2 years. With that said, it has been shown that is safe to return sometime after 6-9 months.

For cartilage restoration procedures, anatomical and physiological healing depend on the technique used. When autogenous or allograft cartilage plugs are used, the rate-limiting step of anatomical healing is the cancellous bone-to-bone healing at the base of the plug. For marrow stimulation or cellular-based restoration procedures, a period of non-weight-bearing is necessary to allow the restoration cells to take hold in the base of the lesion being repaired. Range of motion is usually allowed to avoid stiffness and enable lubrication of the cartilage surfaces.

## Functional readiness (range of motion, strength, agility, endurance, performance)

After strength of tissues and surgical construct are accounted for, both at time zero and through a period of maturation, the next steps along the pathway to return to sport target functional readiness. These steps are the cornerstones of most rehabilitation programs and are the foundational philosophy of how an athlete can safely return to sport post-surgery.

For most musculoskeletal injuries focus on allowing early range of motion within a safe range as defined by the surgeon, and progress the patient to full range of motion as tissue healing and the surgical construct allow. This is followed by muscle activation to prevent atrophy followed by active range of motion, and strengthening against light resistance, leading to full resistance training with the goal of return to symmetric motor strength. Once range of motion and motor power have been regained, a true functional focus can begin with optimisation of endurance, agility and coordination followed by the introduction of sport-specific skills and a gradual progressive return to sport.

The timing of progression is based on the individual athlete and is related to the anatomical and physiological readiness of the tissues. As an example, a patient who underwent ACL reconstructive surgery with meniscus repair might have their weight-bearing restricted or protected for the first 6 weeks to enable healing of the meniscus repair. Simultaneously, flexion may be restricted beyond 90° to prevent loading of the meniscus repair. After 6 weeks, full range of motion may be progressively allowed and strengthening progressed while open-chain quadriceps exercises are avoided for the first 2 months in this clinical scenario in my practice.

As graft maturity allows, strengthening and loading are advanced, but no plyometric loading or hard twisting and cutting is allowed until after 4 months. Return to sport may be delayed for 6–9 months depending on the surgeon's sense of the physiological healing of the tissues. Hamstring grafts and allograft may be protected longer than autograft patellar tendon grafts. Once the athlete has achieved full range of motion, motor control and coordination, strength and endurance, and the team is confident with the timing of the physiological healing of the tissues, functional testing should be performed.

In one study, assessments at 6 months after surgery consisted of knee functional tests (quadriceps index, hamstrings index, and single-leg hop for distance) and 2 self-report questionnaires (International Knee Documentation Committee [IKDC] subjective score and ACL Return-to-Sport After Injury [ACL-RSI] scale). At 1 year after surgery, athletes were classified into the return-to-sport group ($n = 101$) or non-return-to-sport group ($n = 23$) based on self-reported sports activities. In competitive athletes, single leg hop <81% and ACL-RSI scale <55 points at 6 months after surgery were associated with a greater risk of unsuccessful return to sport at 1 year after surgery. Single leg hop and ACL-RSI scale at 6 months could serve as screening tools to identify athletes who have difficulties with returning to sport after ACL reconstruction.[18]

The exact tests included in the functional test assessment may vary from clinic to clinic, but should include a progressive series of reproducible dynamic testing that assesses strength coordination with a series of challenges.

## Psychological readiness

Beyond anatomical, physiological and functional readiness, psychological readiness is a critical factor for successful return to sport, especially at the athlete's previous level. Psychological readiness also plays an important role in safe return to sport, as those with poor confidence have an elevated incidence of recurrent injuries.

In one study of athletes with ACL injuries, 37% did not return to sport. Of these, 65% cited psychological reasons as the cause—often, fear of re-injury specifically.[19] The 12-Item Short Form Health Survey Mental Composite Scale (SF-12 MCS) can predict those at risk of worse outcomes and failure to return to sport after ACL reconstruction: 33% do not return due to fear.[20]

In another study, psychological responses before surgery and in early recovery were associated with returning to pre-injury level of sport at 12 months, suggesting that attention to psychological recovery after ACL injury and reconstruction surgery is warranted. In contrast, clinical screening for maladaptive psychological responses in athletes before and soon after surgery can help to identify athletes at risk of not returning to their pre-injury level of sport by 12 months.[21] An athlete who returns to participation lacking mental readiness, especially in a contact or collision sport, is predisposed for risk of further injury.[22]

> **PRACTICE PEARL**
>
> If you suspect that an athlete is not ready mentally, or lacks confidence to return to sport safely, you should validate the athlete's feelings and take action.

As a clinician, you can support the athlete by listening to them, pointing out their progress in rehabilitation (e.g. greater range of motion), providing emotional support, encouraging them to reach their rehabilitation goals and encouraging positive coping. It may be appropriate to share your own experience and opinions,[23] for example: "I've seen other athletes have some challenges during this post-operative rehabilitation period and then come out the other end with a great result."

## KEY POINTS

- While many sports injuries can and should be treated non-surgically, there are occasions when surgical intervention is required. In many cases, rehabilitation may be trialled prior to surgery.

- Factors related to the injury itself (severity, location, etc.) and the athlete (age, level of competition, etc.) help determine who may benefit most from surgery.

- There is a lack of consensus as to whether surgery is indicated for various musculoskeletal conditions. This is why you should factor in the patient's goals, preferences and values, along with the details of their injury and overall health status.

- When presenting treatment options to an athlete, do not try to convince the athlete, but rather present the options, available evidence, risks and benefits associated with each option and allow them to decide.

- There are inherent risks to any surgery, including bleeding, infection and risks associated with anaesthesia. Post-operative risks include compartment syndrome, blood clots and infection.

- For each type of surgical intervention, there is a weak link. The weak link can be used to guide post-operative rehabilitation, estimate timelines and avoid complications.

- Honest communication between medical staff and athlete is crucial. The athlete should understand what post-operative recovery will look like, a general timeline for return to sport and what they will need to do to reach their post-surgery goals.

- To fully return to participation in sport, a post-operative athlete should be ready physiologically (demonstrating sufficient healing of the injured tissues), functionally (able to perform sport-related tasks proficiently) and psychologically (demonstrating mental and emotional readiness).

## REFERENCES

References for this chapter can be found at www.mhprofessional.com/CSM6e

## ADDITIONAL CONTENT

Scan here to access additional resources for this topic and more provided by the authors

## CHAPTER 27

# Principles of sports injury rehabilitation

with **HÅVARD MOKSNES** and **PHIL GLASGOW**

*Rehabilitation is training in the presence of injury.*

PHIL GLASGOW

## CHAPTER OUTLINE

General principles
Understanding the patient: build a working alliance
Goal setting and targeted interventions
Phases of rehabilitation
Knowing when to progress the exercises
When rehabilitation does not go according to plan

## LEARNING OBJECTIVES

By the end of this chapter you should be able to:

- outline general principles of sports injury rehabilitation
- apply those principles to progress a patient back to their desired level of function
- discuss the goals of each phase in sports injury rehabilitation
- detail strategies for intervening when rehabilitation does not go according to plan.

Sports injury rehabilitation is a dynamic, structured process that aims to:

- restore the injured athlete's function and performance level
- return the athlete to sports participation in a safe and timely manner
- minimise the risk of re-injury.

As previous injury is a prominent risk factor for future injury,[1–3] rehabilitation is a critical aspect of care. In most cases, the goal should be to improve the athlete's physical function to above their pre-injury level.

The foundation of sports injury rehabilitation is a targeted exercise program that is progressed gradually. As outlined in previous chapters (including Chapters 14, 15 and 24), exercise therapy acts at the local tissue level and in the central nervous system. It may be used as a direct injury treatment (mechanotherapy)[4] or to unload injured tissue via altered movement and muscle activation patterns.

It is also important to maintain the athlete's condition as much as possible throughout the rehabilitation process. A model of the parallel priorities of exercise prescription during the rehabilitation process is shown in Figure 27.1.

Exercise prescription, progress and supervision are often performed by a physiotherapist (or similar health professional e.g. sports rehabilitator, trainer, therapist). However, where possible, a broader multidisciplinary team including the sport and exercise physician, orthopaedic surgeon and other sport scientists (e.g. dietitians, strength and conditioning specialists) should collaborate in rehabilitation planning.

The responsibility for implementing the program should be gradually transferred from the clinical team to the strength and conditioning team and coaches in the later phases of rehabilitation. It is critical to engage coaches in all phases of rehabilitation. In the early phases, coaches need to understand the plan and appreciate the functional milestones. In the later phases, they should take an increasingly active role in implementing the program.

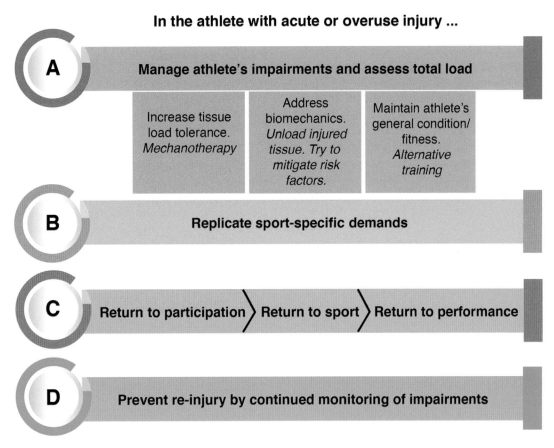

**In the athlete with acute or overuse injury ...**

**A** — Manage athlete's impairments and assess total load

| Increase tissue load tolerance. *Mechanotherapy* | Address biomechanics. *Unload injured tissue. Try to mitigate risk factors.* | Maintain athlete's general condition/ fitness. *Alternative training* |

**B** — Replicate sport-specific demands

**C** — Return to participation ⟩ Return to sport ⟩ Return to performance

**D** — Prevent re-injury by continued monitoring of impairments

**Figure 27.1** A model of the parallel priorities of exercise prescription during sports injury rehabilitation

Active rehabilitation is often supplemented with medical and manual therapies that may enhance the effects of exercise through pain management and improved tissue adaptations (Chapter 24). The success of rehabilitation depends on introducing the most effective intervention at the right time in an adequate dosage.[5] Best practice in sports injury rehabilitation is to progress the patient through phases based on sound clinical reasoning, sequenced functional achievements and the completion of functional milestones.

We use the five-phase framework outlined in this chapter and acknowledge that this is one way of structuring rehabilitation—it is not a recipe. We respect tissue-specific biological healing processes to guide the rehabilitation timeline (e.g. ACL reconstructions cannot gain full strength in a few weeks).

Exercise prescription, nutrition, communication and clinical reasoning are core skills for clinicians involved in rehabilitation of sports injuries. Experienced clinicians follow a clear model to progress rehabilitation, but few theoretical models have been published and even fewer have been tested rigorously.[5]

## GENERAL PRINCIPLES

The primary aim of rehabilitation is to return the athlete to sport with appropriate function and fitness to participate at the desired level with a low risk of re-injury. However, this is sometimes challenging due to the desire of the athlete, coach, parents, management and/or others to return the athlete to high-risk activities prematurely.

Regardless of the circumstance, the medical team is obliged to ensure that the athlete's long-term health is not compromised in the return-to-sport process. Thus, the rehabilitation plan should include predefined sport-specific functional milestones to ensure that the athlete is fit to return to sport with minimal risk of re-injury. Return to sport comprises three phases (Fig. 27.2).

The rehabilitation principles described in this chapter primarily apply to the treatment of acute sports injuries and post-operative musculoskeletal rehabilitation. These rehabilitation processes are usually relatively linear and, for the most part, predictable. The principles can also be applied to overuse injuries. However, because the symptoms of overuse injuries often fluctuate and athletes continue to train and compete with pain/impaired function, athletes may present at different stages of the rehabilitation continuum.[6]

Rehabilitation plans following sports injury are usually separated into distinct phases and include active interventions aimed at addressing body impairments and functional limitations, with the aim of facilitating the athlete's participation in their desired physical activity or sport.[7]

### Effective planning—an essential element

Effective detailed planning is one of the most important aspects of rehabilitation. The plan should integrate accurate anatomical, pathophysiological, biomechanical and sport-specific knowledge with physical training principles. For example, a professional athlete can devote more time to rehabilitation and rest between exercise bouts than an amateur athlete with a demanding work schedule. This will influence the total volume of training that can be tolerated.

Top athletes with day-to-day follow-up can usually progress more rapidly than recreational athletes, who have less frequent encounters with their clinician. Hence, you should create a larger safety buffer when designing rehabilitation programs for non-professionals.

> **PRACTICE PEARL**
>
> When designing a rehabilitation program, you should identify specifically how the injury affects or impairs the athlete's function—considering the sport and their role within it (e.g. their event, discipline or position).

Furthermore, physiological responses to rehabilitation stimuli vary between individuals, making the prediction of recuperation following an exercise more uncertain. Thus, the expected time to recovery differs depending on the injury, intrinsic personal and contextual factors, and the volume of stimuli that can be applied to facilitate tissue healing and recovery.

## UNDERSTANDING THE PATIENT: BUILD A WORKING ALLIANCE

At the outset of the rehabilitation journey, it is important to take time to understand the patient's goals (these may be injury- or performance-related) and to agree what successful rehabilitation looks like for them and the wider performance team, where applicable. The value of taking time to understand the patient's needs and to individualise the rehabilitation process cannot be overstated.

Alarmingly, on average physicians only listen to a patient's concerns for a median of 11 seconds before

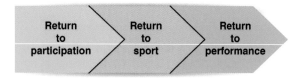

**Figure 27.2** The three elements of the return-to-sport continuum

interrupting.[8] Physiotherapists are no better, interrupting patients after 20–45 seconds depending on the type of question asked.[9]

By carefully listening, clinicians can identify different lanes of information and create a foundation of trust.[10] Taking time to listen to the patient and address their personal agenda helps foster a strong working alliance and can enhance patient satisfaction.[11, 12]

The working alliance (often referred to in healthcare as the therapeutic alliance), first described by Bordin, refers to "the collaboration between the client and therapist built upon the development of an attachment bond alongside a mutual commitment to the goals and task".[13]

The working alliance has a positive effect on outcomes across a range of medical settings.[13] In physiotherapy, it correlates with less pain and disability as well as better physical health, mental health and patient satisfaction.[14–16]

Five practices that promote clinician presence and connection have been identified:

1. *Prepare with intention. (Are you prepared for a meaningful interaction?)* Familiarise yourself with the patient you are about to meet. Create a ritual to focus your attention before a visit.
2. *Listen intently and completely. (What does your patient say when uninterrupted?)* Sit down, lean forward and position yourself to listen. Don't interrupt. Your patient is your most valuable source of information.
3. *Agree on what matters most. (What are your patient's health goals, now and in the future?)* Find out what your patient cares about and incorporate these priorities into the visit agenda.
4. *Connect with the patient's story. (How can you contribute positively to your patient's journey?)* Consider the circumstances that influence your patient's health. Acknowledge your patient's efforts, and celebrate successes.
5. *Explore emotional cues. (What can you learn from the patient's emotions?)* Tune in. Notice, name and validate your patient's emotions to become a trusted partner.[17]

## GOAL SETTING AND TARGETED INTERVENTIONS

Early goal setting and an outline of the rehabilitation plan are important elements that should be addressed in collaboration with the athlete, coach, physiotherapist and other members of the clinical team.[18] In the first meeting between the medical team and the athlete, the key steps should include:

1. obtaining a thorough history, including the current injury, any previous injuries and available resources

2. setting long-term goals
3. striving for an accurate diagnosis, which may be provisional and subject to supplementary investigations
4. identifying key impairments in body structure and function
5. raising potential physiological, psychological and logistical barriers
6. drafting a realistic progress plan that includes functional and measurable milestones.

Identifying the athlete's ultimate goal is usually straightforward—most athletes want to return to competition in sport as quickly as possible. However, expectations of a rapid return may sometimes be unrealistic, and misconceptions can undermine the collaboration and focus of the rehabilitation.

Thus, giving the athlete an early outline of the expected progress with specific short-term goals accompanied by specific tasks will usually build a bond of confidence. Communicating the expected progress plan to coaches, team members, family and sometimes the media usually fosters a collaborative environment for focused rehabilitation.

Physical impairments and limitations are commonly subdivided into the areas of restricted range of motion, motor control and muscle strength. Different injuries will, in combination with previous injuries and fitness status, result in different impairments and limitations. The medical team should analyse the status of the injury and decide to what extent each of the impairments or limitations should be targeted during rehabilitation.

The clinical skill of prioritising exercise interventions throughout rehabilitation has been designated as the "X-factor" in Figure 27.3. Prioritising rehabilitation interventions relies on the ability of the clinician and the broader team to effectively synthesise complex information (via skilled clinical assessment) and identify key limitations to performance as well as barriers to progression. While a large part of the X-factor will be based on sound clinical reasoning, it also involves the clinician's ability to relate to the athlete, to collaborate with other professions, to motivate and guide the athlete, and to educate key personnel.

> **PRACTICE PEARL**
>
> You should clearly indicate that the rehabilitation plan is dynamic—the focus will change depending on the patient's response to the program.

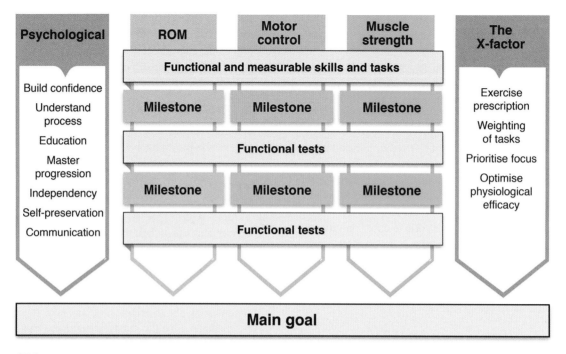

**Figure 27.3** A theoretical model of clinical focus throughout the sports injury rehabilitation process

Endurance and its specific subcomponents may also have to be integrated throughout the phases of rehabilitation. Examples are strength endurance for alpine skiers and speed endurance for footballers. The ability to carry out a specific task or exercise for an extended period of time without a reduction in quality or effort is an important component of the rehabilitation process.

Fatigue has been identified as a risk factor for injury,[17] so ensuring that the athlete is able to maintain good technique under fatigue is essential. Particular attention should be given to enhancing specific subqualities of endurance, such as skill execution under fatigue, as well as other strength and mobility parameters.

## Rehabilitation requires structure and flexibility

Rehabilitation is a dynamic continuum during which the nature and difficulty of exercises are progressed in response to tissue healing and the functional abilities of the athlete. Every athlete is different and rehabilitation should reflect individual needs and the performance consequences of the injury. The multidimensional nature of rehabilitation means organising several concurrent blocks with different goals and milestones.

Many injury rehabilitation protocols tend to be linear in nature, concentrating solely on restoration of strength or flexibility at the expense of wider performance characteristics. Ideally, you should adopt a blended approach that targets a range of components simultaneously. The following questions can be helpful when planning rehabilitation:

- What is happening at a tissue level?
- What outcomes are you trying to achieve with your exercise prescription?
- What is the specific adaptation associated with different exercise types?
- Is this exercise being used primarily to reduce symptoms, stimulate tissue adaptation (tissue capacity) or enhance function (movement capability)?

Restoration of physical qualities affected by injury is usually the central focus of rehabilitation. The four physical pillars of (1) movement quality, (2) movement capacity, (3) movement speed and (4) movement strength and power (Fig. 27.4) mirror those seen in normal training but with one key difference: the focus on improving the quality of injured/pathological tissue.

> **PRACTICE PEARL**
>
> In a sense, rehabilitation can be described as "training in the presence of injury".

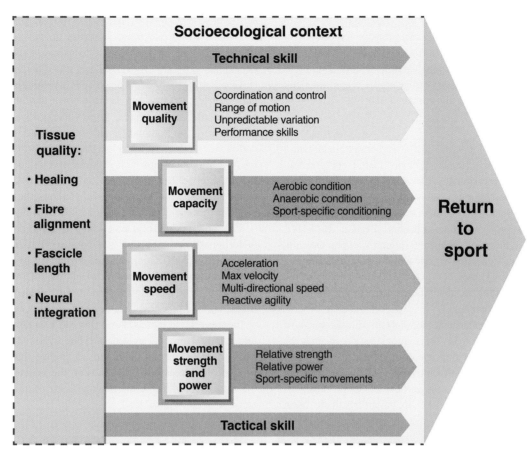

**Figure 27.4** Rehabilitation is the process of restoring tissue quality (the vertical green bar) and re-training movement (the four coloured arrows) while the player maintains their technical and tactical skills (the two grey arrows). This all takes place within the individual's socioecological context (hence the light-green shading across the entire panel between "tissue quality" and "return to sport").

When you guide return to sport you should also consider the technical and tactical aspects of training as well as ensuring psychological readiness (Fig 27.4). And experienced clinicians take contextual (e.g. socioecological) factors into account in the rehabilitation program. For example, the level of competition, the time in the season, specific performance goals, previous injury history as well as the time the athlete is able to commit to the program should all be considered as you build the return-to-sport plan (see green shading in Fig. 27.4).

## PHASES OF REHABILITATION

A five-phase structure can guide the aims and content of the rehabilitation process:

1. acute phase
2. early phase: restore activities of daily living
3. sport-specific phase
4. return-to-training phase
5. return-to-sport phase.

Specific functional milestones and achievement goals will be identified within each phase. Some goals will be primary in a phase, such as achieving full knee extension and quadriceps activation after knee surgery in phase 1. At the same time, preservation of gluteal muscle activation and ankle mobility will be important secondary areas of focus.

Clinicians with different backgrounds, knowledge and experience will choose different exercises and treatments to achieve rehabilitation aims. Although there is now consensus regarding the importance of individually tailored rehabilitation after injury,[19] well-documented rehabilitation guidelines are scarce for most conditions in sports medicine. In addition, treatment algorithms differ between cultures, countries and institutions.

Due to the multidimensional nature of sports rehabilitation, you should be able to manage several parallel focus areas throughout the various phases of rehabilitation, each with different goals and milestones. The relative importance of each focus area will change throughout the rehabilitation process. Progressing active rehabilitation requires continuous evaluation, which is necessary to guarantee a confident and timely return to training and competition.

## 1. Acute phase

In line with the increased focus on active rehabilitation strategies, the traditional acronym PRICE (Protection, Rest, Ice, Compression and Elevation) for the treatment of acute soft-tissue injuries is increasingly being replaced with POLICE (Protection, Optimal Loading, Ice, Compression and Elevation) and more recently, PEACE & LOVE (Protection, Elevation, Avoid anti-inflammatory medication, Compression, Education & Load Optimism, Vascularisation, Exercise) (see Chapter 24).[20] Optimal loading refers to the clinician evaluating the ability of the tissue to withstand and adapt to mechanical load.[21]

The clinical challenge is not only to choose the most effective and safest exercise interventions, but also to apply the interventions in the appropriate dose. Immediate protection and relative rest after an acute injury still play a role, but because of the detrimental effect of inactivity on biological tissues, leading clinicians look to have the athlete begin active movement (optimal loading) as soon as possible. For example, a player may begin hamstring activation exercises (loading) within 24 hours of a hamstring muscle strain depending on the severity of the injury and other factors.

Goal setting in the acute phase should be unidimensional and targeted towards impairments and limitations. For example, after knee ligament surgery, the goals are for the athlete to regain voluntary quadriceps activation towards end-range extension (impairment) and to perform a straight-leg raise without extension lag (limitation). In combination they comprise the functional milestone of controlled active terminal knee extension, which allows the athlete to progress to walking without crutches for short distances.

The ability to perform a slow step-up with good control of terminal knee extension is a common functional goal during early rehabilitation of acute knee injuries (Fig. 27.5). When adequate step-up quality of movement is achieved, the use of crutches can be terminated for all distances. Blanchard and Glasgow have depicted the process for how to progress single exercises and this can be adapted to the rehabilitation process in general (Fig. 27.6).[5] The model describes how you can build and manipulate the exercises to gradually increase the demands on the athlete, while at the same time allowing the healing tissue to adapt to the increase in mechanical load.

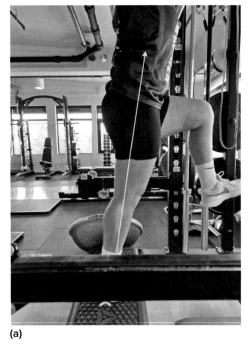
(a)

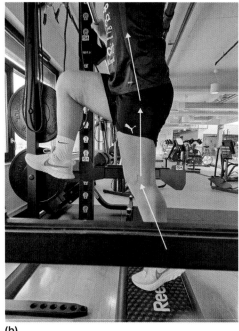
(b)

**Figure 27.5** The ability to perform a slow step-up with good control of terminal knee extension is a common functional goal during early rehabilitation of acute knee injuries: (a) good control on the uninjured side and (b) lack of end-range control on the injured side.

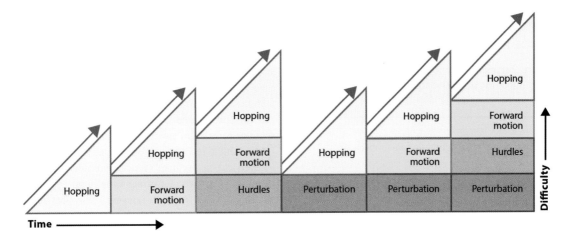

**Figure 27.6** Visual aid to demonstrate a complex rehabilitation progression with undulating tiers using lower limb injury as an example.[5] The horizontal axis represents time and the vertical axis represents difficulty. The clinician adds and subtracts elements of the rehabilitation to progressively challenge the athlete while keeping the overall workload appropriate.
Source: Reproduced from Blanchard S, Glasgow P. A theoretical model to describe progressions and regressions for exercise rehabilitation. *Phys Ther Sport* 2014 Aug;15(3):131–5.

A variety of interventions are available to the clinician in the initial phase. Traditional low-load controlled exercises are at the core of interventions. However, adjunct modalities such as neuromuscular electrical stimulation can help the athlete to regain voluntary muscular control.[22,23] Furthermore, manual therapies can be effective in the recovery of impairments during this phase (see Chapter 24).

## 2. Early phase

The aim of the second phase is to enable the athlete to return to daily activities and basic sport-specific technical movements. Gradually increase the complexity of movements from single joint-controlled actions to more complex tasks including movements through several biomechanical planes.

For example, an overhead athlete who has regained pain-free external rotation in the scapular plane with adequate scapular control in the initial phase will typically progress to mimic the throwing motion at low velocity in the early phase. While the throwing motion will be the primary focus of the rehabilitation program, you should ensure that secondary functions such as contralateral hip stability and ankle range of motion are maintained.

Exercises can be progressed by increasing the:

- number of repetitions
- velocity of the movement or
- frequency (rate) of the exercises.

Furthermore, adding external loads and increasing the complexity of movement will stimulate muscle strength and motor control. Thus, the early phase challenges you to prioritise exercises successfully. Skilled clinicians can keep their eye on several parallel processes at the same time (the X-factor).

Goal setting in this phase will still focus on the remaining impairments, although the main goals are related to addressing functional limitations in activity and improving performance of semi-complex sport-specific movement patterns. Examples of early phase functional milestones for an ACL-injured athlete can be jogging with good form, and the ability to perform single leg hops with full knee extension at take-off and high degrees of knee and hip flexion during landing.[24]

The primary intervention is to continue progressing the therapeutic exercise program. The program will mainly incorporate elements to improve motor control and muscle strength, with additional sessions of cardiovascular training.

When determining the exact nature of cardiovascular training in rehabilitation, ensure that the correct energy system is being trained and that adequate time is allowed for recovery and physiological adaptation. For athletes who are rehabilitating over longer periods of time (i.e. months after ACL reconstruction), the acute:chronic workload ratio should be considered (see Chapter 15).

The nature of training used should involve adequate stress on the injured tissues while simultaneously exercising muscle groups involved in the athlete's sport. Aerobic and anaerobic endurance can be effectively trained using pool-based conditioning or cardiovascular equipment such as a bicycle ergometer, cross-trainer, rowing ergometer and step machine.

**PRACTICE PEARL**

The nature, intensity, duration and work:rest ratio of individual training sessions should reflect sporting demands.

An example of a weekly schedule may consist of:

- two muscle strength sessions
- two motor control session
- two cardiovascular sessions
- one recovery day.

The precise nature of the sessions and the order in which exercises are carried out will be dictated by the clinician's understanding of the sport to which the athlete must return, the effects of the specific impairments and an appreciation of how the prescribed exercise will influence restoration of function.

The clinician must have a good understanding and ability to appropriately modify load and difficulty of the exercises, while still guarding the healing tissue from abrupt forces and overload. Efficient communication with specific cues that facilitate a move from an internal focus of attention to an external focus, in combination with careful explanation and involvement of the athlete, can greatly increase the efficacy and adherence to interventions.[25, 26]

### 3. Sport-specific phase

During the sport-specific phase, you should gradually incorporate activities that relate more closely to the athlete's sport. Attention should be given to the training demands of the sport. Increased focus on the dominant movement patterns, skill execution and expression of physical qualities in a sporting context will guide session content. The following questions may be helpful when planning this phase:

- What are the performance characteristics?
  - Repeated short bursts?
  - Prolonged activity?
  - How long for?
  - Sport-specific skills: reactive/open skills?
- What are the physiological characteristics?
  - Anaerobic dominant?
  - Aerobic dominant?
  - Combination?
- What are the physical characteristics?
  - Predominant muscle groups?
  - Range of movement demands?
  - Strength requirements?

### 4. Return-to-training phase

In this phase, you should guide the athlete towards returning to participation in their sport. More traditional strength and conditioning training can be incorporated in the weekly rehabilitation plan with increased focus on more complexity and velocity. Emphasis should be on a higher rate of force development and introduction of on-field sessions to bring in environmental adaptation.

An athlete recovering from a knee injury can be brought to the field to perform sessions focused on higher speed running, cutting and turning tasks, and include relevant equipment (ball, racquet, skis, etc.). Physical conditioning in the gym will be similar to pre-season training for the specific sport, although a majority of exercises should still be unilaterally focused to stimulate adaptation and reverse any remaining impairments.

Goal setting in this phase will relate to all levels of function. Typically, for lower extremity injuries, muscle strength measurements (impairment) and single-leg hop tests (activity) are compared with the goal of 90% of the uninjured side.[27, 28] Participation goals can include completing specific parts of the team training sessions without symptoms during or after training.

An important task for the clinician will be to monitor the overall load on the healing structures, which again calls for close collaboration and clear communication with coaches and strength and conditioning professionals.

### 5. Return-to-sport phase

Return-to-sport decisions are perennially challenging and require a team approach that focuses on ensuring that function has been adequately restored. To facilitate safe return to sport, it is paramount that functional testing with valid and reliable outcome measures be performed. (See Chapter 23 for more on relevant outcome measures.) Multidimensional sets of tests that evaluate the different layers of function are best.[29-32] However, scientific backing regarding content and cut-off limits for the test batteries is still lacking for most injuries. The return-to-sport process is discussed in Chapter 28.

## KNOWING WHEN TO PROGRESS THE EXERCISES

Due to the multidimensional nature of rehabilitation, you should be able to organise several parallel blocks with different goals and milestones.[33] To progress rehabilitation successfully, you should carefully and continually evaluate the athlete. Rehabilitation programs usually rely on specific physical tests and symptom provocation to inform progression.

The most common clinical outcome measure used to progress rehabilitation is the patient's perception of pain.[34] The level of discomfort tolerated during rehabilitation should be guided by the rationale for the specific exercise. You should be clear whether there is an acceptable level of discomfort during activities or if pain-free function is the goal.

Both may be appropriate but are highly context- and activity-dependent. For example, where the primary goal of the exercise is tissue loading, some discomfort may be acceptable. In contrast, where the focus is on restoring movement quality, it is more appropriate for exercises to be pain-free.

Many different clinical tests can inform progression of rehabilitation. Importantly, no single test is able to determine the ability of an athlete to progress. Rather, progression should be based on an appropriate battery of tests that assess different aspects of function. These will normally include measures of strength (and its subcomponents e.g. eccentric strength, strength endurance, rate of force development), dynamic "functional" tests (hop tests, jump tests, agility tests), sport-specific testing as well as psychological readiness.

Testing for specific injuries and anatomical regions is discussed in the relevant chapters. Throughout rehabilitation it is necessary to continuously communicate closely with the patient to ensure that the program aligns with their functional ability, psychological readiness and specific performance goals.

## Criteria for progression

Criteria for progressing to the next phase include:

- pain
- pathology and/or stage of repair (time-based)
- strength (and subqualities)
- motor control and movement quality
- execution of sport-specific tasks
- limb symmetry
- psychological readiness.

## Prevention of re-injury

All sports injuries with tissue disruption will render the athlete more susceptible to re-injury, even though tissue structure and physical function may be restored after rehabilitation. In spite of the increased attention on and knowledge of rehabilitation of sports injuries, the incidence of re-injury remains high in professional sports.[35,36] The importance of internal risk factors such as previous injury in the prevention of sports injuries has been known for the past 30 years.[37]

Athletes should be monitored for total load when possible. Re-testing of the return-to-competition test battery could be beneficial to detect possible decline in function, as attention to physical training may become secondary to performance in this period. Intervention should be aimed at impairments and functional limitations known to exist as a result of injury, such as altered muscle activation patterns and inadequate landing and cutting strategies.[38,39]

> **PRACTICE PEARL**
>
> Every clinician involved in the rehabilitation of sports injuries must work diligently with the athlete, coach and conditioning professionals to continue targeted individualised prevention training after the athlete has returned to the competitive level.

## WHEN REHABILITATION DOES NOT GO ACCORDING TO PLAN

Sports injury rehabilitation can seem like a straightforward linear process but, as every clinician has experienced, progression does not always go according to plan. Longstanding pain, recurrent effusion, persistent range of motion deficits and muscle inhibition are a few of the most common obstacles. What should you do when progression seems to fail?

A thorough look at the content and volume of the rehabilitation program is usually indicated. Are the interventions targeting the impairments they were intended to target? It is often prudent to follow the athlete through a full session to ensure that proper technique and understanding are present. Experienced clinicians often state that "less is more" and that splitting the original rehabilitation program into two parts is a wise decision.

> **PRACTICE PEARL**
>
> It may be necessary to revisit the diagnosis and the functional assessment.

Symptoms tend to change over time—and not always in a predictable fashion. A step back to address the basic functional impairments is often necessary.

The athlete has performed all sessions, but no improvement can be measured in muscle strength over a period of 6–8 weeks. Ask about nutritional status. Has the athlete lost or gained weight? Is your female athlete's menstrual cycle normal? Has your male athlete experienced reduced libido? Athletes can develop dysfunctional eating habits and an altered body image during rehabilitation. Consider referral to a dietitian experienced with the relative energy deficiency in sport (REDs).[40,41]

Sit down with the athlete and analyse the total load during the week. Is there enough time to recover between sessions? How much load is placed on the healing structures between training sessions? Are there any environmental challenges related to family, friends, facilities or motivation?

Collaborate with the athlete to resolve underlying challenges. Ask open questions and probe their psychological status. A few days off rehabilitation may be a relief to many athletes.

Ask a colleague! A referral back to the physician or orthopaedic surgeon may be indicated. A second opinion from another clinician within the field can often open new doors. Additionally, a multidisciplinary meeting with all parties can adjust and streamline the expectations and responsibilities of each member of the rehabilitation team.

## KEY POINTS

- Planning a sports injury rehabilitation program entails pursuing parallel goals at the same time, while protecting the injured tissue.

- Active exercise is the cornerstone of a sports injury rehabilitation plan and may be complemented with manual or medical therapies.

- Communicating an honest timeline for rehabilitation is important in building trust between athlete and clinician. While many athletes share a goal of returning to sport, clearly defining goals is important.

- Depending on the level of sport, the injured athlete may have daily or only occasional contact with their clinician. An athlete who sees their clinician less frequently may require more of a safety buffer.

- Return to sport is an individual process that requires personalisation. There are frameworks and questions that can guide and tailor the process, rather than relying on an injury-based "recipe" for rehabilitation.

- While pain is the most commonly used criterion in progressing through rehabilitation, validated and reliable tools are available to supplement return-to-sport decisions.

- Even after an athlete returns to sport, they are vulnerable to re-injury and should continue with injury prevention strategies after clearance.

- Return to sport is not always linear in nature. Setbacks are not unusual, and require a re-evaluation of the injury, assessment and/ or rehabilitation plan and possibly additional screening.

## REFERENCES

References for this chapter can be found at www.mhprofessional.com/CSM6e

## ADDITIONAL CONTENT

 Scan here to access additional resources for this topic and more provided by the authors

## CHAPTER 28

# Return to sport

with **KATE YUNG** and **CLARE ARDERN**

*I honestly didn't know if I would be ready for the WNBL [Australian Women's National Basketball League] this season. But I am fitter than I was last year—it's the best I have felt in a long time. The rehab has gone really well, and the club has seen me on court, and they know I am ready. That's why we're here again.*

LAUREN JACKSON (AUSTRALIAN BASKETBALL PLAYER, 7-TIME WNBA ALL STAR, 3-TIME WNBA MOST VALUABLE PLAYER, 3-TIME OLYMPIC SILVER MEDALIST, SPEAKING IN OCTOBER 2023 ABOUT HER RETURN TO PROFESSIONAL BASKETBALL AT THE AGE OF 42 AFTER ACHILLES TENDON SURGERY)

## CHAPTER OUTLINE

The return-to-sport continuum

Progressing from out (injured) to outstanding (performance)

Testing the athlete's readiness to return

Gathering, integrating and synthesising information to support shared return-to-sport decisions

What to work on today to avoid poor return-to-sport outcomes tomorrow

Data science supporting high-quality return-to-sport decisions

## LEARNING OBJECTIVES

By the end of this chapter you should be able to:

- identify the stages of the return-to-sport continuum
- justify the choice of return-to-sport tests
- use a multidimensional, criteria-based approach and shared decision making in the return-to-sport process
- recognise clinical scenarios where shared return-to-sport decision making requires careful consideration
- choose appropriate criteria for interpreting the results of return-to-sport tests.

Returning to sport is a shared process where clinicians, athletes and others, as appropriate (Chapter 4), collaborate to decide where, when, how or if an athlete will transition from injury/illness to reaching their goals for performing in sport.[1-3] Return-to-sport decisions are often complex. Delaying return to sport may mean trading better health for the athlete with worse team performance.[4,5] Yet returning to sport too early raises the risk of re-injury for the athlete.[6-8]

Outside of the elite arena, return-to-sport decisions are governed by the athlete's health and wellbeing. In elite sport, there is often irreconcilable tension between protecting the athlete's health and their need to perform. The available resources (e.g. time, equipment, human resources), personal preferences and clinical approach also inform return-to-sport decisions. Clinicians and athletes weigh the risks and benefits together to share the decision.

## THE RETURN-TO-SPORT CONTINUUM

Instead of a thumbs up (ready to return) or thumbs down (not ready to return), think of return to sport as a continuum starting when the injury/illness is first diagnosed and ending when the athlete reaches their return-to-sport goals (Fig. 28.1).[1] Using a common language when talking about return to sport helps clinicians, athletes and coaches to communicate. There are three critical stages in the return-to-sport continuum:

1. *return to participate:* the athlete participates in rehabilitation, training or sport at a lower level than their return-to-sport goal
2. *return to sport:* the athlete participates without restriction in their sport but is not yet performing at their desired level
3. *return to perform:* the athlete has returned to sport *and* is performing at or above their pre-injury level.

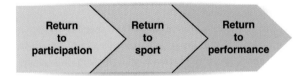

**Figure 28.1** The return-to-sport continuum

The continuum emphasises that return to sport is a dynamic process that requires careful balancing of the benefits and risks to progress to the next stage.[9] Stages in the continuum may overlap, depending on the athlete's capacity and readiness.

## PROGRESSING FROM OUT (INJURED) TO OUTSTANDING (PERFORMANCE)

For an athlete to make progress through the return-to-sport continuum, experienced clinicians support a steady increase in load, and physical and psychological demands. How do you support the athlete to progress from the controlled environment of the rehabilitation room to the increasing complexity of the sports arena? Consider the key areas of the athlete's sport you would like to focus on during the return-to-sport and return-to-performance phases. The areas might include strength and power, or sport-specific skills (e.g. ball-handling). For more ideas, see Figure 27.4 in Chapter 27. Various frameworks describe how you can support return-to-sport progress in different sports and at different times in the continuum.[10-15] These frameworks can help you to structure rehabilitation plans and communicate with athletes and coaches.

To make progress, the athlete moves from training in a closed environment (i.e. static and predictable) to an open environment (i.e. dynamic and changing).[1,16] The control-chaos continuum is a helpful guide in designing and implementing rehabilitation that progresses from a controlled and closed environment (high control, low chaos) to a complex sport environment (low control, high chaos).[13]

In basketball the control-chaos continuum might see players recovering from lower limb injury progress from a high-control training program (e.g. basic dribbling and on-court running) to a high-chaos program (e.g. unrestricted basketball drills with contact).[14] In soccer, an injured player might progress from high-control gym-based physical preparation to high-chaos on-pitch sport-specific conditioning.[17]

To support returning to the typical match/game demands during return to performance, the control–chaos continuum includes examples of how to incorporate strength and power metrics for a range of lower limb injuries.[11]

Listen to two experienced sports physiotherapists, Dr Lionel Chia and Professor Nicola Phillips, explain how they approach planning for return to sport:

Beginning with the end in mind for return to sport, with Dr Lionel Chia

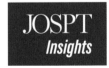

Optimal loading to improve upper limb performance, with Professor Nicola Phillips

## TESTING THE ATHLETE'S READINESS TO RETURN

There are two key reasons why you should consider return-to-sport testing:

1. *To gather information about the athlete's current health and performance status.* Without testing, you are guessing. Key questions you might seek answers to include:

   - Has the injured tissue healed?
   - Have muscle strength and movement control been restored?
   - Is the athlete psychologically prepared to cope with the demands of their sport?

   Key decisions are which tests to choose to evaluate the athlete's current physical and psychological readiness to return to sport, and when to test.

2. *To gather information that will guide the shared decision-making team when predicting a future outcome (prognosis).* Keys questions you might want answers to include:

   - What is the likelihood of another injury?
   - When will the athlete reach their pre-injury performance level?

   After an athlete returns to sport, the risk of a new injury (to either limb) remains elevated for weeks to months.[8, 18-20] In Australian football, the injury risk is highest in the week the athlete returns to sport, and athletes with a history of ACL injury have double the risk of subsequent hamstring injury than their un-injured teammates.[19] New injuries have a similarly negative impact on athletes' health and team performance as the index/primary injury[4, 5, 21, 22] and can wreak a heavy financial toll on sports organisations.[22-26] Having an estimate of the likelihood of a new injury (1) helps the shared decision-making team to make informed return-to-sport decisions, and (2) provides an opportunity to implement strategies (e.g. injury prevention/reduction programs, managing the athlete's match minutes or training load) to minimise the impact of new injuries.

## GATHERING AND SYNTHESISING INFORMATION TO SUPPORT SHARED RETURN-TO-SPORT DECISIONS

Decision frameworks can help support quality return-to-sport decisions because they provide a structured way to organise information.[27] When planning return-to-sport testing, begin with the end in mind:[28]

- What is the athlete's return-to-sport goal?
- What specific domains do you want to test that relate to this goal?
- Which test is appropriate?

Then, use a shared decision-making mindset to improve decision quality by eliminating blind spots (i.e. information you cannot possibly know) such as the athlete's expectations, preferences and values. Work with the athlete (and others, as required) to make decisions together. You need to understand each other's perspectives to better align priorities and values when making decisions.

Box 28.1 illustrates how you might choose return-to-sport tests for a youth athlete with a hamstring strain injury.

### Zoom out: which domains of function to test and how

Experienced clinicians favour criteria-based return-to-sport testing over a time-based approach (i.e. deciding based solely on the time the athlete has spent in rehabilitation).[29-34] When using a criteria-based approach, consider how you will test physical readiness *and* psychological readiness to return to sport.

There are five domains to consider when planning return-to-sport testing:

1. *Clinical assessment:* use your clinical judgment to decide which impairments are appropriate to test. You might choose joint range of motion, muscle strength and length, pain and effusion, depending on the return-to-sport goal (e.g. MHFAKE[35]).

2. *Physical fitness and function:* assess the movements (known as activities and activity limitations in the World Health Organization's International Classification of Function, Disability and Health) that athletes need to perform to reach the return-to-sport goal. You might consider tests that incorporate strength, speed, power, endurance, flexibility, speed and agility (e.g. single-leg hop for distance[36]).

3. *Sport-specific skills:* assess the specific tasks and movements that an athlete executes when participating in their sport (e.g. grand plié through full range of motion and without pain[15]).

4. *Training load:* assess the athlete's accumulated training load and intensity during rehabilitation and compare this with match demand (e.g. evaluate the high-speed running workload for Australian football players[7]).

5. *Psychological readiness:* athletes judge their mental readiness to return to sport based on (i) how they perceive their physical function, (ii) their expectations for recovery and re-injury, (iii) their motivation to return to sport and (iv) their confidence to perform.[37] There are generic- and injury-specific tools for measuring psychological readiness to return to sport (Box 28.2 and Table 28.1).

**BOX 28.1**  Clinical scenario: choosing return-to-sport tests after hamstring injury

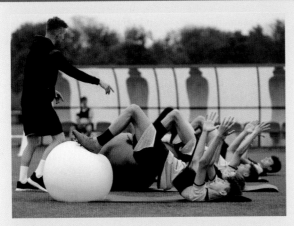

**Figure 28.2** Ben sustained a hamstring strain injury during soccer training
ISTOCK/MATIMIX

Ben (Fig. 28.2) is a promising 16-year-old soccer player who sustained a hamstring strain injury (biceps femoris grade II) during a sprinting session in training 8 weeks ago.

The coach thinks Ben has a high potential for selection in the junior national team for an upcoming international tournament (4 months from today, Fig. 28.3). You are overseeing Ben's treatment from injury and working with him to plan his return to club soccer. This scenario focuses on the return-to-sport tests you might choose when asked whether Ben is ready to return to sport after his injury.

**Step 1. Decide what to test, how and when**
To assess Ben's physical readiness to return to competitive club soccer, you assess the match demands with a particular focus on his playing position as a forward. Based on your analysis of his soccer demands, you decide that testing should aim to address the following key match demands:

- goal kicking
- high-speed running
- sprinting
- field kicking
- changing direction
- accelerating and decelerating
- vertical jumping.

Guided by the recommendations of the Aspetar hamstring protocol, developed by expert sport and exercise clinicians, you consider ways to assess the following factors:

- pain
  - on palpation at rest
  - during strength and flexibility tests
  - during and after training

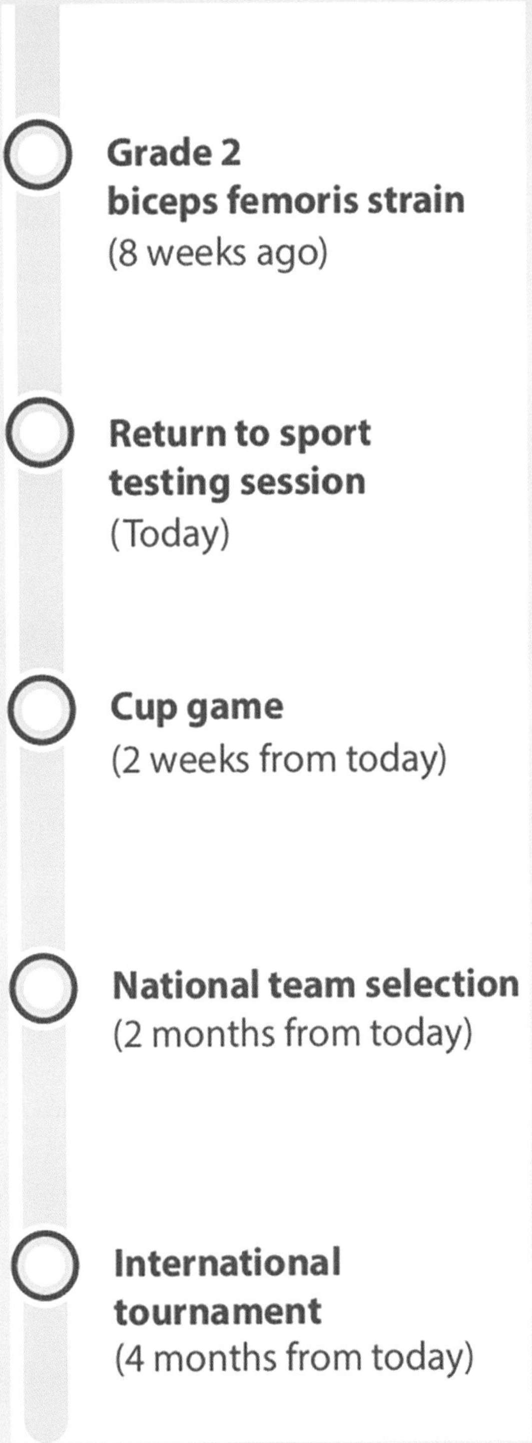

**Grade 2 biceps femoris strain**
(8 weeks ago)

**Return to sport testing session**
(Today)

**Cup game**
(2 weeks from today)

**National team selection**
(2 months from today)

**International tournament**
(4 months from today)

**Figure 28.3** Timeline of Ben's hamstring injury and return-to-sport planning

*continues*

453

- hamstring static flexibility using MHFAKE (maximum hip flexion with active knee extension)
- concentric and eccentric isokinetic strength at 60°/second
- eccentric hamstring strength (using the Nordic hamstring exercise)
- confidence and hamstring dynamic flexibility (using the Askling H-test)
- sport-specific tests
  - repeated sprinting (timed, compared with Ben's pre-season test results)
  - accelerating and decelerating from a sprint (evaluated qualitatively with video + absence of symptoms: pain or tightness)
  - single-leg bridge (pain-free: yes/no)
  - goal kicking and field kicking (pain-free: yes/no; evaluated during team training).

Aspetar hamstring protocol

There are more tests that you could choose but you are balancing the limited time you have with Ben, and this is your list of priority tests.

### Step 2. Consider how you plan testing and make clinical decisions (clinical reasoning)

Acknowledging the potential for bias in the decision-making process, you implement a strategy to enhance decision quality. You write a checklist with all your tests for the session, plan sufficient time to complete the testing and allocate time to write your recommendations for the coaching staff at the end of the session.

Before the testing session with Ben, you also arrange to meet with his coaches and the club's strength and conditioning specialist to (1) discuss Ben's progress and (2) confirm that you have all the information you need from the coaches about the injury and team context (i.e. the big picture).

### Step 3. Contribute to shared decision making

Ben performs well on each of the return-to-sport tests. After the testing session, you coordinate a meeting with Ben, his parents and the club's coaching staff, where you present Ben's results to discuss the next steps. During the meeting, you hear different perspectives: Ben is eager to resume competitive soccer as soon as possible; his parents are concerned about Ben injuring his hamstring again; and as the team has an important cup game in 2 weeks, the coaches are hoping that Ben will be available to play the match.

### Wrap-up: balancing re-injury risk with returning to sport

Ben's parents and coaches are struck by your advice that hamstring injury recurrence rates are highest (and relatively high at 15%) in the first 4 weeks after returning to competition.

While the coaches would have liked to select Ben for the cup game in 2 weeks, everyone agrees that because of his substantial potential for national representation, and his young age, the risk of a recurrence (and the lengthy setback a recurrence would mean) warrant a more careful and gradual return to sport. Ben re-joins training (Fig. 28.4), where he gradually progresses the intensity of his high-speed running and full-force kicking, and complements his on-field training with a tailored gym program. You propose close workload monitoring by the coaching staff and a gradual increase in playing time over the next 4 weeks.

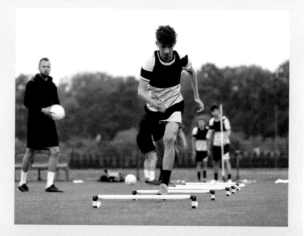

**Figure 28.4** Workload monitoring and shared decision making are key elements in Ben's successful return to sport
ISTOCK/MATIMIX

### Outcome

The shared decision-making team decide on an approach that aims to mitigate risk while gradually re-introducing Ben to competitive play and preparation for the national team selection trials in a few months.

**BOX 28.2** Putting your skills into practice: testing psychological readiness to return to sport after ACL injury

Sara is a 19-year-old amateur handball player (Fig. 28.5) with a non-contact, isolated ACL tear. For the first 3 months after her knee injury, Sara sees a physiotherapist who guides her rehabilitation, focusing on reducing pain and swelling, restoring symmetrical gait and strengthening her quadriceps, hamstrings, calves and gluteal muscles.

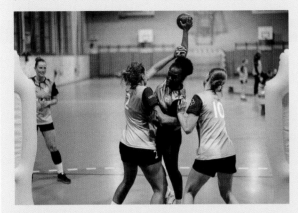

**Figure 28.5** Sara sustained a non-contact, isolated ACL tear while playing handball
ISTOCK/ANCHIY

Unfortunately, Sara experiences recurrent dynamic instability in her injured knee. She is adamant that she wants to return to the handball court, and together with her physiotherapist and orthopaedic surgeon decides that an ACL reconstruction plus active rehabilitation is the most appropriate course of treatment.

Sara's surgery goes well, and she attends regular physiotherapy for the first 3 months postoperatively before she moves interstate to attend university. While at university, Sara struggles to find affordable healthcare, and for the next 2 months (post-operative months 4–6)

she tries to manage and progress her rehabilitation by following the handouts from her previous physiotherapist.

At 6 months after her surgery, Sara has an appointment with you at her university's student-led physiotherapy clinic. She explains her strength training and running program. She has done no hopping or direction change tasks because she is terrified of her knee giving way again.

### Testing Sara's psychological readiness to return to sport

Using a regular monitoring question will give you a quick idea how Sara is feeling each time you see her in the clinic, and before and after introducing a new task (e.g. hopping, jump-land activities, etc.). The score takes less than a minute to collect (Fig. 28.6):

> Question: "How confident do you feel about returning to sport, on a scale of 0 to 10?"

Once Sara is used to answering the question, she can incorporate self-monitoring into her regular training diary, which helps you and Sara to track her progress. Review her training diary at each appointment and work together to identify and discuss any setbacks.

Example: "I see you tried incorporating those direction change drills we practised in the clinic last time. It looks like your confidence was a bit lower than normal in your next training session. What do you think happened?" Focused questionnaires (i.e. psychological readiness patient-reported outcome measures) take longer to complete and are most helpful when used at key transitions on the return-to-sport continuum (e.g. return to running, return to unrestricted training).

Follow-up after Sara's return to sport should check how she feels about her return and her re-injury risk. Consider collecting a psychological readiness patient-reported outcome measure again.

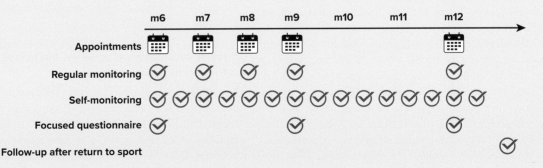

**Figure 28.6** An example of how to monitor an athlete's psychological readiness to return to sport

**TABLE 28.1**   Testing psychological readiness to return to sport

| Examples of generic psychological readiness patient-reported outcome measures | |
| --- | --- |
| Tampa Scale for Kinesiophobia (TSK) (17 items[38] or 11-item short form[39]) | Measures fear of moving Common in chronic pain research |
| Re-injury Anxiety Inventory (RIAI)[40] (28 items) | Measures anxiety about a new sports injury Limited research on its measurement properties |
| Injury Psychological Readiness to Return to Sport after Injury Scale (I-PRRS)[41] (6 items) | Focuses on the athlete's confidence Limited research on its measurement properties |
| **Examples of condition-specific psychological readiness patient-reported outcome measures** | |
| ACL-Return to Sport after Injury (ACL-RSI) scale (12 items[42] or 6-item short form[43]) | Developed for athletes with ACL injury Measures confidence, emotions and risk appraisal Adapted for hip[44] and shoulder[45] complaints Measurement properties are well-studied |
| Knee Self-Efficacy Scale (K-SES)[46] (22 items) | Developed for active people with sports-related knee injury Some questions may not apply to all athletes (e.g. moving around in a small boat, cross-country skiing) Measurement properties are well-studied |

## Zoom in: shared return-to-sport decisions

Historically, the clinician (usually the physician) held the return-to-sport decision-making power—think of this "old-school" approach to decisions as a "gatekeeper".[2,47-51] The clinician's skills are in assessing injury-related criteria, including assessing the state of healing, the risk of re-injury and the risk of short- or long-term problems.[2,52-54] Clinicians have a duty of care to athletes, and a legal and ethical obligation to act to protect the health of athletes. It is important to acknowledge the often-irreconcilable tension between the athlete performing in sport and staying healthy. Shared decision making can help here. See Box 28.3 for an example of shared return-to-sport decision making for an Olympic fencing athlete with an ACL tear.

Clinicians are not the only people who can contribute to return-to-sport decisions. Others, including coaches, can provide important information about non-medical factors and context to consider.[2,9,50,58-61] In a sports setting, the clinician may have dual allegiances, as they do not work exclusively for the injured athlete, but also on behalf of a club, federation or national organisation, for example. In the professional sport setting, clinicians and athletes may feel pressured by their employer to minimise lay-off time and return to sport soon as possible.[62,63]

Shared decision making is considered best practice in medicine (general practice).[1,64,65] In sports and exercise medicine, it usually involves the athlete, clinicians, coaches and others (e.g. parents).[59] Shared decision making respects multiple perspectives, while aiming to minimise disagreement due to conflicting interests. For more on the theory of shared decision making, including adopting a shared decision-making mindset, see Chapter 4. For more on the practice of shared decision making when managing injury and illness, see Chapter 5.

For shared return-to-sport decision making to work well, those "at the table" need to agree on what they consider successful return to sport.[1] Only then can the team decide which information to consider, weigh the benefits and risks, and make a decision.[59,65,66]

### Shared decision making when the health risks of returning to sport are high

Shared decision making is not appropriate for return-to-sport decisions if the athlete and coaches do not have sufficient capacity to make an informed decision. One example is returning to the field immediately after a head impact with potential for concussion. Rules mandating withdrawing the athlete for a minimum period of time and completing concussion testing (such as the head impact assessment rule instituted by World Rugby) protect the athlete's health.

**BOX 28.3** Integrating and interpreting evidence from different sources to support informed return-to-sport decisions

Veronique (Fig. 28.7) is a renowned elite épée fencer who, at the age of 25 years, sustained a right ACL injury with a small radial tear of the medial meniscus during an international tournament. She was her nation's premier fencing athlete, ranked 10th in the world, before her knee injury. You first met Veronique 11 months before the Olympics, when she was anxious about needing to accrue sufficient qualification points. Her right knee is her leading leg for fencing. After spending time talking with Veronique to hear her preferences and goals, and the demands of her sport, and considering the best available evidence together, you used shared decision making to support Veronique as she decided to have an ACL reconstruction.

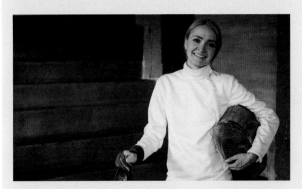

**Figure 28.7** Veronique sustained a right ACL tear during an international fencing tournament
ISTOCK/SILVERKBLACK

Here we document the process of planning return to sport with Veronique, including how the team clinicians might interpret clinical information related to return to sport.

**Applying the return-to-sport continuum to Veronique's progress**
*1. Return to participation (active rehabilitation)*
Veronique's acute rehabilitation followed standard postoperative knee care, prioritising achieving a "quiet knee": managing pain and effusion, restoring strong quadriceps activation, and symmetrical gait. During postoperative week 2, Veronique commenced upper body strengthening and technical training in a seated position. Her training focused on blade disengage (quick and controlled disengages by alternating attacks between high and low lines), circular parries (execute circular parries to defend against attacks from various angles) and target point control (use a target dummy to practise accurate hits).

*2. Return to participation (active rehabilitation + introducing sport-specific exercises)*
After 4 weeks of targeted swelling control and quadriceps activation exercises (including using neuromuscular electrical stimulation[55]), Veronique transitioned to upper body technical training in a static standing position. She continued with her prescribed upper and lower body strengthening regimen, supervised by her physiotherapist and strength and conditioning coach. All training sessions emphasised managing load in a controlled and safe environment, to avoid flare-ups (characterised by swelling) and mitigate injury risks. As Veronique's load tolerance and strength improved, the rehabilitation team gradually introduced slow footwork drills, emphasising control and balance during lunges.

*3. Return to participation (restricted training)*
Two months into rehabilitation, Veronique commenced training in a controlled environment, gradually incorporating footwork into her technical drills. Her footwork drills included lunges and half steps (short movements to adjust distance without fully committing to a forward or backward motion) and later extended to fleches (a swift and aggressive action where the fencer launches into a fast, direct attack), focusing on fluidity and precision. All exercises were conducted with Veronique's coach in a controlled environment. She continued with gym-based strength training, progressing with heavier loads.

*4. Return to sport (unrestricted training, restricted competition)*
At 3 months, Veronique's physical function was sufficient to start running drills, which gradually progressed to incorporate hopping, jumping, landing and cutting movements from 4 months. Veronique's specific fencing training also gradually progressed, incorporating unpredictable elements, allowing for simulated attacks and parries with her coach or a partner. Initially, the attacks and parries had no contact but progressed to allowing contact as Veronique's strength, balance and motor control continued to improve. The objective was to enhance distance control, refine offensive and defensive precision, and reinforce skills. Participating in her first tournament at 5 months after ACL reconstruction (Fig. 28.8), Veronique strategically focused on defensive manoeuvres, avoiding high-risk engagements, and secured a top-16 finish.

*5. Return to sport (unrestricted competition)*
Following thorough clinical (impairment) and function assessments, Veronique received medical clearance at 6 months to fence without any restrictions on her movements.

*continues*

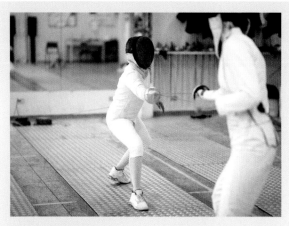

**Figure 28.8** After an intensive strength and movement training program, Veronique returned to fencing at 5 months after ACL reconstruction
ISTOCK/CAPUSKI

### 6. Return to performance

Veronique continued to work on her lower limb strength and control to execute her skills at the level she perceived she was at before her knee injury. She qualified for the Olympics and achieved her best-ever finish in an international competition, showcasing her resilience and determination to recover and perform at her best.

Veronique returned to tournament fencing 5 months after her ACL reconstruction. This is how the team (including you and other clinicians and coaches) could have interpreted and integrated information to support the shared return-to-sport decision.

### Step 1. Assess the risks related to tissue healing

- *Athlete demographics:* relatively young (25 years). Faster recovery than other athletes you have worked with. Practised good sleep hygiene and nutrition habits.
- *Symptoms:* no specific complaints about the wound or swelling; strength and knee range of motion within pre-injury measures.
- *Athlete medical history:* no previous injury to either knee. Right lateral ankle sprain (grade I) 3 months before the ACL injury that healed well. In good general health; not taking any medications.
- *Signs:* no swelling, clinically stable (quiet) knee.
- *Special tests:* negative Lachman test.

### Step 2. Assess the risks related to the sport

- *Sports-specific training capacity:* completed 3 weeks of high-intensity modified training with the coach; no pain or discomfort after training.
- *Type of sport:* épée fencing is a relatively low-contact sport. Each fencing discipline requires specific techniques, footwork and strategies. Foil and sabre emphasise speed,

agility and tactics involving right-of-way; épée focuses on precision and control.
- *Position and demands:* Veronique prefers a defensive style, and relies on strong parries, distance control and counterattacks to capitalise on her opponent's mistakes. This style involves patience, timing and a focus on exploiting openings rather than aggressive attacks. Veronique is right-hand dominant and her right leg is her leading foot, which usually points directly ahead towards her opponent. Most of Veronique's body weight is on her back leg to allow for swift movements and flexibility in engaging or disengaging.
- *Level of competition:* elite athlete; high demands and low margin for taking it easy.
- *Ability/requirement to protect:* Veronique could wear a hinged knee brace as required.
- *Strength and power diagnostics:* concentric quadriceps and hamstrings limb symmetry index were 80%. Single-hop test limb symmetry index was 75%.
- *Psychological readiness:* positive attitude; Veronique was highly motivated to return to fencing. Moderate concern about re-injury (score of 59 on the ACL-RSI scale).

### Step 3. Weigh up the risks and benefits

- *Timing and phase of the season:* the season was about to begin; the approaching Olympics are often a once-in-a-career competition opportunity.
- *Pressure from athlete:* Veronique's desire to compete in the Olympics was very strong.
- *External pressure:* minimal; Veronique's coaches and family were supportive and respected the decisions Veronique made in collaboration with her medical team.
- *Masking the injury:* there were no signs of pain, discomfort or instability.
- *Conflict of interest:* Veronique has sponsorships from a fencing equipment company and a sportswear company, and there was no specific pressure from those companies to return to sport and/or compete before she was ready.

### Decision

Veronique was keen to compete in the competition at 5 months, and you helped her understand the high re-injury risk (limb symmetry index <90%, less than 9 months since surgery) of returning to competition so soon after her surgery.[56, 57]

Based on your input, Veronique chose to modify her competition strategy, prioritising defensive manoeuvres, to protect her knee. Considering her specific circumstances and the specific demands of épée fencing, you and her coaches agreed with Veronique's plan to compete in her first international tournament 5 months after surgery.

You continued to check in with Veronique beyond her return to sport by monitoring her maintenance strength training program, knee symptoms and weekly training loads to help her prepare to compete at the Olympics in the best physical condition possible.

Shared decision making can support exploring the best evidence to inform a return-to-sport decision when there is more than one reasonable option. International cardiology societies have historically advocated for disqualifying athletes with genetic heart disease from competitive sport.[67-69] Yet with appropriate interventions and follow-up, it is possible for some athletes to safely return to sport.[70] Shared decision making is an appropriate way for medical teams to support athletes to balance the risks of a cardiac event with the potential harms that could arise from disqualifying an athlete.[70, 71]

Shared return-to-sport decision making with youth athletes is complex and requires careful planning, especially because there is greater uncertainty of outcome, and youth athletes' life plans are still developing.[72] It is difficult to obtain legally binding informed consent for return-to-sport decisions from a child. Therefore, you should seek and document approval (assent) from the child, irrespective of parent/guardian wishes, *and* obtain consent from the parent(s)/guardian.[72] Consider that youth athletes may place intense pressures on themselves to return to sport.[73] Clinicians and parents/guardians must work together to provide strong psychosocial support for injured youth athletes.[74-76]

## WHAT TO WORK ON TODAY TO AVOID POOR RETURN-TO-SPORT OUTCOMES TOMORROW

Clinicians, athletes and coaches often target the athlete's pre-injury health and fitness level as an important milestone to achieve before return to sport.[1] In this section, we outline four key considerations when choosing return-to-sport tests and criteria to decide whether an athlete is physically and psychologically ready to return to sport.

### Establishing a baseline to inform return-to-sport decisions

If you work in a team environment (or consult with a team), you may have pre-injury physical testing data available from routine pre-season test sessions. These data can help you to:

1. establish a pre-injury "baseline" level of function to target during rehabilitation and when deciding on return-to-sport criteria
2. monitor progress by comparing the athlete's current function with their pre-injury status.

It is challenging to identify and set a trustworthy baseline for different sports settings.[77] The limb symmetry index is often used as a return-to-sport criterion for lower limb injuries. However, even when limb symmetry is achieved, it may not indicate that the athlete has reached a level

sufficient for safe sports participation and performance.[78, 79] It is also questionable whether the uninvolved side is an appropriate benchmark when pre-injury data are unavailable.[77, 80]

Consequently, defining the baseline measure for comparison remains challenging. A well-rounded set of return-to-sport tests will help you overcome some of the challenges of interpreting the test results.[1]

### Deciding on the number of tests to do

So many tests and so much data—how to make sense of all the information? The challenge is to identify which tests will help you efficiently and effectively track the athlete's progress and inform return-to-sport decisions. Having too many tests may simply increase error (e.g. the athlete's performance might decline due to fatigue or reduced motivation) and exhaust resources (staff, time, equipment) without providing helpful information.

Knowing the content validity of a test (is it measuring what you expect it to measure?) and its predictive validity (does a result on the test predict the return-to-sport outcome?)[81] will help you make informed decisions about whether a test can add value to your planning. Validity and reliability are examples of measurement properties—for more information on measurement properties and how to interpret them, see Chapter 23.

### Detecting a meaningful change in the athlete's function

Responsiveness (sometimes called sensitivity) refers to how well a test detects meaningful changes in skill and function.[82] While it is important to track progress, remember that some common clinical tests cannot accurately track recovery after injury.[35, 36, 83] For example, if after a lower limb injury you choose to assess hopping performance, you need to consider that 6-metre timed hop test results may return to the pre-injury baseline (normal) earlier than other single-leg hop test results (single hop for distance, triple hop for distance and crossover hop for distance).[84] Similarly, after a hamstring strain, straight-leg raise results may return to normal earlier than the maximum hip flexion with active knee extension test.[35] It is currently unclear which tests are best for monitoring treatment and rehabilitation progression.[35]

### Detecting a meaningful change in test results

One of the reasons for conducting return-to-sport tests is to assess the athlete's current function, which is a proxy for their progress through the return-to-sport continuum. Statistical tests can indicate whether a change in a

C

return-to-sport test is probably a true change or simply due to chance. Yet a statistical test alone is not sufficient to establish whether a change is clinically meaningful.

The concept of clinical significance qualifies whether a change is noticeable and meaningful to an injured athlete and/or the treating clinician.[85,86] For example, the smallest change required to detect a meaningful change beyond typical error for the 6-metre timed hop test is 13%.[87] For tests where the change required to feel certain of a meaningful change in the athlete's status is unknown, longitudinal tracking may help you to identify a trajectory and facilitate an informed decision.[84]

## DATA SCIENCE SUPPORTING HIGH-QUALITY RETURN-TO-SPORT DECISIONS

Applying technology in the sports and exercise medicine setting can support quality return-to-sport decisions that are tailored to the athlete and based on appropriate criteria. Large volumes of data are routinely collected in rehabilitation, training and competition. Data are collected off and on the field. Off the field in the rehabilitation and training setting, wellness scores and screening tests such as countermovement jump, adductor isometric strength, hamstring isometric and hamstring eccentric strength tests are often used in field team sports.[88-90] On the field, physical output (e.g. running distance), psychological measures and skills metrics (e.g. passing frequency and accuracy) are available.

The clinician's challenge is to interpret something meaningful from the data to underpin high-quality decisions. To effectively integrate all of the information from return-to-sport tests, clinicians may consider collaborating with colleagues in data science[91] to analyse large datasets with new techniques such as machine learning. Professional clubs may employ analysts with specialist knowledge in data science, modelling, statistics and mathematics. These colleagues can play a central role in bridging gaps across disciplines (clinicians, high-performance staff, data scientists) and in coordinating new ways to apply research methods in sport.

## KEY POINTS

- Return to sport is not a single moment in time. It represents a continuum of interrelated and sometimes overlapping stages.

- In returning to sport, the athlete must transition from a high-control/low-chaos rehabilitation setting to a low-control/high-chaos competitive or training setting.

- Return-to-sport testing provides information about the athlete's health and performance, and informs shared decision making.

- Criteria-based decisions about return to sport are preferable to a time-based approach. The criteria to consider include the athlete's clinical assessment, physical fitness, sport-specific skills, training load and psychological readiness.

- Return to sport has evolved from a gatekeeper model, where the clinician makes unilateral decisions about the athlete, to a shared decision-making model, where the athlete's goals and input are valued and respected.

- There are some clinical scenarios in which shared decision making may be inappropriate or requires special consideration.

- In situations where there are multiple treatment options, the best available evidence should be clearly communicated.

- The following should be considered when selecting return-to-sports measures: the value of baseline data, how many tests are required to gather the necessary information, what the return-to-sport criteria are and how to define meaningful change for the athlete.

- Consulting with a data scientist/analyst can help when processing the large amounts of data collected on athletes.

## REFERENCES

References for this chapter can be found at www.mhprofessional.com/CSM6e

## ADDITIONAL CONTENT

 Scan here to access additional resources for this topic and more provided by the authors

C

# Index

## A

absolute load, 233
accelerometers, 175
acceptance and commitment therapy, 160
accurate diagnosis, 293–4
Achilles tendon, 114, 117, 167, 337
  conditions, 432–3
ACL injuries *see* anterior cruciate
    ligament (ACL) injuries
acromioclavicular joint pathology, 199
active insufficiency, 174
active rehabilitation, 440
active tension, 79
Actovegin, 393
acupuncture, 159–60, 385–6
acute and subacute pain, 150–2
acute:chronic workload ratio, 234
acute compartment syndrome, 85
acute injuries, 69
  bone, 71–3
  bursa, 87
  fascia, 85
  fat pads, 88
  fibrocartilage, 75–6
  hyaline cartilage, 74–5
  inflammatory phase, 71
  initial management, 70–1
  joint, 73–4
  ligament, 77
  management, 358–62
    compression, 360–2
    elevation, 362
    ice, 359–60
    optimal loading, 359
    protection, 358
  mechanisms, 69–70
  modifiable *vs* non-modifiable risk
      factors, 70
  muscle, 77–86
  nerve, 87–8
  pathophysiology, 70–1
  skin, 88
  tendon, 86
acute patellar tendinopathy, 29–30
adhesive capsulitis, 336
age, periodic health assessment, 286
agility training, 220
agility T-test, 282
AI *see* artificial intelligence (AI)
alcohol, 245
allodynia, 131
American College of Cardiology, 286
American Heart Association, 286
amitriptyline, 158
analgesics, 386–7

ankle braces, 378–9
  and taping, 271–2
ankle sprains, 377
anterior cruciate ligament (ACL) injuries,
    257, 286, 287, 421, 428–9
  history of, 452
  management, 422
  return to sport, 456, 459
anticonvulsant medication action, 158
antidepressant medication action, 158
antifibrinolytic drug, 84
anti-neuropathic medications, 158
anxiety, 297
aponeurosis, 80
apophysitis, 108
APSQ *see* Athlete Psychological Strain
    Questionnaire (APSQ)
aromatase inhibitors, 115
arthritis (rheumatological
    conditions), 337–8
arthrokinematics, 165
articular cartilage, 75, 109, 363
artificial intelligence (AI), 316, 414
ASBQ *see* Athlete Sleep Behaviour
    Questionnaire (ASBQ)
aseptic bursitis, 87
ASSQ *see* Athlete Sleep Screening
    Questionnaire (ASSQ)
ASSURE model, 411
athlete education, 403–4
  aims and objectives, 411
  ASSURE model, 411
  common topics, 408–10
  communication, 411–12
  conversation, 413
  DISCERN tool, 415
  empathy/emotional intelligence,
      412–13
  evaluation, 416
  exercise prescription, 410
  external learning resources, 414–15
  health belief model, 404–5
  injury prevention programs, 410
  lifestyle factors, 410
  load management, 410
  locus of control theory, 405
  models and frameworks, 404–8
  needs, 408
  Patient Education Materials
      Assessment Tool, 415
  program, 405–9
  reinforce learning, 414
  self-efficacy theory, 405
  sessions, 413
  sport, team and individual's
      culture, 414

success, 416
Theoretical Domains
    Framework, 405–7
theories, 404–8
working programs, 417
Athlete Psychological Strain
    Questionnaire (APSQ), 285
athletes *see also* athlete education
  bone stress injury with, 107
  coach and clinician, 33–4
  examples of PROMs, 351–2
  health case management, 36
  health education for, 47
  home environment, 252
  managing sleep in, 250–2
  mental recovery in, 249–50
  peak isometric torque, 170
  performance, 36–8
  periodic health assessment of *see*
      periodic health assessments
  rapport, 281–2
  readiness to return, 452
  recovery program, 319
  rehabilitation journey, 407
  risk factors, 265
  training load, 229–31
  travel *see* travel
Athlete Sleep Behaviour Questionnaire
    (ASBQ), 250
Athlete Sleep Screening Questionnaire
    (ASSQ), 250
attentive listening, 58–9
autologous blood injections, 396
autonomic dysfunction, 142–3
avulsion fractures, 72
axonotmesis injury, 87

## B

back-foot contact (BFC), 189–91
back injuries, 210–11
ballistic stretching, 226
BAMIC system *see* British Athletics
    Muscle Injury Classification
    (BAMIC) system
baseball, 179–86
baseline testing, 281
benzodiazepines, 393
beverage rehydration index (BHI), 245
BFC *see* back-foot contact (BFC)
BHI *see* beverage rehydration index (BHI)
bike-fitting methods, 193
bio-banding, 268
biomechanics, 107
  concepts in, 165–70
  contact force, 170
  data, 175–6

field, 165
joint moments, 168–9
kinematics, 165–6
kinetics, 166–7
muscle performance
measurement, 170–1
in shoulder injuries, 184–5
swimming, 204
tissues, 171–2
homeostasis and
mechanotherapy, 172–4
strain, 167
biomedical *vs* biopsychosocial model,
147–50
biopsies, 334
biopsychosocial (BPS) model, 139, 148, 293
biomedical *vs*, 147–50
bisphosphonates, 394
blisters, 122–3
blood flow restriction, 366–8
bone, 171, 363–5
acute injuries, 71–3
fractures, 71–3
periosteal contusion, 73
infection, 332
bone stress injuries
apophysitis, 108
biomechanical factors, 97
bone remodelling and, 94–5
cause of, 96
definitions, 92
diagnosis, 99–100
epidemiology, 95
gait retraining, 103
healing, 101
high-risk, 106
load and bone health, 96–9
low-risk, 102–6
management principles, 102–6
nomenclature and pathophysiology,
91–101
osteitis, 108
stages of, 92
bracing, 378–9
breaking pitches, 185
British Athletics Muscle Injury
Classification (BAMIC)
system, 81–2
bruise, 88
bursa, 87, 122

C

calcaneal fat pad, 88
calibration, 322–3
cannabinoids, 395
capability, opportunity, motivation and
behaviour (COM-B) model, 407–8
cardiac screening, 282–3
career development
clinician's journey, 56
common concerns, 63–4

control of, 59–61
empowered workplace, 61–3
goal setting, 57
heart of clinical practice, 56–7
income, 63
KPI development, 58
options, 64
other skills, 58–9
personal and professional
development, 61
relationship marketing, 58
roadblocks, 63
taking opportunities, 63
time management, 58
career sponsor, 60
"catch" position, 200
causal questions, 20
cause–effect relationship, 324
central sensitisation, 129–31
"change-in-load" analysis, 234
chest wall pain, 201–2
chondral injuries, 74–5
chondroitin, 394
chronic exertional compartment
syndrome, 110
chronic fatigue syndrome, 336
chronic periods, 233
chronic sarcoidosis, 337
climbing, 186–8
clinical advisor, 60–1
clinical assessment, 452
diagnosis and sharing, 319–23
disease mechanisms, 322
gathering clinical data, 319
likelihood ratios, 321
positive and negative predictive
values, 320–2
primary goals, 319
prognosis, 322–3
reliability, 320
sensitivity and specificity, 320
three phases of, 319
treatment plan, 324–6
clinical case management, 36
clinical practice, 56–7
demands, 19
clinical reasoning
decisions, prioritise for, 19
evidence-based practice, 17–18
reliability, 20–1
research question, 19–20
shared decision making, 21–2
validity, 21
coach-led programs, 272–5
codeine, 386
cognitive behavioural therapy, 160
cold debriefs, 11
cold therapy, 241
collagen, 395–6
collagen helix, 395
Colles' fracture, 71

colour Doppler ultrasound, 315
COM-B model *see* capability,
opportunity, motivation and
behaviour (COM-B) model
communication, 5, 47
athlete education, 411–12
training, 59
compartment syndrome, 433
complex regional pain syndrome
(CRPS), 143
comprehensive patient history, 319
compression, 101, 243–4, 360–2
computed tomography, 315–16
concentric elbow flexion, 168
concentric exercises, 222
conditioning training, 218
consent, 288
"conservative" pain management,
152–3
construct validity, 346
contact force, 170
content validity, 346
contextual factors, 235
continuing professional
development, 47
contrast therapy, 243
contusion, 84, 88
conventional radiography, 310
Copenhagen Hip and Groin Outcome
Score (HAGOS), 343, 345–7
corked thigh, 84
corticosteroids, 30, 121, 391–2
COSMIN framework, 349
counterirritants, 390
COX-1, 387
COX-2 inhibitors, 388, 389
cramps, 85–6
cricket fast bowling, 188–91
Cronbach's alpha measure, 354
cross-training, 219
cryotherapy, 71, 226, 241, 359, 360
cultural sensitivity, 39
curvilinear motion, 165
cycling, 192–6
knee pain, 192–4
low back pain, 194–5
overuse injuries in, 192
spinal position in, 195
ulnar neuropathy, 195–6

D

decision talk, 25, 29
deep venous thrombosis, 433
delayed/non-united fractures, 73
delayed-onset muscle soreness
(DOMS), 83–4
delayed swelling, 295
depression, 297
de Quervain tenosynovitis, 204
dermatitis, 123
dermatomyositis, 338

descriptive questions, 19–20
diagnosis
    accurate, 293–4
    differential, 297, 304
    function, 295
    instability, 295
    patient history, 294–7
    physical examination, 297–304
    psychological factors, 297
    reproduce patient's symptoms, 298
    tissue, 293
    ultrasound, 314–15
    work and leisure activities, 296
diagnostic utility, 321
dietary protein, 247
dietary sodium/sodium chloride, 245
differential diagnosis, 297, 304, 319
digital ischaemic pressure, 373
direct observation, 416
direct palpation, 99
DISCERN tool, 415
disc herniations, 76
discrimination, 323
disease mechanisms, 322
dislocation, joint injury, 73–4
displaced fractures, 431
distal biceps brachii rupture, 426–7
dorsal rim impaction syndrome,
    197–8
Down syndrome, 331
drill practice, 14
dry needling, 159–60, 383–5
dynamic stretching, 226, 276

E
eating disorders, 297
eccentric elbow flexion, 168–9
eccentric exercises, 222
ECG see electrocardiograph (ECG)
echocardiography, 283
education, 47
    athlete see athlete education
        interventions, 405
    periodic health assessments (PHAs), 281
Ehlers-Danlos syndrome, 330
elbow ulnar collateral ligament tear, 426
electrocardiograph (ECG), 283
electromagnetic therapy, 382–3
electromyography (EMG), 175–6
electrophysical agents, 380–3
electrotherapy, 108
elevation (acute injury management), 362
emergency action plan, 13, 50
EMG see electromyography (EMG)
emotional intelligence, 412–13
empathetic listening, 59
empathy, 412–13
endocrine disorders, 336
endomysium, 77
endurance training, 218–19

enthesitis, 121
enthesopathy, 120–2, 337
epimysium, 77
epiphyseal fracture, 187
equipment, 304
ergonomics, 9
    medical equipment and, 12
erythema nodosum, 337
evidence-based medicine, 17
evidence-based practice, 17–18
    principles of, 17–18
    treatment, 37
exercise-associated muscle cramps, 85, 86
exercise-induced anaphylaxis, 297
exercise-induced hypoalgesia, 365
exercise-induced muscle damage, 247
exercise-induced muscle soreness, 83–4
exercise prescription, 410, 439
exercise rehabilitation, 152, 153
extensor mechanism injuries, 430
external forces, 166
external learning resources, 414–15
external load, 229–30, 236, 410
external stakeholders, 9
extracorporeal shockwave therapy,
    383, 384
extrinsic loads, 70
extrinsic risk factors, 258, 259
eye movement desensitisation and
    reprocessing, 160

F
facio-scapulo-humeral dystrophy, 339
FAI syndrome see femoroacetabular
    impingement syndrome (FAI
    syndrome)
Fartlek training, 219
fascia, 87
fasciotomy, 110
fast-bowling biomechanics, 188–91
fatigue, 185, 200
fat pads, 88
femoroacetabular impingement syndrome
    (FAI syndrome), 428
FFC see front-foot contact (FFC)
fibrocartilage, 75–6
    acute tear, 75–6
    intervertebral disc herniation, 76
fibromyalgia, 336
fibrous septa, 88
"fight or flight" response, 142
finger and hand fractures, 427
finger injuries, 186–7
"fit for purpose/play/performance"
    model, 131–2
flexibility training, 225–6
flexor/extensor finger tendon injury, 427
fluoroquinolones, 115
    antibiotics, 297
force and torque, 167–8

force-velocity relationship, 173, 174
fractures, 71–3
    delayed/non-united, 73
    management, 72–3
Fredericson MRI bone stress injury, 100
freestyle swimming, 205
friction massage, 373–4
front-foot contact (FFC), 189–91
Functional Movement Screen (FMS), 284
functional readiness, 434–5

G
gabapentin, 390
gait retraining, 103
ganglion cysts, 334
genetic disorders, 330–1
giant cell tumours, 333
glenohumeral ligaments, 184
Global DRO see Global Drug Reference
    Online (Global DRO)
Global Drug Reference Online (Global
    DRO), 48, 386
global positioning systems (GPS), 230
glucocorticoids, 115
glucosamine, 394
glyceryl trinitrate, 121
goal setting, 57–8
golf, 196–9
Golgi tendon, 86
GPS see global positioning
    systems (GPS)
graded exercise rehabilitation, 149–50
graded motor imagery, 159
grading muscle injuries, 81
granulomatous diseases, 336–7
GRASP trial, 18
greenstick fracture, 71
growth plate fractures, 72

H
haematoma, 84
    formation, 70
haemochromatosis, 331
Haglund's deformity surgery, 432
HAGOS see Copenhagen Hip and Groin
    Outcome Score (HAGOS)
hamstring injury, 453–4
harvesting knowledge, 56
healing, stress fracture, 102
health belief model, 404–5
healthcare practice, 21
healthcare team, 403
health case management, 36
health leadership, 35
health screening, 47
heart rate monitoring, 232
heating, 241–2
heat therapy, 241
helmets, 269–71
hereditary (genetic) disorders, 330–1

herniation, 76
high-performing clinical teams, 34–6
  responsibilities and communication, 35
  roles, 35
high-risk bone stress injuries, 99–100, 106
hip arthroscopy, 28–9
hip joint, 74
hip pain, 199
"hip pointer" injury, 73
Hoffa's fat pad, 113
home-based exercise therapy program, 18
hook of hamate, 197
hot debriefs, 11
human factors
  concept of, 13
  in sports and exercise medicine, 13–14
    advanced medical information, 14
    cognitive breadth and situational
      awareness, 14
    drill practice, 14
    emergency action plan, 13
    positioning and skill mix relevant, 14
    pre-event "safety huddle", 14
    radio skills, 14
    video technology, 14
hyaline cartilage, 74–5
  injuries, 430–1
hyaluronic acid, 391
hydrostatic pressure, 243, 244
hyperalgesia, 131
hyperpathia, 142
hypertrophic cardiomyopathy, 283
hypertrophy training, 225
hypomobility, 304
hypothenar hammer, 195
hypothesis testing, 346, 347

I
ICC see intraclass correlation
    coefficient (ICC)
ice (acute injury management), 359–60
ice hockey
  body checking policy in, 266
  helmet and facemask, 270
iliotibial band (ITB) syndrome, 192–4
imaging
  artificial intelligence in, 316
  computed tomography, 315–16
  conventional radiography, 310
  habits, 307–10
  magnetic resonance imaging, 310–13
  modalities, 310
  radioisotopic bone scanning, 316
  ultrasound, 314–15
  zero echo time (ZTE), 313
impairment-based language, 412
impingement syndromes, 109
inciting event, 258–9
individualisation (training), 218
individual multiskilling, 35

indoor vs beach volleyball, 213
inflammatory musculoskeletal
    disorders, 337
inflammatory soup, 129
informal leadership, 59
information sources, 19
informed consent, 152
informed decision, 28
infrapatellar fat pad, 88
injury and illness management, 36–8
injury, in sports
  baseball, 179–86
  climbing, 186–8
  cricket fast bowling, 188–91
  cycling, 192–6
  golf, 196–9
  rowing, 199–204
  swimming, 204–8
  tennis, 208–11
  volleyball, 211–13
injury prevention
  basic model, 258
  in coach-led programs, 272–5
  evidence-informed, 272–4
  extrinsic risk factors, 258, 259
  inciting event, 258–9
  intrinsic risk factors, 258
  modifiable risk factors, 258
  non-modifiable risk factors, 258
  personal protective equipment, 268–72
  primary and secondary, 410
  reducing risk, 259–65
  role of playing surfaces in, 276
  science, 257–9
  sport policy and rules, 266–8
  sport-related, 258
  stretching, 276
  surveillance program, 261
Injury-Psychological Readiness to Return
    to Sport (I-PRRS) scale, 343
insertional tendinopathies, 172
insurance medical assessment, 289
integrated performance health management
    and coaching model, 35, 36
interferential stimulation, 382
intermuscular haematomas, 84
internal impingement, 209
internal load, 229–30, 410
internal models, 132–5
internal vs external moment arm, 168
intersection syndrome, 204
interval training, 219
interventional pain management, 158–9
intervertebral disc herniation, 76
intraclass correlation coefficient (ICC),
    347, 348
intramuscular contusions, 84
intrinsic loads, 70
IOC's Sport Mental Health Assessment
    Tool, 285

I-PRRS scale see Injury-Psychological
    Readiness to Return to Sport
    (I-PRRS) scale
isokinetic exercises, 223
isometric exercises, 221, 365
isometric knee extensor torque, 170
isotonic exercises, 221–3
ITB syndrome see iliotibial band (ITB)
    syndrome

J
jet lag, 51
job insecurity, 43
joint
  acute injuries, 73–4
  contact force, 170
  moments, 168–9
  overuse injuries, 109
  techniques, 369–71
joint pain, 332

K
key performance indicators (KPIs),
    57, 58
kinematics, 165–6
kinesiology tape, 376, 377
kinetic chain, 124, 182–3
kinetics, 166–7
knee arthroscopy, for managing
    osteoarthritis 17–18
knee braces, 379
knee injuries in volleyball, 211–12
  extensor mechanism injuries, 430
  surgery, 421–3
Knee Injury and Osteoarthritis Outcome
    Score (KOOS), 345
knee ligament injuries, 267
knee pain, 192–4
KOOS see Knee Injury and Osteoarthritis
    Outcome Score (KOOS)
KOOS-PF, 348–9
KPIs see key performance indicators
    (KPIs)

L
language
  impact of, 156
  learning, 61
laser therapy, 382
lateral epicondylalgia, 208
leading wrist, 196–7
length-tension relationship, 174
ligaments, 73, 77
  overuse injuries, 109
  sprains, 78
  testing, 299
linear biomedical model, 139
linear motion, 165
LIPUS see low-intensity pulsed
    ultrasound (LIPUS)

load management, 229
  analysing training, 233-4
  athlete education, 410
  collecting training, 229-33
  with competitive excellence, 238
  decision making with, 234
  mechanical and physiological
    loads, 230
  remains, 235-8
Load, Optimism, Vascularisation,
  Exercise (LOVE), 71
loads/physical demands, 171, 319
local anaesthetic injections, 390-1
local analgesia, 359
locus of control theory, 405
LOVE see Load, Optimism,
  Vascularisation, Exercise
low back pain, 198-9, 207-8
lower limb fracture repair, 432
low-intensity pulsed ultrasound
  (LIPUS), 380
low-level laser therapy, 382
low-risk bone stress injuries, 99-106, 171
lubricants, 375
lumbar spine injuries, 188
lymphatic drainage, 374

**M**

magnetic resonance imaging (MRI), 307,
  310-13
  clinical points, 313
  erroneous interpretation of, 313
  features and patient benefits, 313
  sequences, 313
maladaptive processes, 158
malignant tumours, 332-4
manipulation (musculoskeletal
  conditions), 369-71
manual therapy, 159-60
manual treatments (musculoskeletal
  conditions), 368-76
Marfan syndrome, 331
"match/fixture density", 233
maximal aerobic speed training, 219
mechanotherapy, 173-4, 362-5
mechanotransduction, 94, 362
medial knee pain, 208
medial tibial stress syndrome, 92, 94
media training, 59
medical equipment, 45
medical team, 45-7
medical travel assessments, 50-1
medications, 158
  and mindfulness, 160
Meeuwisse's models, 258
meniscus injuries, 429-30
mental health screening, 285-6
mental recovery, 248-50
mentors, 45, 60
mesenchymal stem cells, 397
methylprednisolone, 392

microdosing, 236
microloading, 236
microtrauma, 83
mindfulness, 160
mindset, shared decision-making,
  25, 26
minimal detectable change (MDC), 348
mobilisation (musculoskeletal
  conditions), 369-71
modifiable risk factors, 70, 234, 258
moment arms, 169
motor-control training programs, 365-6
mouthguards, 268-9
movement, types of, 165
MRI see magnetic resonance
  imaging (MRI)
multidisciplinary team approach, 57
  high-performing clinical teams, 34-6
  sports and exercise medicine, 33
  teamwork tips, 38-9
  tripartite nucleus, 33-4
multifaceted injury prevention
  program, 265
multisensory perceptual inference, 140
muscle, 363
  acute injuries, 77-86
    acute compartment syndrome, 85
    contusion, 84
    cramps, 85-6
    exercise-induced muscle
      soreness, 83-4
    injury classification, 81
    myositis ossificans, 84
    strain/tear, 77-83
  belly strains, 82
  fibres, 77
  inhibition, 71
  insufficiency, 174
  myofascial pain, 109-10
  overuse injuries, 109-10
muscle disorder, 338-9
muscle performance
  measurement, 170-1
muscular endurance training, 225
musculoskeletal pain, 4, 294
musculoskeletal system, 165, 331
  imaging anatomy of, 307
myofascial pain syndromes, 109-10, 336
myositis ossificans, 84

**N**

negative predictive values, 320-2
neoplasia, 332-4
nerve, 122
  acute injuries, 87-8
neural mechanosensitivity, 298
neural mobilisation techniques, 372-3
neural Thomas test, 302
neurodynamic testing, 299-303
neuromuscular electrical
  stimulation, 381-2

neuropathic pain, 146, 389
neuropraxia, 87-8
neuropsychological testing, 281
neurotags, 132-5
neurotmesis, 87
nocebos, 143-6
nociception, 127-31, 139, 150
non-melanoma skin cancers, 123-4
non-modifiable risk factors, 70, 234, 258
non-organic pain, 139
non-sport-related load, 229
non-steroidal anti-inflammatory drugs
  (NSAIDs), 30, 387-9
  and bone, 388
  and ligament, 388
  and muscle, 388
  and tendon, 388
non-technical factors see human factors
noxious stimulus, 127
NSAIDs see non-steroidal anti-
  inflammatory drugs (NSAIDs)
nutraceuticals, 394-6
nutrition, 244-8, 297, 394-6
  and other lifestyle factors, 160-1
  travel, 51

**O**

Olympic-type weightlifting, 225
omega-3 fatty acids, 161, 394
one-handed backhand technique, 209
open and closed chain exercises, 223
open wounds, 88
opiates/opioids, 158
optimal loading, 359
optimal tennis serve technique, 210
option talk, 25, 28-9
Osgood-Schlatter disease, 108
OSIS see Oxford Shoulder Instability
  scores (OSIS)
Oslo Sports Trauma Research Center
  (OSTRC) questionnaire, 261-3
osteitis, 108
osteoarthritis, 72
osteochondral injuries, 74-5
osteoid osteoma, 333
osteokinematics, 165
osteonecrosis, 394
OSTRC questionnaire see Oslo Sports
  Trauma Research Center (OSTRC)
  questionnaire
overload, 217
overtraining, 296-7
overuse injuries, 261
  articular cartilage, 109
  bone stress injuries see bone stress
    injuries
  bursa, 122
  challenges, 91
  in cycling, 192
  growth-related injuries and, 268
  joints, 109

ligaments, 109
muscle, 109–10
nerve, 122
risk factors, 91
skin, 122–4
tendon, 110–22
Oxford Shoulder Instability scores
(OSIS), 423

**P**

pain, 71, 124, 127, 139, 297 *see also* pain
management
autonomic dysfunction, 142–3
characteristics, 295
comprehensive approach, 136
education, 153
"fit for purpose/play/performance"
model, 132–3
for individual, 140–6
inhibition, 81
internal models, 132–5
neuropathic, 146
other treatment tools, 158–61
persistent, 135–6
placebos and nocebos, 143–6
radicular, 147
resolution, 134
revolution, 154, 155
sensitisation, 141–2
somatic, 146–7
spectrum, 139–40
system hypersensitivity, 131
pain management
acute and subacute, 150–2
biomedical *vs* biopsychosocial model,
147–50
"conservative", 152–3
graded motor imagery, 159
interventional, 158–9
medications, 158
neuropathic, 146
persistent (chronic) pain, 152–7
psychological treatment
approaches, 160
pain-monitoring model, 119
pain relief, 117
palpation, 113, 299
paracetamol, 386
paraesthesia, 88
paratenonitis, 120
parathyroid hormone, 108
partial-body cryotherapy, 241
partner talk, 28
PASS *see* patient acceptable symptoms
state (PASS)
passive insufficiency, 174
passive range of motion testing, 299
passive tension, 79
patellar instability, 431
patellofemoral joint contact force, 170
patellofemoral pain, 376–7

patient acceptable symptoms state
(PASS), 349–50
patient-centred care, 25
Patient Education Materials Assessment
Tool (PEMAT), 415
patient-reported outcome measures
(PROMs), 343
benefits, 344
commonly used, 351–4
construct validity, 346
content validity, 346
cost/licence requirement, 344
score, 349–50
use, 344–9
patients
clinical encounter as relationship, 5
establishing boundaries, 9
practising people skills, 9–10
voice, 3
patient-specific elements, 325
PEACE *see* Protection, Elevation, Avoid
anti-inflammatory medication,
Compression, Education (PEACE)
PEDro scale, 20, 22
PEMAT *see* Patient Education Materials
Assessment Tool (PEMAT)
people skills, 9–11
peptidergic inflammation, 129
peptides, 129
perimysium, 77
periodic health assessments (PHAs),
264–5, 279
age, 286
available resources, 287
baseline testing, 281
consent, 288
current medications and
supplements, 280
education, 281
goals, 287
insurance medical assessment, 289
medical conditions, 280
objectives, 279
perform, 279–86
pre-employment health
assessment, 288–9
screening, 282–6
template, 287–8
timing, 287
periodisation, 217
periosteal contusion, 73
periostitis, 108
peripheral nerve injuries, 87
peripheral sensitisation, 129–31
peripheral vascular disease, 335
persistent (chronic) pain, 152–7
personal and professional
development, 61
personal protective equipment, 268–72
phagocytosis, 70
pharmaceuticals management policy, 11

PHAs *see* periodic health assessments
(PHAs)
physical activity, 38–40
physical examination, 297–304, 319, 329
physical fitness and function, 452
physical injuries, 139
physical performance testing, 416
physical therapy, 423
Pittsburgh Sleep Quality Index
(PSQI), 250
placebos, 143–6
plantar fascia ruptures, 87
plantar pressure sensors, 167
plant-based proteins, 248
platelet-rich plasma, 396–7
plyometric exercises, 119–20, 225
POLICE *see* Protection, Optimal
Loading, Ice, Compression,
Elevation (POLICE)
polymyositis, 338
polyphenols, 395
positive predictive values, 320–2
post-exercise recovery, 241–4
power training, 224–5
prediction models, 322, 324
predictive questions, 20
predictive values, 320–322
pre-employment health assessment, 288–9
pre-event "safety huddle", 14
pregabalin, 390
Prep to Play warm-up program, 274
pressure injuries, 122
pressure wounds, 122
pretend listening, 58
PRICE *see* Protection, Rest, Ice,
Compression and Elevation (PRICE)
primary allodynia, 131
primary hyperalgesia, 131
primary nociceptors, 127, 128
sensitisation of, 129
primary prevention, 257
"primum non nocere", notion of, 9
process, of shared decision making,
25, 34
prognosis, 322–3
prognostic model, 323
prolotherapy, 121, 393
PROMs *see* patient-reported outcome
measures (PROMs)
prophylactic knee bracing, 271
proprioceptive neuromuscular facilitation
stretching, 226
protection (acute injury
management), 358
Protection, Elevation, Avoid anti-
inflammatory medication,
Compression, Education (PEACE),
71, 358, 444
Protection, Optimal Loading, Ice,
Compression, Elevation (POLICE),
71, 358, 444

Protection, Rest, Ice, Compression and Elevation (PRICE), 71, 358, 444
protective equipment, 73
PSQI *see* Pittsburgh Sleep Quality Index (PSQI)
psychological readiness, 435, 452
psychological wellbeing, 244
public health systems, 64
pulley injuries, 187

**Q**

quadriceps tendon, 430
qualitative sensory testing, 142
quinolone antibiotics, 394

**R**

radicular pain, 147
radionuclide bone scanning, 316
range of motion testing, 299
rate of force development, 171
rationale behind load management, 235
real-time ultrasound, 315
recording injuries, 261
recovery
    compression, 243-4
    contrast therapy, 243
    cooling, 241
    heating, 241-2
    hydrostatic pressure, 243
    mental recovery, 248-50
    nutrition, 244-8
    periodisation, 253
    practical strategies, 252-3
    rate and quality, 241
    sleep, 250-2
red flags, 124, 329
    conditions, 330-40
REDs *see* relative energy deficiency in sport (REDs)
referred pain syndromes, 335-6
regional limb dystrophies, 339
regional pain syndromes, 335-6
rehabilitation, 238, 424, 443
    criteria for progression, 447
    exercise, 152, 153
    graded exercise, 149-50
    phases of, 443-6
        acute phase, 443-5
        early phase, 445-6
        return-to-sport phase, 446
        sport-specific phase, 446
    prevention of re-injury, 447
relative energy deficiency in sport (REDs), 61, 98-9
relative load, 233-4
remote posture monitoring system, 195
"repeated bout" effect, 79
research question, 19-20
research *vs* clinical experience, 397-8

resistance training, 220-5
    exercise used in, 221-3
    open and closed chain exercises, 223
    types, 223-5
return-to-sport
    anterior cruciate ligament (ACL) injuries, 455
    continuum, 440, 451
    decisions, 433-5, 440
    outcomes, 459-60
    shared decision making, 452-9
    supporting high-quality, 460
    testing, 452
    testing psychological readiness, 456
RMDQ *see* Roland-Morris Disability Questionnaire (RMDQ)
rock climbers, 188
Roland-Morris Disability Questionnaire (RMDQ), 345
rotational motion, 165
rotator cuff tendinopathy, 293
rowing, 199-204
rugby, preventing tackle injuries in, 266-7
running shoes, 213-14

**S**

SAMPLE forms, 51
scapula
    arm with repeated throwing, 185
    biomechanics in shoulder injuries, 184-5
    in throwing, 183
SCR *see* shoulder counter-rotation (SCR)
SCREEND'EM, 337-9
screening, 51
    cardiac, 282-3
    mental health, 285-6
    periodic health assessment (PHA), 282-6
    for risk factors for future injury, 284-5
    for unknown illnesses, 283
SDC *see* smallest detectable change (SDC)
secondary prevention, 257
secondary/spinal nociceptors, 128
self-efficacy theory, 405
self-treatment of soft tissues, 375
sensitisation
    pain, 141-2
    of primary nociceptors, 129
septic arthritis, 332, 336
serotonin reuptake inhibitors, 389
session rating of perceived exertion (sRPE) method, 230-2
shared decision making, 21-2
    complex elements of, 30
    definition, 25
    mindset, 25, 26
    in practice, 27-30

principles for, 26-7
    process of, 25, 26, 34
    return-to-sport, 452-9
    self-diagnose, 26
    three-talk model of, 25-6
shin splints, 92
short-term management, 236
shoulder counter-rotation (SCR), 190
shoulder impingement and cuff injuries, 425-6
shoulder injuries, 184-5
    baseball, 184-5
    climbing, 187-8
    golf, 198-9
    swimming, 205-7
    tennis, 209-10
    volleyball, 212-13
shoulder instability, 423, 425
    in overhead athletes, 423
shoulder pain, 18
Shoulder Pain and Disability Index (SPADI), 345
shoulder-related pain, 151
SHRed Injuries Soccer warm-up program, 275
significant event analysis, 11
skin, 71
    acute injuries, 88
    blisters, 122-3
    infections, 123-4
    overuse injuries, 122-4
    pressure injuries, 122
skin cancers, 123-4
sleep, 250-2
"sleep audit", 252
sleep medication, 393
slump test, 302
smallest detectable change (SDC), 348
SMART objectives, 57
SMHAT-1 *see* Sport Mental Health Assessment Tool 1 (SMHAT-1)
Smith's fracture, 71
soft-shell padded headgear, 269-71
soft-tissue injuries, 73, 434
soft-tissue therapy, 35, 373-6
somatic pain, 146-7
SPADI *see* Shoulder Pain and Disability Index (SPADI)
specificity (training), 217-18, 320
speed training, 219-20
spondylolysis, 211
sporting teams, working with
    core principles, 44
    mentor, 45
    self-care, 45
    social media, 44-5
    in-season, 48-9
        equipment and consumables, 48-9
        scheduling/planning, 48
        treatment room, 48

off-season, 52–3
  exit screening, 52
  other considerations, 53
  trades, 52–3
pre-season, 45–8
  communication, 47
  continuing professional
    development, 47
  education, 47
  health screening, 47
  medical equipment, 45
  medical team, 45–7
  policies and protocols, 48
  relationships, 47
travel, 49–52
Sport Mental Health Assessment Tool 1
  (SMHAT-1), 285–6
sports
  injury prevention *see* injury
    prevention
  policy and rules, 266–8
  specialisation, 267
sports and exercise medicine
  challenge of, 36
    diagnosis, 37
    individual athlete's needs, 37–8
    treatment, 37
  high-performance teamwork, 38, 40
  human factors in, 13–14
  model, 35–6
  MRI in, 311
  research questions in, 19
  surgery in *see* surgery
  work in, 307
sports injuries, 69, 296
  rehabilitation
    according to plan, 447–8
    exercise prescription during, 439
    exercises, 446–7
    goal setting and targeted
      interventions, 441–3
    phases of, 443–6
    principles, 440
    working alliance, 440–1
  treatment
    acupuncture, 385–6
    acute injury management, 358–62
    autologous blood injections, 396
    bracing, 378–9
    dry needling, 383–5
    electrophysical agents, 380–3
    manual treatments, 368–76
    mesenchymal stem cells, 397
    nutraceuticals and nutrition, 394–6
    platelet-rich plasma, 396–7
    research *vs* clinical
      experience, 397–8
    taping, 376–8
    therapeutic exercise, 362–8
    therapeutic medication, 386–94

sprain/tear, 77
sRPE method *see* session rating of
    perceived exertion (sRPE) method
*Staphylococcus aureus,* 332
static stretching, 226, 276
statins, 115
STOP mnemonic, 11
strain gauges, 170
strain injuries, 82–3
strain/tear, 77–83
strength testing, 299
strength training, 223–4
stress fracture, 91–3, 100–1
  healing, 102
stress shielding, 172–3
stretching, 225, 226, 276
subluxation, joint injury, 73–4
supershoes, 213–14
supervised *vs* home exercises, 18
supraspinatus tendons, 86
surgery
  Achilles tendon conditions, 432–3
  ACL injuries, 428–9
  anatomical/physiological
    readiness, 434
  communication for, 424–5
  distal biceps brachii rupture, 426–7
  elbow ulnar collateral ligament
    tear, 426
  FAI syndrome, 428
  finger and hand fractures, 427
  flexor/extensor finger tendon
    injury, 427–8
  hyaline cartilage injuries, 430–1
  identifying candidates for, 419–21
  indications, 420
  knee injuries, 421–3
  meniscus injuries, 429–30
  patellar instability, 431
  post-surgical complications, 433
  return-to-sport decisions, 433–5
  shoulder impingement and cuff
    injuries, 425–6
  for shoulder instability, 423, 425
  treatment by anatomical
    location, 420
sustained myofascial tension, 373
swelling, 71, 295
swimming, 204–8
sympathetic nervous system, 142, 143
synovial cell sarcoma, 333

**T**
talk therapies, 160
taping, 376–8
team
  multiskilling, 35
  sports, 231–3
  sports physician, 62–3
team (partner) talk, 25

teamwork
  high-performance, 35, 38
  sports and exercise medicine, 40
  tips, 38–9
telemedicine, 35
temazepam, 393
tendinopathies, 91, 110–16, 192
tendons, 86, 171, 363
  compression, 172
  hyaluronic acid, 391
  management principles, 116–22
  overuse injuries, 110–16
  pain/rupture, 116
  rehabilitation, 117, 119
tennis, 208–11
TENS *see* transcutaneous electrical nerve
    stimulation (TENS)
tensioning technique, 372
tertiary prevention, 257
test-retest reliability, 347–8
Theoretical Domains
    Framework, 405–8
therapeutic alliance, 413
therapeutic exercise, 362–8
therapeutic medication, 386–94
therapeutic ultrasound, 380
thermotherapy, 241
three-talk model, shared decision
    making, 25–6
throwing
  arm with repeated throwing, 185
  biomechanics of, 179–83
  scapula, 183
  stride, 179
tibial stress fractures, 101
tissues, 171–2
  diagnosis, 293
  homeostasis, 172–4
  strain, 167
topical NSAIDs, 387
trades, 52
trailing wrist, 197–8
training, 296–7
  agility, 220
  conditioning, 218
  designing program, 227
  endurance, 218–19
  flexibility, 225–6
  principles, 217–18
  resistance, 220–5
  speed, 219–20
training load, 229, 452
tramadol, 386
transcutaneous electrical nerve
    stimulation (TENS), 159–60, 380
Translating Research Into Practice
    (TRiP) database, 22
traumatic bursitis, 87
traumatic fractures, 71
Traumeel, 392–3

travel, 49–52
  accommodation, 49
  arrival, 52
  destination, 49
  emergency action plan, 50
  equipment and logistics, 49–50
  injury prevention, 51
  insurance and indemnity, 51
  jet lag, 51
  journey home, 52
  medical assessments, 50-1
  nutrition, 51
  reconnaissance, 50
  SAMPLE forms, 51
  treatment room, 49
  vaccinations, 49
traveller's diarrhoea, 51
Travell's theory, 109
treatment
  evidence-based practice, 37
  room, 48
  sports and exercise medicine, 37
triamcinolone, 392

tricyclic antidepressants, 389
trigger point model, 109–10
TRiP database *see* Translating
  Research Into Practice (TRiP)
  database
tuberculosis, 336
turmeric, 395
twin peaks model, 142

**U**
ulnar neuropathy, 195–6
ultrasound, 198, 314–15
upper limb neurodynamic test, 303

**V**
vaccinations, 49
vacuum cupping, 375
vitamin D, 395
  deficiencies, 248
volleyball, 211–13
  indoor *vs* beach, 213
  knee injuries, 211–12
  shoulder injuries, 212–13

**W**
WADA *see* World Anti-Doping Agency
  (WADA)
wearable devices, 175
whole-body cryotherapy, 241
wind-up, 179
work and leisure activities, 296
working alliance, 441
work–life balance, 57
World Anti-Doping Agency (WADA),
  280, 386
wrist and forearm injuries, 202–4
wrist pain, 196–8

**Y**
youth American football, 267

**Z**
zero echo time (ZTE) imaging, 313